The Cannabis Health Index

LOGOS PUBLISHING HOUSE

Copyright © 2013 Uwe Blesching, Ph.D.
Published by Logos Publishing House
Berkeley, California.

ISBN-13: 978-0-9823570-3-3

ISBN-10: 0-9823570-3-6

Second Edition: March 2013

Printed in the United States of America

The Cannabis Health Index

How to Achieve Deep(er) Healing of 100 Chronic
Symptoms and Diseases by Linking the Science
of Medical Marijuana with the Art of Mind-Body
Consciousness

Sneak Preview

Welcome to the beginning of an in-depth exploration of the impact of cannabis and consciousness on our growth, health and healing.

KEY CONCEPTS - WHY DO SOME PEOPLE HEAL WHILE OTHERS DON'T?

Whether you are suffering from disease yourself, concerned about someone you love, or simply eager to learn more about health and healing, at some point you will arrive at this pivotal question: Why do some people heal while others don't? This book contains individual chapters for most major diseases or disease groups. In each of these chapters, we address this very question in some detail. A more general answer, and a key premise of this book, is this: chronic exposure to stressful emotions interferes with our body's ability to fight disease and heal injury.

Here's why. Stressful emotions consume vital energy, leaving us depleted. When we encounter an immediate threat -- a wild animal, say, or the edge of a cliff -- our bodies begin to shut down non-essential functions. We divert blood, with all its nutrients, away from the skin (we get pale) and away from the gastro-intestinal organs needed for nurturing. Instead, blood is delivered to the muscles and the heart in an effort to prepare to run away from the perceived threat. This mechanism is life-saving and essential if reversed relatively quickly. However, many of us suffer from chronic stress, which induces the same "shut down" mechanism on a semi-permanent basis. Chronic stress may be caused by any number of things such as a lack of money to pay the bills, a fearful outlook on life in general, a threatening boss, or a difficult, drawn-out divorce. The shut-down mechanism that occurs when we experience intense stress prevents billions of cells that are not strictly essential for immediate survival from relaxing and receiving sufficient nutrients to grow and to thrive. When this shut-down mechanism occurs not just once in a long while, but many times, over and over again, our bodies are left out of balance and vulnerable to disease.

ENTER CANNABINOIDS AND CONSCIOUSNESS - KEY ALLIES IN GROWTH, HEALTH AND HEALING

The human body contains endocannabinoid systems comprised of specific molecules and their matching receptors in almost every vital organ and bodily system, including the immune system, the heart and the brain. Endocannabinoids, that is, cannabinoids produced by our own bodies, may be thought of as "keys" that activate ("unlock") matching receptors. When a receptor is activated (to continue the analogy, "a door is opened"), therapeutic benefits are realized in the mind as well as the rest of the body. Endocannabinoid systems (ECS) relax the mind and help the body restore balance and energy. The function of ECS suggests that for deep and lasting healing to occur, mind and body must be engaged as partners.

To date, five endocannabinoids ("keys" to cannabinoid receptors that are produced by our bodies) have been identified and examined. The first to be discovered, called anandamide, was named after the sanscrit word for bliss. Cannabinoids can also be made outside of the human body: they are found in plants, and can now be produced in laboratories. Cannabis contains over eighty different cannabinoids. Tetrahydrocannabinol, commonly referred to as THC, is the most studied cannabis constituent. THC engages the body and the mind and in so doing often produces shifts in conscious awareness related to patients' healing process. The hypothesis of this book is that it is these shifts in perspective that are responsible for the vast healing potential reported by many cannabis-using patients.

And, while cannabis can certainly be used as a plant ally to activate deep and lasting healing processes, it is important to realize that the ability to heal was always within our bodies. Cannabis is not required to activate this potent healing synergy. It can be activated by consciousness alone.

Studies in the field of mind-body medicine have identified numerous internal mechanisms (frames of mind), which have been linked to the development of certain illness and disease expressions. Most importantly, these mechanisms are subject to interpretation and conscious intervention. In other words, by understanding how unmanaged constricting emotions negatively affect us, we can consciously decide to make the changes that a mild form of an illness seems to invite, or even make the changes that a debilitating disease so often demands.

People that respond with conscious awareness to the invitation or demand of an illness open the door to achieving a natural balance, virility and inherent capacity for generating or re-generating health and healing. The ECS, cannabinoids and consciousness play a vital role in this process. The purpose of this book is to pull together all the available research and provide a practical foundation for the reader to commence his or her own private journey to achieve deep healing and well-being.

Whether you decide to work with cannabis or mind-body consciousness (or both), this book provides a practical basis to understand what keeps us from healing and to set in motion a powerful and natural mechanism for self-healing that no disease can overcome.

Table of Content & Index

Chapter I

Cannabinoid Research
and Deep Healing

When psychological and spiritual aspects are combined with the thoughtful and reflective use of cannabis (or any other healing method), the power of our natural healing abilities multiply. We can then achieve, perhaps for the first time, the kind of deep healing that goes beyond the mere management of symptoms and brings about profound positive changes in the quality of our life.

While medical practitioners have historically considered conditions of "the body" distinct and separate from conditions of "the mind", more and more doctors and other health care practitioners now embrace a different approach. When they prescribe cannabis they intend to heal the mind as well as other body parts, fully cognizant that the two are interdependent.

In order to better understand how the use of cannabis helps patients find heart-opening psychological healing that directly or indirectly influences their physical symptoms, it is useful to review insights from the latest research into cannabis and consciousness.

THE ENDOCANNABINOID SYSTEM (A BRIEF INTRODUCTION)

All mammals have an endocannabinoid system (ECS). The ECS is involved in initiating a host of physiological and psychological changes needed to adjust to ever-changing internal and external environments as well as other functions. This is true from the very beginning of life when ECS signaling determines if a fertilized egg will implant in the uterine wall or not. Throughout our life the ECS produces nurturing responses to injuries and inflammations. It is involved in protective mechanisms against numerous cancers, neurological diseases and nerve damage and it may mitigate changes associated with aging.

The scientific identification of the endocannabinoid system is a relatively recent development that stemmed from research into the cannabis plant, for which it is named.[1] Since then, about ten new studies have been published every month examining the impact of the ECS, its range and complexity.[2] Presumably this is a reflection of the excitement and hope this research has generated in the medical research community, physicians, patients and caregivers.

The ECS is a biological regulatory mechanism that operates much like a lock and key. Understanding the ECS is a critical task if we are to more effectively manage diseases, especially chronic, debilitating diseases for which there is no orthodox cure. For instance, if properly activated, the ECS is capable of suppressing numerous cancers and may be protective against Alzheimer's disease.

In addition to its preventive and protective mechanisms, the ECS balances and strengthens our nervous and immune systems, initiates pain control, and calms inflammation. The ECS initiates neurogenesis[3] (the production of new nerve cells) which is essential to recovery from brain damage, and crucial to protecting nerve cells and enhancing memory function. The ECS increases our ability to try out new perspectives and experiences. When we try new things, we literally change our brain functions for the better in a process called neuroplasticity. Evidence suggests the ECS may be involved in generating subtle but therapeutic shifts in the ways we perceive the world, relate to our internal landscape, think and feel about ourselves, and interact with each other.

The role of the ECS in neurogenesis, neuroplasticity, learning, and opening us to new experiences demonstrates connections between our frame of mind, the development of illness or the expansion of health and well-being. For example, a frame of mind that frequently leads to guilt or shame produces specific negative changes that impact our bodies' ability to defend against pathogens.[4] On the other hand, many cannabis-using patients notice the positive health effects of open-mindedness, creativity, humor, laughter, bliss, acceptance, tolerance, gratitude, and forgiveness despite an often-difficult healing process.

These shifts in frame of mind can be induced by endocannabinoids (cannabinoids produced by the body itself) or by cannabinoids extracted from plants or synthesized in a laboratory. Either way, the ECS can be activated to help us move beyond limiting ways of being and behaving based on past experiences. The ECS can be activated to support movement towards whatever could produce enhanced health and vitality now.

CANNABINOID RECEPTORS

Large numbers of cannabinoid receptors are embedded in specific cell membranes throughout the human body. These receptors can be activated in three ways: by release of the body's own cannabinoids (for example, anandamide), through the introduction of plant-based cannabinoids such as cannabis, or through manufactured cannabinoids such as Dronabinol.

The two most common types of cannabinoid receptors are the CB1 and the CB2 receptors. Scientists suspect there are three more endocannabinoid receptors whose locations and functions will be more fully understood after more research. For the time being, these other receptors are referred to as non-CB1 and non-CB2.

Rather than creating a long list of organs, cells and systems that contain cannabinoid receptors and the diseases they influence, I have generated the following charts to show 1) the specific cannabinoid receptors discovered to date and 2) a list of chronic diseases for which cannabinoid therapy has shown promise.

CANNABINOID RECEPTORS (CHART A)

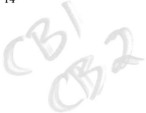

Endocannabinoid receptors influence, modulate or regulate the function of each of the cells, tissues, glands, organs and systems in which they are contained.

CB1 RECEPTORS ARE LOCATED IN CELLS OF THE:

Brain/CNS/Spinal cord (CB1)
Cortical regions (CB1): (neocortex, pyriform cortex, hippocampus , amygdala)
Cerebellum (CB1)
Brainstem (CB1)
Basal ganglia (CB1): globus pallidus, substantia nigra pars, reticulata
Olfactory bulb (CB1)
Thalamus (CB1)
Hypothalamus (CB1): endocrine-brain link
Pituitary gland (CB1)

Thyroid (CB1)

Upper airways (CB1)

Liver (CB1): kupffer cells (macrophage immune cells), hepatocytes (liver cell), hepatic stellate cells (fat storage cell)

Adrenals (CB1)

Ovaries (CB1): gonads and endocrine gland

Uterus (CB1): myometrium

Testes (CB1): gonads and endocrine gland, leydig cells, sperm cells

Prostate (CB1): epithelial and smooth muscle cells

CB1 AND CB2 RECEPTORS ARE LOCATED IN CELLS OF THE:

Eye (CB1 and CB2): retinal pigment epithelial/RPE cells

Heart (CB1 and CB2)

Stomach (CB1 and CB2)

Pancreas (CB1 and CB2)

Digestive tract (CB1 and CB2)

Bone (CB1 and CB2)

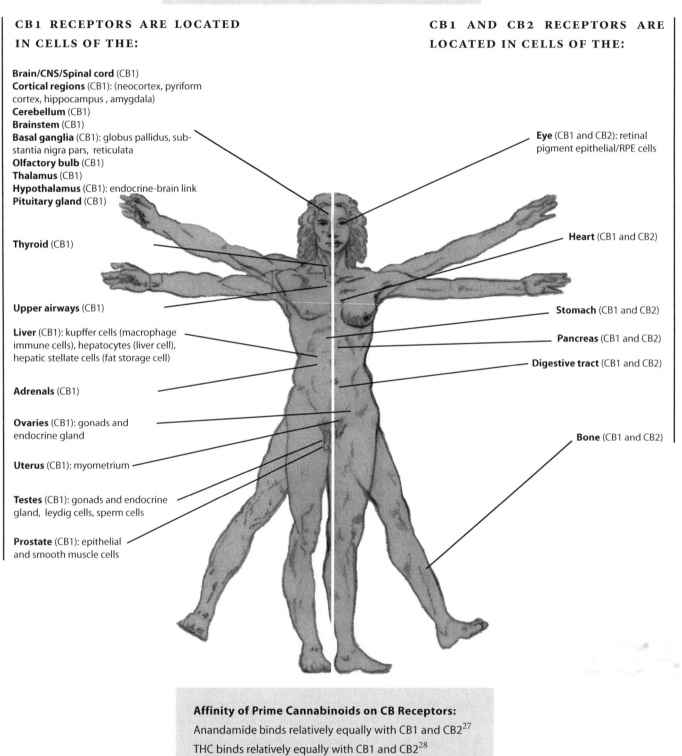

Affinity of Prime Cannabinoids on CB Receptors:
Anandamide binds relatively equally with CB1 and CB2[27]
THC binds relatively equally with CB1 and CB2[28]

For key study references for CB repector site location see footnotes [31] through [46].

CANNABINOID RECEPTORS (CHART B)

CB2 RECEPTORS ARE LOCATED IN THE CELLS OF THE:

Lymphatic/Immune system more specifically cells of the
spleen (CB2)
thymus (CB2)
tonsils (CB2) and the
blood (CB2)
    lymphocytes

NON-CB1 AND NON-CB2 RECEPTORS ARE LOCATED IN CELLS OF THE:

Blood vessels: epithelial cells of arterial blood vessels (non-CB1 and non-CB2)

Non-immune cell CB2 receptors are found in the skin
    keratinocytes

Affinity of Prime Cannabinoids on CB Receptors:

CBD has a greater affinity for CB2[29]

CBN has a greater affinity for CB2[30]

(E)-β-caryophyllene activates CB2

For key study references for CB repector site location see footnotes [31] through [46].

CANNABIS HEALTH INDEX – FOR 100(+) CHRONIC SYMPTOMS & DISEASES

Disease/Symptom	Number of Studies		Total CHI Value
Aging		1	2
Anorexia & Cachexia		11	28
Bacterial Infections		**1**	**1**
Gonorrhea		0	0
MRSA		1	1
Cancer	**Total**	**60**	**107**
Bone Cancer		3	8
Brain Cancer/Glioma/Glioblastoma		9	26
Breast Cancer		6	11
Cervical Cancer		2	2
Colon Cancer (Colorectal)		3	4
Kaposi's sarcoma (See Viral Infections)		2	1
Leukemia and Lymphoma		7	9
Liver Cancer		2	4
Lung Cancer		4	7
Melanoma (Malignant Skin Cancer)		1	1
Pains due to Advanced Cancer (See Pain)		2	10
Pancreatic Cancer		2	4
Prostate Cancer		3	3
Rhabdomyosarcoma		2	1
Skin Cancer (Non-melanoma)		2	11
Thyroid cancer		2	3
Cancer Induced Night Sweats		1	3
Cancer caused by Cannabis?		7	-1
Cardio-Vascular Diseases	**Total**	**12**	**29**
Heart Disease		7	16
Hypertension		2	5
Stroke		3	8
Diabetes		5	11
Eye Diseases	**Total**	**11**	**23**
Age Related Macular Degeneration (ARMD)		1	1
Glaucoma		9	19
Improved Night Vision		1	3
Fever/Temperature Regulation		2	4
Fibromyalgia		3	14
Hemorrhoids		0	0
Inflammatory Diseases	**Total**	**17**	**45**
Arthritis		3	6
Rheumatoid Arthritis		3	10
Atherosclerosis		3	6
Interstitial cystitis		1	3
Gastro-Intestinal Inflammatory Diseases	**Total**	**4**	**15**
Inflammatory Bowel Disease (IBD/IBS)		3	8
Gastro-Esophageal Reflux Disease (GERD)		1	7

Disease/Symptom	Number of Studies		Total CHI Value
Pancreatitis		2	3
Periodontitis		1	2
Injuries	**Total**	**8**	**30**
Post-Surgery Wounds		1	4
Spinal Cord Injuries		5	19
Wound Care		0	0
Insomnia		1	5
Libido Enhancement		1	2
Lung Diseases	**Total**	**12**	**38**
Asthma		7	24
Chronic Obstructive Pulmonary Disease (COPD)		2	3
Cough		3	11
Mental Disorders	**Total**	**24**	**68**
Anxiety		4	14
Autism		0	0
Depression		8	23
Manic-Depressive Disorder/Bipolar Affective Disorder		5	8
Post Traumatic Stress Disorder (PTSD)		3	7
Schizophrenia		4	16
Neurological Diseases	**Total**	**69**	**215**
Neuro-Protection in General		4	11
Alcoholism		4	9
Alzheimer's Disease (AD)		4	10
Amyotrophic Lateral Sclerosis (ALS)		7	19
Epileptic Seizure (Status Epilepticus)		5	13
Huntington's Disease (HD)		5	10
Multiple Sclerosis (MS)		26	91
Parkinson's Disease		4	14
Tourette's Syndrome		10	38
Obstetrical and Gynecological (OBGYN)	**Total**	**5**	**11**
Endometriosis		2	5
Menstrual Pain		2	3
Morning Sickness		1	3
Osteoporosis		3	5
Pain	**Total**	**14**	**50**
Chronic non-malignant pains (CNMP)		2	5
Migraines		3	10
Neuropathies (in general)		5	15
Neuropathies (AIDS related)		2	10
Pains (due to advanced cancer)		2	10
Prion Diseases/Creutzfeldt – Jacob Disease (CJD)		1	3
Sickle Cell Disease (SCD)		2	5
Skin Diseases		4	11
Viral Infections	**Total**	**12**	**27**
Cold and Flu		0	0

Disease/Symptom	Number of Studies		Total CHI Value
Cough		3	10
Hepatitis		3	8
Herpes Virus		3	5
HIV/AIDS in General		1	3
Kaposi's Sarcoma		2	1
Vomiting	**Total**	**27**	**111**
Chemotherapy Induced Nausea and Vomiting		24	104
Motion Sickness		2	4
Morning Sickness		1	3
	Total Number: 306		**Total CHI Value: 845**

CANNABIS HEALTH INDEX (BIG GROUPS BY NUMBER OF STUDIES)

Disease/Symptom	Number of Studies	Total CHI Value
Neurological Diseases	69	215
Cancer	60	107
Vomiting	27	111
Mental Disorders	24	68
Pain	14	50
Inflammatory Diseases	14	40
Bacterial and Viral Infections	13	28
Cardio-Vascular Diseases	12	29
Lung Diseases	12	38
Eye Diseases	11	23
Anorexia & Cachexia	11	28
Injuries	8	30
Diabetes	5	11
Obstetrical and Gynecological (OBGYN)	5	11
Skin Diseases	4	11
Fibromyalgia	3	14

CANNABIS HEALTH INDEX (BIG GROUPS BY HIGHEST CHI)

Disease/Symptom	Number of Studies	Total CHI Value
Neurological Diseases	69	215
Vomiting	27	111
Cancer	60	107
Mental Disorders	24	68
Pain	14	50
Inflammatory Diseases	14	40
Lung Diseases	12	38
Injuries	8	30
Cardio-Vascular Diseases	12	29
Anorexia & Cachexia	11	28
Bacterial and Viral Infections	13	28
Eye Diseases	11	23
Fibromyalgia	3	14

Disease/Symptom	Number of Studies	Total CHI Value
Skin Diseases	4	11
Diabetes	5	11
Obstetrical and Gynecological (OBGYN)	5	11

For those who prefer a visual representation of the Cannabis Health Index (CHI) rather than charts and numbers: Here on this page CHI is represented by honeycombs and shades of grey. One honycomb represents one study conducted on the disease listed and the darker the shade of grey the higher the overall CHI score.

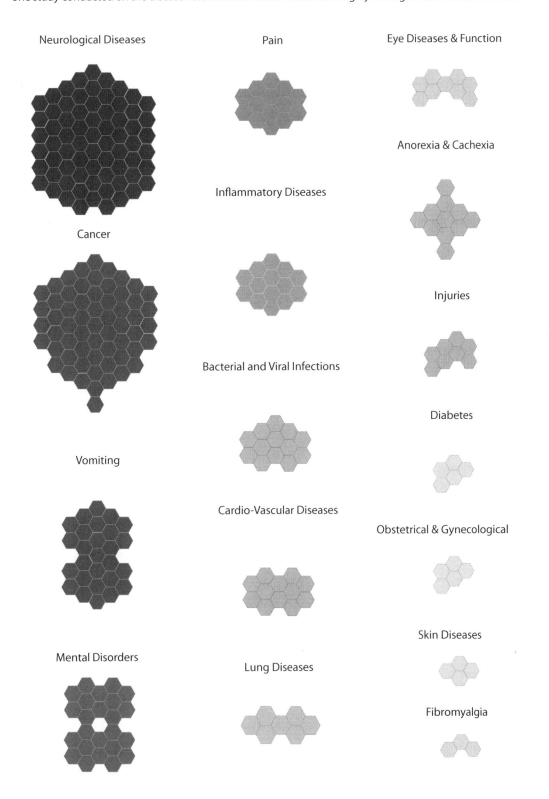

CANNABINOIDS (IN GENERAL)

If cannabinoid receptors function as a lock, cannabinoids are the key. Scientific knowledge of cannabis and its most potent constituents is expanding exponentially, reflective of the far-reaching implications for human health and medicine. Cannabis has repeatedly demonstrated profound therapeutic efficacy for multiple conditions, many of which you will find in the index. A search in the US National Library of Medicine using the single keyword "cannabinoids" currently yields over 15,000 studies.[5] Worldwide, millions of patients rely on cannabis or cannabinoid prescriptions to maintain health and well-being and mitigate the assault of chronic degenerative illness or the terrible adverse effects of allopathic treatments such as chemotherapy. Hundreds of medical and scientific organizations support the use of medical marijuana including Kaiser Permanente, the California Medical Association and the American Nurses Association. Even the conservative American Medical Association now supports research on cannabis for medicinal use.

This support from the medical community is hardly surprising considering the level of frustration felt by a large number of physicians and health care providers faced with no adequate and safe treatment options for the many chronic degenerative diseases listed in the index.

One of the plant's many astounding capabilities is that it simultaneously relaxes and stimulates the autonomic nervous system. Cannabinoids induce these changes by enhancing and balancing individual cellular function as well as that of the whole organism. This occurs in the mind as well as elsewhere in the body. Marijuana's constituents enhance left-brain and right-brain functioning, inducing an expanded state of consciousness which embraces logic and intuition, individuality and oneness, thought and feeling.

To date, over 80 cannabis-based cannabinoids have been isolated and researchers are beginning to look at other plant constituents such as terpenoids as important co-factors in inducing therapeutic effects.[6]

FOUR PRIME CANNABINOIDS (AEA, THC, CBD, AND (E)-BCP)

ANANDAMIDE - AEA (PRODUCED BY THE BODY)

The discovery of the "Bliss Molecule" anandamide[7] in the nineties was a major scientific breakthrough that led to a better understanding of the interaction between cannabinoids and the endocannabinoid system of the human body. Like all other cannabinoids, anandamide is a "key" molecule. It fits relatively equally into both CB1 and CB2 receptors ("locks").[8] Once the connection is made, the lock opens and a signal is generated. At that point, numerous physiological as well as mental and emotional changes take place. For instance, anandamide enhances pleasure,[9] may be involved in mitigating episodes of acute schizophrenia,[10] destroys numerous types of cancers[11,12,13] and soothes coughs.[14]

Five distinct endocannabinoids have been identified.

Anandamide (N-arachidonoylethanolamide) - (AEA)

2-arachidonoyl glycerol - (2-AG)

2-arachidonoyl-glyceryl-ether - (Noladin ether)

O-arachidonoyl-ethanolamine (Virodhamine)

N-arachidonoyl-dopamine - (NADA)

TETRAHYDROCANNABINOL - THC (SOURCED IN CANNABIS)

Under a microscope, tetrahydrocannabinol (THC) looks like a sticky liquid crystal when warm and a glass-like solid when cool. It is the primary mind-altering constituent of marijuana, and is responsible for generating complex changes that occur physically as well as mentally and emotionally.

The chemical structure of THC was first determined in 1964 by Raphael Mechoulam and Yechiel Gaoni who isolated the compound from hashish at an Israeli University. It is without a doubt the most studied cannabis constituent. However, despite this vast knowledge base, this unique molecule keeps surprising scientists as new information about its vast influence on human physiology and psychology comes to light.

Like anandamide, THC binds equally well to both CB1 and CB2 receptors[15] and thus initiates a host of therapeutic changes in both the central nervous system (CB1) and in the immune system (CB2). It is interesting to note that changes in our frame of mind similarly effect our central nervous system and immune system.

Whenever applicable, the therapeutic impact of THC is examined in the discussion of specific diseases in this book. Rather than repeat information included elsewhere, I'd like to mention a highly significant discovery relevant to the number one killer in the United States: Heart Disease.

THC may protect the heart from damage and may mitigate damage from an infarction (heart attack). Recent discoveries have isolated several mechanisms by which THC demonstrates heart protective abilities. While these latest insights are still in their beginning stages it is likely that the way we will treat acute and chronic heart disease in the future will change as a result: THC reduced heart attack size in mice;[16] THC may protect heart cells against damage from hypoxia by induction of nitric oxide, in a sense THC preparing heart cells to better withstand hypoxia (poor perfusion of heart cells and a direct cause of heart attacks);[17] THC is neuroprotective via CB1;[18] THC causes bronchodilation (enlargement of the airways leading to increased air supply -- a key problem in heart disease);[19,20,21,22,23,24] THC causes weight gain and an increase in walking distance in chronic obstructive pulmonary disease (COPD).[25]

Synthetic drugs containing THC include Sativex, Dronabinol, Marinol, and Nabilone. These pharmaceuticals are approved by the FDA and are used to treat a large number of conditions some of which include AIDS related anorexia/cachexia, nausea and vomiting secondary to chemotherapy cancer treatments, neurological disorders, inflammatory conditions, and PTSD.

With the exception of Sativex, which is essentially a plant derived tincture, pharmaceuticals that contain THC do not contain any of the other biologically active components of cannabis that may play an important therapeutic role in the human body.

Plant-based THC content varies by cannabis strain, and varies depending upon whether it is fresh or dried (and if dried, its age), and whether it is grown indoors or outdoors. Some strains may be especially potent in THC while others may only contain trace amounts. Fresh cannabis contains THC in the form of THC-carboxylic-acid, which is considered only minutely psychoactive. Once dried however, the chemical composition of THC-acid changes, and it becomes decarboxylated through heat (as it dries or when it is burned). Once devoid of its carboxyl group, THC becomes psychoactive. Talk to your local medical dispensary for information on the THC profiles of current strains.

THC content decreases over time and is affected by UV-light, heat, and exposure to moisture. Indoor cultivation follows a three-month cycle while outdoor cultivation follows an annual or biannual cycle. Indoor crops tend to contain a markedly higher THC content than outdoor crops.

CANNABIDIOL - CBD (SOURCED IN CANNABIS)

Sourced in cannabis, cannabidiol (CBD) is a non-psychoactive cannabinoid. CBD has a greater affinity for CB2 receptors than CB1 receptors[26] but much of its therapeutic influence stems from its ability to suppress the enzyme (fatty acid amide hydrolase or FAAH) that breaks down anandamide thus keeping "the Bliss Molecule" active at higher concentrations and for a longer duration. At the same time, CBD tames the psychoactive influence of THC allowing patients to focus on THC's other therapeutic powers at higher concentrations.

While the full complexity of how CBD interacts with the body's endocannabinoid system is yet to be revealed, numerous studies have shown that CBD effects diseases of both the mind and the body, particularly neurological diseases, inflammatory illness and cancer.

More specifically, CBD is considered a very promising agent with the highest prospect for therapeutic use in the treatment of neurodegenerative illness.[27,28,29,30] An oil based solution of CBD has been documented as effective for pediatric patients suffering from epileptic seizures who failed to respond to traditional pharmaceutical anti-seizure medications.[31] CBD may also be useful in preventing nerve damage associated with alcohol poisoning.[32]

In addition to providing neuroprotection, CBD appears to calm autonomic responses to stress (such as rapid heart rates) by engaging receptors that select serotonin to achieve a calming effect.[33] Cannabidiol's therapeutic potential in psychological disorders is based on its antipsychotic,[34] anxiolytic, and antidepressant effects.[35] CBD is able to reduce symptoms of acute paranoid schizophrenia as well as the pharmaceutical drug amisulpride which (unlike CBD) has significant adverse side-effects.[36]

CBD has been shown to have a clear and measurable therapeutic impact on inflammatory and anti-inflammatory regulation mechanisms[37] such as in inflammatory bowel disease,[38,39,40] arthritis,[41] peridontitis,[42] and atherosclerosis.[43]

As regards cancer, CBD is able to produce significant antitumor activity both in vitro and in vivo.[44] Further, CBD has been shown to selectively produce oxidative stress in cancer cells thus producing apoptosis (cancer cell suicide) without impacting normal cells.[45,46]

E-β-CARYOPHYLLENE (PRIMARILY SOURCED IN SPICE PLANTS)

An international group of researchers from Switzerland, Germany, Italy and the U.S. (2008, 2012) reported that certain plants, most notably spice produc-

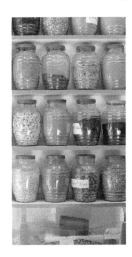

ing plants, contain a functional non-psychoactive CB2 agonist called (E)-β-caryophyllene or (E)-BCP. Scientists suggest that activation of CB2 receptors via this newly discovered dietary plant-based cannabinoid might present a new and additional therapeutic strategy in the treatment of a multitude of diseases associated with inflammation and oxidative stress, both underlying factors in a host of different pathologies.[47,48] Additional research has shown that β-caryophyllene may also protect against microbes, pain and cancer.[49]

This food-based cannabinoid is fully accepted by the U.S. Government with the FDA's seal of approval and key β-caryophyllene containing organic spices are relatively easy to obtain. Spices that contain β-caryophyllene include: black and white Ashanti (West African) peppers, Indian bay-leaf, alligator pepper, basil, cinnamon, rosemary, caraway, black pepper, Mexican oregano, and clove.

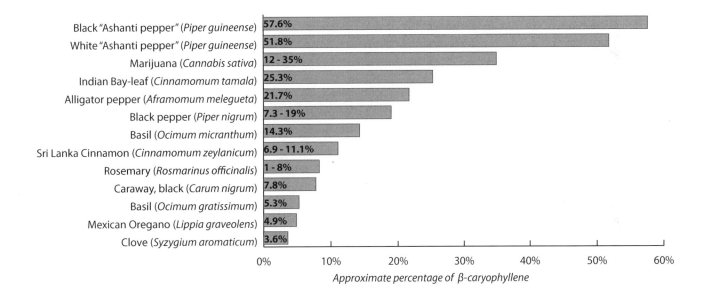

Black "Ashanti pepper" (*Piper guineense*) 57.6%
White "Ashanti pepper" (*Piper guineense*) 51.8%
Marijuana (*Cannabis sativa*) 12 - 35%
Indian Bay-leaf (*Cinnamomum tamala*) 25.3%
Alligator pepper (*Aframomum melegueta*) 21.7%
Black pepper (*Piper nigrum*) 7.3 - 19%
Basil (*Ocimum micranthum*) 14.3%
Sri Lanka Cinnamon (*Cinnamomum zeylanicum*) 6.9 - 11.1%
Rosemary (*Rosmarinus officinalis*) 1 - 8%
Caraway, black (*Carum nigrum*) 7.8%
Basil (*Ocimum gratissimum*) 5.3%
Mexican Oregano (*Lippia graveolens*) 4.9%
Clove (*Syzygium aromaticum*) 3.6%

Approximate percentage of β-caryophyllene

BLACK AND WHITE "ASHANTI PEPPERS" (PIPER GUINEENSE): The β-caryophyllene content contained in test samples of Black Ashanti pepper was 58% and in White Ashanti pepper 52%.[50] In comparison, the β-caryophyllene content in a sample of cannabis sativa ranges from 12 to 35%.[51] These peppers also have antibacterial properties against E. coli and Staphylococcus aureus.

INDIAN BAY-LEAF (CINNAMOMUM TAMALA): The β-caryophyllene content of a tested sample was 25%.[52] In addition, Indian Bay-leaf, a prominent herb in Ayurvedic traditions, exhibits proven anti-oxidant and anti-diabetic properties.[53]

GRAINS OF PARADISE (AFRAMOMUM MELEGUETA): The β-caryophyllene content measured in this spice was 22%.[54] Additional medicinal uses and properties supported by scientific studies include the promotion of wound healing by cell membrane support.[55] It is also an anti-oxidant,[56] anti-inflammatory,[57] analgesic,[58] molluscicidal (destroys snails),[59] anti-diarrheal agent,[60,61] anti-microbial agent[62] and may enhance sexual interest and function.[63]

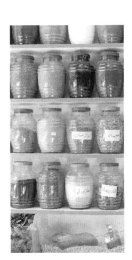

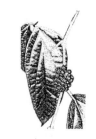

Piper guineense

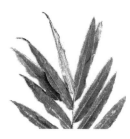

Cannabis sativa

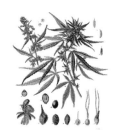

Cinnamomum tamala

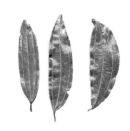

Aframomum melegueta

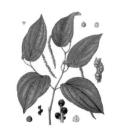

Piper nigrum

BLACK PEPPER (PIPER NIGRUM): Samples of black pepper yielded a β-caryophyllene content ranging between 7% -19%.[64] Scientific studies have documented additional medicinal benefits including anti-bacterial properties,[65] use as a protective agent against colon cancer,[66] and anti-oxidant activity.[67]

AFRICAN BASIL (OCIMUM MICRANTHUM): This type of basil typically contains β-caryophyllene content of 14%.[68] There are many varieties of basil with similar constituents. However, not all species have been fully explored. The medicinal uses and properties of Ocimum basilicum, a form of basil commonly used world-wide, has antimicrobial (giardia) properties, may assist in dyspepsia and high blood pressure (diuretic), is potentially effective against cholera-induced diarrhea, has anti-viral activity against herpes virus I and II, adenoviruses, hepatitis B virus and the RNA viruses (coxsackievirus B1 and enterovirus 71), is an anti-bacterial for middle ear infections and has anti-inflammatory properties.[69]

SRI LANKA CINNAMON (CINNAMOMUM ZEYLANICUM): A sample of Sri Lanka (Ceylon) Cinnamon contained 7–11% β-caryophyllene when tested.[70] Other medicinal uses and properties supported by scientific studies include improved fat and sugar metabolism, a possible treatment for high blood pressure, antioxidant properties, broad-spectrum antibiotic properties, and the ability to cure mite infestation in animals.[71]

ROSEMARY (ROSMARINUS OFFICINALIS): Approximately 1% and 8% of β-caryophyllene was contained in two different samples of rosemary.[72] Medicinal uses and properties supported by scientific studies include use of rosemary as an anti-microbial (bacteria, fungi), to treat dyspepsia (digestive complaints), to promote circulation, as a radio protective, to possibly prevent skin cancer tumors and other kinds of tumors, as an anti-inflammatory, and in the prevention and treatment of diabetic, cardiovascular, and other neurodegenerative diseases.[73]

CARAWAY, BLACK (CARUM NIGRUM): Levels of β-caryophyllene in a sample of black caraway were measured at 8%.[74] Essential oil of carum nigrum has demonstrated potent anti-oxidant, antibacterial and antifungal properties.[75]

BASIL (OCIMUM GRATISSIMUM): β-caryophyllene content in a sample of this type of basil was measured at 5%.[76] See also African Basil, above. Basil has shown protective gastro-intestinal abilities[77] and antibacterial properties against E. coli and Staphylococcus aureus.[78]

MEXICAN OREGANO (LIPPIA GRAVEOLENS): The β-caryophyllene content in a sample of Mexican oregano was measured at 5%.[79] This herb, commonly used in Mexican traditional healing, has demonstrated abilities to inhibit acyclovir resistant herpes virus in the laboratory.[80]

CLOVE (SYZYGIUM AROMATICUM): A sample of clove contained almost 4% β-caryophyllene.[81] Studies have shown the essential oil of clove to work as an analgesic, anti-inflammatory, antioxidant, anti-microbial, anti-fungal, anti-viral (herpes simplex –HSV I&II and hepatitis C), anti-bacterial (including a several of the multi-drug resistant Staphylococcus epidermidis), anti-cancer, cancer protective (skin and lung), anti-diabetic, and insect repellant. It contains aphrodisiac properties. A cream from clove works as an effective treatment for chronic anal fissures.[82]

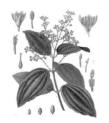

Cinnamomum zeylanicum

CANNABIS

Numerous good books have been written on the history of cannabis and its place among the people and cultures of the world, so I will keep this section brief and relevant to healing. There are hundreds of varieties of cannabis with similar appearance and characteristics. With the exception of Antarctica, the species grows on every continent.

For our purposes two basic distinctions are of importance. First, the name hemp is used to indicate extremely low or non-psychoactive cannabis species. And, while hemp plants are a good source of nutrition (e.g. essential fatty acids), the medicinal property of hempseed oil is limited to some mild anti-inflammatory properties. Hemp is a legal crop in numerous countries and used for food, drink, fiber, oil, paper, building materials, erosion control, fuel, biodegradable plastics, and a multitude of other uses.

Secondly, medicinal cannabis species consist of two basic species, cannabis sativa and cannabis indica. Both are psychoactive and both contain the cannabinoids required to engage the endocannabinoid system for specific therapeutic purposes. These two strains look different and contain different ratios of the primary cannabinoids, which is relevant when selecting a strain for specific therapeutic purposes.

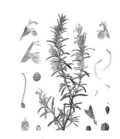

Rosmarinus officinalis

Indica plants tend to be short and stalky, with wider leaves than sativas, which usually grow longer, higher and display a finer leaf structure. More important however, indicas and sativas produce different THC:CBD/CBN ratios. These ratios are important, because the ratio determines the degree to which the balancing properties of the whole plant's constituents are additive or cancel each other out.

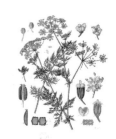

Carum nigrum

Sativa: Higher THC to Lower CBD/CBN Ratio	Indica: Lower THC to Higher CBD/CBN Ratio
Generally stimulating, energizing, uplifting	Generally sedating, relaxing, grounding
Generally more mental/emotional	Generally more physical
Usually more extrovert	Usually more introvert
Best for daytime use	Better after work is done, bedtime
Increases alertness	Sleeping aid
Consider with depression	Consider with anxiety
Pain relief, muscle relaxant	Pain relief, muscle relaxant
THC binds both CB1 and CB2 receptors	CBD has a greater affinity for CB2

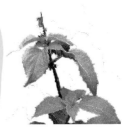

Ocimum gratissimum

Many cannabis-using patients use the plant not only as medicine, but as a means to seek a deeper and longer lasting healing. The cannabis induced "high" is employed to explore our frame of mind associated with illness and disease, to reach a deeper understanding, gently accept oneself and initiate nurturing changes that support health and healing and desired levels of energy.

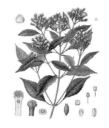

Syzygium aromaticum

A carefully balanced and finely tuned body and mind can more easily surpass ordinary states of consciousness and open doors to spiritual dimensions of reality. Ascetics of India and modern urban shamans alike consider this dance of expanding consciousness between plant and human a literal infusion of spirit. The ingestion, topical application or inhalation of marijuana is employed as a tool to learn and explore, and to seek knowledge, insights and spiritual revelations about the self in an ever-expanding and mysterious universe. And it is precisely this infusion of spirit with its vibrancy, aliveness and enthusiasm that ultimately allows for a renewed sense of health and well-being.

In one sense, the cannabis-using patient reaching for deeper healing is not dissimilar to who use the plant to access realms that are beyond the comprehension and imagination of ordinary consciousness. Those who use the plant as a spiritual practice echo a tradition which dates back to ancient times. Some of the wandering yogis of India and Nepal and the Sadhus -- ascetics who have dedicated their life to explore the ineffable presence of God -- use cannabis as a means to this end. To Rastafarians, "the herb is the key to new understanding of the self, the universe, and God. It is the vehicle to cosmic consciousness."[83] Ancient Scythians used cannabis to produce trance states, divination,[84] delight and joy.[85] According to the Bible,[86] God instructs Moses to make holy anointing oil containing keneh bosem (cannabis)[87] to "…anoint Aaron and his sons, sanctifying them as priests to Me." The Egyptian Ebers papyrus, which documents medical practices dating from 3400 BC,[88] describes the use of cannabis ground in honey as a remedy for vaginal illness.[89]

"Unlike many of the drugs we prescribe every day, marijuana has never been proven to cause a fatal overdose."
- Joycelyn Elders, MD, former US Surgeon General

Even though cannabis has more proven therapeutic applications than any other plant in the world, working with cannabis is by no means a panacea. However, combining an informed and responsible use of cannabis by engaging mind–body medicine, we open a door to a new and potent synergy of healing that can take our healing journey to new depths, far beyond temporary relief or mere cessation of symptoms. We might discover places of profound understanding, combined with a deep sense of empathy. Perhaps it will show up as a newly-found freedom, rooted in responsibility without blame. The journey might reveal a love emerging from an ancient hatred, or the lifting of a humiliating shame that was crushing our spirit. Or we may surprise ourselves by the emergence of a tender intimacy that transcends the lingering sensation of worthlessness like dew in the morning fog.

IS CANNABIS SAFE?

WHO SHOULD NOT USE CANNABIS?

As with any medicine that affects the mind and the body, cannabis evokes numerous concerns and questions worthy of examination. Chief among them is the potential for adverse effects. Does the use of marijuana lead to addiction? How does the use of the plant affect the development of adolescents, or the developing fetus in pregnant women? Concerns about fertility are raised. The smoking of plant material and its effect on the lungs are another commonly expressed concern. What about the plants impact on the heart, or the development of cancer? Some studies have suggested that marijuana may be implicated as a co-factor in developing schizophrenia, or cause traffic accidents from irresponsible use. Could smoking pot encourage use of other illegal and/or dangerous "recreational" drugs (an idea known as The Gateway Theory)? Lastly, is it possible to overdose on cannabis?

Without going into the social, historical and political aspects of cannabis, I will attempt to briefly address these reasonable health concerns in descending order. I used to judge a drug by the harmful impact it had on the people I treated as an Emergency Medical Technician and the frequency with which people needed to call 911 due to drug use. The number one drug responsible for generating 911 emergency calls is nicotine contained in tobacco cigarettes, due to the lasting and serious damage smoking causes, followed closely by alcohol abuse. Next comes heroin, stimulants (cocaine, crack, methamphetamine, diet pills), and PCP, respectively.

On the other side of the spectrum are occasional calls to 911 related to use of psychogenic substances such as LSD, ecstasy or psilocybin. During my 20 years working in emergency services, I can barely recall an incident in which someone called 911 for cannabis use alone. However, many studies show large numbers of cannabis-related visits to the ER. Upon closer examination, it is clear that the majority of such visits were due to cannabis used in combination with other drugs, or incidences of people experiencing anxiety. Government statistics seem to echo my experience.

According to several U.S. government sources, there were zero deaths due to the exclusive use of cannabis in the periods studied which range from January, 1997 through June, 2005.[90,91] (Deaths in which cannabis was one of several drugs used are not counted here.) In contrast, recent CDC estimates suggest that on average, tobacco (particularly cigarette smoking) claimed 110,750 lives per year from 2000 to 2004.[92] The average number of alcohol-related fatalities per year was estimated at 75,766 in 2001.[93]

Commonly noted effects of cannabis include euphoria, relaxation, intensification of sensory experiences, infectious laughter and talkativeness, increased appetite, and "feeling stoned." Adverse effects include reduced attention span, red sclera (reddening of the normally white part of the eyes), dry mouth, and decreased cognitive and motor skills. Other rare side-effects, more common when ingested or when used at higher than the subjective therapeutic dose, include ataxia (unsteady gait), aphasia (inability to speak clearly), unusual perceptions of all senses, including hallucinations, anxiety (though this can be addressed by reassurance), slight increase in heart rate, subtle shifts in blood pressure depending on the position of the body, and panic (moderated by reassurance) upon first ever use.

In the context of addiction, both opponents and proponents of medical marijuana have numerous studies to support their arguments. However, one distinction is usually agreed upon. If dependency occurs, it is an addiction in psychological terms rather than in the physical realm, as is the case with many other substances, such as tobacco, alcohol or heroin. The large numbers of people enrolled in drug treatment centers is often cited to substantiate claims that the plant is psychologically addictive. This overlooks the reality that many court judges do not believe marijuana users should go to jail, but as they are bound to uphold present laws, they are left with no other option but to mandate drug treatment instead of jail or prison time.

Compared to pharmaceuticals, some of which have a more significant addiction potential, cannabis carries a considerably reduced risk of adverse side-effects (including death). An FDA report compared marijuana to 17 common FDA-approved pharmaceutical drugs used to treat similar symptoms and conditions. Their findings make a compelling argument for medical marijuana. Between 1997 and 2005, no deaths were attributed to the exclusive use of cannabis while the FDA recorded 10,008 deaths due to the 17 FDA-approved pharmaceutical drugs in the study.[94]

If you are concerned about developing a dependence on cannabis, you may reduce this potential risk by infusing mindfulness into your process of healing and/or using raw preparations of cannabis which have little or no psychoactive effect.

> *Walter had sexual performance anxiety. The use of cannabis reduced his anxiety and otherwise enhanced his sensual experience. Rather than becoming dependent on the use of the plant each time he wished to engage in sexual activity, he used the cannabis-induced state of mind to explore the deeper causes for his anxiety and took corrective action, which eventually cured his anxiety and eliminated his need for cannabis.*

When it comes to fertility, to the developing fetus or to the still physically developing adolescent, the use of any mind-body altering substance is cause for concern. As before, various studies are cited as evidence by those on both sides of this issue. No long-term studies examining the exclusive use of cannabis on fertility, the fetus and adolescents have been conducted. Instead, people enrolled in most studies were exposed to other substances, thus complicating the overall picture.

However, a study conducted at Duke University[95] which collected subjective observational data from New Zealand residents over a period of about 38 years[96] concluded that while cannabis use by adults has no effect on intelligence, "cannabis dependency" in adolescents (defined by the authors as continued use despite major health, social, and/or legal problems related to its use) may contribute to reduced IQ test scores later in life. The study has limitations: data was described subjectively, the study had a small sample size (17% or 153 people fit the authors' dependency definition), and only some factors that may alter IQ were considered in the analysis. Still, no other study to-date has examined the impact of adolescent use of cannabis on intelligence measured over time. Until more is known, it is advisable to assume a possible correlation.

Whenever plant matter is burned, smoke is released, and with it potentially harmful particles. However, the largest population-based case-controlled study ever conducted of cannabis-only use yielded somewhat counter-intuitive results. For the 2,252 people studied in a Los Angeles, California study, smoking (only) cannabis was found to be mildly lung-protective, and was not associated with an increased risk of lung cancer.[97]

Cannabis oil produces therapeutic effects in patients with chronic obstructive pulmonary disease (a serious lung disorder) and asthma. (See also the chapter on lung disease.) To minimize any potential risk of negative consequences to one's lungs, some people use vaporizers to inhale cannabis rather than smoking cannabis wrapped in paper. Use of a vaporizer eliminates the inhalation of carbon compounds from burned paper. An infused oil or alcohol-based tincture can also be used to address symptoms related to lung diseases.

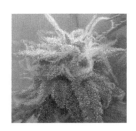

Endocannabinoid receptors are present in the heart, and thus are involved in regulating heart function. THC can increase one's heart rate, but not to a dangerous extent. Furthermore, numerous studies have shown that THC, CBD and CBN have potentially potent cardio-protective properties. (See the chapter on heart disease.) And in the context of cancer, cannabis' constituents have demonstrated remarkable abilities to produce apoptosis (cancer cell death) in a great variety of cancer manifestations. (See also the chapter on cancer.)

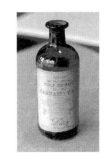

Observational studies have concluded that ingesting cannabis as an adolescent may increase one's risk of developing schizophrenia later in life. While cannabis is not itself a causal factor for schizophrenia, in some instances it may be a co-factor. Based on the current evidence, it would be prudent for adolescents or young adults with a known family history of psychosis or schizophrenia to stay away from cannabis or any other mind-altering substance, especially speed-based drugs such as cocaine or methamphetamines. (See also the chapter on mental disorders–schizophrenia.)

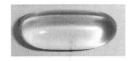

The controversial gateway theory suggests that adolescents who experiment with cannabis are more likely to subsequently try, and become addicted to, other illicit drugs. While the gateway theory has never attempted to address therapeutic uses of legally obtained medicine, the suggestion that even short-term cannabis use could lead to addiction to other drugs still lingers in many peoples' minds. In fact, a recent study of over 4,000 cannabis smokers concluded that cannabis use leads to a decrease in the use of alcohol, tobacco and hard drugs.[98]

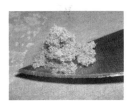

Can cannabis kill you? A laboratory study conducted in 1973 reported the median lethal dose of oral THC in rats as 800–1900 mg/kg, depending on the sex and genetic strain of the animal.[99] If body weight is used as the sole criteria, this study suggests that 200 grams of herb per kilogram of body weight is required to approach a lethal dose in humans. Accordingly, a person weighing 70 kg, or 154 lbs., would need to consume 14 kg of herb to approach a fatal dose. A 2004 study was much more conservative, and stated "628 kg of cannabis would have to be smoked in 15 min. to induce a lethal effect."[100]

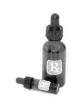

Another area of concern for some is the possibility that external toxins or biological pathogens could be present on the cannabis plant, particularly pesticides or aspergillus fungus. The presence of pesticides on any consumed plant material may increase the body's toxic load, and can contribute in numerous and unpredictable ways to ill health, but can easily be eliminated by purchasing or growing organic cannabis. Aspergillus is a mold that grows on many agricultural products throughout the world and is a common contaminant of bread, potatoes and peanuts. Because cannabis is not regulated, growers do not routinely test for aspergillus nor report concentration amounts as is required for, say, peanut growers. Patients with an already depressed immune system could be particularly vulnerable to any negative effects of aspergillus fungus-contaminated cannabis. Use caution to determine the presence of the fungus on any plant product before consumption. Many cannabis patients believe that heating cannabis at temperatures of 300°F (~149°C) for a period of 5 minutes will kill the pathogen but I have not been able to find any studies to verify this suggestion. However, one study suggested that aspergillus fungus was not present in any samples of ten medicinal herbs dried and stored with a water activity of less than 0.81 in temperature ranges of 25 +/- 2°C (77 +/- 3.6 °F),[101] highlighting the importance of proper drying practices.

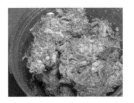

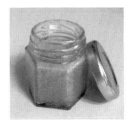

30

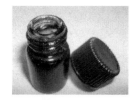

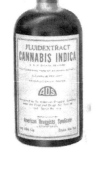

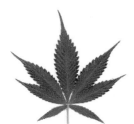

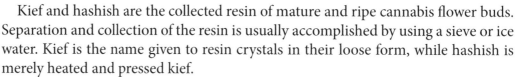

In summary, the bottom line is that extensive evidence indicates that cannabis is neither dangerous nor harmless. Consideration of its medicinal use should include a risk versus benefit analysis, focused on the specific therapeutic needs and health challenges of the individual in question. This book is written and organized in order to facilitate exactly that.

FORMS OF CANNABIS

Cannabis is used medicinally in many forms. Most often, patients utilize dried buds, flowers and leaves of the cannabis plant. To minimize inhalation of burned carbon products, many patients prefer the use of a vaporizer to heat the plant material to a precise temperature that will evaporate the cannabinoids just below the burning point of the plant matter.

Cannabis can be cooked into other foods such as a cookie, brownie or savory dishes. Cannabis is usually added to recipes in the form of an herbed butter, infused oils or tinctures. A dropper may be used to measure medicine precisely and thereby stay within an established optimum therapeutic window.

Fresh cannabis leaf is consumed by many self-growing patients as a salad mixed with other greens. Fresh, raw leaves can also be juiced; this is often diluted with other vegetable juices to disguise its bitter taste. Fresh cannabis contains CBD and THC in their acid forms. As THC is not psychoactive in this form, fresh, raw cannabis is ideal for patients advised to consume large quantities of CBD for its numerous therapeutic and preventative purposes. While studies are underway to determine the therapeutic value of raw cannabis, to-date only physician case studies and patient testimonials are available.

Kief and hashish are the collected resin of mature and ripe cannabis flower buds. Separation and collection of the resin is usually accomplished by using a sieve or ice water. Kief is the name given to resin crystals in their loose form, while hashish is merely heated and pressed kief.

Alcohol or glycerin may be used as a medium to dissolve plant material and produce a tincture useful in oral or topical preparations. This is often called "green dragon". Tinctures extracted using alcohol, glycerin or oil form the basis of various medicinal creams, balms, and lotions. Alternatively, hemp oil, almond oil or coconut oil (preferably of the virgin, organic, variety) may be mixed with cannabis as an additive to create topical skin creams and food products.

Solvents such as hexane, butane or isopropyl alcohol may be employed to dissolve the ingredients of cannabis. While this method produces the highest concentration of cannabinoids, it is also dangerous due to the flammability of the solvents. Explosions have lead to serious injuries and deaths. Also, solvent residue may linger in the concentrate and add a toxic material to the medicine.

MODES OF ADMINISTRATION

Cannabis may be eaten raw, cooked into other foods, drunk as juice, inhaled after vaporization, smoked in a pipe, wrapped in paper and smoked, or rubbed into the skin. It is not safe to drive or operate heavy machinery after taking any psychoactive form of cannabis.

Pharmaceutical prescription cannabinoids:

Dronabinol

Nabilone

Sativex

Rimonabant (no longer available)

If you receive a prescription from your doctor for medical marijuana, your doctor will probably recommend a preferred method for taking your medicine. Medical marijuana dispensaries typically have literature available and staff prepared to teach new patients how to correctly use medical marijuana as prescribed. Your local pharmacist can also discuss derivatives of cannabinoids in pill or liquid form with you if you are unsure how to follow your doctor's instructions.

Inhalation of cannabinoids via vaporization quickly reaches the bloodstream and effects are often experienced in minutes or even seconds. However, effects are of a shorter duration than other modes of administration.

If eaten, it may take forty-five minutes to an hour-and-a-half for cannabis to be absorbed through the gastrointestinal tract. The effects of consumed cannabis thus tend to be delayed, last much longer, and are noticeably different compared to the effects of inhalation. Some patients who want to deliver cannabinoids to the lower half of the intestinal tract use suction-bulbs filled with cannabis-infused oils inserted into the rectum similar to a suppository.

Any favorite recipes can be fortified with cannabis-infused oil, or an alcohol-based tincture that supports your specific needs. Add the oil or tincture after the cooking process is completed, and at the right dose specific to your therapeutic window.

Infused oils or tinctures often come in dropper bottles, which allow for precise dosing. As always, start slowly with a few drops, and wait at least one hour to feel the effect. Then slowly increase the dosage by a couple of drops, repeating the process until you have achieved the desired therapeutic effect. Many patients start with 3 or 4 drops and work from there. The oil or tinctures can easily be made at home or bought at most dispensaries. Since most products are not standardized, you may need to repeat the process each time you make or purchase a new bottle.

Topical creams are used to deliver medicine to specific and isolated problem areas. Absorption rates may be similar to that of ingestion but tend to be less systematic and more local.

WORKING WITH CANNABIS/CONSCIOUSNESS TO REACH FOR DEEPER HEALING

Once you have determined the appropriate therapeutic window or dose that is right for you, allow yourself to explore the feelings that are connected to the symptom or disease you are working to heal. In particular, try to focus on how you feel about anything your illness is preventing you from doing.

Think of these feelings as the needle of a compass that points to underlying issues that require your attention. Often, at this point of the process, patients report the emergence of a memory or a related scenario. Sometimes several memories or scenarios emerge, but, not unlike layers of an onion, show an emotional connection or similarity, and thus reveal a theme that may be important to notice on your journey to health and well-being.

Like many others who have used this method for deeper healing, you may become (more) aware of some internal resistance to getting better. Under the influence of cannabis or through engaging a spirit of gentle mindfulness, you may find, to your surprise, that you are fully able and willing to forgive yourself for any resistance present. This is an excellent start.

Synthetic cannabinoids primarily used in research.

CB1 agonists:

CP 55,940 (is equally strong at CB1 and CB2 receptors)

HU 210 (primarily CB1)

HU239 (Ajulemic acid) a potential CB1 agonist

WIN 55212-2 (binds with both but stronger at CB1)

CB1 antagonists:

SR141716A (Rimonabant)

AM251

CB2 agonists:

AM1241

CP 50556-1 CP 55,940

JWH-015 JWH-133 JWH-300 JWH-359 JWH-361

GW-405,833 (primarily CB2)

WIN 55212-2

CB2 antagonists:

SR144528 (blocks both but much stronger at CB2)

AM630

You may discover that merely being with whatever emotions or resistance surface, no matter how unpleasant or difficult it at first seems, is the beginning of true healing. Once you have discharged blocked emotional energy, you will be able to identify the beliefs, attitudes and choices that are contributing to your ill-health and which need to be replaced.

Focusing on how you feel about anything your illness is preventing you from doing can be thought of as the needle of a compass that points to the underlying issues that require your attention.

Additionally, you might find yourself intrigued by your own higher intelligence at work. Think of your symptoms as messengers trying to communicate what needs to happen so that you can thrive, reclaim your health, and persist in the loving and learning you have come here to do.

The next chapter, "Consciousness and Deep Healing", will provide more specific and in-depth insights experienced during altered states excursions, whether induced by cannabis or other meditative shifts in awareness.

SUMMARY

- **The endocannabinoid system is a bridge between the body and mind.**
- **Bodies make their own cannabinoids to regulate, regain or maintain a healthy body and mind.**
- **Cannabinoid sources: our body, cannabis, certain spice plants and man-made.**
- **The endocannabinoid system is involved in healing 100(+) chronic symptoms and stubborn diseases.**
- **Cannabinoids are essential to life, health, and well-being.**
- **Cannabis is neither dangerous nor harmless.**

1 Matsuda LA, Lolait SJ, Brownstein MJ, Young AC, Bonner TI. *Structure of a cannabinoid receptor and functional expression of the cloned cDNA.* 1990. Nature 346: 561–564.

2 June 2, 2012 PubMed Search for the keyword "*Endocannabinoid system*" yielded 2393 published scientific experiments.

3 Susanne A Wolf1,2*, Anika Bick-Sander1, Klaus Fabel4, Perla Leal-Galicia4, Svantje Tauber2, Gerardo Ramirez-Rodriguez1,3, Anke Müller1, Andre Melnik2, Tim P Waltinger2, Oliver Ullrich2 and Gerd Kempermann1,4* *Cannabinoid receptor CB1 mediates baseline and activity-induced survival of new neurons in adult hippocampal neurogenesis.* 1Max Delbrück Center for Molecular Medicine (MDC) Berlin-Buch, and Volkswagenstiftung Research Group, Department of Experimental Neurology, Charité University Medicine, Berlin, Germany. 2Institute of Anatomy, University of Zurich, Zurich, Switzerland. 3National Institute of Psychiatry "Ramón de la Fuente Muñiz", Neuropharmacology Department, Calz. México-Xochimilco 101, 14370 México, D.F. México. 4CRTD - Center for Regenerative Therapies Dresden, Dresden, Germany. Cell Communication and Signaling 2010, 8:12

4 Sally S. Dickerson, MA, Margaret E. Kemeny, PhD, Najib Aziz, MD, Kevin H. Kim, PhD and John L. Fahey, MD. *Immunological Effects of Induced Shame and Guilt.* Department of Psychology (S.S.D., M.E.K., K.H.K.), Cousins Center for Psychoneuroimmunology (S.S.D., M.E.K. J.L.F.), Department of Psychiatry and Biobehavioral Sciences (M.E.K.), Center for Interdisciplinary Research in Immunology and Disease (N.A., J.L.F.), and Department of Microbiology and Immunology (J.L.F.), University of California, Los Angeles, CA. M.E.K. is now at the Department of Psychiatry/Health Psychology program, University of California, San Francisco. K.H.K. is now at the Department of Psychology in Education, University of Pittsburgh. Psychosomatic Medicine 66:124-131 (2004).

5 June 2, 2012 PubMed Search for the keyword "*Cannabinoid*" yielded 15,015 published scientific studies.

6 Russo EB. *Taming THC: potential cannabis synergy and phytocannabinoid-terpenoid entourage effects*. GW Pharmaceuticals, Salisbury, Wiltshire, UK. Br J Pharmacol. 2011 Aug;163(7):1344-64.

7 Mechoulam R, Ben-Shabat S, Hanus L, Ligumsky M, Kaminski NE, Schatz AR et al. *Identification of an endogenous 2-monoglyceride, present in canine gut, that binds to cannabinoid receptors*. 1995. Biochem Pharmacol 50: 83–90.

8 Felder CC, Joyce KE, Briley EM, Mansouri J, Mackie K, Blond O, Lai Y, Ma AL, Mitchell RL. *Comparison of the pharmacology and signal transduction of the human cannabinoid CB1 and CB2 receptors*. Laboratory of Cell Biology, National Institute of Mental Health, Bethesda, Maryland 20892, USA. Mol Pharmacol. 1995 Sep;48(3):443-50.

9 Osei-Hyiaman D, DePetrillo M, Pacher P, Liu J, Radaeva S, Bátkai S, Harvey-White J, Mackie K, Offertáler L, Wang L, Kunos G. *Endocannabinoid activation at hepatic CB1 receptors stimulates fatty acid synthesis and contributes to diet-induced obesity*. National Institute on Alcohol Abuse & Alcoholism, NIH, Bethesda, Maryland 20892, USA. J Clin Invest. 2005 May;115(5):1298-305.

10 Giuffrida A, Leweke FM, Gerth CW, Schreiber D, Koethe D, Faulhaber J, Klosterkotter J, Piomelli D. *Cerebrospinal anandamide levels are elevated in acute schizophrenia and are inversely correlated with psychotic symptoms*. Department of Pharmacology, University of California, Irvine, CA, USA. Neuropsychopharmacology. 2004 Nov;29(11):2108-14.

11 Mauro Maccarrone, Tatiana Lorenzon, Monica Bari, Gerry Melino and Alessandro Finazzi-Agrò. *Anandamide Induces Apoptosis in Human Cells via Vanilloid Receptors: Evidence for a Role of Cannabinoid Receptors*. Istituto Superiore di Sanità (III AIDS Program), by Ministero dell'Università e della Ricerca Scientifica e Tecnologica, Rome October 13, 2000 The Journal of Biological Chemistry, 275, 31938-31945.

12 Cozzolino R, Calì G, Bifulco M, Laccetti P. *A metabolically stable analogue of anandamide, Met-F-AEA, inhibits human thyroid carcinoma cell lines by activation of apoptosis*. Department of Structural and Functional Biology, University of Naples Federico II, 80126 Naples, Italy. cozzolino1@interfree.it Invest New Drugs. 2010 Apr;28(2):115-23.

13 Dominique Melck, Luciano De Petrocellis, Pierangelo Orlando, Tiziana Bisogno, Chiara Laezza, Maurizio Bifulco and Vincenzo Di Marzo. *Suppression of Nerve Growth Factor Trk Receptors and Prolactin Receptors by Endocannabinoids Leads to Inhibition of Human Breast and Prostate Cancer Cell Proliferation*. Istituto per la Chimica di Molecole di Interesse Biologico (D.M., T.B., V.D.M.), Istituto di Cibernetica (L.D.P.), and Istituto di Biochimica delle Proteine ed Enzimologia (P.O.), Consiglio Nazionale delle Ricerche, 80072 Arco Felice (NA); and Centro di Endocrinologia e Oncologia Sperimentale, Consiglio Nazionale delle Ricerche, and Dipartimento di Biologia e Patologia Cellulare e Molecolare, Università di Napoli Federico II (C.L., M.B.), 80131 Naples, Italy. Endocrinology, 2000. Vol. 141, No. 1 118-126.

14 United States Patent Application 20060013777. Kind Code A1. Piomelli; Daniele January 19, 2006. Assignee: The Regents of the University of California. Filed September 12, 2005.

15 Michael D. Roth. Pharmacology: *Marijuana and your heart*. Division of Pulmonary and Critical Care, Department of Medicine, CHS 37-131, David Geffen School of Medicine, University of California, Los Angeles, California 90095-1690, USA. Nature 434, 708-709 (7 April 2005).

16 Hayakawa K, Mishima K, Abe K, Hasebe N, Takamatsu F, Yasuda H, Ikeda T, Inui K, Egashira N, Iwasaki K, Fujiwara M. *Cannabidiol prevents infarction via the non-CB1 cannabinoid receptor mechanism*. Department of Neuropharmacology, Faculty of Pharmaceutical Sciences, Fukuoka University, Nanakuma 8-19-1, Fukuoka City, Fukuoka, 814-0180, Japan. Neuroreport. 2004 Oct 25;15(15):2381-5.

17 Shmist YA, Goncharov I, Eichler M, Shneyvays V, Isaac A, Vogel Z, Shainberg A. *Delta-9-tetrahydrocannabinol protects cardiac cells from hypoxia via CB2 receptor activation and nitric oxide production*. Faculty of Life Sciences, Bar-Ilan University, Ramat-Gan, Israel. Mol Cell Biochem. 2006 Feb;283(1-2):75-83.

18 Hayakawa K, Mishima K, Abe K, Hasebe N, Takamatsu F, Yasuda H, Ikeda T, Inui K, Egashira N, Iwasaki K, Fujiwara M. *Cannabidiol prevents infarction via the non-CB1 cannabinoid receptor mechanism*. Department of Neurop-

harmacology, Faculty of Pharmaceutical Sciences, Fukuoka University, Nanakuma 8-19-1, Fukuoka City, Fukuoka, 814-0180, Japan. Neuroreport. 2004 Oct 25;15(15):2381-5.

19 Tashkin DP, Shapiro BJ, Frank IM. *Acute effects of smoked marijuana and oral delta9-tetrahydrocannabinol on specific airway conductance in asthmatic subjects.* Am Rev Respir Dis. 1974 Apr;109(4):420-8.

20 Tashkin DP, Shapiro BJ, Lee YE, Harper CE. *Effects of smoked marijuana in experimentally induced asthma.* Am Rev Respir Dis. 1975 Sep;112(3):377-86.

21 Williams SJ, Hartley JP, Graham JD. *Bronchodilator effect of delta1-tetrahydrocannabinol administered by aerosol of asthmatic patients.* Thorax 1976;31(6):720-723.

22 Tashkin DP, Reiss S, Shapiro BJ, Calvarese B, Olsen JL, Lodge JW. *Bronchial effects of aerosolized delta 9-tetrahydrocannabinol in healthy and asthmatic subjects.* Am Rev Respir Dis. 1977 Jan;115(1):57-65.

23 Hartley JP, Nogrady SG, Seaton A. *Bronchodilator effect of delta1-tetrahydrocannabinol.* Br J Clin Pharmacol. 1978 Jun;5(6):523-5.

24 Gong H Jr, Tashkin DP, Calvarese B. *Comparison of bronchial effects of nabilone and terbutaline in healthy and asthmatic subjects.* Journal of Clinical Pharmacology 1983;23(4):127-133.

25 Karl-Christian Bergmann. *Dronabinol - eine mögliche neue Therapieoption bei COPD-Patienten mit pulmonaler Kachexie.* Presentation at the 2005 Conference of the German Society for Pneumology, Berlin, 17 March 2005. Karl-Christian Bergmann, Allergie- und Asthmaklinik, Bad Lippspringe, Germany.

26 Mechoulam R, Peters M, Murillo-Rodriguez E, Hanuš LO. *"Cannabidiol--recent advances".* Department of Medicinal Chemistry and Natural Products, Hebrew University Medical Faculty, Jerusalem 91120, Israel. Chemistry & biodiversity, August 2007. 4 (8): 1678–92.

27 Iuvone T, Esposito G, De Filippis D, Scuderi C, Steardo L. *Cannabidiol: a promising drug for neurodegenerative disorders?* Department of Experimental Pharmacology, Faculty of Pharmacy, University of Naples Federico II, Via D. Montesano 49, Naples, Italy. CNS Neurosci Ther. 2009 Winter;15(1):65-75.

28 Sagredo O, Ramos JA, Decio A, Mechoulam R, Fernández-Ruiz J. *Cannabidiol reduced the striatal atrophy caused 3-nitropropionic acid in vivo by mechanisms independent of the activation of cannabinoid, vanilloid TRPV1 and adenosine A2A receptors.* Departamento de Bioquímica y Biología Molecular III, Universidad Complutense, 28040-Madrid, Spain. Eur J Neurosci. 2007 Aug;26(4):843-51.

29 Fernández-Ruiz J, Moreno-Martet M, Rodríguez-Cueto C, Palomo-Garo C, Gómez-Cañas M, Valdeolivas S, Guaza C, Romero J, Guzmán M, Mechoulam R, Ramos JA. *Prospects for cannabinoid therapies in basal ganglia disorders.* Departamento de Bioquímica y Biología Molecular III, Instituto Universitario de Investigación en Neuroquímica, Facultad de Medicina, Universidad Complutense, Madrid, Spain. Br J Pharmacol. 2011 Aug;163(7):1365-78.

30 Reuven Sandyk, Paul Consroe, Lawrence Z. Stern, and Stuart R. Snider, Tucson, AZ. *EFFECTS OF CANNABIDIOL IN HUNTINGTON'S DISEASE.* Neurology 36 (Suppl 1) April 1986 p. 342.

31 Pelliccia A, Grassi G, Romano A, Crocchialo P. Treatment with CBD in oily solution of drug-resistant paediatric epilepsies. 9-10 September, 2005 Congress on Cannabis and the Cannabinoids, Leiden, The Netherlands: International Association for Cannabis as Medicine, p. 14. in cooperation with Institute of Biology, Pharmacognosy/Metabolomics, Leiden University. Office of Medicinal Cannabis, Ministry of Health, Welfare and Sports. II Facoltà di Medicina, Università "La Sapienza", 00100 Rome, Italy, Istituto Sperimentale Colture Industriali, Sezione di Rovigo, Italy, American University of Rome, 00100, Italy.

32 Carol Hamelink1, Aidan Hampson1, David A. Wink, Lee E. Eiden and Robert L. Eskay. *Comparison of Cannabidiol, Antioxidants, and Diuretics in Reversing Binge Ethanol-Induced Neurotoxicity.* Section on Molecular Neuroscience, Laboratory of Cellular and Molecular Regulation, National Institute of Mental Health (C.H., A.H., L.E.E.); Section of Neurochemistry and Neuroendocrinology, Laboratory of Clinical Studies, National Institute on Alcohol Abuse and Alcoholism (R.L.E.); and Radiology and Biology Branch, National Cancer Institute (D.A.W.), National Institutes of Health, Bethesda, Maryland. JPET August 2005 vol. 314 no. 2 780-788.

33 Resstel LB, Tavares RF, Lisboa SF, Joca SR, Corrêa FM, Guimarães FS. 5-HT receptors are involved in the canna-bidiol-induced attenuation of behavioural and cardiovascular responses to acute restraint stress in rats. Department of Pharmacology, School of Medicine of Ribeirão Preto, University of São Paulo, Ribeirão Preto, SP, Brazil. leoresstel@yahoo.com.br Br J Pharmacol. 2009 Jan;156(1):181-8.

34 Parolaro D, Realini N, Vigano D, Guidali C, Rubino T. *The endocannabinoid system and psychiatric disorders.* DBSF and Neuroscience Center, University of Insubria, Via A. da Giussano 10, 21052 Busto Arsizio (Varese), Italy. Exp Neurol. 2010 Jul;224(1):3-14

35 Crippa JA, Zuardi AW, Hallak JE. *Therapeutical use of the cannabinoids in psychiatry.* Departamento de Neuro-ciências e Ciências do Comportamento, Faculdade de Medicina de Ribeirão Preto, Universidade de São Paulo, Ribeirão Preto, SP, Brasil. Rev Bras Psiquiatr. 2010 May;32 Suppl 1:S56-66.

36 F.M. Leweke1, D. Koethe1, F. Pahlisch1, 2, D. Schreiber1, 2, C.W. Gerth1, B.M. Nolden1, J. Klosterkötter1, M. Hellmich3 and D. Piomelli2 S39-02 *Antipsychotic effects of cannabidiol.* 1Dept. of Psychiatry and Psychotherapy, University of Cologne, Cologne, Germany. 2Depts. of Pharmacology and Biological Chemistry, University of California, Irvine, USA. 3Institute for Medical Statistics, Informatics, and Epidemiology, University of Cologne, Cologne, Germany. European Psychiatry. Volume 24, Supplement 1, 2009, Page S207.

37 Weiss L, Zeira M, Reich S, Slavin S, Raz I, Mechoulam R, Gallily R. *Cannabidiol arrests onset of autoimmune dia-betes in NOD mice.* Department of Bone Marrow Transplantation and Cancer Immunotherapy, Hadassah Hebrew University Hospital, Jerusalem 91120, Israel. lolaw@hadassa.org.il Neuropharmacology. 2008 Jan;54(1):244-9.

38 R Capasso,1 F Borrelli,1 G Aviello,1 B Romano,1 C Scalisi,1,2 F Capasso,1 and A Izzo1* *Cannabidiol, extracted from Cannabis sativa, selectively inhibits inflammatory hypermotility in mice.* 1Department of Experimental Phar-macology, University of Naples Federico II and Endocannabinoid Research Group, Naples, Italy. *Author for cor-respondence: Email: aaizzo@unina.it 2Current address: Human Physiology Section, Department of Experimen-tal Medicine, University of Palermo, corso Tukory 129, 90134 Palermo, Italy. Br J Pharmacol. 2008 July; 154(5): 1001–1008.

39 R Capasso,1 F Borrelli,1 G Aviello,1 B Romano,1 C Scalisi,1,2 F Capasso,1 and A Izzo1* *Cannabidiol, extracted from Cannabis sativa, selectively inhibits inflammatory hypermotility in mice.* 1Department of Experimental Phar-macology, University of Naples Federico II and Endocannabinoid Research Group, Naples, Italy. *Author for cor-respondence: Email: aaizzo@unina.it 2Current address: Human Physiology Section, Department of Experimen-tal Medicine, University of Palermo, corso Tukory 129, 90134 Palermo, Italy. Br J Pharmacol. 2008 July; 154(5): 1001–1008.

40 R Capasso,1 F Borrelli,1 G Aviello,1 B Romano,1 C Scalisi,1,2 F Capasso,1 and A Izzo1* *Cannabidiol, extracted from Cannabis sativa, selectively inhibits inflammatory hypermotility in mice.* 1Department of Experimental Phar-macology, University of Naples Federico II and Endocannabinoid Research Group, Naples, Italy. *Author for cor-respondence: Email: aaizzo@unina.it 2Current address: Human Physiology Section, Department of Experimen-tal Medicine, University of Palermo, corso Tukory 129, 90134 Palermo, Italy. Br J Pharmacol. 2008 July; 154(5): 1001–1008.

41 A. M. Malfait,*† R. Gallily,†‡ P. F. Sumariwalla,* A. S. Malik,* E. Andreakos,* R. Mechoulam,‡ and M. Feld-mann*§ *The nonpsychoactive cannabis constituent cannabidiol is an oral anti-arthritic therapeutic in murine collagen-induced arthritis.* *Kennedy Institute of Rheumatology, 1 Aspenlea Road, Hammersmith, London W6 8LH, United Kingdom; and ‡Hebrew University, Hadassah Medical School, P.O.B. 12272, Jerusalem 91120, Israel. †A.M.M. and R.G. contributed equally to this work. Edited by Anthony Cerami, The Kenneth S. Warren Laboratories, Tarrytown, NY. Proc Natl Acad Sci U S A. 2000 August 15; 97(17): 9561–9566.

42 Napimoga MH, Benatti BB, Lima FO, Alves PM, Campos AC, Pena-Dos-Santos DR, Severino FP, Cunha FQ, Guimarães FS. *Cannabidiol decreases bone resorption by inhibiting RANK/RANKL expression and pro-inflammatory cytokines during experimental periodontitis in rats.* Laboratory of Molecular Biology, University of Uberaba, Brazil. Int Immunopharmacol. 2009 Feb;9(2):216-22.

43 Takeda S, Usami N, Yamamoto I, Watanabe K. *Cannabidiol-2',6'-Dimethyl Ether, a Cannabidiol Derivative, Is a Highly Potent and Selective 15 Lipoxygenase Inhibitor.* Department of Hygienic Chemistry, Faculty of Phar-maceutical Sciences, Hokuriku University, Ho-3 Kanagawa-machi, Kanazawa, Japan. Drug Metab Dispos. 2009 Aug;37(8):1733-7.

44 Paola Massi, Angelo Vaccani, Stefania Ceruti, Arianna Colombo, Maria P. Abbracchio and Daniela Parolaro. *Antitumor Effects of Cannabidiol, a Nonpsychoactive Cannabinoid, on Human Glioma Cell Lines.* Department of Pharmacology, Chemotherapy and Toxicology (P.M., A.C.), and Department of Pharmacological Sciences, School of Pharmacy, and Center of Excellence for Neurodegenerative Diseases, University of Milan, Milan, Italy (S.C., M.P.A.); and Department of Structural and Functional Biology, Pharmacology Unit and Center of Neuroscience, University of Insubria, Busto Arsizio (Varese), Italy (A.V., D.P.) JPET March 2004 vol. 308 no. 3 838-845.

45 Massi P, Vaccani A, Bianchessi S, Costa B, Macchi P, Parolaro D. *The non-psychoactive cannabidiol triggers caspase activation and oxidative stress in human glioma cells.* Department of Pharmacology, Chemotherapy and Medical Toxicology, University of Milan, via Vanvitelli 32, 20129 Milan, Italy. Cell Mol Life Sci. 2006 Sep;63(17):2057-66.

46 Marcu JP, Christian RT, Lau D, Zielinski AJ, Horowitz MP, Lee J, Pakdel A, Allison J, Limbad C, Moore DH, Yount GL, Desprez PY, McAllister SD. *Cannabidiol Enhances the Inhibitory Effects of {Delta}9-Tetrahydrocannabinol on Human Glioblastoma Cell Proliferation and Survival.* California Pacific Medical Center Research Institute, San Francisco, California 94107, USA. Mol Cancer Ther, 6. Januar 2010.

47 Gertsch J, Leonti M, Raduner S, Racz I, Chen JZ, Xie XQ, Altmann KH, Karsak M, Zimmer A. Beta-caryophyllene is a dietary cannabinoid. Institute of Pharmaceutical Sciences, Department of Chemistry and Applied Biosciences, Eidgenössische Technische Hochschule (ETH) Zurich, 8092 Zürich, Switzerland. Proc Natl Acad Sci U S A. 2008 Jul 1;105(26):9099-104.

48 Béla Horvátha, Partha Mukhopadhyaya, Malek Kechrida, Vivek Patela, Gali Tanchiana, David A. Winkb, Jürg Gertschc, Pál Pachera. *β-Caryophyllene ameliorates cisplatin-induced nephrotoxicity in a cannabinoid 2 receptor-dependent manner.* a Laboratory of Physiologic Studies, National Institute on Alcohol Abuse and Alcoholism, National Institutes of Health, Bethesda, MD 20892, USA. b Radiation Biology Branch, National Cancer Institute, National Institutes of Health, Bethesda, MD 20892, USA. c Institute of Biochemistry and Molecular Medicine, University of Bern, 3012 Bern, Switzerland. Free Radical Biology and Medicine. Volume 52, Issue 8, 15 April 2012, Pages 1325–133.

49 Legault J. Pichette A. *Potentiating effect of beta-caryophellene on anticancer activity of alpha-humulene isocaryophellene and palitaxel.* Laboratoire LASEVE, Université du Québec à Chicoutimi, Chicoutimi, Québec, Canada. J Pharm Pharmacol 2007 Dec;59(12):1643-7.

50 Jirovetz L, Buchbauer G, Ngassoum MB, Geissler M. *Aroma compound analysis of Piper nigrum and Piper guineense essential oils from Cameroon using solid-phase microextraction-gas chromatography, solid-phase microextraction-gas chromatography-mass spectrometry and olfactometry.* Institute of Pharmaceutical Chemistry, University of Vienna, Althanstrasse 14, A-1090 Vienna, Austria. J Chromatogr A. 2002 Nov 8;976(1-2):265-75.

51 Gertsch J, Leonti M, Raduner S, Racz I, Chen JZ, Xie XQ, Altmann KH, Karsak M, Zimmer A. *Beta-caryophyllene is a dietary cannabinoid.* Institute of Pharmaceutical Sciences, Department of Chemistry and Applied Biosciences, Eidgenössische Technische Hochschule (ETH) Zurich, 8092 Zürich, Switzerland. Proc Natl Acad Sci U S A. 2008 Jul 1;105(26):9099-104.

52 Aftab Ahmed1, M. Iqbal Choudhary2, Afgan Farooq2, Betül Demirci3, Fatih Demirci3, K. Hüsnü Can Başer3, *Essential oil constituents of the spice Cinnamomum tamala (Ham.) Nees & Eberm.* 1Institute of Chemistry, University of the Punjab, Lahore, Pakistan. 2International Center for Chemical Sciences, H.E.J. Research Institute of Chemistry, University of Karachi, Karachi-75270, Pakistan. 3Anadolu University, Medicinal and Aromatic Plant and Drug Research Centre (TBAM), 26470-Eskişehir, Turkey. Flavour and Fragrance Journal. Volume 15, Issue 6, pages 388–390, November/December 2000.

53 Vineeta Singh,1 Atul Kumar Gupta,1 S. P. Singh,2 and Anil Kumar1 *Direct Analysis in Real Time by Mass Spectrometric Technique for Determining the Variation in Metabolite Profiles of Cinnamomum tamala Nees and Eberm Genotypes.* 1Department of Molecular Biology & Genetic Engineering, College of Basic Sciences and Humanities, G. B. Pant University of Agriculture and Technology, Uttarakhand, Pantnagar 263145, India2Department of Pharmacology & Toxicology, College of Veterinary Science, G. B. Pant University of Agriculture and Technology, Uttarakhand, Pantnagar 263145, India. The Scientific World JournalVolume 2012 (2012), Article ID 549265, 6 pages.

54 E. O. Ajaiyeoba1, O. Ekundayo2, *Essential oil constituents of Aframomum melegueta (Roscoe) K. Schum. seeds (alligator pepper) from Nigeria.* 1Department of Pharmacognosy, Faculty of Pharmacy, University of Ibadan, Ibadan, Nigeria. 2Department of Chemistry, University of Ibadan, Ibadan, Nigeria. Flavour and Fragrance Journal. Volume

14, Issue 2, pages 109–111, March/April 1999.

55 Umukoro S, Ashorobi BR. *Further pharmacological studies on aqueous seed extract of Aframomum melegueta in rats.* Department of Pharmacology and Therapeutics, College of Medicine, University of Ibadan, Nigeria. J Ethnopharmacol. 2008 Feb 12;115(3):489-93.

56 Ibid.

57 Umukoro S, Ashorobi RB. *Further studies on the antinociceptive action of aqueous seed extract of Aframomum melegueta.* Department of Pharmacology and Therapeutics, University of Ibadan, Ibadan, Nigeria. umusolo@yahoo.com J Ethnopharmacol. 2007 Feb 12;109(3):501-4.

58 Ibid.

59 Ndamukong KJ, Ntonifor NN, Mbuh J, Atemnkeng AF, Akam MT. *Molluscicidal activity of some Cameroonian plants on Bulinus species.* Department of Administrative Affairs, University of Buea, Cameroon. East Afr Med J. 2006 Mar;83(3):102-9.

60 Umukoro, S., Ashorobi, R. B. *Pharmacological evaluation of the antidiarrhoeal activity of Aframomum melegueta seed extract.* Department of Pharmacology, College of Medicine, University of Lagos, P.M.B. 12003, Lagos, Nigeria. West African Journal of Pharmacology and Drug Research, 2004, (Vol. 19).

61 Umukoro, S., Ashorobi, R. B. *Effect of Aframomum melegueta seed extract on castor oil-induced diarrhea.* Department of Pharmacology, College of Medicine, University of Lagos, Nigeria. Pharmaceutical biology (Pharm. biol.) ISSN 1388-0209 2005, vol. 43, no4, pp. 330-333 [4 page(s) (article)] (17 ref.)

62 Konning GH, Agyare C, Ennison B. *Antimicrobial activity of some medicinal plants from Ghana.* Department of Pharmaceutics, Faculty of Pharmacy, Kwame Nkrumah University of Science and Technology, Kumasi, Ghana. Fitoterapia. 2004 Jan;75(1):65-7

63 Kamtchouing P, Mbongue GY, Dimo T, Watcho P, Jatsa HB, Sokeng SD. *Effects of Aframomum melegueta and Piper guineense on sexual behaviour of male rats.* Laboratoire de Physiologie Animale, Faculté des Sciences, Université de Yaoundé I, Yaoundé, Cameroun. mbongue@yahoo.com Behav Pharmacol. 2002 May;13(3):243-7.

64 Jirovetz L, Buchbauer G, Ngassoum MB, Geissler M. *Aroma compound analysis of Piper nigrum and Piper guineense essential oils from Cameroon using solid-phase microextraction-gas chromatography, solid-phase microextraction-gas chromatography-mass spectrometry and olfactometry.* Institute of Pharmaceutical Chemistry, University of Vienna, Althanstrasse 14, A-1090 Vienna, Austria. J Chromatogr A. 2002 Nov 8;976(1-2):265-75.

65 Chaudhry NM, Tariq P. *Bactericidal activity of black pepper, bay leaf, aniseed and coriander against oral isolates.* University of Karachi, Pakistan. ak J Pharm Sci. 2006 Jul;19(3):214-8.

66 Nalini N, Manju V, Menon VP. *Effect of spices on lipid metabolism in 1,2-dimethylhydrazine-induced rat colon carcinogenesis.* Annamalai University, Annamalainagar, Tamilnadu, India. J Med Food. 2006 Summer;9(2):237-45.

67 Gülçin I. *The antioxidant and radical scavenging activities of black pepper (Piper nigrum) seeds.* Department of Chemistry, Atatürk University, Faculty of Science and Arts, TR-25240, Erzurum, Turkey. Int J Food Sci Nutr. 2005 Nov;56(7):491-9.

68 Silva, Matos, Lopes, F. Silva, Holanda. *Composition of essential oils from three Ocimum species obtained by steam and microwave distillation and supercritical CO2 extraction .* Departamento de Química Analítica e Fisico-Química Departamento de Química Orgânica. Inorgânica, Centro de Ciências, Laboratório de Produtos Naturais, Universidade Federal do Ceará, CEP 60.021-970, Fortaleza-Ce, Brazil.

69 U. Blesching, Ph.D. *Spicy Healing: A Global Guide to Growing and Using Spices for Food and Medicine.* Logos Publishing, Berkeley. 2009. Second Edition.

70 Pran N Kaul1, Arun K Bhattacharya1, Bhaskaruni R Rajeswara Rao1, Kodakandla V Syamasundar2, Sriniva-

saiyer Ramesh2 V*olatile constituents of essential oils isolated from different parts of cinnamon (Cinnamomum zeylanicum Blume).* 1Central Institute of Medicinal and Aromatic Plants, Field Station, Boduppal, Uppal (PO), Hyderabad 500 039, India. 2CIMAP, Field Station, Allalasandra, GKVK (PO), Bangalore 560 065, IndiaJournal of the Science of Food and Agriculture. Volume 83, Issue 1, pages 53–55, 1 January 2003

71 U. Blesching, Ph.D. *Spicy Healing: A Global Guide to Growing and Using Spices for Food and Medicine.* Logos Publishing, Berkeley. 2009.

72 R. Jamshidi, Z. Afzali and D. Afzali. *Chemical Composition of Hydrodistillation Essential Oil of Rosemary in Different Origins in Iran and Comparison with Other Countries.* Islamic Azad University, Bardsir Branch, Bardsir, Iran. International Center for Science, High Technology and Environmental Sciences, Kerman, Iran. American-Eurasian J. Agric. & Environ. Sci., 5 (1): 78-81, 2009

73 U. Blesching, Ph.D. *Spicy Healing: A Global Guide to Growing and Using Spices for Food and Medicine.* Logos Publishing, Berkeley. 2009. Second Edition.

74 Singh G, Marimuthu P, de Heluani CS, Catalan CA. *Antioxidant and biocidal activities of Carum nigrum (seed) essential oil, oleoresin, and their selected components.* Chemistry Department, D.D.U. Gorakhpur University, Gorakhpur 273009, India. J Agric Food Chem. 2006 Jan 11;54(1):174-81.

75 Singh G, Marimuthu P, de Heluani CS, Catalan CA. *Antioxidant and biocidal activities of Carum nigrum (seed) essential oil, oleoresin, and their selected components.* Chemistry Department, D.D.U. Gorakhpur University, Gorakhpur 273009, India. J Agric Food Chem. 2006 Jan 11;54(1):174-81.

76 Silva, Matos, Lopes, F. Silva, Holanda. *Composition of essential oils from three Ocimum species obtained by steam and microwave distillation and supercritical CO2 extraction.* Departamento de Química Analítica e Fisico-Química Departamento de Química Orgânica. Inorgânica, Centro de Ciências, Laboratório de Produtos Naturais, Universidade Federal do Ceará, CEP 60.021-970, Fortaleza-Ce, Brazil.

77 P.A. Akah , Lucy John-Africa and C.S. Nworu , 2007. *Gastro-Protective Properties of the Leaf Extracts of Ocimum gratissimum L. Against Experimental Ulcers in Rat.* International Journal of Pharmacology, 3: 461-467.

78 Nwinyi, Obinna C.1, Chinedu, Nwodo S. 1, Ajani, Olayinka O. 2, Ikpo Chinwe.O2 and Ogunniran, Kehinde O.2 *Antibacterial effects of extracts of Ocimum gratissimum and piper guineense on Escherichia coli and Staphylococcus aureus.* 1 Department of Biological Sciences, College of Science and Technology, Covenant University. KM 10 Idioroko Road, Canaanland, PMB 1023 Ota, Ogun State, Nigeria. 2 Department of Chemistry, College of Science and Technology, Covenant University, Km 10 Idiroko Road, PMB 1023, Ota, Ogun State, Nigeria. African Journal of Food Science Vol. 3(3). pp. 077-081, March, 2009.

79 L. M. Calvo-Irabien, J. A. Yam-Puc, G. Dzib, F. Escalante-Erosa, L. M. Peña-Rodriguez. *Effect of Postharvest Drying on the Composition of Mexican Oregano (Lippia graveolens) Essential Oil.* Journal of Herbs, Spices & Medicinal Plants Vol. 15, Iss. 3, 2009

80 Marciele Ribas Pilau, Sydney Hartz Alves, Rudi Weiblen, Sandra Arenhart, Ana Paula Cueto, Luciane Teresinha Lovato. *Antivaral Activity of the Lippia Graveolens (Mexican Oregano) Essential Oil and its Main Compound Carvacrol against Human and Animal Viruses.* Brazilian Journal of Microbiology (2011) 42:1616-1624.

81 Alma, M. Hakkı; Ertaş, Murat; Nitz, Siegfrie; Kollmannsberger, Hubert. *Chemical composition and content of essential oil from the bud of cultivated Turkish clove.* BioResources (Raleigh, North Carolina, USA: North Carolina State University) 2 (2): 265–269.

82 U. Blesching, Ph.D. *Spicy Healing: A Global Guide to Growing and Using Spices for Food and Medicine.* Logos Publishing, Berkeley. 2009. Second Edition.

83 Leonard E. Barrett, Sr. *The Rastafarians.* Beacon Press. Massachusetts 1988. Page #255.

84 J.Harmatta: *"Scythians"* in UNESCO Collection of History of Humanity - Volume III: From the Seventh Century BC to the Seventh Century AD. Routledge/ UNESCO. 1996. Page # 182.

85 Herodotus. *The Histories of Herodotus*. Book IV, 72. Written in the Fifth Century B.C. Published by A. Knopf 1910 by Everyman's Library.

86 *Exodus*, Chapter 30, 30:22 – 30:33

87 Kaplan, Aryeh. *The Living Torah*. New York. Page # 442.

88 The Ebers Papyrus was dated by a reference to the reign of Imhotep to circa 1530 B.C. but other references in the text suggest thatit was copied from the original text dating to circa 3,000B.C.

89 *Ebers Papyrus 821* (96, 7 - 96, 8) SmSmt-Pflanze, zerreiben in Honig, eingießen in ihre Scheide. Das bedeutet eine Zusammenziehung (der Gebärmutter).

90 ProCon.org Medical Marijuana. *Deaths from Marijuana v. 17 FDA-Approved Drug*. (Jan. 1, 1997 to June 30, 2005). http://medicalmarijuana.procon.org/view.resource.php?resourceID=000145

91 U.S. Department of Health and Human Services. *Substance Abuse and Mental Health Services Administration. Mortality Data From the Drug Abuse Warning Network, 2002*. See page18, table H and page 24 where it states: "… marijuana is rarely the only drug involved in a drug abuse death. Thus, in many MSA's, the proportion of marijuana involved cases labeled as "one drug" (i.e., marijuana only) will be zero or nearly zero."

92 CDC, MMWR. *Smoking-Attributable Mortality, Years of Potential Life Lost, and Productivity Losses --- United States, 2000—2004*. November 14, 2008 / 57(45);1226-1228.

93 CDC, MMWR. *Alcohol-Attributable Deaths and Years of Potential Life Lost --- United States, 2001. September 24, 2004 / 53(37);866-870.*

94 ProCon.org *Medical Marijuana. Deaths from Marijuana v. 17 FDA-Approved Drug*. (Jan. 1, 1997 to June 30, 2005).

95 Meier MH, Caspi A, Ambler A, Harrington H, Houts R, Keefe RS, McDonald K, Ward A, Poulton R, Moffitt TE. Meier MH, Caspi A, Ambler A, Harrington H, Houts R, Keefe RS, McDonald K, Ward A, Poulton R, Moffitt TE. P*ersistent cannabis users show neuropsychological decline from childhood to midlife*. Duke Transdisciplinary Prevention Research Center, Center for Child and Family Policy, Department of Psychology and Neuroscience, and Institute for Genome Sciences and Policy, Duke University, Durham, NC 27708. Proc Natl Acad Sci U S A. 2012 Oct 2;109(40):E2657-64.

96 Silva P, Stanton W. *From Child to Adult: The Dunedin Multidisciplinary Health and Development Study*. New York, NY: Oxford University Press; 1996.

97Hashibe M, Morgenstern H, Cui Y, Tashkin DP, Zhang ZF, Cozen W, Mack TM, Greenland S. *Marijuana use and the risk of lung and upper aerodigestive tract cancers: results of a population-based case-control study*. IARC, Lyon, France. Cancer Epidemiol Biomarkers Prev. 2006 Oct;15(10):1829-34.

98 Thomas J O'Connell1 and Ché B Bou-Matar2 *Long term marijuana users seeking medical cannabis in California (2001–2007): demographics, social characteristics, patterns of cannabis and other drug use of 4117 applicants*. 1 Private medical practice, Oakland, CA, USA. 2 Private consultant, Mountain View, CA, USA. Harm Reduction Journal 2007, 4:16

99 Thompson GR, Rosenkrantz H, Schaeppi UH, Braude MC. *Comparison of acute oral toxicity of cannabinoids in rats, dogs and monkeys*. Toxicol Appl Pharmacol 1973; 25:363–72.

100 Gregory T. Carter, Patrick Weydt, Muraco Kyashna-Tocha and Donald Abrams. *Medicinal Cannabis: Rational guidelines for Dosing*. Idrugs 2004. &(5):464-470.

101 Kulshrestha R, Gupta CP, Shukla G, Kundu MG, Bhatnagar SP, Katiyar CK. *The effect of water activity and storage temperature on the growth of Aspergillus flavus in medicinal herbs*. Ranbaxy Laboratories Limited, Gurgaon, (Haryana), India. Planta Med. 2008 Aug;74(10):1308-15.

ABOUT THE AUTHOR AND MY INTEREST IN THIS TOPIC

When I was a boy a terrible accident occurred in my home in a little suburb of Dortmund, Germany. This accident took the life of a relative and cracked my heart. Little did I know that this traumatic experience would become a formative event. It propelled me to become very adept at managing traumatic events and to be curious about the influence of consciousness on health and well-being.

After getting drafted into the military, I completed my pre-med requirements in Germany and was placed on the waiting list for a medical school. While waiting, I took the opportunity to travel. When I came to San Francisco, I fell in love with this enigmatic city and its people, so much so that I decided to stay. Medical school in the U.S. proved prohibitively expensive, so a friend suggested I consider work in Emergency Medical Services (EMS). After a bit of research I enrolled at Stanford University, training to become a Mobile Intensive Care Paramedic.

Initially, I worked as a paramedic in Oakland and San Francisco for a private company, but I quickly got hired in the same capacity by the San Francisco Department of Public Health. After serving for about ten years, the Paramedic Division got absorbed into the S.F. Fire Department, and we became cross-trained to function in both roles, as emergency medical workers and firefighters.

I approached my EMS work with an almost counter-phobic attitude to trauma. Other emergency workers often referred to this common experience among rescue workers as an adrenalin rush akin to thrill-seeking. After many years of working this way, I started to sustain injuries, and to experience the long-term psychological effects of such a frame of mind. Symptoms of post-traumatic stress disorder (PTSD) appeared: an inexplicable sense of guilt and irritability, anxiety, impatience, hypervigilance, and emotional numbness. After an initial phase of denial I got some help, in part, from our famous plant ally and I began to explore my symptoms more closely. Eventually my emotional reality revealed an interesting connection to the accident at home from long ago.

My uncle had used a high-speed carbide blade cutter to remove some piping in the ceiling. Somehow he slipped and the blade cut his skull exposing his eye and brain. I called 911, and returned to the basement where my uncle lay dying in his father's arms. I stood at the edge of the door, but did not dare look around the corner, and instead listened to his last tender words whispered to his dad. Finally, after what appeared an eternity, the ambulance arrived and took my uncle to the hospital where he succumbed to his injuries.

As I worked through the emotional complexities of my PTSD, I eventually realized that I felt that I had done something wrong and was being rightfully punished because I did not help my uncle. As a result of this irrational guilt, I had somehow come to believe that I had contributed to my uncle's death and was trying to make up for it by living on the edge of an adrenalin-centered life, rescue after rescue, and it was now taking a toll on my body and mind.

When I came to accept that I was an adrenalin junkie trying to numb myself from the emotional impact of a belief that I was flawed based on something that happened long ago, my symptoms began to lighten a bit. I learned to embrace and accept emotions and thoughts I had never welcomed before. However, the big shift came for me when I replaced the belief system that demanded punishment for mistakes, real or imagined. With it came the new thought that what kept me from entering the room where my uncle lay dying was not my weakness or a flaw but an intuitive respect for the last intimate moment between a father and his dying son.

With this shift in my belief, I noticed changes in my emotional reality at work. I felt more empathy, compassion, and deeper respect and curiosity for what might be going on at a deeper level for those of us challenged with acute or chronic events and illnesses. Thereafter, in the daily kaleidoscope of emergency calls, instead of responding with anxious adrenalin-packed emotions, a new consciousness, awareness and mindfulness became my best tools to address the challenges of each unique emergency I encountered.

Concurrently and on the way to my Ph.D., I studied health care in the U.S., Cuba, Ghana, and other countries around the world. I wanted to learn more about the conscious use of the mind in various healing practices, and how it could be used in chronic and acute situations to improve one's healing. One of the things I learned from many shifts as a paramedic on the streets of San Francisco, from Bone-Setters in Accra, from the Yerberos in Havana, and from homeopaths and orthodox physicians alike, was that a participatory consciousness[1] infused into the healing process in the form of expectation[2] or belief can deepen healing.

While I eventually left the emergency medical services field, I continued to focus on this connection between the mind and the body in the context of health and healing. From that fateful day in the basement of my family's home, to the thousands of patients I had the privilege to serve, I have come to deeply care about realizing our optimal health potential through the use of awareness and other natural healing practices. I have written this book to share with you my conviction that conscious awareness, whether plant-induced or the result of mindfulness, is essential to our well-being and a critical factor in mind–body medicine.

Chapter II

Consciousness Research
and Deep Healing

CANNABINOIDS AND CONSCIOUS AWARENESS – A TWO-WAY STREET

Research on cannabinoids naturally produced by the body demonstrates a prominent link between frame of mind and the development of illness and disease. This link is further elucidated by research from the field of body-mind medicine. A wealth of study data helps us understand how constricting or outdated mental and emotional material may give rise to illness and disease. To reach for deeper healing, rather than mere momentary relief of symptoms, we must learn to activate our naturally occurring endocannabinoid system and utilize insights from body-mind medicine.

For instance, chronic fears and anxieties can make us sick and shorten our life. Pharmaceutical antidepressants may induce relaxation, but will not increase one's conscious awareness of underlying issues. In contrast, cannabis does more than induce relaxation. It brings revelation and insight as the psyche brings forth formerly unconscious material relevant to our healing process.

Similarly, being prone to constricting emotions (negative affect) can make us vulnerable to diseases, while a tendency toward expansive emotions (positive affect) can protect us from getting sick.[3] Marijuana is famous for suspending negative affect (pessimism, anxiety, anger, fear, hurt, pain, intolerance, hopelessness) and for helping us re-discover and maintain positive affect (laughter, optimism, happiness, gratitude, tolerance, compassion, hope).

Many patients have learned and applied insights gained via their cannabis regimen. As a result, some have taken their healing journeys to a new and profound level evidenced by a reduced need for medicine in any form or shape. Other patients have healed a chronic wound by adding a meaningful spiritual dimension to their life. Still others have achieved a complete cure even though orthodox medicine had no solution to offer them.

Cannabis brings to the surface otherwise hidden material which might seem intolerable in our normal frame of mind.[4]

> *Jonathan, a man in his fifties, didn't remember ever feeling anything for his mother but intolerance, scorn and impatience tempered by an occasional indulgence. In a state of relaxed and expanded awareness, he felt himself cry, child-like, "I want my mama, I want my mama." Once the previously unacceptable feelings of needing his mama when he was a child re-entered his awareness, Jonathan began to develop safer, deeper and more meaningful relationships whereas previously his fear of intimacy led only to unsafe, shallow connections with women.*

To better understand the interplay between our psychology, behavior and the development of illness, it is perhaps useful to examine a recent contribution by pharmacologist Candice Pert, Ph.D. and developmental cell biologist Bruce Lipton, Ph.D. In his book *The Biology of Belief*, Lipton[5] suggests that each of the trillion cells working in concert to provide balance and well-being in the human body have self-receptors in their membrane.[6] It is these receptors that know the difference between a virus, bacteria and the body's own structures. A mismatch in self-receptors can trigger a severe immune response, such as the dreaded rejection of a transplanted organ, which is needed to sustain life.

It is these cellular self-receptors that demonstrate that our mind is omnipresent in a trillion cellular membranes, all connected with each other and operating in concert. This may explain how the impact of nonphysical influences, such as suppressed emotions, can induce signals throughout the body at a cellular level that generate the transcription of disease-producing proteins instead of those involved in the production of health.

Pert echoes Lipton's findings in more depth and detail, in her book *Molecules of Emotions: The Science Behind Body-Mind Medicine*. Similarly, one of her key findings shows that intelligence is present in each cell of the body, and that the dance between emotions and molecules is indeed a two-way street. Pert's discoveries of a two-way communication between the environment (physical or nonphysical) and the production of either health-supporting or disease-producing molecules is further supported by research conducted in the field of epigenetics.

Epigenetics is a new and still-evolving term, generally used to describe environmental signals (epigenator) that initiate change in genetic expressions without changing the DNA sequence. These changes are specifically initiated by environmental signals, via a direct pathway into the cellular nucleus. Once the signal is received, an intra-cellular epigenetic initiator determines the precise location in the nucleus for the pathway, and an epigenetic maintainer sustains the change through succeeding generations.[7] In other words, an environmental signal (physical or nonphysical) begins a two-way communication with the human body at a cellular level that produces a switch that either turns a gene on or off. This switch can be inherited by future generations.

Since our mental and emotional architecture is part of the environment that sends constant signals to our body, and vice versa, the implications for Mind–Body medicine are significant. Epigenetics may provide a basis for better understanding the results of clinical trials which indicate that chronically suppressed or repressed emotions exacerbate a variety of medical conditions such as hypertension,[8,9] cardiovascular disease,[10] and breast cancer11 and thus eventually reduce life expectancy.[12]

Reasons for suppressing an emotion vary. Danger, inability to cope, protective mechanisms, feeling overwhelmed, societal judgments, taboos, personal beliefs, and the need to function with a singular focus are examples of motivating factors for temporary or long-term suppression of emotion(s). To express anger in the wrong situation can be dangerous, and even life-threatening. Children who are abused often do not have the opportunity or safety required to process their emotional traumas until they reach maturity and acquire the resources needed to handle and heal their emotional wounds.

> *Consider the following story of a 43 year-old African American woman who was suffering from chronic and severe hypertension, with complications that could not be controlled even with aggressive pharmaceutical interventions.13 There was no reported stress or distress, other than that associated with her blood pressure. Despite taking multiple blood pressure medications for a decade, her hypertension remained dangerously uncontrollable.*
>
> *Then, after an apparently normal conversation with her nephew, she began having recurring nightmares of a man approaching her from behind and grabbing her. She was woken from these nightmares by the sound of her own screaming. She became terrified to go to bed. Her physician asked her if a man had ever attacked her in reality. Hesitantly, the patient reported that since the nightmares had begun, she started to recall fragmented memories of rape by her uncle. She remembered telling only her father, who promised, "I'll take care of it, Baby," but never did. The rapist had long ago left the family and she had largely suppressed her memory of him for 30 years…until seeing her now-grown nephew, who resembled his father (her rapist), triggered the emergence of the emotional experience of the attack. Previously, she had remembered bits and pieces of the rape, but was always numb and void of any affect about it.*
>
> *Now, however, she was very upset recalling the event, and kept repeating, "He hurt me, he hurt me." She agreed to counseling and after several sessions also revealed that her abusive ex-husband attempted to strangle her while her father, whom she adored, was present though once again he did nothing to protect her. In subsequent sessions, the emotional intensity of her memories intensified. For the first time, the patient reported feeling powerless, betrayed, and rageful toward her uncle and her father. By processing her emotions, she began to identify less as a victim and recognize a reality in which she has a hand in controlling her life. These changes were followed by a physiological response, with a dramatic and sustained improvement in her blood pressure. Over a period of 18 months, the patient's blood pressure returned to normal despite a gradual reduction of pharmaceuticals. There was no recurrence of the nightmares.*

We need to face what we are thinking and experiencing and to tolerate the initial discomfort of doing so if we are to make significant change. —Alistair Cunningham, O.C., Ph.D., C.Psych.

PRONENESS TO NEGATIVE AFFECT

Besides the damaging effects of repressed or suppressed emotion, being prone to negative emotions (e.g. shame, guilt, anger, fear) has also been demonstrated to diminish health and well-being. More specifically, studies have shown that persistent experiences of negative emotions and stressful experiences can worsen chronic degenerative diseases through the increase in the production of pro-inflammatory cytokines (cell-signaling protein molecules), which increase inflammation activity associated with aging, cardiovascular disease, osteoporosis, arthritis, type 2 diabetes, certain cancers, Alzheimer's disease, frailty, and functional decline, as well as periodontal disease.[14] A team of California researchers similarly discovered that the emotions of shame and guilt produce specific immunological changes in tumor necrosis factor-α receptor levels (sTNFαRII), an indicator of pro-inflammatory cytokine activity.[15]

At this point, it is important to remember that constricting emotions are not themselves harmful to our health provided they are expressed and let go of appropriately. Long-standing habits (for example, binge drinking when upset) and entrenched ways of thinking (for example, making catastrophic predictions) that generally result in unresolved difficult or constricting emotions have been proven to negatively impact health. The opposite is true for long-standing habits (daily exercise) and entrenched ways of thinking (seeing the best in people) that generally result in pleasant or expansive emotions: these positively impact your health.

A Word about Emotions

Generally speaking, all appropriately expressed emotions are healthy. Anger, while normally seen as a negative emotion, can certainly be destructive, but it can also bring about positive change. The constricting emotion of fear can paralyze a life, but it can save one from falling off the edge of a cliff. Hopelessness can kill or give birth to determination. Worthlessness can imprison or produce compassion, blame can fuel violence toward others, and it can demonstrate what matters. Conversely, the expansive and positive emotion of love can be a true wonder to behold, but can also be used to control or smother another. Hope can sustain life in difficult times, or can maintain a negative influence. Trust can propel a positive reality, while inappropriate trust can destroy it.

However, three types of emotions, guilt, martyrdom and harbored (righteous, fanatical) anger tend to have only negative health consequences. Guilt seeks purification through punishment, and martyrdom involves torture and horrific death. Harbored emotions are emotions that are recycled as soon as they have been expressed, and as such are never released and continue to impact the body and the mind negatively.

PRONENESS TO POSITIVE AFFECT

While we all welcome emotions that make us feel good, the idea that what feels good may in this case be good for us warrants investigation. Psychologist Barbara Fredrickson makes an evolutionary argument that positive feelings broaden minds and serve as valuable resources during times of hardship.[16]

Until recently, the exact mechanism by which positive emotions support physical health and contribute to healing was not well understood. However, a study published in 2005 by researchers from London showed that positive emotions such as happiness can lower cortisol levels, reduce heart rate, and decrease fibrinogen stress responses.[17] The beneficial physiological results of positive emotions were further confirmed by a recent Harvard experiment that demonstrated that curiosity and hope decrease the likelihood of developing hypertension.[18]

Positive emotional experiences have also been associated with longevity. One study reviewed autobiographical material of 180 Catholic nuns, and compared this to the length of each nun's life. Researchers found that "positive emotional content reported in early-life autobiographies were [sic] strongly associated with longevity six decades later."[19] Study results were confirmed by another large population study from Texas, which concluded that "positive affect seems to protect individuals against physical declines in old age."[20]

REPLACING CHRONIC NEGATIVE AFFECT
WITH THE HABIT OF POSITIVE AFFECT

Within the proper therapeutic window, that is, a carefully measured dose selected with each patient's unique situation in mind, cannabis may assist patients who wish to transform their overall outlook on life. Similarly, happiness research has identified numerous ways in which positive emotions support health and contribute to healing. And, while we are still learning to better understand the intricate workings of how it all fits together, we know enough from the fields of medicine and psychology to draw important conclusions with practical ramifications. While there are a myriad of ways to produce deep and profound change in one's outlook, the following specific suggestions are presented for your consideration: Taking Ownership of Where We Are: Self-Acceptance, Conscious Choice, Reaching for Gratitude and Happiness, Practicing Forgiveness, and Changing Belief(s).

TAKING OWNERSHIP OF WHERE WE ARE: SELF-ACCEPTANCE

When we lack conscious ownership of thoughts and emotions that we have labeled intolerable or unacceptable, we spend a significant amount of energy engaged in avoidance mechanisms. For example, we may try to avoid unacknowledged emotions by bingeing on "comfort" foods which in fact make us ill, or reaching for any behavior or substance which acts like an emotional painkiller or numbing agent.

> It is the willingness to embrace the present moment, rather than avoid it, that allows us to change ourselves and so transcend our experience.

This expenditure of energy on avoidance techniques often results in exhaustion, a constricting sensation in the physical body and in our emotional experience. And, this misspent energy has real consequences for our health and vitality.

To reverse the damaging influence of our avoidance strategies, and the loss of vital energy that comes with it, it is important to begin by accepting where we are, no matter where we find ourselves.[21] We need to find ways to accept and honor ourselves when we are swimming in self-pity, entitlement, envy, hostility, grief, despair, loneliness, shame, or any thought or emotional state we have previously labeled intolerable or unacceptable. We don't have to linger in this emotional state, but in order to shift our experience we must first accept where we are. Studies have shown that honest self-expression, alone or with a close and trusted friend(s), reduces both the frequency and the intensity of seemingly intolerable states of mind.

With time and a bit of practice, embracing our present condition can make it easier to tolerate even the most unwelcome situations. We may even begin to notice a shift in attitude from aversion to curiosity. It is this willingness to embrace the present moment, rather than avoid it, that, combined with a sense of wonder, allows us to change ourselves and so transcend our experience.

At the age of 37, Jill Bolte Taylor, a Harvard-educated brain scientist, suffered a serious stroke and simultaneously entered a state of extraordinary consciousness. Bleeding from a ruptured vessel in the left side of her brain caused her to lose numerous left-brain functions (the ability to "walk, talk, read, write or recall any of my life"). After her stroke, she experienced cognitive shifts between the two sides of her brain. She lived two realities, as different as day and night. After a recovery process that took eight years, she wrote a book about her experience.[22]

Perhaps for the first time in medical history, a brain researcher was able to examine first-hand the right and left hemispheres of the brain, and then explain the subjective experience of each side of the brain. Taylor writes of the two halves of her brain as two cognitive minds with distinct personalities.

The left-brain is all about logic, time, method, details, categorizing, and the internal voice of our individual self-perception as separate from others; it is always concerned about what happened in the past, and based on the past is trying to connect and project what's going to happen in the future. During her stroke, it was this part of her brain that was becoming more and more disabled.

Taylor describes her experience: "My brain chatter went completely silent. [....] It was as if someone had taken a remote control and pushed the mute button. [....] I could not define where I began and where I ended. [....] I was captivated by the magnificence of the energy around me. [....] I felt enormous and expansive. [....] Any stress related to my job was gone. [....] I lost 37 years of emotional baggage. [....] In the wisdom of my dementia, I understood that this body was, by the magnificence of its design, a precious and fragile gift. It was clear to me that it functioned like a portal through which the energy of who I am can manifest here. I wondered how I could have spent so many years in this construct of life and never realize I was just visiting."[23]

In contrast with the left, the right-brain is concerned with intuition, feeling, emotions, energy, oneness, and connection; it lives exclusively in the present moment, unconcerned about the past or the future. The right half "thinks" in pictures; the left, in words. The right perceives the input from our senses as a tapestry of energy (sounds, sights, smells, sensations, taste, and movement).

Taylor described her right-brain experience, now uninhibited by the left-brain, in this way: "I am an energy being connected to the energy all around me through the consciousness of my right hemisphere. We are energy beings connected to one another through the consciousness of our right hemispheres as one human family. And right here, right now, we are all brothers and sisters on this planet, here to make the world a better place. And in this moment we are perfect. We are whole. And we are beautiful."[24]

Taylor called her cognitive shift to the right the euphoric nirvana of the right brain. When thinking with her right hemisphere, she experienced a complete sense of timeless well-being and peace. However, it was a switch back to the logical, sequential left that allowed her to recognize that she was having a stroke and ultimately enabled her to call for help.

Taylor's experience highlights the differences between the two sides of the brain, and in so doing shows the capabilities of each.

She posits the question "Who are we? We are the life force, power of the universe, with manual dexterity and two cognitive minds. And we have the power to choose, moment by moment, who and how we want to be in the world. Right here, right now, I can step into the consciousness of my right hemisphere where we are–I am–the life force power of the universe, and the life force power of the 50 trillion beautiful molecular geniuses that make up my form. At one with all, that is. Or I can choose to step into the consciousness of my left hemisphere, where I become a single individual, a solid, separate from the flow, separate from you. I am Dr. Jill Bolte Taylor, intellectual, neuroanatomist. These are the 'we' inside of me."[25]

> Right here, right now, I can step into the consciousness of my right hemisphere where we are–I am–the life force power of the universe, and the life force power of the 50 trillion beautiful molecular geniuses that make up my form. — Dr. Jill Bolte Taylor

Taylor's descriptions during her state of extraordinary consciousness may sound somewhat familiar to some cannabis patients. A similar cognitive shift to the right hemisphere occurs often during cannabis treatments, such as experiences of reduced stress or lack of stress, and intense sensations of peace and relaxation, even when aware of otherwise intolerable memories. Furthermore, increases in creativity, enhanced sensation of colors, sounds, taste, transcending life moments, feelings of connectedness to all of life, a sense of belonging where we are, gratitude, and an enhanced ability to empathically understand and forgive transgression may all be indicative of a shift in consciousness to the right brain.

This shift to the right can be learned and achieved without the traumatic experience of a stroke and without the use of cannabis. Several books have been written on the subject, examining the scientific understanding of left and right brain activity, and suggesting techniques and exercises to shift consciousness to the right. One of the more popular books is called *Drawing on the Right Side of the Brain*, by Betty Edwards.

GRATITUDE AND HAPPINESS

Gratitude is a valuable tool to change the tendency to have one's life experiences colored by negative affect.[26] This was facilitated by a simple gratitude exercise in which patients at the University of California – Davis' Medical Center for Neuromuscular Disease Clinic were instructed to write down five things they were grateful for every day, using no more than one sentence to describe each item. After two months, researchers noted a heightened sense of well-being, more hours of sleep, and reduced pain compared to a control group who were asked to write one sentence about a grudge or a neutral emotional event on a daily basis.

Experiencing and expressing gratitude enhances positive affect and results in other measurable benefits, too. Study participants have reported increases in optimism, happiness, fewer physical symptoms, positive states of alertness, greater attentiveness and determination, high energy, positive moods, feeling connected to others, increased empathy towards others, improved sleep, and more positive attitudes toward their family.

FORGIVENESS

Negative affect, such as blame and sustained hostilities directed at others, has been shown in numerous studies to negatively impact mental and physical well-being. In one experimental study, 287 surviving heart attack patients were followed and examined seven weeks after the attack and again after a period of eight years. Patients who reported they had learned something from their experience were significantly less at risk for a second heart attack compared to patients who believed that others had caused their heart attack.[27] Similarly, these results were confirmed by a meta-analysis of 45 independent studies that found hostility is an independent risk factor for coronary heart disease.[28]

Recent psychological inquiries have attempted to evaluate whether a chronic need for revenge, blame or hostility is itself a pathology. If we were to treat the need for revenge as a disease, could we not reason that learning to forgive is the ideal treatment?

Psychoneuroendocrinology, the study of the interplay between emotions and hormones, has shown that hormone profiles respond to forgiveness.[29,30] In one study, merely imagining forgiving an offender produced measurable improvements in heart rate and blood pressure compared to study participants who were instructed to imagine not forgiving them.[31]

Beyond the physiological benefits of forgiving someone or oneself, studies have shown that forgiveness has other clear and measurable health benefits such as reductions in hopelessness, defensiveness, blame, revenge, anxiety and depression as well as increases in optimism, self-efficacy, self-acceptance, and one's perceived level of social and emotional support. Forgiveness is also associated with the preservation of supportive and close relationships, greater satisfaction in life, transcendent consciousness and spiritual connection.[32,33,34]

BELIEF

Which came first, the chicken or the egg? When it comes to belief and experience, it seems that the same question may apply. Our thoughts and feelings shift in a new direction when specific underlying belief(s) are challenged and changed.[35] It may help to think of life's experiences as the multidimensional manifestation of our beliefs, or, to put it differently, experiences can be considered our beliefs in motion. Experience tends to change when we make a fundamental shift in belief, choose a new path, or make a profound decision, which leads to a new way of seeing the world.

Belief is a subjective conviction in a truth or trust in the existence of something without rigorous proof.

Ayaan Hirsi Ali,[36] a Somali feminist, was raised as a Muslim fundamentalist. She describes her thoughts and feelings as a young woman, steeped in her family's culture, living on the horn of Africa. Hirsi thought of Westerners and non-Muslims as infidels, and felt that their eternal punishment in the afterlife was just and right. She accepted the subservient roles of women, and thought of female genital mutilation (FGM) as normal and religiously justifiable.

It was not until she began to critically examine her religion, her socialization, her way of life and its impact on women and men alike that her adopted belief(s) began to erode and be replaced by new ones. She noticed that as her fundamental belief system shifted, so did her thoughts and feelings. She served a term as a Member of Parliament in Holland, and now writes and talks about her change of heart, beliefs, and the new set of feelings and thoughts that were generated by them. Ali has continued to make appearances on television, talk shows, and panel discussions where she highlights her changes. Ali now defends equality between the sexes, advocates for human rights and access to education, and vehemently opposes the practice of genital mutilation. She argues with a palpable conviction against the views, beliefs, and practices of many traditional Muslims, clerics and politicians. Ali not only challenges the tenets of Islam, she focuses particularly on its impact on girls and women in the Muslim World and Muslim families who have migrated into Europe or the US.

Ali is only one example of a public figure who demonstrates the connection between belief and experience. Examine any person who has had a change of heart, and you will likely discover an underlying belief that also changed. In health and in healing, it is important to realize that beliefs are not right or wrong. Beliefs are powerful, and have real physiological consequences that range from physical alterations, as in female genital mutilations, to specific habitual affects and their resultant influence on our bodies. It is with this in mind that we might want to make changes in belief(s) to support life, and dismiss those that hurt life.

Researchers argue that, initially, beliefs are passed on by parents or significant caregivers and are readily received and accepted by the early developing psyche. Consider Bruce Lipton, Ph.D., author of Developmental Cell Biology, who explores this connection with a puzzle: "Why do we need to teach children how to swim when practical experiences from water births have shown that all children, when born into water, have the innate ability to swim instinctively and without much effort, just like any other mammal?" Lipton posits that children have been given a set of negative beliefs about water by their parents or caretakers, which in turn produces feelings of fear, trepidation and ultimately the very real inability to swim safely and easily until it is re-learned. During the learning process of how to swim, the kids will learn, little by little, to again believe that they can swim with ease and without harm, but it takes time to change their minds and reset their internal architecture.

> While a traumatic or painful event may cause great stress to an organism, the chronic stress resulting from the meaning, negative interpretation and unhealthy beliefs we often attach to the original event is potentially more debilitating that the original trauma.

Researchers have noted that while a traumatic or painful event may cause great stress to an organism, the chronic stress resulting from the meaning, negative interpretation and unhealthy beliefs we often attach to the original event is potentially more debilitating that the original trauma. Take the deep-seated and common belief that "the world is a scary place" which itself produces chronic fear, aggression, hostility and a paranoid outlook on the world as a 'dog eat dog,' 'might is right,' 'winner takes all' environment where competition and domination are forever on the horizon. People with significant fear-based belief(s) will often try to control their environment and the people in it. One of several expressions of a fear-based belief structure is commonly referred to as a type A personality, which numerous studies have shown to be involved in the genesis of coronary artery disease (CAD).

Another example of real physiological changes stemming from belief-based negative affect comes from research conducted on patients suffering from post-traumatic stress disorder (PTSD). A meta-analysis of available neuroimaging research suggests real and measurable physiological changes in the limbic system in patients with PTSD; changes occur in the amygdala, the part of the brain responsible for processing fear, the medial prefrontal cortex, involved in decision making, and the hippocampus, the storage site of long-term memories. During episodes of activated PTSD the hippocampus is diminished in size, and reductions in neuronal integrity and functional integrity are evident. The medial prefrontal cortex also appears to shrink in size during symptomatic PTSD, and is less responsive than usual. Finally, neuroimaging research reveals heightened amygdala responsivity during PTSD symptomatic states.[37]

Associated emotional symptoms of PTSD include profound lack of interest in anything, feelings of emptiness, hopelessness, helplessness, worthlessness, shame, emotional numbness, distrust, inexplicable fear, anxiety, impatience, irritability and hostility. People with PTSD often exhibit paranoid behavior with hypervigilance, lost memories, a passive affect, withdrawal from regular activities, fits of anger with little or no provocation, lack of focus, insomnia, difficulties rising in the morning, fitful sleep with sweating, nightmares, generalized weakness or fatigue, flashbacks, and avoidance of anything associated with the traumatic event. Avoidance strategies can themselves become an additional problem for patients with PTSD. The compounding effect of detachment from actual or potential social supports and unhealthy attempts to reduce tension through substance abuse, overeating, cutting, or unsafe sexual practices can make recovery especially challenging.

The therapeutic benefits of leveraging a patient's belief system to support healing have been examined in recent years in many research studies. It seems that placebos (sugar pills) are just as therapeutic as standard pharmaceutical treatment for a wide variety of diseases.[38,39] While this may turn out to be bad news for pharmaceutical companies, it also highlights the impact of belief on disease, health and healing.

Simply put, emotionally expressive people with a tendency for positive affect are significantly healthier and live longer than people who have a tendency to suppress their feelings or are prone to "negative" emotions.

Consciously engaging or increasing the body's own healing abilities may be accomplished by enlisting specific belief(s). In the case of placebos, this entails believing that the provided treatment will be effective. Though the placebo itself is not therapeutic, taking the placebo with the expectation of healing may enhance and focus the self-regenerating powers of the body, mind and spirit. For the purpose of healing, it may or may not matter whether a belief is factually correct or not. The emotional state that results from one's belief determines the impact

> It does not matter if a belief is right or wrong. What matters is that they can have real consequences on our health and well-being.

of the treatment on one's health. Beliefs can heal or hurt. Fortunately, we can choose to nourish or banish any beliefs we attach to a particular treatment. In this way, we are in control of the results. Some beliefs are difficult to challenge and change, while others are not.

Jim used to like tofu. He had learned from his mother, an avid vegetarian, that soy was good for you and healthy. When Jim was finishing his last year at a premed college, he came across an in-depth research article written by a prominent scientist and expert in nutrition, published in a journal he had come to trust, that explained in compelling terms why soy is not good for you. Jim changed his mind and chose to avoid soy products. His thoughts and feelings were almost instantly different about tofu and other soy products.

Let's look at another example.

Sarah grew up with her grandparents. When her grandfather was angry, he gave Sarah the silent treatment or left, slamming the door on his way out. Sarah was scared and felt terribly guilty after such incidents. Sarah's grandfather instilled in her the belief that "anger is scary and that expressing anger is dangerous and unsafe." As a result, she avoided anger at all costs. While her suppression of anger may have been a useful survival mechanism in her childhood, later in life her anger aversion became a liability.

Sarah's anger aversion attracted abusive relationships, with anger appearing to come at her from seemingly everywhere but herself. Emotionally, she felt always on edge and drained of vitality, and her body felt tense, rigid, and sometimes numb. By the age of thirty-five, she was taking prescription medications for chronic anxiety and high blood pressure.

After unpleasant adverse effects from pharmaceutical medications, Sarah obtained a prescription for cannabis. Her blood pressure dropped almost instantly. More important to her, for the first time in a long time, Sarah felt at ease. "It was like the plant put me in touch with a part of my mind that was fully capable of being relaxed and unencumbered by my normally anxious internal mode of being. I loved this unexpected and much-needed break. But the biggest kicker was that I noticed myself feeling angry as I was thinking of my boyfriend. I noticed a constricting sensation in my body, but I wasn't scared. Instead it was just sort of okay. One moment it was there, and I felt it; then it dissipated like smoke in the wind. I have since been able to repeat the same experience of feeling my anger even when I'm not using cannabis. Perhaps it's been a long time coming, but I do believe now that it is okay to feel angry."

These examples illustrate the importance of expanding our experiential repertoire. By having "new" and "positive" experiences, we learn what this feels like, and then we are able to replicate the feeling in other areas and aspects of our emotional life.

For almost everybody, it's natural to want to experience some emotions and avoid others. Most people are well aware of how to produce certain emotional states. We play this record, and we feel energized and ready to keep driving on the long road to our destination. We'll pray or meditate, and our mind becomes calm and serene.

Most people also know how to avoid, at least for a while, those feelings they do not wish to feel. Addictions in many forms and shapes begin most often as an attempt to control and conquer unwanted feelings, and to force desired feelings onto the stage of consciousness. A person may think "I am tired of feeling insecure–where is my cocaine? I want confidence now." Or perhaps, "I have been treated unjustly. Where is my vodka so that I can make all of this go away?"

My drug of choice was adrenaline. It worked for a long time to keep pesky repressed emotions at bay while producing a thrill I found enjoyable. But, like with any drug, over time I needed more and more just to maintain the status quo. Maintaining a fearful worldview was helpful to me in my quest to continually squeeze more adrenalin from my adrenal glands. Being in the midst of trauma made it easy for me to maintain the view that the world was a scary place. To produce more adrenaline when I was not working, it was helpful to add anxiety into the mix. I became inundated with so much adrenaline that my adrenal glands were exhausted, which in turn increased my symptoms of post-traumatic stress disorder, irritability, mood swings, feeling cold, run down and tired all the time.

Whatever our drug of choice, such attempts to manipulate our internal state in order to avoid unpleasant emotions succeed only for a short while, if at all, after which more effort (drug) is again required. Therapists of all persuasions know very well that external means will often strengthen the presence of the unwanted feelings, and raise the chemical threshold needed to avoid them. This dynamic is often at the core of addiction, leading to a vicious downward spiral of continuous struggle and constant conflict. While the drug user believes the drug gives them a degree of control over their emotions, in fact they are locked into an unending struggle for dominance with no end in sight.

Every belief has impact.

When we continually use avoidance strategies such as thrill seeking, alcohol, drugs, or sex we may become dependent on these substances or activities to feel okay about ourselves. At some point, we need these substances just to feel "normal".

If, however, we take another approach and take an inventory of our emotional habits and core beliefs(s), we can begin to make more permanent changes. We begin by approaching our current feelings with curiosity and, if possible, even a sense of admiration. When we acknowledge and eventually accept our feelings as part of ourselves (our current selves), we are owning our present emotional reality. This leads to a healing emotional release, increased self-respect and possibly some insight into where these emotions originated.

The point of origin of a particular emotion may be an experience or a belief(s). It may be a reaction to a recent event or sourced in a memory from long ago. The emotional discovery process may take us through several layers, like the rings of an onion, but ultimately it will lead us to a point of origin. By exploring that origin, we can become more aware and mindful of any beliefs attached to a particular feeling.

Once the belief is made conscious, we can begin to replace it with a newer belief that produces a healthier internal architecture of thoughts and feelings, and the resultant healthier physiological responses.

The trauma of witnessing the accidental death of my uncle did damage. Guilt and shame, albeit repressed and hidden in the recesses of my mind, motivated me to be better prepared in the future. As a child I was aware only of the resolve to become able to handle trauma and emergencies, and the hope that I would one day feel right as rain again. The emotions which I could not process as a kid ultimately surfaced twenty-five years later as PTSD. There it was again, my old companion, my guilt and a bit of shame oozing through the crack of a "broken heart," old actors in a new play on another continent. However, unlike when I was a kid with few resources, I was now better equipped and prepared to "dance with my shadow." I now had resources and friends (plant and other) to help reconfigure an old chapter of my life by infusing a bit of conscious awareness.

Once I learned to accept rather than reject these "ugly emotions," I began to change a bit, and so did my perception of the world around me. The changes be-

came more pronounced when I directly challenged the belief that "mistakes must be punished," and "there is something wrong with me." Why couldn't mistakes be forgiven? Maybe I was mistaken in thinking that I was flawed! Over time, my self-talk turned more positive, and a bit of light, instead of darkness, started streaming through the figurative cracks of my heart. And, while a lot of change has taken place, I suspect I will find still deeper layers of meaning in the future.

In the context of health and healing, it is important to understand that beliefs are not right or wrong, good or bad. Beliefs are just recipes for various emotional responses, each of which have physiological consequences.

Consider beginning your journey by taking on a left-brain task: Without the use of cannabis, examine the meaning, logic, details and sequence of past events, as well as their influence on future expectations.

A suggested reading list is provided at the end of this chapter for readers who would like to learn more about how to identify unhealthy or life-draining beliefs and replace them with healthy and life-sustaining ones. You may also benefit from an internet search using keywords such as "change belief techniques."

DISEASE AS MESSAGE

In the paradigm of 'Disease is a Message,' symptoms or diagnosed diseases are a request or demand for change. Here, the symptoms, or more specifically the feeling we have about our symptoms and what they keep us from doing contain a message about the direction of change we need to take in order to heal.

Focused awareness, whether facilitated by cannabis or some other method, can provide a Rosetta Stone of sorts, that is, a guide for decoding the messages and feedback hidden in our illness.

Hilary was stressed and somewhat overwhelmed with the demands in her life. She had stepped on a nail and it hurt so badly that she had to really be careful about how she placed her foot. After ingesting a carefully dosed edible portion of cannabis, she began to relax, slow down and just be with her discomforts, both physical and emotional. Hilary felt instantly better, her breathing became deep and calming, and she realized that she needed to slow down. Then she remembered that a week earlier she had gotten a speeding ticket on her way to running some errands. She smiled at herself for missing the initial feedback and message that cost her $156 and was strangely grateful to the ache in her foot. Hilary resolved to slow down.

The interplay of the conscious mind and physiological feedback can serve as a reminder and sensitizing agent to pay attention to messages long before they manifest as highly undesirable symptoms. When initial messages are not acknowledged or responded to, the message may be repeated at a greater volume, that is, with a growing intensity. As the saying goes, an ounce of prevention is worth a pound of cure.

Disease allows us to experience physically that which has previously been repressed psychologically.

Sometimes, disease allows us to experience physically any unfinished psychological work. For instance, suppressed material such as emotions continuously wander ghost-like between the body and the mind's conscious, subconscious, and unconscious realms. In this sense, suppressed emotions are similar to the elusive nature of most chronic diseases such as hypertension or cancer.

When we are finally ready to respond to the demand for change, it is paramount to interpret and understand the message correctly. If the message indicates that we must express emotions we have labeled "unacceptable" or face memories we have repressed, then this is the corrective action required to alter the internal landscape of our psyche. Traumatic memories may surface from the unconscious and be perceived in a cathartic, corrective, and therapeutic fashion. Through this process, unwanted, unwarranted, unhealthy, or conflicting beliefs -- and their negative impact on vitality, aliveness, health, and well-being -- may finally be seen and recognized as such by the conscious mind.

The insights resulting from these inner changes can reduce or end self-defeating tendencies and negative patterns that otherwise may lock disease in place. Real healing can then occur, healing that transcends a mere cessation of adverse symptoms and encompasses a spiritual dimension as well.

Self-respect grows as one's ability to face and deconstruct old emotional material expands. Self-esteem develops from the careful attention paid to the message and feedback of the disease. Connecting with the meaning of illness can lead to a greater appreciation and connection with our body and the life all around us.

In each disease chapter of this book, the 'Disease as Message' theme is explored in a section called Exploring Mind-Body Consciousness.

RESISTANCE TO HEALING AND USING ILLNESS TO MANIPULATE

When resistance to healing is present, a part of the self attributes something positive to the presence of the disease. Perhaps the most difficult thing to do in deep healing is to examine the reasons why you might not want to heal…or, if you're honest with yourself, aren't eager to be completely well this very minute. A reluctance to completely heal could be a reflection of your yearning for attention from others, a belief that you deserve punishment, misplaced family loyalties, fear of loss, or an idea like "as long as I am sick she will never leave me." Perhaps your illness has become an identity or a way of

> If someone wishes for good health, one must first ask oneself if he is ready to do away with the reasons for his illness. Only then is it possible to help him.— Attributed to Hippocrates

life, a way to get your needs met, or a means to feel special, feel in control, or justify fanatical anger (that is, anger which is righteous, harbored, recycled, and punishing). Perhaps you see your illness as a way to avoid something such as unwanted responsibilities, difficult emotions or the judgment of others.

If this reluctance to fully heal is not addressed and resolved, you will consciously or unconsciously nourish the disease rather than yourself.

> *Emily was on vacation in Mexico with her sister Jane and her two nieces. As soon as they got to the beach resort Emily came down with a terrible cold and cough. She was unable to participate in any activities and became confined to her room. Emily was a body-mind therapist so she tried to understand the message of the cough. It did not take her long to determine that her cough was keeping Jane and her kids at a distance. She noticed that she felt angry when coughing. She realized that she did not want to be on vacation with kids but out of misplaced family loyalties had allowed herself to agree to something she*

did not really want to do. Once she recognized that she had been using her cough to symbolically bark at her sister and her nieces, Emily also realized that her anger was misplaced. She allowed herself to gently feel her frustration and her anger at the situation and at herself for not respecting her preferences for the kind of vacation she really wanted. As her anger dissipated, she began to let it be okay that she'd messed up. She forgave herself, and within a day or two her symptoms diminished sufficiently that she was able to make something of her remaining time with her family at the lovely tropical beach resort. She had, however, learned her lesson. Future vacations were planned and executed based on respecting what she really wanted, free of obligation.

While this chapter has hinted that the message of one's disease often requires examination of suppressed material, this is not the only possible scenario. Sometimes the material that demands expression was never repressed. Some patients talk in terms of past-life influences or life-lessons. Others have discovered that, for them, the illness was related to the release of toxins that sometimes occurs when deep and profound internal changes are realized. Yet others have experienced transformations (e.g. a state of extraordinary consciousness) or rediscovered the potency of their attachment to a collective identity (e.g. an intense commitment to sharing a group's/tribe's/family's experience) as part of their very private and subjective healing experience.

SUMMARY:

- **Both cannabinoids and consciousness engage the body and the mind simultaneously. This facilitates shifts in awareness important to deep healing.**
- **Suppressed or repressed emotions can make us sick and shorten our lives. They can be found and released, and this is part of the work of getting better.**
- **Constricting emotions are not themselves harmful to our health, provided they are expressed and let go of appropriately.**
- **Being prone to expressing expansive or positive emotions strengthens the immune system, improves quality of life and contributes to longevity.**
- **To reverse the damaging influence of our avoidance strategies, and the loss of vital energy that comes with it, it is important to begin by accepting where we are, no matter where we find ourselves.**
- **"We have the power to choose, moment by moment, who and how we want to be in the world." – Jill Bolte Taylor, Ph.D.**
- **Research has shown that experiencing and expressing gratitude enhances positive affect and results in measurable benefits.**
- **Merely imagining forgiving an offender produced measurable improvements in heart rate and blood pressure in a scientific study.**
- **Beliefs are not right or wrong, but in the area of health they have real and measurable physiological consequences. We get to choose.**
- **Disease is a message. Once the message is answered, resistance to healing is dissolved. We approach every symptom or disease with resistance initially. Owning, forgiving and releasing the resistance speeds recovery.**

Suggested Reading List on the Topic of Changing Beliefs:

Richard Bandler and John Grinder. *Neuro-linguistic Programming (NLP). The Structure of Magic, Vol. 1: A Book About Language and Therapy.* Science and Behavior Books; 1 edition (January 1, 1975)

Richard Bandler and John Grinder. *Frogs into Princes: Neuro Linguistic Programming.* Real People Press (1989)

Stephen LaBerge, Ph.D. *Lucid dreaming.* Ballantine Books (November 13, 1991)

Sidney Rosen. *Ericksonian Hypnosis. My Voice Will Go with You: The Teaching Tales of Milton H. Erickson.* W. W. Norton & Company (March 17, 1991).

1 Simon J. Griffin, MSc, DM,1 Ann-Louise Kinmonth, MSc, MD,1 Marijcke W. M. Veltman, PhD,1 Susan Gillard, MSc,1 Julie Grant, BSc,2 and Moira Stewart, PhD2 *Effect on Health-Related Outcomes of Interventions to Alter the Interaction Between Patients and Practitioners: A Systematic Review of Trials.* 1General Practice and Primary Care Research Unit, Department of Public Health and Primary Care, Institute of Public Health, Cambridge, UK. 2Department of Family Medicine, University of Western Ontario, London, Ontario, Canada. Ann Fam Med. 2004 November; 2(6): 595–608.

2 Zubieta JK, Bueller JA, Jackson LR, Scott DJ, Xu Y, Koeppe RA, Nichols TE, Stohler CS. *Placebo effects mediated by endogenous opioid activity on mu-opioid receptors.* Department of Psychiatry, Mental Health Research Institute, The University of Michigan, Ann Arbor, Michigan 48109-0720, USA. J Neurosci. 2005 Aug 24;25(34):7754-62.

3 Kiecolt-Glaser JK, McGuire L, Robles TF, Glaser R. *Emotions, morbidity, and mortality: new perspectives from psychoneuroimmunology.* Department of Psychiatry The Ohio State University College of Medicine, 1670 Upham Drive, Columbus, Ohio 43210, USA. Annu Rev Psychol. 2002;53:83-107.

4 L.S. Kubie M.D., and S. Margolin M.D. *The Therapeutic Role of Drugs in the Process of Repression, Dissociation and Synthesis.* New York Neurological Institute, and the Department of Neurology, College of Physicians and Surgeons, Colombia University New York. Psychosomatic Medicine May 1, 1945 vol. 7 no. 3 147-151.

5 Bruce H. Lipton Ph.D. *The Biology of Belief: Unleashing the Power of Consciousness, Matter, & Miracles.* Hay House (September 15, 2008).

6 Leremy A. Colf1, 3, Alexander J. Bankovich1, 3, Nicole A. Hanick1, Natalie A. Bowerman2, Lindsay L. Jones2, David M. Kranz2 and K. Christopher Garcia1 *How a Single T Cell Receptor Recognizes Both Self and Foreign MHC.* 1 Howard Hughes Medical Institute, Departments of Molecular and Cellular Physiology, and Structural Biology, Stanford University School of Medicine, Stanford, CA 94305, USA 2 Department of Biochemistry, University of Illinois at Urbana-Champaign, Urbana, IL 61801, USA. Cell, Volume 129, Issue 1, 135-146, 6 April 2007.

7 Shelley L. Berger1,5, Tony Kouzarides2,5, Ramin Shiekhattar3,5 and Ali Shilatifard4,5 *An operational definition of epigenetics.* 1Department of Cell and Developmental Biology, University of Pennsylvania, Philadelphia, Pennsylvania 19104, USA; 2Gurdon Institute and Department of Pathology, Cambridge CB2 1QN, United Kingdom; 3Wistar Institute, Philadelphia, Pennsylvania 19104, USA; 4Stowers Institute for Medical Research, Kansas City, Missouri 64110, US. Genes & Dev. 2009. 23: 781-783.

8 Kahn HA, Medalie JH, Neufeld HN, Riss E, Gouldbourt U. *The incidence of hypertension and associated factors: the Israeli ischemic heart disease study.* Hadassah Medical Organization, Jerusalem, Israel, the Ministry of Health, Jerusalem, Israel and the National Heart and Lung Institute, Bethesda, Maryland, USA. Am Heart J 1972; 84: 171–82.

9 Cottington EM, Mathews KA, Talbott E, Kuller LH. *Occupational stress, suppressed anger, and hypertension.* Psychosom Med 1986; 48: 249–60.

10 Kahn HA, Medalie JH, Neufeld HN, Riss E, Gouldbourt U. *The incidence of hypertension and associated factors: the Israeli ischemic heart disease study.* Hadassah Medical Organization, Jerusalem, Israel, the Ministry of Health, Jerusalem, Israel and the National Heart and Lung Institute, Bethesda, Maryland, USA. Am Heart J 1972; 84: 171–82.

11 Pettingale KW, Greer S, Tee DEH. *Serum IgA and emotional expression in breast cancer patients.* Faith Courtauld Unit for Human Studies in Cancer, King's College Hospital Medical School, Denmark Hill, London S.E.5., England. J Psychosom Med 1977; 21: 395–9.

12 Ernest Harburg, PhD, Mara Julius, ScD, Niko Kaciroti, PhD, Lillian Gleiberman, PhD and M. Anthony Schork, PhD. *Expressive/Suppressive Anger-Coping Responses, Gender, and Types of Mortality: a 17-Year Follow-Up* (Tecumseh, Michigan, 1971–1988). Department of Epidemiology, School of Public Health (E.H., M.J.), Biostatistics, School of Public Health (M.A.S.), Psychology (E.H.), Internal Medicine (L.G.), and the Center for Human Growth and Development (N.K.), University of Michigan, Ann Arbor, Michigan. Psychosomatic Medicine 65:588-597 (2003).

13 SJ Mann and M Delon. *Improved hypertension control after disclosure of decades-old trauma.* Cardiovascular Center, New York Hospital--Cornell Medical Center, New York 10021, USA. Psychosomatic Medicine, Vol 57, Issue 5 501-505.

14 Kiecolt-Glaser JK, McGuire L, Robles TF, Glaser R. *Emotions, morbidity, and mortality: new perspectives from psychoneuroimmunology.* Department of Psychiatry The Ohio State University College of Medicine, 1670 Upham Drive, Columbus, Ohio 43210, USA. Annu Rev Psychol. 2002;53:83-107.

15 Sally S. Dickerson, MA, Margaret E. Kemeny, PhD, Najib Aziz, MD, Kevin H. Kim, PhD and John L. Fahey, MD. *Immunological Effects of Induced Shame and Guilt.* Department of Psychology (S.S.D., M.E.K., K.H.K.), Cousins Center for Psychoneuroimmunology (S.S.D., M.E.K. J.L.F.), Department of Psychiatry and Biobehavioral Sciences (M.E.K.), Center for Interdisciplinary Research in Immunology and Disease (N.A., J.L.F.), and Department of Microbiology and Immunology (J.L.F.), University of California, Los Angeles, CA. M.E.K. is now at the Department of Psychiatry/Health Psychology program, University of California, San Francisco. K.H.K. is now at the Department of Psychology in Education, University of Pittsburgh. Psychosomatic Medicine 66:124-131 (2004).

16 Barbara Fredrickson. *The Value of Positive Emotions: The emerging science of positive psychology is coming to understand why it's good to feel good.* American Scientist. July-August 2003 Volume 91, Number 4 Page: 330.

17 Steptoe A, Wardle J, Marmot M. *Positive affect and health-related neuroendocrine, cardiovascular, and inflammatory processes.* International Centre for Health and Society, Department of Epidemiology and Public Health, University College London, London WC1E 6BT, United Kingdom. Edited by Bruce S. McEwen, The Rockefeller University, New York, NY. Proc Natl Acad Sci U S A 2005;102:6508–12.

18 Richman LS, Kubzansky L, Maselko J, Kawachi I, Choo P, Bauer M. *Positive emotion and health: going beyond the negative.* Department of Society, Human Development, and Health, Harvard School of Public Health, Cambridge, MA, USA. Health Psychol. 2005 Jul;24(4):422-9.

19 Danner DD, Snowdon DA, Friesen WV. *Positive emotions in early life and longevity: findings from the nun study.* Department of Preventive Medicine and Sanders-Brown Center on Aging, College of Medicine, University of Kentucky, Lexington 40536-0230, USA. Pers Soc Psychol. 2001 May;80(5):804-13.

20 Ostir GV, Markides KS, Black SA, Goodwin JS. *Emotional well-being predicts subsequent functional independence and survival.* Department of Preventive Medicine and Community Health, University of Texas Medical Branch, Galveston 77555-0460, USA. J Am Geriatr Soc. 2000 May;48(5):473-8.

21 Alastair J Cunningham, O.C., Ph.D., C.Psych. Kimberly Watson, M.A. *"How psychological therapy may prolong survival in cancer patients: new evidence and a simple theory"* Ontario Cancer Institute. 610 University Avenue, Suite 10/502B Toronto, ON, Canada, M5G 2M9.

22 Jill Bolte Taylor, Ph.D. *My Stroke of Insight: A Brain Scientist's Personal Journey.* 2008. Viking Penguin.

23 From 'Jill Bolte Taylor's Stroke of Insight' at TED.com

24 Ibid.

25 Ibid.

26 Robert A. Emmons, University of Miami and Michael E. McCullough, University of Miami. *Counting Blessings Versus Burdens: An Experimental Investigation of Gratitude and Subjective Well-Being in Daily Life.* Journal of Personality and Social Psychology 2003, Vol. 84, No. 2, 377–389.

27 Affleck, G., Tennen, H., Croog, S., & Levine, S. (1987). *Causal attributions, perceived benefits and morbidity after heart attack: An 8 year study.* Journal of Consulting and Clinical Psychology, 55, 29-35.

28 Miller, T. Q., Smith, T. W., Turner, C. W., Guijarro, M. L., & Hallet, A. J. (1996). *A meta-analytic review of research on hostility and physical health.* Psychological Bulletin, 119, 322-348.

29 Benjamin A. Tabak a, Michael E. McCullough a, Angela Szeto a, Armando J. Mendez b, Philip M. McCabe a. *Oxytocin indexes relational distress following interpersonal harms in women.* a. Department of Psychology and Behavioral Medicine Research Center, University of Miami, Coral Gables, FL, United States b. Diabetes Research Institute at the University of Miami Miller School of Medicine, Miami, FL, United States. Psychoneuroendocrinology (2011)36,115—122.

30 Berry, J. W., & Worthington, E. L., Jr. (2001). *Forgivingness, relationship quality, stress while imagining relationship events, and physical and mental health.* Journal of Counseling Psychology, 48, 447-455.

31 Witvliet, C. V., Ludwig, T. E., & Bauer, D. J. (2002). *Please forgive me: Transgressors' emotions and physiology during imagery of seeking forgiveness and victim responses.* Journal of Psychology and Christianity, 21, 219-233.

32 Thoresen, C. E., Harris, A. H. S., & Luskin, F. *Forgiveness: Theory, research, and practice* (pp. 254-280). New York: Guilford Press. (2000).

33 Greenwald, D. F., & Harder, D. W. (1994). *Sustaining fantasies and psychopathology in a normal sample.* Journal of Clinical Psychology, 50, 707-710.

34 Giacomo Bono , Michael E. McCullough. *Positive Responses to Benefit and Harm: Bringing Forgiveness and Gratitude Into Cognitive Psychotherapy.* University of Miami. Journal of Cognitive Psychotherapy: An International Quarterly. Volume 20, Number 2 • 2006.

35 U. Blesching. Unpublished Master Thesis. *Emotional Authorship.* June 2001. Western Institute for Social Research, Berkeley.

36 For more information on Ayaan Hirsi Ali go to her website at: http://theahafoundation.org/

37 Shin LM, Rauch SL, Pitman RK. *Amygdala, medial prefrontal cortex, and hippocampal function in PTSD.* Department of Psychology, Tufts University, 490 Boston Avenue, Medford, MA 02155, USA. Ann N Y Acad Sci. 2006 Jul;1071:67-79.

38 Ted J. Kaptchuk1,2*, Elizabeth Friedlander1, John M. Kelley3,4, M. Norma Sanchez1, Efi Kokkotou1, Joyce P. Singer2, Magda Kowalczykowski1, Franklin G. Miller5, Irving Kirsch6, Anthony J. Lembo1. Placebos without Deception: *A Randomized Controlled Trial in Irritable Bowel Syndrome.* 1 Beth Israel Deaconess Medical Center, Harvard Medical School, Boston, Massachusetts, United States of America, 2 Osher Research Center, Harvard Medical School, Boston, Massachusetts, United States of America, 3 Psychology Department, Endicott College, Beverly, Massachusetts, United States of America, 4 Massachusetts General Hospital, Harvard Medical School, Boston, Massachusetts, United States of America, 5 Department of Bioethics, National Institutes of Health, Bethesda, Maryland, United States of America, 6 Department of Psychology, University of Hull, Hull, United Kingdom. PLoS ONE 5(12): e15591. doi:10.1371/journal.pone.0015591

39 Ted J Kaptchuk, associate professor of medicine1, John M Kelley, assistant professor of psychology and statistics2, Lisa A Conboy, instructor of medicine1, Roger B Davis, associate professor of medicine and biostatistics3, Catherine E Kerr, instructor of medicine1, Eric E Jacobson, lecturer4, Irving Kirsch, professor of psychology5, Rosa N Schyner, research associate1, Bong Hyun Nam, research fellow1, Long T Nguyen, research fellow1, Min Park, research coordinator1, Andrea L Rivers, research coordinator1, Claire McManus, research coordinator1, Efi Kokkotou, assistant professor of medicine3, Douglas A Drossman, professor of medicine6, Peter Goldman, professor emeritus 7, Anthony J Lembo, assistant professor of medicine3 *Components of placebo effect: randomised controlled trial in patients with irritable bowel syndrome.* BMJ 336 : 999 doi: 10.1136/bmj.39524.439618.25 (Published 3 April 2008).

Chapter III

How to Use this Book

ORGANIZATION OF THIS BOOK

The purpose of this book is two-fold: 1) to provide readers with the information they need to make informed choices that truly serve their healing process, in particular an annotated review of the scientific evidence for using cannabis for specific diseases and conditions, and 2) to introduce the reader to essential concepts of body-mind consciousness as they relate to disease, health and healing. The central part of this book, The Cannabis Health Index (CHI), reviews scientific literature on the use of cannabis to treat over 100 illnesses (or groups of illnesses), one disease (or disease group) at a time. Please note that this is not intended to be a comprehensive list of all major diseases and conditions! Only diseases and conditions for which cannabis is an effective or promising treatment are included here.

The information provided for each disease or disease group follows a consistent format. Beneath the chapter header, you will see an overall Cannabis Health Index numerical score for that disease or condition. This scoring system is fully explained in the paragraphs below. Please be sure that you read Measuring Efficacy prior to diving into the disease-specific sections so that you understand how this rating scale works and what it means.

Each disease-specific section begins with a succinct description of the disease in everyday language. This is followed by a discussion of the evidence-base for integrating cannabis into the treatment plan. This annotated summary of scientific research is summarized in a table that lists the publication date, research location, key results, and CHI score assigned to each study.

The second part of each disease-specific section attempts to bridge the gap between allopathic medical practice and a mind-body consciousness approach. Here you will find practical suggestions and thought-provoking material to help discern any psychological or environmental issues that may underlie or impact your disease progression and healing process. Subsections include *Exploring Mind-Body Consciousness, Powerful Questions, Aggravating Factors, Healing Factors, Suggested Blessings, Suggested Affirmations, Anecdotes, Strain-specific Considerations, Form-specific Considerations,* and a *Take Notice* Section featuring CB2 activating spices and other supportive measures.

Measuring Efficacy: the Cannabis Health Index

WHAT IS A CHI SCORE?

Doctors and health practitioners are taught how to decipher medical research, but general readers are not. Even the intrepid reader prepared to wade through acronyms and statistical tables may not know how to evaluate conflicting results from different types of studies. The CHI Score is designed to do this for you. The CHI Score is a rating system that takes into account both the type of research study (which impacts the reliability of a study's conclusions) and the study's findings, which may be positively associated with medical use of cannabis (that is, the study reports that cannabis is a viable treatment) or negatively associated with it (the study says it doesn't work).

Each study discussed is scored based on its scope and the type of methodology used in the study, and then this number is multiplied by +1 if the study concluded that cannabis was effective, or multiplied by -1 if the study concluded that cannabis was ineffective. Studies with inconclusive or mixed results may be included in the text for your reference, but do not contribute to the overall disease CHI Score. Please note that efficacy (effectiveness) is not rated along a continuum; for our purposes here study results are categorized simply as positive or negative, that is finding cannabis to be effective or ineffective. Finally, all of the scores for individual studies included in the analysis of a disease (group) are added together to create an overall disease CHI Score.

You may think of the disease CHI Score as one indicator of both the volume and the direction of research studies available on the subject of cannabis to treat a particular disease.

IMPORTANCE OF THE TYPE OF RESEARCH STUDY

Not all study types and designs, and their respective findings, translate equally well into practically useful insights. The scientific method informs and guides basic research and experiments. Different types of research studies attempt to test hypotheses, for example, that cannabis is an effective treatment for multiple sclerosis. Within medical research, double-blind, placebo-controlled, human clinical trials provide the strongest degree of evidence (that is, are deemed most likely to determine the truth). Studies that review and compare available published research are also highly respected, strong pieces of evidence. Less convincing, respectively, are human case studies and case studies of individual clinical experiences, animal experiments, and laboratory studies. In this book, values are assigned to reviewed research studies that reflect the intrinsic strength of evidence associated with each type of study.

POSSIBLE CHI SCORES

Type of Study	CHI
Double-blind and/or placebo and/or cross-over controlled human trial	5
Meta-analysis (review of available studies)	4
Human case studies, and clinical experiences	3
Animal studies	2
Laboratory studies	1

When comparing CHI values for one disease versus another, it is important to realize that the values are relative to the available academic literature. A lower value does not necessarily mean that cannabis is a less effective treatment. On the other hand, a higher CHI value does indicate not just a greater knowledge base, but also a higher degree of scientific certainty that medical marijuana is beneficial for treating a specific disease (or disease group).

A score of 4 or 5 for a particular study means that there is solid evidence that cannabis may be a useful treatment. If it is relevant to your health issues, you may wish to share this citation with your doctor for his or her review.

A score of 2 or 3 for a particular study means that while more research needs to be done, it is plausible that cannabis could be a useful treatment. While this is not conclusive evidence, you may still want to discuss these studies with your doctor, particularly if you have concerns about the effectiveness and/or safety of other methods available to you.

A score of 0 suggests that study results were mixed or inconclusive.

A score of any negative number suggests that cannabis was found to be ineffective or lacking any significant benefit. A score of -2 or -3, for example, would suggest that a study concluded that cannabis was not an effective treatment, but the study design was not especially rigorous, either.

A score of -4 or -5 suggests that a rigorous, credible study found cannabis to be an ineffective treatment for this condition.

This book concentrates only on diseases and conditions for which cannabis shows promise, so it should not surprise you that you will rarely see negative CHI scores. However, you may see negative as well as positive scores for individual studies if various studies reached different conclusions. Published studies were extracted from MEDLINE, the U.S. National Library of Medicine's bibliographic database for further review based on inclusion criteria that included a focus on the influence of the endocannabinoid system, cannabis and/or cannabinoids on symptoms and diseases listed in the Cannabis Health Index.

Please note that a high disease score reflects the amount of available published research to a much larger extent than it reflects the degree of efficacy of cannabis to treat disease. The disease score is a simple sum of all the individual study scores for that disease, so higher numbers indicate a large amount of research has been conducted for that disease.

Exploring Mind–Body Consciousness

Mind–Body Consciousness is merely being aware that mind and body always work together, even though it sometimes appears that we are more focused on one or the other. Part of exploring our mind–body territory is evident in the habitual and natural tendency of humans to search for meaning in everything we experience. It may be part of what makes the mysteries and wonders of life so real to us. This is true for the big questions: "Why am I here?" "What is the meaning of life?" "Does God exist? And, this is also true for the little questions, such as when we ponder the shape of clouds and declare that they look like a bunny or a flower. Our natural search for meaning is omnipresent, and it also applies to getting sick. "Why did I get this disease?" "What is the meaning of my symptom(s)?" This book is, in part, an exploration in search of the meaning of illness.

Many of the diseases examined in this publication escape orthodox medicine's explanations and may even be labeled "incurable", and yet they are often alleviated by the application of cannabinoids, a substance that crosses the body–mind barrier. This book follows the plant's lead and explores possible metaphysical underpinnings of disease (mental-emotional-spiritual) reported by patients, physicians and researchers alike.

The mind-body material (psychosomatic considerations) in this book are based on a meta-analysis of relevant literature, scientific study results, reported case studies, practitioners' reports, patient support groups, studies from the fields of psychology,[1] psychohistory,[2] psychoncology,[3] psychoendocrinology,[4] epigenetics,[5] psychoneuroimmunology[6] and insights from cannabis-using people who work with states of extraordinary consciousness to answer the challenges of illness and infirmity. The material is also informed by my experience in emergency medicine, phytopharmacology,[7] patient consultations and homeopathic medicine.

> Many of the diseases examined in this publication escape orthodox medicine's explanations and may even be labeled "incurable", and yet they are often alleviated by the application of cannabinoids, a substance that crosses the body–mind barrier.

In its most potent form, working with mind–body consciousness is predicated on the hypothesis that one is fully responsible for one's experience. Misunderstood and misused, the concept can be applied to assign blame and judgment, which naturally add insult to injury. However, when applied properly it can be used to learn, discover, and embrace the psychosomatic underpinning of disease, and thus begin a very personal and self-empowering journey towards health and well-being.

To begin working in mind–body territory, it's helpful to remember that it is a very subjective process. While the potential meaning or message embedded in symptoms and illness will be unique to each person, common patterns often emerge. The loss of function experienced by those suffering from a particular disease has some individual variation but many obvious patterns and commonalities exist. Far less homogenous is the emotional response individuals have to this loss of function, the meaning they ascribe to the illness, and their path of recovery from it. Two cannabis-using people may have the same symptoms of stiff and painful knee joints, diagnosed by their physicians as arthritis, but find different avenues to answer the individualized message their pain carries.

> *When David allowed himself to relax and sink into the knee pain it brought images and memories of old hurts and grievances from long ago to the surface of his mind.*
>
> *On the other hand Jennifer, who presented with exactly the same physical symptoms, discovered in her process of embracing her knee pain that for her the message had to do with being inflexible.*
>
> *Both heeded their respective messages, and received relief. David accepted his ancient grievances, and worked with forgiveness until the stiffness went*

away. Jennifer did not notice her pain diminish until she made a conscious decision to be more flexible whenever she found herself adopting a rigid or righteous posture in her thinking or in conversation with others.

Cannabis-using people who have been successful in bringing about a deep and profound healing have often reported a common process. They use their symptoms as a map to chart their journey from one place of awareness and understanding to another until they arrive at meaning and serenity. By embracing or "being with" their feelings, they have discovered some internal construct that contained a meaningful connection related to their disease or symptom formation. Similarly, patients who incorporate mindfulness in their healing regimen report that in exploring mind–body territory they become the captain of their experiences. How they feel about a symptom or an illness is itself an important navigational instrument, which can bring the normally hidden to the forefront of the mind. Once aware of the connection, the next step is to answer the message or the feedback delivered by the disease or symptom.

No book or publication can encompass the full range of scenarios in which a "disease message" is heard and answered productively. However, you can begin to enhance your own aliveness, enthusiasm, and well-being by putting into action the recommendations in the section entitled, *Replacing Chronic Negative Affect with Tendencies for Positive Affect."*

POWERFUL QUESTIONS

People are like fingerprints or snowflakes in that we are unique. Human beings have their own set of questions to explore, including those raised by the crisis of a mild, acute, or debilitating illness. However, there are common threads that may weave through the internal architecture of a manifest disease. The questions used in the *Exploring Mind–Body Consciousness* section of each disease chapter attempt to address these common threads. You could ponder them during meditation, or engage the plant's help to examine them together.

The exploration of these questions, or your own versions of them, makes it possible to look through your unique veil of misery and pain to discover what lies beyond. The learning that can take place on the fulcrum between life and death, between body and mind, between doing and being, can play an integral part in health and healing.

AGGRAVATING FACTORS/HEALING FACTORS

These headings indicate a summary of psychosomatic study results and other key indicators associated with aggravating or ameliorating elements related to each disease.

SUGGESTED BLESSINGS

Some people like to engage the spiritual, by whatever name or form they may hold dear. One way to engage something larger than ourselves is to ask for a blessing to seed new, healthier thoughts and feelings as part of our daily health routines. This section suggests sample blessings to spur your own imagination.

SUGGESTED AFFIRMATIONS

Thoughts and words affect the immune system. We can be imprisoned by our own words and thoughts, or we can use them to set us free. For those people who like to work with carefully and consciously chosen words to support their health and healing, this section suggests affirmations directly related to the possible internal architecture of each illness described.

ANECDOTES (IN ITALICS)

Although this book emphasizes scientific findings and evidence-based methods, some readers may have difficulty relating to mind-body healing without personal accounts to put these findings in context. Where personal accounts have been included, the names and context of the cases have been altered. Healing journeys are often complex and multi-layered. Due to space constraints, the examples chosen are necessarily simplified, focusing on only one, or at best a handful, of key elements in a person's experience of using cannabis and/or consciousness to foster their health and healing.

Jim had been a Deacon at his church for many years. He was an active member of an organization committed to retaining the traditional definition of marriage as the joining of a man and a woman. He was very vocal and emotionally charged whenever the topic came up. To Jim, homosexuality was wrong, and his church agreed. He was quite vocal and proud of expressing his righteous indignation and anger at those who disagreed with him. He freely spent the emotional charge of his convictions when an opportunity presented itself. When the moment passed, he recycled his anger for the next time the topic might appear on the horizon of his mind.

Jim had liver cancer. A couple of years ago he had undergone surgery, and he was just beginning a new course of chemotherapy. Just when the vomiting got so bad it seemed intolerable, his hospital roommate Daryl offered to share a joint with him. Not knowing what else to do, Jim accepted. It reduced his nausea to a manageable level. He looked over and saw Daryl holding Hank's hand. He noticed the care and tenderness between them, and looked upon them both with compassion. Jim felt grateful and very puzzled by his change of demeanor.

While Jim's change of heart about homosexuality did not last, for a brief time his nausea and vomiting – and his lack of compassion for others – had subsided. It took some time for him to connect the dots between his change of mind and the change in his symptoms. Jim would not know until many months later that this fateful meeting with Daryl had been the conscious beginning of his particular healing journey. To answer the message of his illness, Jim had to learn to accept some things about himself that previously made him shrivel in disgust and shame. He had to challenge and change certain age-old beliefs, and to find a way to meet the demand for a new life. Eventually, Jim rose to the occasion, and has now joined the ranks of cancer survivors.

STRAIN-SPECIFIC CONSIDERATIONS

Sativas and indicas as well as their respective dominant hybrids present with a different cannabinoid profile. Sativas and sativa dominant strains present with a higher THC to CBD ratio when compared to indicas or indica dominant strains. THC binds with both CB1 and CB2 receptors while CBD has a greater affinity for CB2.

In general, if you require focused CB1 activation, select a strain with a higher THC to CBN ratio, namely sativas or sativa-dominant hybrids. On the other hand, if you are trying to enhance CB2 activation, select an indica or indica-dominant strain with a lower THC to CBD ratio thus favoring CB2 expression.

A CBD-rich cannabis plant strain is ideal for the treatment of anxiety with CBD's sedating, relaxing, and grounding properties. Most cannabis dispensaries will have a laboratory-tested cannabinoid profile available for each of the strains they carry. Any strain that produces a CBD profile of more than 3% is considered CBD-dense and can be used to target a specific therapeutic need such as anxiety. The likely choice would be an indica or indica-heavy hybrid.

FORM-SPECIFIC CONSIDERATIONS

To fine-tune therapeutic effects, in addition to carefully selecting the ideal strain of cannabis with the most appropriate ratios, also consider the "method of administration", meaning how you take your medicine. There are several options.

In fresh and raw cannabis leaf, CBD and THC cannabinoids exist as CBD-acid and THC-acid, both of which are non-psychoactive in the raw state. Once the plant cannabinoids become heated, dried or stored, decarboxylation takes place, changing the molecular structure and its resultant properties. While CBD remains non-psychoactive after decarboxylation, THC-acid becomes THC, the main psychoactive molecule in cannabis, which limits the maximum potential dose accordingly.

William L. Courtney, M.D., a physician who has been working with dietary raw cannabis, considers fresh and raw cannabis leaf an especially rich form of CBD, further increasing CBD influence potential. Courtney suggests that unheated large cannabis leaf or leaf juice can be tolerated at doses 60 times higher than when cannabis is heated. The juice tastes bitter and can be diluted with another vegetable juice at a ratio of 1:10. Mix one part cannabis juice with nine parts vegetable juice to mask the taste. Ten to twenty large fan leaves juiced daily is a commonly recommended dose.

Additionally, research is beginning to show that raw plant THC-acid has unique and potent therapeutic properties of its own and does not make users "high". Dutch scientists' research suggests that raw THC-acid inhibits tumor necrosis factor alpha (TNF-α) levels,[8] which have become associated with the promotion of inflammation and the overall regulation of specific immune responses.

Raw, fresh cannabis leaf medicine allows patients to benefit from cannabis' potent therapeutic properties without altering their state of consciousness. Thus they remain able to safely operate heavy machinery, drive to and from work, and make delicate decisions.

TAKE NOTICE

The efficacy of ancient healing practice using spices as medicine has been confirmed by the recent scientific discoveries of β-caryophellene – a common food-based cannabinoid fully accepted by the Food and Drug Administration (FDA). β-caryophyllene contained in specific exotic spices activate the endocannabinoid system via CB2, which makes these spices a potentially novel form of treatment available to everyone. These food-based cannabinoids can activate CB2 receptors for therapeutic purposes. Used in conjunction with cannabis, a synergy of beneficial effects may result.

> β-caryophyllene contained in specific exotic spices activate the endocannabinoid system via CB2, which makes these spices a potentially novel form of treatment available to everyone.

It is well known that ingesting cannabis enhances taste and smell and stimulates the appetite. It is less well known that your spice rack, a treasure chest of wondrous culinary delights, is also an inexpensive natural pharmacy. Research has shown that β-caryophyllene protects against microbes, inflammation, oxidative stress, pain and cancer.[9]

In addition to listing relevant CB2 activating β-caryophyllene containing spice plants this section focuses on knowing how to select and use medicinal spices, whether you do so alone or in combination with an appropriate strain of cannabis for your unique healing journey.

While the spice, herbal, and nutritional information in this publication are primarily based on western herbal philosophies, you can choose how and how much to include them as building blocks in your overall therapeutic regimen.

The spices and plant products listed here are based mainly on the prior research I conducted on the medicinal benefits of spice, published in the book *Spicy Healing - A Global Guide to Growing and Using Spices for Food and Medicine*. Many more spices with therapeutic potential are available than are discussed in this text.

It's important to realize that while scientific studies are available to highlight certain therapeutic potentials, and while the time-proven use of spice for health and healing speaks of its general efficacy and safety, their use should not be construed as a silver bullet that will cure all ailments. Spices can, however, be helpful for bringing an awareness or mindfulness to how we prepare and enjoy food, and encourage us to make food choices based on their impact to our health.

Those using Ayurvedic prescriptions based on the three Doshas (body-types) or working with Five Element considerations can further fine-tune the potential effectiveness of food and recipe choices with the information provided here. Suggested spices can easily be added or subtracted from most meals. If you have an interest in growing your own spices, you will find resources and guidance in *Spicy Healing* for that as well. Growing instructions are also available for free on the website www.spicyhealing.com

The "TAKE NOTICE" section may also report on other natural therapeutic possibilities related to the particular illness in question.

So, in summary, each disease or symptom listed in this index includes a section that is organized to direct your attention to the following sequence of possibly helpful considerations:

THE CANNABIS HEALTH INDEX (CHI)
EXPLORING MIND–BODY CONSCIOUSNESS
POWERFUL QUESTIONS
AGGRAVATING FACTORS
HEALING FACTORS
SUGGESTED BLESSING
SUGGESTED AFFIRMATION
ANECDOTE
STRAIN AND FORM SPECIFIC CONSIDERATIONS
TAKE NOTICE:

Hopefully, this book will be a useful tool for you, or perhaps for your friends, clients and/or loved ones on the journey toward greater health and deeper awareness of the power of mind-body healing. We can exercise the power to create and to promote our health in the midst of these explorations. In doing so, we can dissolve issues, release whatever needs releasing, gain new perspectives, try new beliefs and the new set of feelings they induce, make healthier choices, and walk our own unique path to better health and healing. Some manage to do it instantly as in spontaneous remission, while others embark on a more gradual, slower pace.

Where we go from here is up to us.

1 Psychology literally refers to the study of soul and spirit, but in its modern use is the study of mind and behavior.

2 Psychohistory is the study of historical motivation.

3 Psychoncology is the study of the relationship between cancer and psychology.

4 Psychoendocrinology is the study of the relationship between cancer and hormones.

5 Epigenetics is a new and still evolving term used to describe environmental signals that initiate change in genetic expressions without changing the DNA sequence.

6 Psychoneuroimmunology is the study of the relationship between psychology and immunity.

7 Phytopharmacology is the study of plant constituents and their impact on the human physiology.

8 Kitty C.M. Verhoeckxa, c, , , Henrie A.A.J. Korthoutb, A.P. van Meeteren-Kreikampa, Karl A. Ehlerta, Mei Wangb, Jan van der Greefa, c, Richard J.T. Rodenburgd, Renger F. Witkampa *Unheated Cannabis sativa extracts and its major compound THC-acid have potential immuno-modulating properties not mediated by CB1 and CB2 receptor coupled pathways.* a TNO Pharma, Utrechtseweg 48, P.O. Box 360, 3700AJ Zeist, The Netherlands b TNO Quality of Life, Zernikedreef 9, P.O Box 2215, 2333 CK Leiden, The Netherlands c Leiden University, Leiden/Amsterdam Center for Drug Research, P.O. Box 9502, 2300 RA Leiden, The Netherlands d Radboud University Nijmegen Medical Center, P.O. Box 9101, 6500 HB Nijmegen, The Netherlands. International Immunopharmacology Volume 6, Issue 4, April 2006, Pages 656–665.

9 Legault J. Pichette A. *Potentiating effect of beta-caryophellene on anticancer activity of alpha-humulene isocaryophellene and palitaxel.* J Pharm Pharmacol 2007 Dec;59(12):1643-7.

DISCLAIMER

Any use of the information contained in this book is at the reader's discretion. The ideas, concepts and suggestions contained in this publication are not intended as a substitute for consulting with your physician. The reader is strongly advised to work closely with the legally authorized health care professional of his or her choice when considering any information contained herein. While every effort has been made to make sure that the information contained in this book is complete and accurate, the author, editors, or publishers do not guarantee the accuracy of the information contained in this book. The author, editors, and publishers specifically disclaim any and all liability arising directly or indirectly from the use and/or application of any information (visual or written) presented in this book, or excerpts from it in any other form or publications.

The Cannabis Health Index

Aging

NUMBER OF STUDIES: 1

CHI VALUE: 2

Scientists do not yet have a thorough understanding of the physiological mechanism of aging. Various theories have been proposed to explain the loss of cellular integrity that we recognize as aging (wrinkles, age-spots or decline in physical and mental function). Such theories largely focus on the cumulative effects of exposure to radiation, toxins or pathogens contributing to mutation in cellular DNA over time.

Specifically, the following are believed to be causal agents in the process of aging: accumulation of toxins, the long-term effect of ionizing radiation, changes in hormone profiles, damage from exposure to free radicals (oxidative stressors), exposure to parasites, fungi, bacteria, viruses or other pathogens; shortening of the end strings of DNA (called telomeres) which occurs with each cell division, and the accumulation of senescent (older) cells.

ANTI-AGING

Animal studies have shown that longevity is achievable through external means such as modest caloric restriction. These decade-old findings were confirmed by a recent study in which scientists proposed a potential mechanism underlying the inverse relationship between calories and longevity. Researchers observed that a reduction of cellular sugar (glucose) caused an increase in free radicals. While we ordinarily think of free radicals as damaging, in this case cells responded rapidly to the reduction of glucose by producing an enzyme (catalase). This enzyme breaks down the radical before it causes any damage. The researchers theorized that it is this enhanced mechanism in response to the presence of free radicals that explains the longer life-span of test animals fed less food (but not so much less as to be malnourished).[1] It would appear that repetitive, low stress exposure to free radicals might have anti-aging effects. If this theory is correct, the use of high doses of antioxidants to "fight" aging may be counterproductive.

Other life extension research has focused on the potential of specific nutritional supplements. Alpha lipoic acid, in conjunction with acetyl-L-carnitine, has demonstrated protective abilities from perceived effects of aging in animal studies.[2] Telomerase, an enzyme thought to prevent the shortening of telomeres (the end string of DNA), seems to hold some promise as an anti-aging supplement. Similarly, a recent Mayo Clinic study found that typical signs of aging were not observed in mice whose senescent cells were eliminated.[3] (Senescent cells tend to aggregate in aging tissue and cause chronic low-grade inflammation.) However, it is important to note that these results have not been confirmed with human subjects.

CANNABIS AND AGING

Scientists from Columbus University in Ohio discovered that the synthetic cannabinoid WIN-55,212-2 (WIN-2) can enhance cognition and have an anti-inflammatory effect in older rats.[4] This effect found in animals has not yet been confirmed in humans.

STUDY SUMMARY:

Drugs	Type of Study	Key Results	CHI
WIN 55,212-2	Animal study	Potential anti- inflammatory and cognitive-enhancing effect in aged rats.[4]	2

Total CHI Value 2

STRAIN AND FORM SPECIFIC CONSIDERATIONS

The synthetic cannabinoid WIN 55212-2 binds more securely ("with higher affinity") to CB2 receptors than CB1 receptors,[5] which suggests that the CB2 receptor may be more important for the desirable anti-inflammatory and cognitive-enhancing effects seen in older rats in the Columbus study.

Similarly, non-psychoactive cannabidiol (CBD) has a greater affinity for CB2 receptors. Indicas and indica-dominant hybrids generally present with a lower THC:CBD ratio when compared to sativa-based strains, thus favoring CB2 signaling.

Raw, fresh cannabis leaf or juice contains CBD and THC in the form of THC-acid and CBD-acid, which can be consumed in larger quantities, since THC in that state is considered non-psychoactive.

EXPLORING MIND–BODY CONSCIOUSNESS

SUGGESTED BLESSING:

May I learn the wonders of the world.

May I love in ways I have never loved before.

The secrets of longevity will be difficult to discover for those of us who look at aging as failure. Those who believe that old-age is ugly will miss the opportunity to discover new depths of beauty that cannot be found in the polished exterior of the 'body perfect' but in ever-deeper dimensions of consciousness. If we think aging is the enemy, we will miss out on befriending life, and will forego the adventure that comes with lasting friendships.

While its significance varies between cultures, aging is regarded by most modern societies as something to be feared and avoided. Corporations exploit and reinforce societal ideals of beauty and youth in order to increase demand for their products, elevating the mythical 'body perfect' in the process. If accepted blindly, these unrealistic archetypes supplant the rich flavors and fabrics of a deeper and richer experience that could otherwise be there and one that only age, the very thing we are taught to fear, can bestow.

The field of medical psychosomatics is concerned with the impact of social, psychological, and behavioral factors on bodily processes and quality of life. Psychosomatic research has expanded knowledge of the specific physiological components of aging. "Positive affect seems to protect individuals against physical declines in old age."[6] "Longevity was associated with being conscientious, emotionally stable, and active."[7] "Positive emotional content reported in early-life autobiographies were strongly associated with longevity six decades later."[8]

Combining the perspectives of different medical disciplines makes it possible to understand various elements of aging better and even shift our attitude toward aging. This new perspective focuses on deeper and broader experiences of life itself. Insights from medical, nutritional, and food sciences can be integrated with knowledge of how our belief systems, thoughts, feelings, choices, decisions, and attitudes impact our health and quality of life.

Now instead of looking at aging as failure, we can see that with each experience, -- each day, each year that passes -- we have an opportunity to learn more, to love more, and explore more of the interactive dance that is our awareness of the world.

We can now see the beauty of experience that only age can bestow. Instead of functioning merely as a body, we can become more aware of previously unexplored dimensions of consciousness.

The more we release repressed or suppressed emotions, the better we understand our tendencies to focus on the negative or previous experience of feeling lousy. By understanding how frequent fear or any other chronically constricting emotions hinder our healing process we may more easily identify how our frame of mind, consciously or otherwise, interferes with our health. The more we challenge faulty beliefs that support disease at the core of each illness, the better able we are to reverse the damage. The more access we gain to our subconscious mind, and the more we explore the sliver of the unconscious at the edge of mindfulness, the more multidimensional we can become.

Change may come slowly and incrementally, almost invisibly, but every action to bring more consciousness to the healing process enhances our essential capacity for wisdom. Wisdom comes from the cumulative experience of conscious living, not simply the passage of time.

QUESTIONS

Think of 8 to 10 words or phrases that mean "getting older"?
Are you eagerly looking forward to your own "old age"? Why or why not?
What does it mean to be old?
What negative beliefs do you have about aging?
Can you replace these negative beliefs with more positive beliefs?
What does it mean to be an elder?
How do I want to return to the source of all life: as an infant or as a wise person?

AGGRAVATING FACTORS

Negative judgments about aging and old people, hating signs of aging (wrinkles, age-spots), lack of care, emotional instability, and inactivity. Aging clichés have become clichés by repetition. Each alone, but especially together, reveals much of society's negative programming and individual negative self-talk related to aging. "You cannot teach an old dog new tricks" implies we cannot learn when we are older. "Dirty old man" insinuates that it is unnatural for an older man to be sexually active. An "old wives tale" dismisses the wisdom of older women. "If the devil can't come him-

---

SUGGESTED AFFIRMATION:

I allow my wonder, my love and my wisdom to show my true age.

My age has been changing since the day I was born; every day I get better at embracing continual change.

Aging takes a lot of courage, so the task can only be given to those with a lot of life experience.

self, he will send an old woman" suggests that an older woman cannot be trusted.

HEALING FACTORS

Wonder about the experiences beneath the signs of age, curiosity about the potential value/wisdom behind the signs of aging, conscientiousness, emotional stability, staying active. Positive aging beliefs: "It is never too late to learn." "Wisdom bestows age." "It's never too late to have a happy childhood." "Death is the ultimate healer of any physical ailment."

TAKE NOTICE

AGE-SPOTS • (E)-β-CARYOPHYLLENE

AGE-SPOTS

Cannabis-using patients have reported that a daily drop of cannabis-infused hemp or coconut-oil applied to moles and age spots have resulted in the reappearance of normal tissue in time periods ranging between three weeks and three months. Here is an example from one of my own moles.

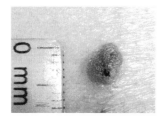 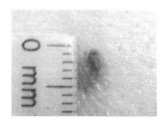 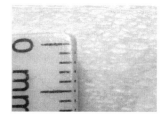

(E)-β-CARYOPHYLLENE

(E)-β-Caryophyllene or (E)-BCP is a FDA-approved dietary plant-cannabinoid that activates CB2 receptor sites and initiates potent anti-inflammatory actions and protection form oxidative stress,[9,10] both potential underlying factors in aging. Spice plants known to contain significant amounts of (E)-BCP in descending order include: BLACK "ASHANTI PEPPER" (PIPER GUINEENSE), WHITE "ASHANTI PEPPER" (PIPER GUINEENSE), INDIAN BAY-LEAF (CINNAMOMUM TAMALA), ALLIGATOR PEPPER (AFRAMOMUM MELEGUETA), BASIL (OCIMUM MICRANTHUM), SRI LANKA CINNAMON (CINNAMOMUM ZEYLANICUM), ROSEMARY (ROSMARINUS OFFICINALIS), BLACK CARAWAY (CARUM NIGRUM), BLACK PEPPER (PIPER NIGRUM), BASIL (OCIMUM GRATISSIMUM), MEXICAN OREGANO (LIPPIA GRAVEOLENS), AND CLOVE (SYZYGIUM AROMATICUM).

1 Schulz TJ, Zarse K, Voigt A, Urban N, Birringer M, Ristow M. *Glucose restriction extends Caenorhabditis elegans life span by inducing mitochondrial respiration and increasing oxidative stress.* Department of Human Nutrition, Institute of Nutrition, University of Jena, D-07743 Jena, Germany. Cell Metab. 2007 Oct;6(4):280-93.

2 Aliev G, Liu J, Shenk JC, Fischbach K, Pacheco GJ, Chen SG, Obrenovich ME, Ward WF, Richardson AG,

Smith MA, Gasimov E, Perry G, Ames BN. *Neuronal mitochondrial amelioration by feeding acetyl-L-carnitine and lipoic acid to aged rats.* Department of Biology, University of Texas at San Antonio, 78249, USA. J Cell Mol Med. 2009 Feb;13(2):320-33.

3 Darren J. Baker, Tobias Wijshake, Tamar Tchkonia, Nathan K. LeBrasseur, Bennett G. Childs, Bart van de Sluis, James L. Kirkland & Jan M. van Deursen. *Clearance of p16Ink4a-positive senescent cells delays ageing-associated disorders.* Nature 2011. Published online 02 November 2011.

4 Marchalant Y, Brothers HM, Norman GJ, Karelina K, DeVries AC, Wenk GL. *Cannabinoids attenuate the effects of aging upon neuroinflammation and neurogenesis.* Department of Psychology, The Ohio State University, Columbus, 43210, USA. Neurobiol Dis. 2009 May;34(2):300-7.

5 Felder CC, Joyce KE, Briley EM, Mansouri J, Mackie K, Blond O, Lai Y, Ma AL, Mitchell RL. *Comparison of the pharmacology and signal transduction of the human cannabinoid CB1 and CB2 receptors.* Laboratory of Cell Biology, National Institute of Mental Health, Bethesda, Maryland 20892, USA. Mol Pharmacol. 1995 Sep;48(3):443-50.

6 Ostir GV, Markides KS, Black SA, Goodwin JS. *Emotional well-being predicts subsequent functional independence and survival.* Department of Preventive Medicine and Community Health, University of Texas Medical Branch, Galveston 77555-0460, USA. J Am Geriatr Soc. 2000 May;48(5):473-8.

7 Antonio Terracciano, PhD, Corinna E. Löckenhoff, PhD, Alan B. Zonderman, PhD, Luigi Ferrucci, MD, PhD and Paul T. Costa, Jr, PhD. *Personality Predictors of Longevity: Activity, Emotional Stability, and Conscientiousness.* National Institute on Aging, National Institutes of Health, Department of Health and Human Services, Baltimore, Maryland. Psychosomatic Medicine 70:621-627 (2008).

8 Danner DD, Snowdon DA, Friesen WV. *Positive emotions in early life and longevity: findings from the nun study.* Department of Preventive Medicine and Sanders-Brown Center on Aging College of Medicine, University of Kentucky, Lexington 40536-0230, USA. Pers Soc Psychol. 2001 May;80(5):804-13.

9 Béla Horvátha, Partha Mukhopadhyaya, Malek Kechrida, Vivek Patela, Gali Tanchiana, David A. Winkb, Jürg Gertschc, Pál Pachera. *β-Caryophyllene ameliorates cisplatin-induced nephrotoxicity in a cannabinoid 2 receptor-dependent manner.* a Laboratory of Physiologic Studies, National Institute on Alcohol Abuse and Alcoholism, National Institutes of Health, Bethesda, MD 20892, USA. b Radiation Biology Branch, National Cancer Institute, National Institutes of Health, Bethesda, MD 20892, USA. c Institute of Biochemistry and Molecular Medicine, University of Bern, 3012 Bern, Switzerland. Free Radical Biology and Medicine. Volume 52, Issue 8, 15 April 2012, Pages 1325–133.

10 Gertsch J, Leonti M, Raduner S, Racz I, Chen JZ, Xie XQ, Altmann KH, Karsak M, Zimmer A. *Beta-caryophyllene is a dietary cannabinoid.* Institute of Pharmaceutical Sciences, Department of Chemistry and Applied Biosciences, Eidgenössische Technische Hochschule (ETH) Zurich, 8092 Zürich, Switzerland. Proc Natl Acad Sci U S A. 2008 Jul 1;105(26):9099-104.

Anorexia & Cachexia

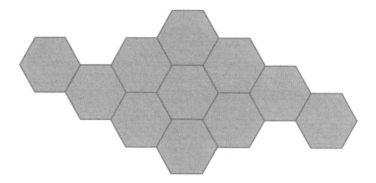

NUMBER OF STUDIES 11

COMBINED CHI VALUE: 28

Anorexia is a lack or loss of appetite leading to weight-loss of fat and muscle tissues. Anorexia nervosa (AN) is a lack of interest in, or a refusal to eat sufficient food and nutrients to maintain a healthy body weight due to psychological reasons. AN is distinct from bulimia nervosa which is defined as binge eating followed by purging or laxative abuse. Cachexia, also called wasting syndrome, refers to a loss of body mass that cannot be replaced through nutrition. It presents as generalized weakness, overall poor health, malnutrition and emaciation. Cachexia is usually a secondary condition in chronic destructive diseases such as end-stage cancer, AIDS, terminal tuberculosis, Multiple Sclerosis, or chronic obstructive pulmonary diseases such as emphysema.

Patients with progressive or late-stage cancer who experience weight loss due to limited appetite, nausea and increased weakness are suffering from Cancer-Related Anorexia-Cachexia. AIDS-Related Anorexia is defined as a lack or loss of appetite leading to weight-loss of fat and muscle tissues due to appetite depressing disease progressions.

CANNABIS AND ANOREXIA

Cannabis has been mentioned as an effective plant remedy to stimulate appetite and weight gain in almost every culture and medical tradition. Building on this traditional knowledge, many scientific studies have evaluated the evidence base for various uses of cannabis in allopathic medicine. It has been discovered that cannabinoids play a part in modulating the desire to eat. Most studies have focused on cannabis and anorexia in the context of cancer, AIDS, and Alzheimer's Disease. In general, study results indicate that cannabinoids are effective in reducing anorexia in AIDS and Alzheimer's patients.

Results for cancer patients with anorexia were more mixed. Cancer anorexia studies reported that cannabis is relatively safe, but usage under the individual study protocols produced some positive and some neutral reports of efficacy. For example, in a 2006 Swiss study, 164 cancer patients were divided into three groups and given a 6-week course of cannabis extract, oral THC, or a placebo to evaluate differences in Cancer-Related Anorexia-Cachexia Syndrome. The results of this randomized, double-blind, placebo-controlled clinical trial showed no difference in appetite or quality of life between cannabis, THC, and placebo. No reports of toxicity were noted.[1]

An animal-based experiment conducted in Madrid and published in 2002 provided scientists with the initial evidence that peripheral endocannabinoid (CB1) receptors play a complex role in the regulation of eating.[2] In a 2007 study conducted in St. Louis, Missouri, 29 senior long-term care patients suffering from weight loss were treated with oral doses of dronabinol. Over a period of twelve weeks study participants gained an average of almost 8 pounds.[3]

Based on earlier studies that established that endocannabinoid CB1 receptors as related to eating behavior, scientists in New York examined the possibility of reducing appetite by influencing CB1 receptors. Results showed that reducing CB1 expression does in fact produce a reduction of appetite. Thus CB1 blockers may warrant further exploration as a possible novel weight-loss product.[4]

CANNABIS AND CACHEXIA

One hundred and seventeen people living with HIV/AIDS and suffering from loss of appetite and weight loss were enrolled in a 3-to-12 month trial based in Orlando, Florida. During this trial, people were given regular oral doses of dronabinol. Researchers reported that the majority of study participants' appetites quickly improved and weight loss was reduced.[5]

A researcher from the University of Liverpool in England summarized the scientific basis for treating cachexia with cannabinoids this way: "…considerable research has examined endocannabinoid involvement in appetite, eating behavior and body weight regulation. It is now confirmed that endocannabinoids, acting at brain CB1 cannabinoid receptors, stimulate appetite and ingestive behaviours. [….] Moreover, there is strong evidence of an endocannabinoid role in energy metabolism and fuel storage."[6]

CANNABIS AND AIDS-RELATED ANOREXIA-CACHEXIA

Inspired by scientific evidence that oral cannabinoid-containing medications reduce chemotherapy-induced nausea as well as AIDS wasting syndrome, researchers hypothesized that cannabinoids might also mitigate the severe side effects of antiviral therapy used to treat Hepatitis C. In a study conducted in Ottawa, Canada in 2009, researchers found 64% of patients undergoing interferon-ribavirin therapy experienced improvements in their symptoms when also administered cannabinoids.[7]

A Tulsa, Oklahoma study followed 139 patients with AIDS, half of whom received dronabinol as treatment. Patients rated their appetite, mood, and nausea 3 times a week. The group receiving dronabinol reported increases in appetite (38% vs. 8% for placebo), improvement in mood (10% vs. -2% for placebo), and decreased nausea (20% vs. 7% for placebo). Body weight was stable in those patients receiving dronabinol, while recipients receiving a placebo had a mean loss of 8.8 pounds (or 0.4 kg). The authors of the study concluded: "dronabinol was found to be safe and effective for anorexia associated with weight loss in patients with AIDS." Further, these excellent results were achieved without significant adverse effects. Researchers Beal et al reported "side effects were mostly mild to moderate in severity (euphoria, dizziness, thinking abnormalities)."[8]

CANNABIS AND CANCER-RELATED ANOREXIA-CACHEXIA

Cancer anorexia studies generally report that cannabinoids are relatively safe and use produces both positive and neutral effects.

Scientists in Toronto, Canada collected data from 82 cancer patients who received nabilone for 53 days for cancer-related pain and other symptoms. Their study results, published in 2006, indicated a potential therapeutic benefit in cancer related anorexia with improvement seen in pain levels, nausea, depression, anxiety, insomnia, and night sweats.[9]

A study in Cleveland, Ohio evaluated the impact of tetrahydrocannabinol (THC) on cancer patients with anorexia. The patients were given 2.5 mg of THC orally, three times per day, one hour after a meal for 4 weeks. Of the 18 patients who completed the course, 13 reported an increase in appetite. The study authors concluded: "THC is an effective appetite stimulant in patients with advanced cancer. It is well tolerated at low doses."[10]

A study of dronabinol used to treat patients with symptomatic HIV infections and/or cancer was conducted in Somerville, New Jersey. Researchers found that "…dronabinol caused weight gain in seven of ten patients with symptomatic HIV infection. In both HIV and cancer patients, dronabinol improved appetite at a dose which was well tolerated for chronic administration."[11]

STUDY SUMMARY:

Drugs	Type of Study	Published Year, Place, and Key Results	CHI
Oral cannabinoid-containing medications	Human trial conducted on patients with hepatitis C	2008 – Ottawa, Canada: May stabilize weight loss during interferon-ribavirin therapy in chronic hepatitis C patients[33]	3
Dronabinol	Human Trial on 29 senior long-term care patients suffering from weight loss	2007 – Saint Louis, MO : Average weight gain of 8 lbs. in long term care patients[27]	3
Dronabinol (isomer of THC)	117 people living with HIV/AIDS	2007 – Orlando, Florida: Improved appetite, weight gain and reduction of nausea[31]	3
Cannabis extract containing 2.5 mg THC and 1mg CBD, or THC 2.5mg or placebo twice daily for 6 weeks	164 cancer patients	2006 – St. Gallen, Switzerland: No difference in appetite, quality of life between cannabis, THC and placebo. No reports of toxicity[28]	0
Nabilone	82 cancer patients	2006 – Toronto, Canada: Reduction in pain, nausea, depression, anxiety, insomnia and night sweats. Drowsiness, tiredness, appetite, and well-being remained the same but decreased in control group[35]	3
Studied the effects of reducing CB1 expression	Animal study (mice)	2005 – Columbia, New York: Endocannabinoids (CB1) receptors are involved in appetite[29]	2

Drugs	Type of Study	Published Year, Place, and Key Results	CHI
Endocannabinoid acting at brain CB1 cannabinoid receptors studied	Analysis	2005 – Liverpool, United Kingdom: CB1 endocannabinoids receptors stimulate appetite and ingestive behaviours. Moreover, there is strong evidence of an endocannabinoid role in energy metabolism and fuel storage[32]	1
Anandamide and other cannabinoid agonists	Animal study (rats)	2002 – Madrid, Spain: Endocannabinoid (CB1) system modulates feeding[30]	2
2.5 mg of dronabinol twice daily, or placebo	139 people living with AIDS	1995 – Tulsa, Oklahoma: Increased appetite, mood and weight gains with reduction of nausea[34]	5
THC 2.5 mg three times daily	18 cancer patients	1994 – Cleveland, Ohio: 13 patients reported an improvement in appetite[36]	3
Dronabinol	HIV and cancer patients	1991 – Somerville, N.J.: Dronabinol improved appetite in both cancer and HIV patients[37]	3

Total CHI Value   28

STRAIN SPECIFIC CONSIDERATIONS

Cannabis constituents are well-known for their ability to induce appetite, reduce nausea, vomiting, and for gently lifting energy of body and mind, thereby addressing both physiological and psychological system needs. Cannabinoids, acting at brain CB1 cannabinoid receptors (especially anandamide and THC), stimulate appetite and ingestive behaviors. Most anorexia/cachexia research has been done on patients with Alzheimer's disease, AIDS and cancer. Study results have shown that the cannabinoid THC increases appetite, reduces nausea, and increases weight gain. Cannabis-using anorexia and/or cachexia patients often prefer sativa strains of cannabis with higher concentrations of tetrahydrocannabinol (THC) relative to cannabidiol (CBD) and cannabinol (CBN). Or, patients may seek isolated synthetic THC medication also available by prescription.

However, patients' individual needs and preferences vary.

> *Patrick, a 48 year-old cancer patient, had suffered from cachexia for over a year, following a course in chemotherapy. His case was centered in the mental or emotional arena, causing him stress and resulting physiological symptoms. He discovered that an indica strain, which he found generally more sedating, relaxing and grounding than other strains though it still contained all the key cannabinoids, was an effective choice for him to increase his appetite.*

EXPLORING MIND–BODY CONSCIOUSNESS

Researchers in North Carolina enrolled 753 female patients diagnosed with anorexia nervosa (AN) to discover possible underlying causes. Results showed that exposure to abuse resulting in post-traumatic stress disorder (PTSD) was a significant co-factor (13.7%) in developing AN. 103 women who met the DSM-IV criteria for PTSD had suffered mostly sexual abuse during childhood or as an adult.[12]

To examine possible personality traits or temperaments of people suffering from AN, Australian scientists examined a prior study that followed 1,002 same-sex female twins in which one twin had AN but the other did not. Results showed that those with AN are prone to an elevated need for order, reward dependence, an elevated concern over mistakes, very high personal standards, and constant doubt about their actions (perfectionism).[13]

Researchers from Munich, Germany and San Diego, California discovered that AN patients, perhaps similarly to autistics, are not able to normally recognize and respond to different facial emotional expressions. The authors write: "Differences in brain dynamics might contribute to difficulties in the correct recognition of facially-expressed emotions, deficits in social functioning, and in turn the maintenance of eating disorders."[14]

A person suffering from AN without an underlying physical pathology may deny any suggestion that s/he is underweight because of an overwhelming false perception of the self as overweight. Here, belief has significant health consequences. Extreme self-loathing may also result in the rejection of any nurturing influences. Intense guilt, with its demand for punishment, has a similar effect.

Lack of appetite, as well as nausea/vomiting after eating even small amounts, may be related to fear or dread of an emotion or experience.

QUESTIONS

Can I find a way to embrace my emotional experience (not my disease)?

If I were to let myself sink into the heart of fear, what would I find there?

How can I make any feeling a safe experience for me?

If weakness is the result of constant self-judgment, what is the source of my strength?

Can I accept and forgive myself for getting in the habit of self-judgment and negative self-talk?

Do I fully understand that human perfection is, by definition, unachievable?

Can I accept and forgive myself for the mistakes I've made?

How might I discover any false beliefs, conscious or unconscious, that influence my unhealthy behavior?

See also chapters on AIDS and CANCER.

AGGRAVATING FACTORS

Traumatic events, abuse, sexual abuse, PTSD, perfectionism, shame, self-loathing, guilt, difficulty recognizing and responding to different facial expressions can aggravate any of the diseases and conditions described in this chapter.

HEALING FACTORS

Factors that can aid and speed your recovery include healing prior traumatic events and abuse, allowing shame to be lifted by something larger than ourselves, meditating on how to return shame to the source from whence it came without harming anyone, and nurturing yourself with self-acceptance, forgiveness, and gratitude.

TAKE NOTICE

Cannabis-infused oils or tinctures can easily be added to your favorite recipes to suit your specific dietary requirements. As needed, please also review these chapters: CANCER, AIDS, LUNG DISEASES, AND MENTAL DISORDERS.

ANISE • BASIL • CARDAMON • CINNAMON • FENNEL • GARLIC • GINGER • ROSEMARY • TURMERIC

ANISE: Scientists have tested Brazilian curandeiros' age-old herbal medicinal practices of using anise to cure digestive difficulties resulting from gas or overeating, cramps and nervous stomach. A University of São Paulo study confirmed the use of anise as an antispasmodic agent.[15]

BASIL: An infusion of basil tea relieves symptoms of abdominal discomfort due to gas. As a diuretic, it treats high blood pressure.[16]

CARDAMON: Cardamon is a drug approved by the German Commission E in the treatment of dyspeptic complaints (digestive difficulty).[17] These findings echo the time-proven Unani and Ayurvedic application of cardamon as a treatment in certain gastrointestinal diseases.

CINNAMON: In Cuba, a cinnamon infusion is prescribed to stimulate appetite and the immune system in patients with tendencies toward bacterial and fungal infections.[18] The German Commission E, a government program to evaluate the safety and efficacy of herbal medicine, approved cinnamon for the treatment of: "loss of appetite, dyspeptic complaints such as mild spasms of the gastrointestinal tract, bloating, flatulence."[19]

FENNEL: Veterinary scientists from Afyon, Turkey confirmed some of fennel's time-proven applications such as its beneficial use as a treatment for certain digestive problems.[20] Another study from Turkey concluded that the essential oil of fennel protected rats from chemically induced liver damage,[21] lending further credibility to fennel's reputation as a useful agent for gastro-intestinal disorders.

GARLIC: Garlic is one of Cuba's most versatile herbs and may help in cases of anorexia or cachexia by acting as an overall tonic, and by preventing and treating infections caused by bacteria, fungi, viruses and parasites.[22]

GINGER: Ginger supports natural appetite by functioning as an anti-emetic (morning sickness, sea sickness, post-surgery sickness), analgesic, anti-inflammatory, anti-oxidant, anti-bacterial (Helicobacter pylori), stomach ulcer preventative, and hepatoprotective agent (protects the liver).[23]

ROSEMARY: An infusion of rosemary leaves is used in Cuba to treat liver and gall bladder complaints, and is also used to reduce spasms due to gas and flatulence.[24] The German Commission E has approved rosemary for "internal dyspeptic complaints."

TURMERIC: Almost considered a wonder drug with a broad therapeutic potential. To date, numerous studies have been conducted on the plant's constituents and gut health.[25] The German Commission E has approved turmeric in the treatment of digestive difficulties with a dose range of 1.5 – 3gm daily.[26]

1 Strasser F, Luftner D, Possinger K, Ernst G, Ruhstaller T, Meissner W, Ko YD, Schnelle M, Reif M, Cerny T. *Comparison of orally administered cannabis extract and delta-9 tetrahydrocannabinol in treating patients with cancer-related ANOREXIA-cachexia syndrome: a multicenter, phase III, randomized, double-blind, placebo-controlled clinical trial from the Cannabis-in-Cachexia-Study-Group.* ABHPM, Oncology and Palliative Medicine, Section of Oncology/Hematology, Department Internal Medicine, Cantonal Hospital, Rorschacherstrasse, 9007 St Gallen, Switzerland; e-mail: florian.strasser@kssg.ch. J Clin Oncol 2006;24(21):3394-400.

2 Gómez R, Navarro M, Ferrer B, Trigo JM, Bilbao A, Del Arco I, Cippitelli A, Nava F, Piomelli D, Rodríguez de Fonseca F. *A peripheral mechanism for CB1 cannabinoid receptor-dependent modulation of feeding.* University Institute of Drug Dependencies, Department of Psychobiology, University Complutense of Madrid, Madrid 28223, Spain. J Neurosci. 2002 Nov1;22(21):9612-7.

3 Wilson MM, Philpot C, Morley JE. *Anorexia of aging in long term care: is dronabinol an effective appetite stimulant? - a pilot study.* M.M.G. Wilson, MRCP, Division of Geriatric Medicine, Saint Louis University, 1402, S. Grand Blvd, Rm M238, St Louis, MO 63104, Tel: (314) 977-8404, Fax: (314) 977-8409, Email: wilsonmg@slu.edu. J Nutr Health Aging. 2007 Mar-Apr;11(2):195-8.

4 Jo YH, Chen YJ, Chua SC Jr, Talmage DA, Role LW. *Integration of endocannabinoid and leptin signaling in an appetite-related neural circuit.* Department of Pathology and Cell Biology, Center for Neurobiology and Behavior, Columbia University, College of Physicians and Surgeons, New York, New York 10032, USA. yjo@aecom.yu.edu Neuron. 2005 Dec 22;48(6):1055-66.

5 Dejesus E, Rodwick BM, Bowers D, Cohen CJ, Pearce D. Use of Dronabinol Improves Appetite and Reverses Weight Loss in HIV/AIDS-Infected Patients. Orlando Immunology Center, Orlando, Florida, edejesus@oicorlando.com. J Int Assoc Physicians AIDS Care 2007;6(2):95-100.

6 Kirkham TC. Endocannabinoids in the regulation of appetite and body weight. School of Psychology, University of Liverpool, Liverpool, England. t.c.kirkham@liverpool.ac.uk Behav Pharmacol. 2005 Sep;16(5-6):297-313.

7 Costiniuk CT, Mills E, Cooper CL. *Evaluation of oral cannabinoid-containing medications for the management of interferon and ribavirin-induced anorexia, nausea and weight loss in patients treated for chronic hepatitis C virus.* Department of Internal Medicine, University of Ottawa, Ottawa, Canada. Can J Gastroenterol. 2008 Apr;22(4):376-80.

8 Beal JE, Olson R, Laubenstein L, Morales JO, Bellman P, Yangco B, Lefkowitz L, Plasse TF, Shepard KV. *Dronabinol as a treatment for anorexia associated with weight loss in patients with AIDS.* St. John's Hospital, Tulsa, Oklahoma, USA. Journal of Pain and Symptom Management 1995;10(2):89-97

9 *The synthetic cannabinoid nabilone improves pain and symptom management in cancer patients.* University of Toronto; William Osler Health Center, Toronto, Canada. Presented at the San Antonio Breast Cancer Symposium on 15 December 2006.

10 Nelson K, Walsh D, Deeter P, Sheehan F. *A phase II study of delta-9-tetrahydrocannabinol for appetite stimulation in cancer-associated anorexia.* Palliative Care Program, Cleveland Clinic Foundation Ohio. Journal of Palliative Care 1994;10(1):14-18.

11 Plasse TF, Gorter RW, Krasnow SH, Lane M, Shepard KV, Wadleigh RG. *Recent clinical experience with dronabinol.* UNIMED, Inc., Somerville, NJ 08876. Pharmacol Biochem Behav. 1991 Nov;40(3):695-700.

12 Mae Lynn Reyes-Rodríguez, PhD, Ann Von Holle, MS, Teresa Frances Ulman, PhD, Laura M Thornton, PhD, Kelly L. Klump, PhD, Harry Brandt, MD, Steve Crawford, MD, Manfred M. Fichter, MD, Katherine A. Halmi, MD, Thomas Huber, MD, Craig Johnson, PhD, Ian Jones, MD, Allan S. Kaplan, MD, FRCP(C), James E. Mitchell, MD, Michael Strober, PhD, Janet Treasure, MD, D. Blake Woodside, MD, Wade H. Berrettini, MD, Walter H. Kaye, MD and Cynthia M. Bulik, PhD. *Posttraumatic Stress Disorder in Anorexia Nervosa.* Department of Psychiatry (M.L.R.-R., A.V.H., T.F.U., L.M.T., C.M.B.), University of North Carolina, Chapel Hill, North Carolina; Department of Psychology (K.L.K.), Michigan State University, East Lansing, Michigan; Department of Psychiatry (H.B., S.C.), University of Maryland School of Medicine, Baltimore, Maryland; Klinik Roseneck, Hospital for Behavioral Medicine (M.M.F.), Prien; and University of Munich (LMU), Munich, Germany; New York Presbyterian Hospital-Westchester Division (K.A.H.), Weill Medical College of Cornell University, White Plains, New York; Klinik am Korso (T.H.), Bad Oeynhausen, Germany; Eating Recovery Center (C.J.), Denver, Colorado; Medical Research Council Center for Neuropsychiatric Genetics and Genomisc (I.J.), Chardiff, United Kingdom; Center of Addiction and Mental Health (A.S.K.), Toronto, Canada; Department of Psychiatry, (A.S.K., D.B.W.) University of Toronto; and Department of Psychiatry (D.B.W.), Toronto General Hospital, University Health Network, Toronto, Canada; Neuropsychiatric Research Institute and Department of Clinical Neuroscience (J.E.M.), University of North Dakota School of Medicine and Health Sciences, Fargo, North Dakota; Department of Psychiatry and Biobehavioral Sciences (M.S.), David Geffen School of Medicine, University of California at Los Angeles, Los Angeles, California; Department of Academic Psychiatry (J.T.), Kings College London, London, United Kingdom; Department of Psychiatry (W.H.B.), University of Pennsylvania, Philadelphia, Pennsylvania; Department of Psychiatry (W.H.K.), University of California at San Diego, San Diego, California; and Department of Nutrition (C.M.B.), University of North Carolina, Chapel Hill, North Carolina. Psychosomatic Medicine July 2011 vol. 73 no. 6 491-497

13 Tracey D. Wade, PhD, Marika Tiggemann, PhD, Cynthia M. Bulik, PhD, Christopher G. Fairburn, FMedSci, Naomi R. Wray, PhD and Nicholas G. Martin, PhD. *Shared Temperament Risk Factors for Anorexia Nervosa: A Twin Study.* School of Psychology (T.D.W., M.T.), Flinders University, South Australia, Australia; Department of Psychiatry and Nutrition (C.M.B.), University of North Carolina at Chapel Hill, Chapel Hill, North Carolina; Department of Psychiatry (C.G.F.), Oxford University, Warneford Hospital, Oxford, United Kingdom; and Department of Genetic Epidemiology (N.R.W., N.G.M.), Queensland Institute of Medical Research, Australia. Psychosomatic Medicine 70:239-244 (2008).

14 Olga Pollatos, MD, PhD, Beate M. Herbert, PhD, Rainer Schandry, PhD and Klaus Gramann, PhD. *Impaired Central Processing of Emotional Faces in Anorexia Nervosa.* Departments of Neurology (O.P.) and Psychology (O.P., R.S.), Ludwig-Maximilians-University of Munich, Germany; Department of Clinical and Cognitive Neuroscience (B.M.H.), University of Heidelberg, Central Institute of Mental Health; and Swartz Center for Computational Neuroscience (K.G.), Institute for Neural Computation, University of California, San Diego, California. Psychosomatic Medicine 70:701-708 (2008).

15 Tirapelli CR, de Andrade CR, Cassano AO, De Souza FA, Ambrosio SR, da Costa FB, de Oliveira AM. *Antispasmodic and relaxant effects of the hidroalcoholic extract of Pimpinella anisum (Apiaceae) on rat anococcygeus smooth muscle.* Departamento de Enfermagem Psiquiátrica e Ciências Humanas, Escola de Enfermagem de Ribeirão Preto, Ribeirão Preto, Universidade de São Paulo, Ribeirão Preto, Brazil. J Ethnopharmacol. 2007 Mar 1;110(1):23-9.

16 *Therapeutic Guide to Plant Pharmaceuticals and Honey Pharmaceuticals (Guia Terapeutica Dispensarial de Fitofarmacos y Apifarmacos)* - Ministerio de Salud Publica, Ciudad de La Habana - Republica de Cuba 1992). Cuban Ministry of Public Health, Havana.

17 *Monographien der E-Kommission (Phyto-Therapie) (380 monographs). A therapeutic guide to herbal medicine evaluating the safety and efficacy of herbs for licensed medical prescribing in Germany.* Published between 1984 and 1994 in the Bundesanzeiger (official publication by the Federal Republic of Germany).

18 *Therapeutic Guide to Plant Pharmaceuticals and Honey Pharmaceuticals (Guia Terapeutica Dispensarial de Fitofarmacos y Apifarmacos)* - Ministerio de Salud Publica, Ciudad de La Habana - Republica de Cuba 1992). Cuban Ministry of Public Health, Havana.

19 *Monographien der E-Kommission (Phyto-Therapie) (380 monographs). A therapeutic guide to herbal medicine evaluating the safety and efficacy of herbs for licensed medical prescribing in Germany.* Published between 1984 and 1994 in the Bundesanzeiger (official publication by the Federal Republic of Germany).

20 Birdane FM, Cemek M, Birdane YO, Gülçin I, Büyükokurolu ME. *Beneficial effects of Foeniculum vulgare on*

ethanol-induced acute gastric mucosal injury in rats. Department of Pharmacology, Faculty of Veterinary Medicine, Afyon Kocatepe University, Afyon, Turkey. World J Gastroenterol. 2007 Jan 28;13(4):607-11.

21 Ozbek H, Ura S, Dülger H, Bayram I, Tuncer I, Oztürk G, Oztürk A. *Hepatoprotective effect of Foeniculum vulgare essential oil.* Yüzüncü Yil University, Faculty of Medicine, Department of Pharmacology, Van 65300, Turkey. Fitoterapia. 2003 Apr;74(3):317-9.

22 *Therapeutic Guide to Plant Pharmaceuticals and Honey Pharmaceuticals (Guia Terapeutica Dispensarial de Fitofarmacos y Apifarmacos)* - Ministerio de Salud Publica, Ciudad de La Habana - Republica de Cuba 1992). Cuban Ministry of Public Health, Havana.

23 Uwe Blesching. *Spicy Healing: A Global Guide to Growing and Using spices for Food and Medicine.* Logos Publishing. Berkeley, California. 2nd Edition 2009.

24 *Therapeutic Guide to Plant Pharmaceuticals and Honey Pharmaceuticals (Guia Terapeutica Dispensarial de Fitofarmacos y Apifarmacos)* - Ministerio de Salud Publica, Ciudad de La Habana - Republica de Cuba 1992). Cuban Ministry of Public Health, Havana.

25 Goel A, Kunnumakkara AB, Aggarwal BB. *Curcumin as "Curecumin": From kitchen to clinic.* Gastrointestinal Cancer Research Laboratory, Department of Internal Medicine, Charles A. Sammons Cancer Center and Baylor Research Institute, Baylor University Medical Center, Dallas, TX, United States. Biochem Pharmacol. 2007 Aug 19.

26 *Monographien der E-Kommission (Phyto-Therapie) (380 monographs). A therapeutic guide to herbal medicine evaluating the safety and efficacy of herbs for licensed medical prescribing in Germany.* Published between 1984 and 1994 in the Bundesanzeiger (official publication by the Federal Republic of Germany).

Bacterial & Viral Infections

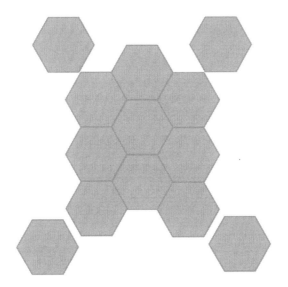

COMBINED NUMBER OF STUDIES: 13

COMBINED CHI VALUE: 29

Western medicine has determined that the diseases listed in the left column of the table below are caused by viruses. Antibiotics are useless in fighting a viral disease, but may work to eliminate bacterial infections such as those listed in the right column.

Viral Infections	Bacterial Infections
Chicken pox	Anthrax
Colds (parainfluenza virus)	Chlamydia
Conjunctivitis (pink eye)	Cholera
Croup (parainfluenza virus)	Conjunctivitis (can also be viral)
Dengue fever	Escherichia coli (aka E. Coli)
Ebola	Diphtheria
Epstein-barr (a herpes virus)	Dysentery
Encephalitis	Gonorrhea
Flu (influenza virus)	Helicobacter pylori (stomach ulcers)
Hepatitis A,B,C (inflammation of the liver)	Legionnaire's disease
Human papilloma virus (HPV)	Leptospirosis
Herpes simplex virus (HSV 1&2)	Leprosy
Kaposi's sarcoma (herpes virus 8)	Meningitis (bacterial)
Measles (Rubella virus)	Pneumonia
Meningitis (inflammation of the lining of the brain and spinal cord)	Rocky Mountain Spotted Fever
	Salmonella
Mumps virus	Staphylococcus
Myocarditis (inflammation of the heart muscle)	Streptococcus
Polio virus	Syphilis
Rabies virus	Tuberculosis
Reye syndrome (influenza virus)	Typhoid
Rubella virus	Urinary tract infections (UTI)
Shingles (herpes zoster virus)	Yersinia pestis (Bubonic and Pneumonic plague)
Smallpox virus	
Yellow fever virus	

Bacterial & Viral Infections

Gonorrhea

NO MODERN STUDIES AVAILABLE

Gonorrhea is caused by gonococcus or neisseria gonorrhea bacteria. It is usually sexually transmitted, though an infected mother can also transmit the disease to an infant during birth. Gonorrhea symptoms in infants are mostly limited to infections of the eyes. In adults, gonorrhea affects the mucus membranes of the genitals, reproductive organs, the anus or the throat. It is estimated that about 1 in 10 males and 5 in 10 females show no or very mild physical symptoms of the disease. Early symptoms of the disease usually occur within the first week after exposure but may present up to 30 days after infection.

Early symptoms in women are usually milder than in males, and include burning or painful sensation when urinating, unusual vaginal discharge (sometimes with an odor), and spotting or bleeding between menstrual cycles. If the disease remains undetected and untreated in females, gonorrhea may progress over time and manifest years later as pelvic inflammatory disease (PID), abscesses along the affected mucus membranes, damage to the reproductive organs and an increased risk for ectopic pregnancies and infertility.

Early symptoms in males include penile discharge (white, yellowish) and painful, burning urination. If allowed to progress, gonorrhea may move deeper into the tissue of the genitals and affect the male reproductive organs causing inflammation of the epididymis and testicles with associated pain and swelling of the groin and scrotum. Untreated gonorrhea can cause infertility in men as well as women.

Both sexes may experience rectal or throat infections of gonorrhea. While rectal infection may produce no symptoms, rectal discharge, anal itching, and pain during bowel movements may be present. Throat infections may also be asymptomatic, or they may cause sore throat, swollen tonsils and discharge at the site of the infected tissue.

Fever and chills, as well as joint aches, may be present from the onset of infection or only after the initial symptoms have passed. In the latter stages of the disease gonorrheal arthritis may develop causing pain in the wrist, knee, and ankle joints.

A urine test or a swab sample from the affected mucus membranes, examined under a microscope, can determine if gonorrhea is present. Both orthodox and holistic doctors recognize that if one sexually transmitted disease is present, others may be also, so testing for other sexually transmitted diseases is usually recommended. When gonorrhea is suspect-

---

How do Scientists determine the cause of a disease?

The answer, in part, is what scientists call Koch's Postulates. In the late 1800's, a virologist named Robert Koch created a set of criteria helpful for identifying a causal relationship between a microbe and a disease. His four primary criteria are not absolute truths, though they continue to inform scientific inquiry today. The criteria are:

1. The microorganism must be found in abundance in all organisms suffering from the disease, but should not be found in healthy organisms.

2. The microorganism must be isolated from a diseased organism and grown in pure culture.

3. The cultured microorganism should cause disease when introduced into a healthy organism.

4. The microorganism must be re-isolated from the inoculated, diseased experimental host and identified as being identical to the original specific causative agent.

ed, Chlamydia and HIV screens are also routinely conducted.

Orthodox medical treatment uses antibiotics exclusively to eliminate the bacteria. While penicillin was initially advertised as able to cure gonorrhea in 4 hours, today it and most other antibiotics are generally ineffective. The bacteria have become resistant and easily survive most antibiotic treatments. For that reason, treatment guidelines of the U.S. Center for Disease Control recommend cephalosporin antibiotics to treat all gonococcal infections.[1] Gonorrhea may soon become a 'superbug' infection, resistant to all known antibiotics. As a consequence, there is global interest in the search for new and effective remedies for gonorrhea.

CANNABIS AND GONORRHEA

Five major cannabinoids (THC, CBD, CBG, CBC, and CBN) have been discovered to be potent against bacteria, including multi-drug-resistant bacteria, most notably methicillin-resistant staphylococcus aureus (MRSA).[2] However, the precise mechanism of their antiseptic effect is still under study. While cannabinoids have been effective in treating MRSA in laboratory settings, no studies are available examining the potential antibacterial impact of cannabinoids on the gonorrhea bacterium.

However, Muslim and Indian Ayurvedic physicians have applied the diuretic, sedative, and anti-inflammatory properties of cannabis to treat cystitis and gonorrhea.[3] Prior to the discovery of penicillin, cannabidiolic acids were commonly prescribed for bacterial infections such as gonorrhea. An 1892 treatment guideline describes the use of cannabis to treat gonorrhea: "it lessens the discharge, inflammation, burning pains, and restlessness, and allays chordee (downward curvature of the penis)."[4] Cannabis was apparently applied as a tincture, extract, or tannate (a salt made from cannabidiolic acids). As late as 1935, a cannabis preparation was sold in the U.S. in the form of pills to be dissolved in clean water and injected into the urethra using a pipette.[5] A Japanese team of scientists recently discovered (2008) that CBD-acid selectively inhibits COX-2, an enzyme responsible for inflammation and pain in general.[6]

STRAIN AND FORM SPECIFIC CONSIDERATIONS

The major cannabinoids, THC, CBD, CBG, CBC, and CBN are present in both sativa and indica, the primary strains of cannabis. Non-psychoactive CBD-acid is present in relatively high concentrations in raw, fresh cannabis flower, leaf, and juice. CBD activates CB2 receptors in immune cells and may play a part in modulating immune responses. It is important to remember that to date no studies are available examining the potential antibacterial impact of cannabinoids on the gonorrhea bacterium.

EXPLORING MIND–BODY CONSCIOUSNESS

Sexually transmitted disease is not exclusively a physiological problem. The field of mind-body medicine examines mental and emotional factors that can make individuals vulnerable to disease, unable to recognize disease, unwilling to request treatment, or even predisposed to spreading disease. A lack of social responsibility

SUGGESTED BLESSING:

May you realize that your genitals are essentially good, healthy, natural, beautiful, and a necessity for all of life.

SUGGESTED AFFIRMATION:

I am an adult and I celebrate my sexuality freely and with harm to none.

may be associated with a lack of self-care or empathy for others. Unhealthy body image or post-traumatic stress disorder following sexual assault can lead people to disassociate during sex or ignore entire regions of their body.

While understanding how STDs are mechanically transmitted is important, it is also important to consider conscious and unconscious mental and emotional factors that impact the genesis, transmission, progression and outcome of disease. Individuals often do not know that they are infected with a STD, or even how or when they were exposed to it. But sometimes individuals know that they are infected and continue to have unprotected sex anyway, spreading the disease to others. A drug addict with an STD may trade sex for drugs, oblivious to the damage this causes to herself and others when her next "fix" is her only priority. An assault victim may refuse to get treatment for an STD, insisting that the pain in his genitals is less onerous than a doctor's physical exam and the admission that he was unable to defend himself. A distorted self-concept based on unresolved childhood shame may induce an adult to validate their (perceived) "worthlessness" by repeatedly taking excessive risks in the sexual arena.

Guilt, fear and shame figure prominently in the emotional context of STDs. Our sexuality and the meanings and value that we attach to it are very complex, and significantly influenced by religious, cultural, family and personal circumstances. It should come as no surprise then that conflicts between these perspectives and our own, or conflicting desires within us, can lead to "cognitive dissonance" or discomfort and stress. Stress gives rise to an internal environment in which the body becomes vulnerable to disease. Many pathogens involved in STDs are found in a dormant state within the body under normal circumstances, and are given an opportunity to activate when the body is under stress and therefore vulnerable.

"There is light and there is shadow on the mountain of Aphrodite from whence life came."[7] The light is the pleasure, the intimacy, the fun, the beauty, and the embrace of primal creative energy. In the shadow we find the guilt, the shame, the blame, and the controls and judgments bringing pain onto the self or others. It is estimated that more than half of all people will have a sexually transmitted disease (STD) at some point during their lifetime.[8] The remainder are able to stay healthy. Our beliefs about ourselves, beliefs about our bodies, beliefs about the validity of our choices and beliefs about our prospects for happiness all interact with the physical functioning of our bodies (and any diseases and discomforts we face). Our thoughts impact our emotions; our emotions impact our actions; our actions impact our health; our health impacts our thoughts, and so on. The pursuit of excellent health may be the same path that allows us to calm our fears and increase our access to and experience of love.

THE POWER OF QUESTIONS

Do you consider sex natural and "good", or something dirty and wrong?
Do you know what constitutes safer sex?
Have you thought through what level of risk is acceptable to you?
Do you engage in unsafe sex?
Do you use alcohol or other drugs to give you "permission" to be sexual?
Do you use alcohol or other drugs to give you "permission" to take risks you other-

wise would not?

What sexual situations scare you?

When you experience sexual difficulties, how do you react?

How do you deal with difficult emotions (for example, anger or shame) accompanied by arousal?

Do you struggle with "unacceptable" sexual desires or thoughts?

When have you felt guilty about your sexual conduct?

When have you felt ashamed by your own behavior?

When have you felt ashamed of your body's appearance or response to sexual attention?

Are there sexual acts you think should be punished? Who would be served by such punishment?

Do you harbor shame or guilt about having a STD?

Does fear of contracting STDs prevent you from experiencing a fully satisfying sex life?

Are you willing to explore your sexual desires?

Are you willing to explore the sexual desires of your partner(s)?

Can you find a way to own and release your fears, resentments, guilt and shame appropriately?

Do you find guilt a useful and welcome signal that your desires and values are in conflict? Or are you sickened and paralyzed by chronic guilt?

How can you set sexual boundaries to protect yourself and others?

How can you increase the love and intimacy in your life?

AGGRAVATING FACTORS

Sexual guilt with its demand for purification through punishment, sex without care, sex without love, sex without intimacy, taking emotional manipulations or payoffs that come with sexual guilt such as the lack of principles related to sex, entitlements around sex, righteous angers around sex, suppressed emotions around sex: fears, anxieties, angers, shame, self-pity.

HEALING FACTORS

Develop healthy principles around sex and abide by them on a consistent basis. Discover and replace all beliefs that initiate guilt, fear or shame around sex. Find a way to release guilt, fear, anger, and shame around sex without hurting yourself or others. Consider adding care and love to balance lust and desire.

TAKE NOTICE

COCONUT • (E)-β-CARYOPHYLLENE CONTAINING SPICES

COCONUT: In this laboratory study from Iceland researchers discovered that medium chain fatty acids, but especially capric acid ($C_{10}H_{20}O_2$), worked effectively in killing all strains of Neisseria gonorrhea.[9] Another laboratory study from the island determined how well medium chain fatty acids destroy or inhibit the growth of other groups of bacteria. Both lauric acid and capric acid showed strong antibacterial abilities.[10] Again, researchers demonstrated another aspect of lauric and capric acids' broad anti-microbial properties in the laboratory; this time against a fungus associated with yeast infections.[11] Lauric acid and capric acid were also found to effectively inactivate Chlamydia in the laboratory. This suggests that these two fatty acids, found in relatively high concentrations in coconut milk and coconut oil, may play a role in the prevention of this particular bacterial infection as well.[12]

(E)-β-CARYOPHYLLENE: (E)-β-Caryophyllene or (E)-BCP is a fully FDA-approved dietary cannabinoid that activates CB2 receptor sites and initiates potent anti-inflammatory actions and protection form oxidative stress, both common associated factors in pathogen-based inflammations. Spice plants known to contain significant amounts of (E)-BCP in descending order include: BLACK "ASHANTI PEPPER" (PIPER GUINEENSE), WHITE "ASHANTI PEPPER" (PIPER GUINEENSE), INDIAN BAY-LEAF (CINNAMOMUM TAMALA), ALLIGATOR PEPPER (AFRAMOMUM MELEGUETA), BASIL (OCIMUM MICRANTHUM), SRI LANKA CINNAMON (CINNAMOMUM ZEYLANICUM), ROSEMARY (ROSMARINUS OFFICINALIS), BLACK CARAWAY (CARUM NIGRUM), BLACK PEPPER (PIPER NIGRUM), BASIL (OCIMUM GRATISSIMUM), MEXICAN OREGANO (LIPPIA GRAVEOLENS), AND CLOVE (SYZYGIUM AROMATICUM).

1 Centers for Disease Control and Prevention 1600 Clifton Rd. Atlanta, GA 30333, USA. *Sexually Transmitted Diseases (STDs). Antibiotic Resistant Gonorrhea. Only one remaining class of antibiotics is recommended for the treatment of gonorrhea.* Page last updated: September 2, 2010. http://www.cdc.gov/std/gonorrhea/arg/default.htm

2 Giovanni Appendino, Simon Gibbons, Anna Giana, Alberto Pagani, Gianpaolo Grassi, Michael Stavri, Eileen Smith and M. Mukhlesur Rahman. *Antibacterial Cannabinoids from Cannabis sativa: A Structure–Activity Study.* Dipartimento di Scienze Chimiche, Alimentari, Farmaceutiche e Farmacologiche, Universit del Piemonte Orientale, Via Bovio 6, 28100 Novara, Italy, Consorzio per lo Studio dei Metaboliti Secondari (CSMS), Viale S. Ignazio 13, 09123 Cagliari, Italy, Centre for Pharmacognosy and Phytotherapy, The School of Pharmacy, University of London, 29-39 Brunswick Square, London WC1N 1AX, U.K., and CRA-CIN Centro di Ricerca per le Colture Industriali, Sede distaccata di Rovigo, Via Amendola 82, 45100 Rovigo, Italy. J. Nat. Prod., 2008, 71 (8), pp 1427–1430.

3 Mia Touw. *The Religious and Medicinal Uses of Cannabis in China, India and Tibet.* Journal of Psychoactive Drugs. Vol. 13(1) Jan-Mar, 1981.

4 Sam'l O. L. Potter, M.A., M.D., M.R.C.P. (Lond,) *A Compend of Materia Medica and Therapeutics and Prescription Writing; with especial references to the physiological actions of drugs.* Based on the last revision of the U.S. Pharmacopeia. Fifth Edition. P.Blakiston, Son & Co., Philadelphia, 1012 Walnut St. 1892. Page #124.

5 Advertised in the 1935 sales/price booklet. CANNABINE Comp. Mfg. By Chicago Pharmacal Co. 5547 E. Ravenswood Ave. Chicago, U.S.A.

6 Takeda S, Misawa K, Yamamoto I, Watanabe K. *Cannabidiolic acid as a selective cyclooxygenase-2 inhibitory component in cannabis.* Organization for Frontier Research in Preventive Pharmaceutical Sciences, Hokuriku University, Kanazawa, Japan. Drug Metab Dispos. 2008 Sep;36(9):1917-21.

7 Uwe Blesching, Ph.D. *Spicy Healing: A Global Guide to Growing and Using Spice for Food and Medicine.* Logos Publishing. Berkeley, California. Second Edition. 2009.

8 Koutsky L. *Epidemiology of genital human papillomavirus infection.* 1997. American Journal of Medicine, 102(5A), 3-8.

9 Bergsson G, Steingrímsson O, Thormar H. In vitro susceptibilities of Neisseria gonorrhoeae to fatty acids and monoglycerides. Institute of Biology, University of Iceland. gudmunb@rhi.hi.is Antimicrob Agents Chemother. 1999 Nov;43(11):2790-2.

10 Bergsson G, Arnfinnsson J, Steingrímsson O, Thormar H. Killing of Gram-positive cocci by fatty acids and monoglycerides. Institute of Biology, University of Iceland, Reykjavik. gudmunb@hi.is APMIS. 2001 Oct;109(10):670-8.

11 Bergsson G, Arnfinnsson J, Steingrímsson O , Thormar H. In vitro killing of Candida albicans by fatty acids and monoglycerides. Institute of Biology, University of Iceland, Reykjavik, Iceland. gudmunb@hi.is Antimicrob Agents Chemother. 2001 Nov; 45(11):3209-12.

12 Bergsson G, Arnfinnsson J, Karlsson SM, Steingrímsson O, Thormar H. In vitro inactivation of Chlamydia trachomatis by fatty acids and monoglycerides. Institute of Biology, University of Iceland, Reykjavik, Iceland. Antimicrob Agents Chemother. 1998 Sep;42(9):2290-4.

Bacterial & Viral Infections

Methicillin-resistant Staphylococcus Aureus (MRSA)

NUMBER OF STUDIES 1

CHI VALUE: 1

Certain strains of staphylococcus, an otherwise common bacterium, have developed a resistance to the usual antibiotic pharmaceuticals, which is the reason they are also referred to as 'superbugs,' or Multi-drug Resistant Staphylococcus Aureus (MRSA). People with weakened immune systems, chronic open wounds, surgical implants, and exposure the bacteria are its most likely victims. The bacteria are spread via close skin-to-skin contact, contaminated items and surfaces, crowded living conditions, and poor hygiene.

Many of the MRSA infections are acquired in hospitals, nursing homes, and prisons. Hospitals isolate infected patients disinfect medical tools and the environment to reduce the risk of public health hazards. If an infection occurs, treatments with standard antibiotics are ineffective, making this microbe a potentially deadly agent. Infections are usually limited to the skin, where they commonly form abscesses, but in severe cases can affect internal organs, leading to sepsis and death.

If a strong suspicion exists that MRSA may be involved, a specific test is performed to determine the exact strains present. The test may take several days to complete, and given that in some cases disease progression is very rapid (2-3 days after first sign of topical symptoms) presumptive treatments are strongly recommended by the allopathic community. However, the problem is discerning which of the few remaining antibiotics, if any, are still able to kill the bacteria. Clinical trials are currently underway to develop updated guidelines on treatment options.

CANNABIS AND MRSA

Various cannabinoids have antibacterial properties, but the mechanism through which the plant constituents are able to destroy even antibiotic resistant bacteria remains elusive. An international group of scientists conducted a laboratory experiment where researchers examined five major cannabinoids (cannabidiol, cannabichromene, cannabigerol, Δ9-tetrahydrocannabinol, and cannabinol) and their effectiveness against MSRA. Result showed potent activity against a variety of methicillin-resistant Staphylococcus aureus (MRSA) strains of current clinical relevance.[1]

STUDY SUMMARY

Drugs	Type of Study	Published Year, Place, and Key Results	CHI
CBD, CBC, CBG, THC and CBN.	Laboratory	2008 - Multi-center international study: All five major cannabinoids showed potent activity against a variety of MRSA.[1]	1

Total CHI Value 1

STRAIN SPECIFIC CONSIDERATIONS

Both indicas and sativas flowers contain five major cannabinoids (cannabidiol, cannabichromene, cannabigerol, Δ9-tetrahydrocannabinol, and cannabinol). Possible synergistic effects of using complete cannabinoid profiles against MRSA have not yet been tested.

EXPLORING MIND–BODY CONSCIOUSNESS

While MRSA has been known to affect the bloodstream, lungs, and urinary tract, its primary target is the skin, possibly suggesting an underlying vulnerability connected to image and identity. The rapid destructiveness of MRSA suggests an extreme defenselessness against something that is literally eating at the patient.

See also SKIN DISEASE and SKIN CANCER.

QUESTIONS

What is eating me?
Where, or with whom, do I feel completely defenseless?

TAKE NOTICE

GARLIC • ESSENTIAL OILS • MAGGOT DEBRIDEMENT THERAPY

GARLIC: A laboratory study in London, England has confirmed that allicin, a major antibacterial component of garlic, is a very effective defense against MRSA.[2] This result was confirmed by another study conducted on mice infected with MRSA, which concluded that the garlic extract, diallyl sulphide and diallyl disulphide possessed multiple protective functions against MRSA infection.[3] Reports from case studies conducted by Dr. Cutler, a member of the research team which conducted the laboratory test, have shown that topical and internal use of allicin (provided by Allicin International) has cured patients infected with MRSA.

ESSENTIAL OILS: Using topical applications, highly volatile essential oils and extracts have been studied in an attempt to find ways to mitigate MRSA. Researchers discovered that grapefruit seed extract (Citricidal) together with geranium oil showed the greatest anti-bacterial effects against MRSA, while a combination of geranium and tea tree oil was most active against the Oxford strain (methicillin-sensitive S. aureus).[4] Another study discovered that the multiple constituents of the essential oils of peppermint, spearmint, and Japanese mint exhibited properties that inhibited the growth of several different kinds of disease-causing bacteria, including MRSA.[5] Essential tea tree oil

SUGGESTED BLESSING:

May I find ways to release the helplessness no matter what it's source.

SUGGESTED AFFIRMATION:

I allow all that eats at me from the inside to dissipate like dew on a warm summer morning breeze.

I can transcend any punishment with forgiveness.

was discovered to be very effective in vitro (laboratory) against MRSA.[6] Other studies confirm similar results of essential oils used to treat MRSA, including lavender, lemongrass, cinnamon, melissa, and mountain savory (satureja cuneifolia Ten.), a common fragrant plant frequently used as a spice and herbal tea in Turkey.

Warning: Essential oils are usually used externally. As with all essential oils, do not rub on mouth, nose or near the eyes, especially those of infants or children. Gagging and throat spasms may occur. Be extra careful when pregnant; any systemic allergic reaction may affect the fetus. You may want to use a small amount and test on a small skin area, then wait a few hours to see if an allergic reaction occurs. Discontinue use if reddening, swelling or pain on site occurs. If you want to try again, dilute it with some other non-essential carrier oil first.

MAGGOT DEBRIDEMENT THERAPY (MDT): Sterile maggot debridement therapy has proven an effective way to clean infected skin wounds, abscesses, ulcers, infected tissue, and necrotic or gangrene tissue.[7] Besides cleaning the infected area maggots also disinfect the wounded tissue and stimulate wound healing. While the antibacterial effect of maggot therapy is not systemic, MRSA is effectively killed in the topical area of application.

1 Giovanni Appendino, Simon Gibbons, Anna Giana, Alberto Pagani, Gianpaolo Grassi, Michael Stavri, Eileen Smith and M. Mukhlesur Rahman. *Antibacterial Cannabinoids from Cannabis sativa: A Structure–Activity Study.* Dipartimento di Scienze Chimiche, Alimentari, Farmaceutiche e Farmacologiche, Universit del Piemonte Orientale, Via Bovio 6, 28100 Novara, Italy, Consorzio per lo Studio dei Metaboliti Secondari (CSMS), Viale S. Ignazio 13, 09123 Cagliari, Italy, Centre for Pharmacognosy and Phytotherapy, The School of Pharmacy, University of London, 29-39 Brunswick Square, London WC1N 1AX, U.K., and CRA-CIN Centro di Ricerca per le Colture Industriali, Sede distaccata di Rovigo, Via Amendola 82, 45100 Rovigo, Italy. J. Nat. Prod., 2008, 71 (8), pp 1427–1430.

2 Cutler RR, Wilson P. *Antibacterial activity of a new, stable, aqueous extract of allicin against methicillin-resistant Staphylococcus aureus.* University of East London, School of Health and Bioscience, Stratford Campus, Romford Road, London E15 4LZ, UK. r.cutler@uel.ac.uk Br J Biomed Sci. 2004;61(2):71-4.

3 Tsao SM, Hsu CC, Yin MC. *Garlic extract and two diallyl sulphides inhibit methicillin-resistant Staphylococcus aureus infection in BALB/cA mice.* Department of Infection, Chungshan Medical University Hospital, Taiwan, ROC. J Antimicrob Chemother. 2003 Dec;52(6):974-80.

4 Edwards-Jones V, Buck R, Shawcross SG, Dawson MM, Dunn K. *The effect of essential oils on methicillin-resistant Staphylococcus aureus using a dressing model.* Department of Biological Sciences, the Manchester Metropolitan University, Chester Street, Manchester, M15GD, UK. v.e.jones@mmu.ac.u Burns. 2004 Dec;30(8):772-7.

5 Imai H, Osawa K, Yasuda H, Hamashima H, Arai T, Sasatsu M. *Inhibition by the essential oils of peppermint and spearmint of the growth of pathogenic bacteria.* Functional Foods Section, Central Laboratory, Lotte Company Ltd, Urawa, Saitama, Japan. Microbios. 2001;106 Suppl 1:31-9.

6 Hada T, Furuse S, Matsumoto Y, Hamashima H, Masuda K, Shiojima K, Arai T, Sasatsu M. *Comparison of the effects in vitro of tea tree oil and plaunotol on methicillin-susceptible and methicillin-resistant strains of Staphylococcus aureus.* Department of Microbiology, Showa Pharmaceutical University, Machida, Tokyo, Japan. Microbios. 2001;106 Suppl 2:133-41.

7 Bowling FL, Salgami EV, Boulton AJ. *Larval therapy: a novel treatment in eliminating methicillin-resistant Staphylococcus aureus from diabetic foot ulcers.* University Department of Medicine and Diabetes, Manchester Royal Infirmary, Oxford Road, Manchester M13 9WL, U.K. frank.bowling@manchester.ac.uk Diabetes Care. 2007 Feb;30(2):370-1.

Viral Infections

Virus is a Latin word, that means slime or juice. Modern medicine has identified hundreds of different viruses. Some are completely harmless, while others can cause specific diseases in the plant, animal, and human kingdoms. Viruses are extremely small and omnipresent. The biggest virus is about the same size as the tiniest bacterium. In comparison to the smallest of all bacteria, a virus is generally the size of a grain of sand next to a skyscraper.

A dormant (sleeping/inactive) virus is described as a simple organism that basically consists of DNA, RNA (a chemical blueprint of itself), and a protective protein (protein is usually a mixture of several elements, like carbon, oxygen, nitrogen, sulfur, and phosphorus). It seems to want but one thing, and that is to make more of itself. Based on a yet-to-be-discovered signal, the virus "wakes up" and begins to develop when it comes across a vulnerable host cell.

The virus either attaches itself to the host cell or enters the host cell. Once attached or inside, it tells the cell to stop doing what it has been doing, namely maintaining your well-being, health, and healing, and instead tells the cell to produce the elements the virus needs to make more of itself. In the case of many viruses, when a copy has been made, it bursts out of the host cell, destroying the host cell in the process. When this occurs a million times over, viruses make people sick or even sometimes kill them.

However, the immune system, the police department of the body, is extremely smart, and if healthy and strong it is more than capable of fighting viruses. For example, many viruses are inactivated or destroyed by a body temperature slightly more than normal. Thus, fever is an effective immune system defense to a viral invasion.

The immune system also produces antibodies and sensitized cells (virus- fighting police) that are made specifically to destroy a specific virus. These police circulate throughout the body long after the virus has been destroyed, keeping the body safe and protected. If the same virus reenters the body, for example the chicken pox virus, the person will not get sick with chicken pox a second time. One is usually immune for life.

EXPLORING MIND–BODY CONSCIOUSNESS

A review and analysis of psychosomatic studies published since 1939 shows that negative emotions, hostility and stressful experiences directly influence pro-inflammatory cytokine production which is associated with slower healing and acceleration of age-related illness.[1,2]

In every epidemic, there are people who do not get ill. While it is clear that pathogens such as viruses play a part in the contraction of disease, pathogens are not the sole cause of disease. Mental-emotional states directly affect the immune system. Mental-emotional states may induce a susceptibility or vulnerability to disease, or instead may initiate a formidable defense and rapid immune response. They

SUGGESTED

BLESSING:

May you begin the process of expanding already-present strengths and abilities.

May you also find new depths of gratitude, love, and trust in yourself and those who are truly trustworthy.

thus play a critical role in determining whether or not an individual will get sick.

Infectious agents are more likely to result in disease whenever negative affect is present, because negative emotional and mental states are resource intensive and deplete the reserves that protect immunity. So we are at greater risk of disease whenever we experience chronic lack of support, insecurity, mistrustfulness, fear, mental or emotional defenselessness, defensiveness, victimization, powerlessness, or a violation of personal boundaries. Conversely, a balanced and powerful immunity results from the experience of emotional support, safety, and security, trust, love, intimacy, functional coping mechanisms, confidence, and belief in one's inner strength and abilities.

TAKE NOTICE

ACACIA • BASIL • CARDAMOM • CLOVE • COCONUT • TURMERIC • (E)-β-CARYOPHYLLENE CONTAINING SPICES

ACACIA: A study from Mumbai, presented at the 8th International Congress on Drug Therapy in HIV Infection, indicated that the aqueous extract of acacia pods is effective in-vitro against the viral enzyme reverse transcriptase.[3]

BASIL: Basil has been used in Traditional Chinese Medicine for thousands of years. Now researchers from the island nation of Taiwan have taken a closer look at the possible anti-viral properties of basil extract and several of basil's specific compounds against DNA viruses, herpes virus, adenoviruses, hepatitis B virus, and the RNA viruses (coxsackievirus B1 and enterovirus 71). The results showed that: "…crude aqueous and ethanolic extracts of basil (ocimum basilicum) and selected purified components, namely apigenin, linalool, and ursolic acid, exhibit a broad spectrum of antiviral activity. Of these compounds, ursolic acid showed the strongest activity against HSV-1 … whereas apigenin showed the highest activity against HSV-2…"[4]

CARDAMON: At the University of Cincinnati College of Medicine, scientists looked at cineole, a major constituent of cardamon, in the context of treating vaginal herpes infections in mice, and determined that sufficient evidence exists to warrant more research, using this compound as a possibly promising natural treatment modality.[5]

CLOVE: In a series of experiments, virologists from the Toyama Medical and Pharmaceutical University in Sugitani, Japan determined that eugenine, a compound purified from the extracts of clove, inhibits viral DNA synthesis in several strains of herpes (I & II), including acyclovir-phosphonoacetic acid-resistant HSV-I.[6]

A Tunisian study reported in the National Library of Medicine determined that essential oil of clove extracts to have anti-viral (herpes simplex –HSV and hepatitis C), and anti-bacterial (including several of the multi-drug resistant Staphylococcus epidermidis) properties.[7]

COCONUT: The authors of a study from Staten Island, New York state: "Lipids can inactivate enveloped viruses, bacteria, fungi, and protozoa." By adding medium chain fatty acids (MCFA) to HIV-infected blood products, the researchers learned that they could reduce the virus concentration by a very large number. Further, the scientists expect that MCFA "...may potentially be used as combination of spermicidal and virucidal agents."[8]

A crude extract of cocos nucifera L. husk fiber demonstrated inhibitory activity against acyclovir-resistant herpes simplex virus type 1 (HSV-1-ACVr).[9]

TURMERIC: Researchers tested the hypothesis that curcumin, the main active constituent in turmeric, would block viral infection and gene expression of HSV-1 by inhibiting promoters of herpes gene expression. Results showed that curcumin significantly decreased HSV-1 infectivity and IE gene expression.[10]

(E)-β-CARYOPHYLLENE: (E)-β-Caryophyllene or (E)-BCP is a fully FDA-approved dietary cannabinoid that activates CB2 receptor sites and initiates potent anti-inflammatory actions and protection form oxidative stress, both commonly associated factors in pathogen-based inflammations. Spice plants known to contain significant amounts of (E)-BCP in descending order include: BLACK "ASHANTI PEPPER" (PIPER GUINEENSE), WHITE "ASHANTI PEPPER" (PIPER GUINEENSE), INDIAN BAY-LEAF (CINNAMOMUM TAMALA), ALLIGATOR PEPPER (AFRAMOMUM MELEGUETA), BASIL (OCIMUM MICRANTHUM), SRI LANKA CINNAMON (CINNAMOMUM ZEYLANICUM), ROSEMARY (ROSMARINUS OFFICINALIS), BLACK CARAWAY (CARUM NIGRUM), BLACK PEPPER (PIPER NIGRUM), BASIL (OCIMUM GRATISSIMUM), MEXICAN OREGANO (LIPPIA GRAVEOLENS), AND CLOVE (SYZYGIUM AROMATICUM).

1 Janice K. Kiecolt-Glaser, PhD, Lynanne McGuire, PhD, Theodore F. Robles, BS and Ronald Glaser, PhD. *Psychoneuroimmunology and Psychosomatic Medicine: Back to the Future.* Departments of Psychiatry (J.K-G., L.M., T.F.R.), Molecular Virology, Immunology, and Medical Genetics (R.G.), and Psychology (T.F.R.), Ohio State University, and Ohio State Institute for Behavioral Medicine Research (J.K-G., R.G.), Columbus, OH. Psychosomatic Medicine 64:15-28 (2002).

2 Kiecolt-Glaser JK, Loving TJ, Stowell JR, Malarkey WB, Lemeshow S, Dickinson SL, Glaser R. *Hostile marital interactions, proinflammatory cytokine production, and wound healing.* Department of Psychiatry, Institute for Behavioral Medicine Research, Ohio State University College of Medicine, 1670 Upham Drive, Columbus, OH 43210, USA. Arch Gen Psychiatry. 2005 Dec;62(12):1377-84.

3 Tabassum A Khan, Pratima A Tatke, Satish Y Gabhe. *Evaluation of Aqueous Extract of Babool Pods for in Vitro Anti-HIV Activity.* Pharmacy, C.U. Shah College of Pharmacy, Mumbai, Maharashtra, India. Int Cong Drug Therapy HIV 2006 Nov 12-16;8: Abstract No. P399.

4 Chiang LC, Ng LT, Cheng PW, Chiang W, Lin CC. *Antiviral activities of extracts and selected pure constituents of Ocimum basilicum.* Department of Microbiology, Kaohsiung Medical University, Kaohsiung, Taiwan. Clin Exp Pharmacol Physiol. 2005 Oct;32(10):811-6.

5 Bourne KZ, Bourne N, Reising SF, Stanberry LR. *Plant products as topical microbicide candidates: assessment of in vitro and in vivo activity against herpes simplex virus type 2.* Children's Hospital Research Foundation, Department of Pediatrics, University of Cincinnati College of Medicine, OH 45229-3039, USA. Antiviral Res. 1999 Jul;42(3):219-26.

6 Kurokawa M, Hozumi T, Basnet P, Nakano M, Kadota S, Namba T, Kawana T, Shiraki K. *Purification and characterization of eugeniin as an anti-herpesvirus compound from Geum japonicum and Syzygium aromaticum.* Virology, Toyama Medical and Pharmaceutical University, Sugitani, Toyama 930-01, Japan. J Pharmacol Exp Ther. 1998 Feb;284(2):728-35.

7 Chaieb K, Hajlaoui H, Zmantar T, Kahla-Nakbi AB, Rouabhia M, Mahdouani K, Bakhrouf A. *The chemical composition and biological activity of clove essential oil, Eugenia caryophyllata (Syzigium aromaticum L. Myrtaceae): a short review.* Laboratoire d'Analyses, Traitement et Valorisation des Polluants de l'Environnement et des Produits, Faculté de Pharmacie, rue Avicenne 5000 Monastir, Tunisie. Phytother Res. 2007 Jun;21(6):501-6.

8 Isaacs CE, Kim KS, Thormar H. *Inactivation of enveloped viruses in human bodily fluids by purified lipids.* Department of Developmental Biochemistry, New York State Institute for Basic Research in Developmental Disabilities, Staten Island 10314. Ann N Y Acad Sci. 1994 Jun 6;724:457-64.

9 Esquenazi D, Wigg MD, Miranda MM, Rodrigues HM, Tostes JB, Rozental S, da Silva AJ, Alviano CS. *Antimicrobial and antiviral activities of polyphenolics from Cocos nucifera Linn. (Palmae) husk fiber extract.* Laboratório de Biologia Celular de Fungos, Instituto de Biofísica Carlos Chagas Filho, Universidade Federal do Rio de Janeiro, 21941-590, Ilha do Fundão, Rio de Janeiro, RJ, Brazil. Res Microbiol. 2002 Dec;153(10):647-52.

10 Kutluay SB, Doroghazi J, Roemer ME, Triezenberg SJ. *Curcumin inhibits herpes simplex virus immediate-early gene expression by a mechanism independent of p300/CBP histone acetyltransferase activity.* Graduate Program in Cell and Molecular Biology, Michigan State University, East Lansing, MI 48824, USA. Virology. 2008 Apr 10;373(2):239-47.

Bacterial & Viral Infections
Colds and Flu

According to orthodox medicine, all common colds as well as all types of flu are caused by viral infections. There are hundreds of known and ever-mutating cold and flu viruses. However, during every flu outbreak in history there have been many people who did not get sick even when sufficiently exposed, so one must consider susceptibility as being a major contributing factor to whether a person falls sick or not. While the allopathic model is aware that people with lower immunity are more vulnerable to becoming sick, it has concentrated research primarily on microbes rather than susceptibility. The allopathic model has no cure for either colds or flu.

Many signs and symptoms of colds and flu tend to represent themselves in a similar fashion. A cold usually affects only the nose and throat, and is associated with a low-grade fever. Flu may have the same symptoms, but the symptoms are usually more sudden, severe, and include a cough, higher fevers, muscle aches, headaches, fatigue, and the addition of aches and pains. While most colds and flu are self-correcting, it is prudent to get help from a licensed health care practitioner when the following symptoms are present: loss of consciousness, disorientation, seizures, vomiting or diarrhea with an inability to regain fluids, fevers over 102° F (39° C), a bloody cough or stool, sustained fever over several days, or inability to walk.

According to the World Health Organization, flu epidemics occur every year during fall and winter in temperate regions (regions without extreme heat or cold). "Worldwide, these annual epidemics result in about three to five million cases of severe illness, and about 250,000 to 500,000 deaths. Most deaths associated with influenza in industrialized countries occur among people age 65 or older. In some tropical countries, influenza viruses circulate throughout the year, with one or two peaks during rainy seasons."[1]

Other diseases that may look like a cold or flu but require different treatment approaches include: asthma, pneumonia, bronchitis, sinusitis, allergies, strep throat, tuberculosis, emphysema, and chronic obstructive pulmonary diseases (COPD).

COMMON ALLOPATHIC TREATMENT

Decongestants are a group of medications from a long list of vasoconstrictors, from A-Actifed through Z-Zephrex, for example. Decongestants constrict blood vessels, and are targeted mainly to reduce the swelling of mucus membranes in the nose. Common side effects may include rebound congestion (the cold actually takes longer to heal), restlessness, dizziness, insomnia, raised blood pressure, and an increased heart rate.

Antihistamines (for example Allegra, Benadryl, Claritin or Seldane) are ineffective treatments for colds. A prominent medical text puts it plainly: "despite early claims and persistent popular belief, histamine-blocking drugs (antihistamines) are without value in combating the common cold."[2] Common side effects, such as blurred vision, dry mouth, dry eyes, constipation, confusion, or sexual dysfunction are related to the anticholinergic properties of antihistamines which block the effects of acetylcholine. Acetylcholine is a substance involved in the function of the parasympathetic nervous system. A suppression of the parasympathetic nervous system produces an increase in heart rate and less production of digestive juices, tears, sweat, or saliva.

Cough suppressants containing opiates (for example, codeine), reduce the reflex to cough up undesirable materials. They are, in most cases, counterproductive to what the body needs to do to rid itself of mucus, phlegm, and the materials encased in them. The most common side effects of cough suppressants are constipation, dizziness, sedation, nausea, and vomiting. Opiates may be habit-forming and can produce respiratory depression ranging from mild hypoxia to respiratory arrest.

Expectorants (such as Robitussin) are drugs that are supposed to assist in the loosening, thinning, and bringing up of phlegm. However, a sufficient amount of water may be a better expectorant, and avoids all their possible side-effects: allergic reaction, dizziness, nausea, vomiting, abdominal discomforts, headache, or a rash.

In 1997, U.S. poison control centers were contacted a total of 110,870 times about cases involving pharmacological cold and cough preparations. 22,073 patients had to be treated in a health care facility, and fourteen people died.[3]

Prescription antiviral medication, such as amantadine, rimantadine, oseltamivir (Tamiflu), and zanamivir are approved in the U.S. for the treatment of flu. Each has a set of potential side effects.[4] The CDC lists the side effects of amantadine and rimantadine as nervousness, anxiety, difficulty concentrating, lightheadedness, and gastrointestinal side effects like nausea and loss of appetite. Among some other persons with long-term illnesses, more serious side-effects, such as delirium, hallucinations, agitation, and seizures can occur. For zanamivir, the CDC lists side-effects such as decreased respiratory function and bronchospasm, diarrhea, nausea, sinusitis, nasal infections, bronchitis, cough, headache, and dizziness. Finally, the side-effects of oseltamivir, (Tamiflu) include nausea, vomiting, and psychotic self-destructive behavior.

Antipyretics (fever reducing) medications such as Acetaminophen (Tylenol and many others) are commonly used to battle a cold or flu. This pharmaceutical medication is broken down in the liver and can cause liver damage and death. Acetaminophen overuse causes about 56,000 emergency room visits and 26,000 hospitalizations yearly, with approximately 500 of these cases ending in death.[5] Aspirin is another very commonly used pharmacological medication used to reduce fever and pain. Side-effects include internal bleeding and liver damage, just two examples. People under twenty years old should not take or be given aspirin products in conjunction with fever because aspirin is linked to Reye's syndrome, a potentially fatal condition.

Antibiotics are still commonly prescribed to treat the common cold or flu. Since, according to the allopathic model, both the cold and the flu are caused by viruses, and antibiotics only kill bacteria, there is no way antibiotics can help cure these diseases or speed up natural healing. Physicians usually justify prescribing antibiotics for cold and flu as a means to prevent bacterial infections such as pneumonia. However, among the many side-effects of antibiotics is making a person more susceptible to a dangerous bacterial super-infection, such as a pneumonia, which nowadays is often resistant to the antibiotic the person is taking. The Public Citizen's Health Research Group reports that "in 1983, more than 51% of the more than three million patients who saw doctors for treatment of the common cold were given an unnecessary prescription for an antibiotic."[6]

Allopathic doctors also prescribe steroidal inhaler and/or systemic steroids. Potential side-effects include growth interference in children, weight gain, high blood pressure, stomach ulcers, pancreatitis and hyperglycemia, osteoporosis, and muscular weakness.

Flu vaccines are made from last year's viral strain. By the time it hits the shelves, the virus blamed for this years "outbreak" is a different mutated kind, rendering the promise of immunity questionable. Furthermore, long-term studies on the other potential effects of flu vaccines and their various ingredients have not been conducted, and their safety cannot be clearly determined as of yet. The decision to be vaccinated or not is yours, and yours alone. If you decide to receive a vaccination, look for any unusual signs or symptoms such as a high fever and/or changes in behavior. Signs of a serious allergic or anaphylactic reaction include shortness of breath, hives, paleness, weakness, a fast heartbeat, low blood pressure, dizziness and/or swelling of the throat. Other conditions to watch for are seizures, more common in the presence of a high fever, and especially in children under the age of three.

You can report cases of vaccine side-effects to your doctor, nurse practitioner, nurse, or public health department and file a Vaccine Adverse Event Reporting System (VAERS) form, or call VAERS yourself at 1-800-822-7967.[7]

CANNABIS AND COLDS/FLU

While not a remedy for colds or flu per se, cannabinoids may be useful in alleviating the cough and fever often associated with colds and flu.

EXPLORING MIND–BODY CONSCIOUSNESS

While the Grace and Graham study referenced earlier focused on vasomotor rhinitis (stuffy or runny nose not caused by allergies or infection), the psychosomatic similarities warrant inclusion of their findings in this section on colds as well. The researchers examined the psychosomatic underpinning of 12 patients with stuffy and runny nose diagnosed as rhinitis, and discovered that symptoms occurred when a patient was faced with a life situation they wished would just go away, or wished someone else would take responsibility for and make it disappear, or felt avoidance would be the best course for them. Typical statements were: "I wanted them to go away." "I didn't want anything to do with it." "I wanted to blot it all out; I wanted to build a wall between me and him." "I wanted to hole up for the winter." "I wanted to go to bed and pull the sheets over my head." Grace and Graham concluded that: "The reaction of the respiratory mucous membrane to a noxious agent is to exclude it by swelling of the membrane with consequent narrowing of the passageway, and to dilute it and wash it out by hypersecretion."[8]

Another experiment used 334 healthy volunteers between 18 and 54 years, who were assessed for their tendency to experience positive as well as negative emotions. Each was exposed to cold viruses and monitored in quarantine for the development of the symptoms of a common cold. Those who had tendencies to experience positive emotions had a significantly greater resistance to developing a cold.[9]

In cases of colds and flu, the body may become a metaphorical stage on which

SUGGESTED BLESSING:

May you slow down and stand still for a while.

Allow yourself to downshift your mind, take a deep breath and relax.

to act out various themes of dis-ease. This "lack of ease" may be the consequence of limiting beliefs such as "The glass is half empty rather than half full", "I don't want anything to change!", "I'll probably get sick because it's the cold season", simply feeling overwhelmed, or all of the above. Likewise, when the fulfillment of a dream becomes a burden, we are ill at ease. ("I wanted this job, but in dealing with the daily grind I have forgotten how great it is to have a job." Or, "I always wanted children, but all this nursing, teaching, and driving means I am constantly exhausted.") During difficult times, it is easy to simply forget to feel grateful. Then here comes fall and winter, and they offer an easy solution – "catch a cold." Now I can cough and sneeze my way into a break from it all.

The season's change, daylight changes, and the air takes on a different feel in each season. Life is change. However, change, in the minds of many, is not considered a friend and is often greeted with great dislike. In such cases, even a simple change in our routines may lead to irritation, anxiety, and attempts to wrestle with and dominate reality. Drained and overwhelmed by attempts to control the inevitable, one may want to curl up in bed, attempting to avoid dealing with change altogether.

The annual anxiety about getting sick during the "cold and flu season" may also contribute to lowered immunity to cold and flu viruses that otherwise would be easily handled by our immune system. Here, catching cold actually means release from the clutches of anxiety of getting sick. To many, the actual cold is preferable to constant anxiety.

It is interesting to note that those people who stay healthy undermine the collective belief in a cold and flu season. In fact, looking at the numbers, those that stay healthy are in the majority. In the U.S., it is estimated that about 1 in 4 will catch a cold, but 3 out of 4 will not. The estimates for flu are similar. 1 out of 10 Americans will catch a flu, but 9 out of 10 will stay healthy.

QUESTIONS

Have any of my fulfilled dreams become a burden?
Has the tedium of my daily routine eroded my gratitude?
Where is my glass "half empty" rather than half full?
Where am I feeling overwhelmed?
In what situations or circumstances am I change averse?
Am I giving my power away to the cold season?

TAKE NOTICE

ANISE • COCONUT • FENNEL • GARLIC • MYRRH • OREGANO

ANISE: Cuban physicians use the fruit (fresh or dried) of anise as an expectorant. It is used to treat coughs and sore throats as well as general low immunity.[10]

Scientists from Mashhad, Iran, discovered a possible mechanism that may explain why many traditional healers have been using anise extracts and oils in the treatment of certain respiratory ailments. Anise extracts and essential oils possess bronchodilatory (opens the upper airways) qualities derived from possible antihistamine-like properties.[11]

COCONUT: The authors of this study from Staten Island, New York, state: "Lipids can inactivate enveloped viruses, bacteria, fungi, and protozoa." The scientists expect that MCFA "...may potentially be used as virucidal agents."[12]

FENNEL: Fennel seeds and oil are approved for the treatment of: "Catarrh of the upper respiratory tract."[13]

GARLIC: Garlic is one of Cuba's most versatile herbs. A syrup made from garlic is utilized to treat colds, coughs and flu.[14]

MYRRH: Approved by the German Commission E for the topical treatment of mucus membrane inflammation such as in sore throats during episodes of cold or cough.[15]

OREGANO: Scientists from the Department of Pharmacology and Biochemistry at the University of Medicine discovered that tea of oregano may be effective in treating certain respiratory illness.[16]

1 World Health Organiztion (WHO). Media Center. *Influenza (seasonal).* Fact sheet No. 211. April 2009.

2 *Goodman & Gilman's The Pharmacological Basis of Therapeutics.* Tenth Edition. 2001.

3 Toby L. Litovitz, M.D., Wendy Klein-Schwartz, Pharm. D., MPH., K. Sophia Dyer, M.D., Micheal Shannon, MD., MPH., Shannon Lee, BSPharm., CSPI, Meggan Power. *Annual Report of the American Association of Poison Control Centers Toxic Exposure Surveillance System 1997.*

4 May 19, 2007. http://www.cdc.gov/flu/protect/antiviral/sideeffects.htm

5 Nourjah P, Ahmad SR, Karwoski C, Willy M. *Estimates of acetaminophen (Paracetomal)-associated overdoses in the United States.* Office of Drug Safety, Division of Drug Risk Evaluation, Center for Drug Evaluation and Research, Food and Drug Administration, Silver Spring, Maryland 20993, USA. Pharmacoepidemiol Drug Saf. 2006 Jun;15(6):398-405.

6 Sidney M. Wolfe, M.D. *Antibiotics.* Public Citizen's Health Research Group. Washington, DC. Health Letter. 1989;5(7):1-5.

7 A relatively unknown fact is that: As of April 12, 2005, 11,302 (4,689 autism/thimerosal and 6,613 non-autism/thimerosal) claims have been filed and compensation totaling over $1.5 billion has been awarded to 1,910 families. Currently, the program covers the following vaccines: diphtheria, tetanus, pertussis (DTP, DTaP, DT, TT, or Td), measles, mumps, rubella (MMR or any components), polio (OPV or IPV), hepatitis B, hepatitis A, Haemophilus influenzae type b (Hib), varicella (chicken pox), rotavirus, and pneumococcal conjugate. As of July 1, 2005, trivalent influenza vaccines will be covered under the VICP (Vaccine Injury Compensation Program). VAERS, P.O. Box 1100, Rockville, Maryland 20849-1100, Phone: 1-800-822-7967

8 William J. Grace, M.D. and David T. Graham, M.D. *Relationship of Specific Attitudes and Emotions to Certain Bodily Diseases.* Dept. of Medicine, of the New York Hospital-Cornell Medical Center. Psychosomatic Medicine July 1, 1952 vol. 14 no. 4 243-251.

9 Sheldon Cohen, PhD, William J. Doyle, PhD, Ronald B. Turner, MD, Cuneyt M. Alper, MD and David P. Skoner, MD. *Emotional Style and Susceptibility to the Common Cold.* Department of Psychology (S.C.), Carnegie Mellon University, Pittsburgh; Departments of Otolaryngology (W.J.D., C.M.A.) and Pediatrics (D.P.S.) Children's Hospital of Pittsburgh and the University of Pittsburgh School of Medicine, Pittsburgh, Pennsylvania; and the Department of Pediatrics (R.B.T.), Medical University of South Carolina, Charleston, South Carolina (now at the University of Virginia Health Sciences Center, Charlottesville, Virginia). Psychosomatic Medicine 65:652-657 (2003).

10 Therapeutic Guide to Plant Pharmaceuticals and Honey Pharmaceuticals (*Guia Terapeutica Dispensarial de Fitofarmacos y Apifarmacos* - Ministerio de Salud Publica, Ciudad de La Habana - Republica de Cuba 1992). Cuban Ministry of Public Health, Havana.

11 Boskabady MH, Ramazani-Assari M. *Relaxant effect of Pimpinella anisum on isolated guinea pig tracheal chains and its possible mechanism(s).* Department of Physiology, Ghaem Medical Centre, Mashhad University of Medical Sciences, 91735, Mashhad, Iran. J Ethnopharmacol. 2001 Jan;74(1):83-8.

12 Isaacs CE, Kim KS, Thormar H. *Inactivation of enveloped viruses in human bodily fluids by purified lipids.* Department of Developmental Biochemistry, New York State Institute for Basic Research in Developmental Disabilities, Staten Island 10314. Ann N Y Acad Sci. 1994 Jun 6;724:457-64.

13 *Monographien der E-Kommission* (Phyto-Therapie) (380 monographs). A therapeutic guide to herbal medicine evaluating the safety and efficacy of herbs for licensed medical prescribing in Germany. Published between 1984 and 1994 in the Bundesanzeiger (official publication by the Federal Republic of Germany). Copies of the monographs are available at the Heilpflanzen-Welt Bibliothek: http://buecher.heilpflanzen-welt.de/BGA-Commission-E-Monographs/

14 Therapeutic Guide to Plant Pharmaceuticals and Honey Pharmaceuticals *(Guia Terapeutica Dispensarial de Fitofarmacos y Apifarmacos* - Ministerio de Salud Publica, Ciudad de La Habana - Republica de Cuba 1992). Cuban Ministry of Public Health, Havana.

15 *Monographien der E-Kommission* (Phyto-Therapie) (380 monographs). A therapeutic guide to herbal medicine evaluating the safety and efficacy of herbs for licensed medical prescribing in Germany. Published between 1984 and 1994 in the Bundesanzeiger (official publication by the Federal Republic of Germany). Copies of the monographs are available at the Heilpflanzen-Welt Bibliothek: http://buecher.heilpflanzen-welt.de/BGA-Commission-E-Monographs/

16 Ivanova D, Gerova D, Chervenkov T, Yankova T. *Polyphenols and antioxidant capacity of Bulgarian medicinal plants.* Department of Pharmacology and Biochemistry, University of Medicine Varna, 55 Marin Drinov Street, 9002 Varna, Bulgaria. J Ethnopharmacol. 2005 Jan 4;96(1-2):145-50.

Bacterial & Viral Infections
Cough

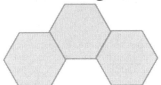

NUMBER OF STUDIES: 3

COMBINED CHI VALUE: 10

While human physiology allows us to cough consciously, most coughs are sudden and involuntary reflexes designed to clear the upper airways of mucus, phlegm, microbes, irritants, or foreign bodies. Differentiations of coughs include onset, duration, and dry, productive, chronic, or tic coughs (psychogenic). The most common cause for a sudden onset cough is a virus-based infection. Antibiotics are useless in these cases, as are antihistamines. While most coughs will simply take their course, and are by nature self-limiting, certain complications or conditions may warrant a treatment. A cough remedy may be helpful if symptoms include severe pain, cough-induced insomnia, fainting, vomiting, incontinence, hernias, or tissue damage of the rib cage.

No cure exists within the orthodox model of medicine. For the past two hundred years of modern medicine, opiates have been its most effective antitussive. However, adverse effects are common, as is the possibility of addiction or abuse.

CANNABIS AND COUGH

The anti-inflammatory, anti-spasmotic, and bronchodialation properties of cannabis all may play a part in the therapeutic impact of the herb as an antitussive. An analysis conducted in 2006 by the University of California in conjunction with the U.S. Federal Government indicated that the immediate impact of smoking cannabis is bronchodilation. The abstract filed with the US patent office states: "The invention discloses the existence of cannabinoid receptors in the airways, which are functionally linked to inhibition of cough. Locally-acting cannabinoid agents can be administered to the airways of a subject to ameliorate cough, without causing the psychoactive effects characteristic of systemically administered cannabinoids. In addition, locally or systemically administered cannabinoid inactivation inhibitors can also be used to ameliorate cough. The present invention also defines conditions under which cannabinoid agents can be administered to produce anti-tussive effects devoid of bronchial constriction." The patent application also states that: "The Government may have certain rights in this invention."[1]

While the abstract is also concerned that the long-term use of the plant might contribute to respiratory symptoms such as coughing, the review acknowledged that these symptoms might also be caused by other factors, such as tobacco. This possibility is highlighted by the discoveries made in Vancouver: "Smoking both tobacco and marijuana synergistically increased the risk of respiratory symptoms and COPD (chronic obstructive pulmonary disease). Smoking only marijuana was not associated with an increased risk of respiratory symptoms or COPD."[2]

Studies have shown that THC opens the upper airways and ameliorates coughing. However, smoke of any kind may cause cough, spasm, reduced lung function, or disease over long periods of time. Intravenous THC is anti-tussive in animal experiments, but has not been tested in humans. Vaporizers that heat cannabis to 350°F do not burn the plant material or produce smoke, yet released THC and other cannabinoids may mitigate the irritation of smoke. The efficacy of taking cannabis infused oils by mouth has yet to be studied. However, oromucosal sprays have been invented (UC Berkeley, US Government 2006) and can be purchased in various forms at some dispensaries. The government patent states: "The present invention unexpectedly achieves the…desired anti-tussive effects without the dysphoric side effects and habit-forming properties characteristic of centrally acting cannabimimetic or opiate drugs."[3] The researchers believe their invention to work via CB1 receptors.

STUDY SUMMARY:

Drugs	Type of Study	Published Year, Place, and Key Results	CHI
Smoked cannabis	Meta-analysis including 34 studies	2007 – Multi-institutional research team: Short-term use produces bronchodilation. Long-term use effects are inconclusive.[4]	4
Cannabinoids (incl. anandamide, THC)	Analysis	2006 – UC Berkeley, US Government: Locally acting cannabinoid agents can be administered to the airways of a subject to ameliorate cough.[5]	4
THC Intravenously	Animal study (cats)	1976 – Wallace Laboratories, Cranbury, N.J. US: THC is antitussive.[6]	2

Total CHI Value   10

STRAIN SPECIFIC CONSIDERATIONS

Anandamide and THC both bind with CB1 and CB2 receptors relatively equally. Sativa and sativa-prominent hybrids tend to present with a higher THC:CBD profile, thus presenting a relatively balanced activation, but favoring CB1.

EXPLORING MIND–BODY CONSCIOUSNESS

Coughing is a survival mechanism that by nature is a self-correcting mechanism and a means to draw one's attention. Other people nearby, especially those who care, will pay attention to a person with a sudden cough. The natural question is "Are you okay?"

However, coughing is also a means to keep people at a distance. Communicating the danger of infection: "Stay away." In a sense, coughing may represent a push – pull, as if to say "Notice me, but do not come too close."

QUESTIONS

What is stuck in my throat that needs to be expressed?
Who do I want to pay attention to me?

SUGGESTED BLESSING:

May you find a way to express yourself with ease and fun, so as to draw only positive attention and care.

May our flowers soothe, relax, and open you to the knowledge that you are loved and the certainty that your message has been heard.

Who would I like to keep at a distance?
Why do I need to be noticed?
Who is not listening to me?
Where do I feel I have not been heard?
What is not communicated until I shout it out?

ANECDOTE

Emily was on vacation in Mexico with her sister Jane and her two nieces. As soon as they got to the beach resort, Emily came down with a terrible cold and cough. She was unable to participate in any of the activities and was confined to her room. Emily was a body-mind therapist and began trying to understand the message of the cough. It did not take her long to feel that her cough was keeping Jane and her kids at a distance. She noticed that she felt angry when coughing. She realized that she did not want to be on vacation with kids, but out of misplaced family loyalties had allowed herself to agree to something that she did not really want to do. Once she realized that she had been using her cough to bark at her sister and her nieces, Emily also saw her misplaced anger. She allowed herself to gently feel her frustration and her anger at the situation, and at herself for not respecting her own preferences. As the anger dissipated, she began to let it be okay that she'd messed up. She forgave herself, and within a day or two her symptoms diminished to the point where she felt good enough to still make something of her time with her family at a lovely tropical beach resort. She had, however, learned her lesson. Future vacations were planned and executed based on respecting what she really wanted, free of obligation.

TAKE NOTICE

See supporting herbs in chapter on COLDS & FLU.

1 United States Patent Application 20060013777. Kind Code A1. Piomelli; Daniele January 19, 2006. Assignee: The Regents of the University of California. Filed September 12, 2005.

2 Tan WC, Lo C, Jong A, Xing L, Fitzgerald MJ, Vollmer WM, Buist SA, Sin DD; Vancouver Burden of Obstructive Lung Disease (BOLD) Research Group. *Marijuana and chronic obstructive lung disease: a population-based study.* iCapture Centre for Cardiovascular and Pulmonary Research, St. Paul's Hospital and the University of British Columbia, Vancouver, Canada. wtan@mrl.ubc.ca CMAJ. 2009 Apr 14;180(8):814-20.

3 United States Patent Application 20060013777. Kind Code A1. Piomelli; Daniele January 19, 2006. Assignee: The Regents of the University of California. Filed September 12, 2005.

4 Jeanette M. Tetrault, MD; Kristina Crothers, MD; Brent A. Moore, PhD; Reena Mehra, MD, MS; John Concato, MD, MS, MPH; David A. Fiellin, MD. *Effects of Marijuana Smoking on Pulmonary Function and Respiratory Complications. A Systematic Review.* Clinical Epidemiology Research Center, Department of Veterans Affairs Connecticut Healthcare System, West Haven Veterans Affairs Medical Center, West Haven, Conn (Drs Tetrault and Concato); Departments of Medicine (Drs Tetrault, Crothers, Concato, and Fiellin) and Psychiatry (Dr Moore), Yale University School of Medicine, New Haven, Conn; and Department of Medicine, Case Western University School of Medicine, Cleveland, Ohio (Dr Mehra). Arch Intern Med. 2007;167(3):221-228.

5 United States Patent Application 20060013777. Kind Code A1. Piomelli; Daniele January 19, 2006. Assignee: The Regents of the University of California. Filed September 12, 2005.

6 Gordon R, Gordon RJ, Sofia D. *Antitussive activity of some naturally occurring cannabinoids in anesthetized cats.* Wallace Laboratories, Half Acre Road, Cranbury, N.J. 08512, U.S.A. Eur J Pharmacol. 1976 Feb;35(2):309-13.

Bacterial & Viral Infections
Hepatitis

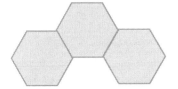

NUMBER OF STUDIES: 3

COMBINED CHI VALUE: 8

The liver is a vital and large organ located in the upper right side of the abdomen. It is the largest gland of the body, and plays a major part in a complex set of life maintaining bodily functions. The liver excretes bile stored in the gallbladder used for digestion. It is a major bodily filter ridding the body of toxic substances whether natural or chemical. It breaks down hormones and hemoglobin, and stores iron and other substances and vitamins A, D and B12. Liver cells participate in the production of glycogen, which functions as a rapid energy reserve and aids in maintaining blood volumes and clotting ability. There is no substitute for the liver. If the liver fails and is not replaced by a suitable donated liver, death results.

Hepatitis is inflammation of the liver, and is characterized as acute or chronic. Acute hepatitis usually lasts no more than a couple of months. Chronic hepatitis can be a life-long debilitating disease. Most commonly, the liver becomes inflamed as a result of the hepatic viruses A, B, C, D, or E, which are a major health problem worldwide. Viral hepatitis is contagious, while non-viral forms of hepatitis are not. However, toxins, alcohol, and many pharmacological medications such as acetaminophen or ibuprofen can also produce hepatitis. Other viruses, such as those causing yellow fever or bacterial infections like leptospirosis can affect the liver and cause inflammation. Hepatitis can also occur after ingesting poisonous mushrooms, or result from an autoimmune disease in which the body's own immune system attacks the liver.

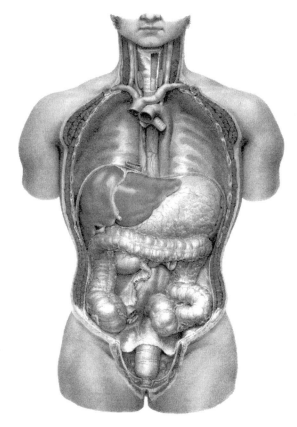

Signs and symptoms vary from one person to another and include increased generalized weakness, decreased energy levels, loss of appetite, nausea, vomiting, diarrhea, clay-colored bowel movements, pain in the joints or muscles, and headaches. Symptoms may progress to include the presence of dark urine, the yellowing of the sclera (white of the eyes) or jaundice (yellowing of the skin). Tenderness or pain in the region of the liver and enlarged spleen and lymph nodes may also be present. The general disease development of hepatitis is two-fold. The patient may go through an acute phase, then recover and gain life-long immunity (in the case of hepatitis A). Or, the illness may progress into a chronic debilitating form, leading to cirrhosis (scarring of the liver), liver cancer, and/or pre-mature death.

Within orthodox medicine, no treatment exists to destroy the hepatitis virus. Treatment focuses on supporting the body through different stages of the illness. Some of the most common pharmaceutical medications used in the management of hepatitis include immune globulin, interferon, and ribavirin. Sometimes liver transplants can sustain life.

Type	Transmission Route	Diagnosis by	Orthodox Treatment	Severity
Hepatitis A virus (HAV)	Infected fecal-oral route	Hepatitis A-specific blood test	No cure; once recovered person has life-long immunity.	Most people recover.
Hepatitis B virus (HBV)	Contact with infected bodily fluids	Hepatitis B-specific blood test	No cure	Most people recover, but for some people it can become chronic.
Hepatitis C virus (HCV)	Contact with infected blood	Hepatitis C-specific blood test	No cure	Most likely to become chronic.

CANNABIS AND HEPATITIS

Cannabinoids have demonstrated the ability to minimize the common side effects of the most common pharmaceutical treatment regimen which uses interferon and ribavirin, thus facilitating compliance with the full dose and length of the recommended treatment. In addition to mitigating adverse effects, a Colombia University study (2008) demonstrated that cannabinoids are themselves able to inhibit the virus.

STUDY SUMMARY:

Drugs	Type of Study	Published Year, Place, and Key Results	CHI
THC, anandamide	Animal study (murine)	2008 – Colombia University, New York. Multi-institutional research team: THC and anandamide and a lack of FAAH, an enzyme that breaks down anandamide, inhibits hepatitis.[1]	2
THC and nabilone	21 patients with hepatitis C undergoing interferon and ribavirin therapy	2008 – University of Ottawa, Ottawa, Canada: Oral THC and nabilone reduce nausea, vomiting, improve appetite.[2]	3
Cannabis	71 Recovering substance users with Hep. C	2006 – Department of Medicine, University of California - San Francisco: Cannabis users were able to maintain adherence to the challenging medication regimen.[3]	3

Total CHI Value 8

STRAIN SPECIFIC CONSIDERATIONS

The primary cannabinoids tested in the context of hepatitis, or as an adjunct treatment to pharmaceutical treatment of hepatitis, were THC, anandamide, nabilone, and whole plant cannabis. THC and anandamide bind relatively equally to CB1 and CB2 receptors. Nabilone is a synthetic cannabinoid similar to THC, and whole plant cannabis, depending on strain, binds to CB1 and CB2 receptors but at different ratios.

Sativas and sativa-dominant strains tend to have a higher THC:CBD ratio.

EXPLORING MIND–BODY CONSCIOUSNESS

The liver acts like a major filter, and is capable of ridding the body of physical toxins. When the liver tissue is infected and inflamed, its ability to break down toxins is diminished. As the toxic load increases, liver function continues to be impaired, ultimately producing the peculiar signs and symptoms of hepatitis.

This particular detoxification function of the liver may be mirrored in the mental-emotional realm by the accumulation of the toxins represented by unexpressed or harbored angers, resentment, rage, and fury, and also by long-standing and unresolved fears, angst, and anxieties.

Some patients completely recover and even gain life-long immunity, while others struggle with the chronic forms of hepatitis for long periods or even the rest of their lives. This fork in the road suggests that some transcend underlying issues more rapidly, while others do not.

QUESTIONS

Do I have long-standing feelings that are clogging me up and remain unprocessed?
Are a heavy load of negative feelings making me toxic?
Which emotions that I regularly experience might lead to toxic build-up?

TAKE NOTICE

BASIL • CLOVE • SAFFRON

BASIL: Basil has been used in Traditional Chinese Medicine for thousands of years. Now researchers from the island nation of Taiwan have taken a closer look at the possible anti-viral properties of basil extract. They found that extracts of basil (ocimum basilicum) exhibit a broad spectrum of antiviral activity, including combatting hepatitis B.[4]

CLOVE: A Tunesian study determined essential oil of clove extracts to have antiviral effects against Hepatitis C.[5]

SAFFRON: Crocus sativus L. or Saffron may poccess anti cancer activity including against hepatitis.[6]

SUGGESTED BLESSING:

May you find, feel and release all emotions hidden in the recesses of your mind.

May you uproot the beliefs from which they sprang.

May you succeed in seeding new and healing beliefs and attitudes.

SUGGESTED AFFIRMATION:

I embrace all my feelings with appropriate intensity and harm no one.

I can find the belief(s) which produced chronic anger or fear, and replace them with belief(s) that generate long-lasting love and wellbeing.

1 Venkatesh L. Hegde, Shweta Hegde, Benjamin F. Cravatt, Lorne J. Hofseth, Mitzi Nagarkatti and Prakash S. Nagarkatti. *Attenuation of Experimental Autoimmune Hepatitis by Exogenous and Endogenous Cannabinoids: Involvement of Regulatory T Cells.* Department of Pathology, Microbiology, and Immunology, School of Medicine, University of South Carolina, Columbia, South Carolina (V.L.H., S.H., M.N., P.S.N.); The Skaggs Institute for Chemical Biology and Departments of Cell Biology and Chemistry, The Scripps Research Institute, La Jolla, California (B.F.C.); and Department of Pharmaceutical and Biomedical Sciences, College of Pharmacy, University of South Carolina, Columbia, South Carolina (L.J.H.). Molecular Pharmacology July 2008 vol. 74 no. 1 20-33.

2 Costiniuk CT, Mills E, Cooper CL. *Evaluation of oral cannabinoid-containing medications for the management of interferon and ribavirin-induced anorexia, nausea and weight loss in patients treated for chronic hepatitis C*

virus. University of Ottawa, Ottawa, Canada. Can J Gastroenterol. 2008 Apr;22(4):376-80.

3 Diana L. Sylvestre a, Barry J. Clementsb and Yvonne Malibub b. *Cannabis use improves retention and virological outcomes in patients treated for hepatitis C.* a Department of Medicine, University of California, San Francisco, California, USA and b Organization to Achieve Solutions in Substance-Abuse (OASIS), Oakland, California, USA. Eur J Gastroenterol Hepatol. 2006 Oct;18(10):1057-63.

4 Chiang LC, Ng LT, Cheng PW, Chiang W, Lin CC. *Antiviral activities of extracts and selected pure constituents of Ocimum basilicum.* Department of Microbiology, Kaohsiung Medical University, Kaohsiung, Taiwan. Clin Exp Pharmacol Physiol. 2005 Oct;32(10):811-6.

5 Chaieb K, Hajlaoui H, Zmantar T, Kahla-Nakbi AB, Rouabhia M, Mahdouani K, Bakhrouf A. *The chemical composition and biological activity of clove essential oil, Eugenia caryophyllata (Syzigium aromaticum L. Myrtaceae): a short review.* Laboratoire d'Analyses, Traitement et Valorisation des Polluants de l'Environnement et des Produits, Faculté de Pharmacie, rue Avicenne 5000 Monastir, Tunisie. Phytother Res. 2007 Jun;21(6):501-6.

6 Deng Y, Guo ZG, Zeng ZL, Wang Z. *Studies on the pharmacological effects of saffron(Crocus sativus L.)--a review.* Dept. of Chemical Engineering, Tsinghua University, Beijing 100084, China. Zhongguo Zhong Yao Za Zhi. 2002 Aug;27(8):565-8.

Bacterial & Viral Infections
Herpes Virus

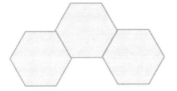

NUMBER OF STUDIES: 3

CHI VALUE: 5

Herpes is a very common virus that belongs to the same family as the chicken pox virus. There are currently eight known herpes viruses. According to orthodox medicine, all herpes viruses can exist in the body without any outward sign or symptom until a period of depressed immunity suddenly results in an outbreak. Oral herpes (cold sores or fever blisters) called HSV-1 usually appears above the waist in contrast to genital herpes (HSV-2). While HSV I and II are relatively benign physically, they often take a profound toll on the patient's emotional well-being.

No orthodox cure exists. A common allopathic treatment to "manage" herpes is Zovirax (Acyclovir). Side-effects may include nausea and/or vomiting, diarrhea, dizziness, anorexia, fatigue, swelling of the skin, skin rashes, leg pains, sore throat, and paresthesia (feeling of numbness). A month's supply for the maximum recommended dose costs about $870.

CANNABIS AND HERPES

A study conducted on humans in Münster, Germany (2010) confirmed that topical cannabinoids significantly reduce nerve pain after a flareup of the herpes virus. Both laboratory experiments from Tampa ((2004) and Johnson City (1980) showed that THC has the ability to interfere with replication of the herpes virus even in instances related to the genesis of cancer.

STUDY SUMMARY:

Drugs	Type of Study	Published Year, Place, and Key Results	CHI
Cannabinoid containing cream	Human	2010 – Münster, Germany: Majority of patients experienced pain reduction by over 80%.[1]	3
THC	Laboratory	2004 – University of South Florida, US: THC specifically targets viral and/or cellular mechanisms required for replication.[2]	1
THC	Laboratory	1980 – Johnson City, TN, U.S.: Herpes simplex I and II failed to replicate when introduced to dishes containing human cell cultures treated with THC.[3]	1

Total CHI Value 5

STRAIN SPECIFIC CONSIDERATIONS

THC binds with CB1 and CB2 receptors relatively equally. Sativas and sativa dominant hybrids have a higher THC:CBD ratio.

A study published by the American Psychosomatic Society acknowledges prior reports of precipitating emotional or psychic trauma as a component in herpes breakouts. In particular, the study focused on a patient with repeating outbreaks of HSV-I who was "… able to consciously associate a relationship between the outbreak of the skin lesions and the existence of repressed hostility."[4]

Guilt, with its demand for punishment and purification through suffering, is not benign. Guilt is damaging to oneself and to others. People who believe it is not acceptable to feel angry may be conscious only of guilt. However, since feeling angry is part of the human experience, where is the anger going to go? In the case of herpes, the unexpressed anger may shift into the physical realm. Herpes sores on the lips may represent guilt associated with affection, expressing affection, or one's inability to tell the truth, while herpes sores on the genitals may represent guilt associated with sexual activity and pleasures.

Herpes sores on the lips is punishing, forcing distance and halting kisses, a physical display of affection and intimacy whose loss impacts both members of a couple. Herpes sores on the genitals are also punishing, denying oneself and the other the experience of sexual fun, pleasure, and intimacy. In both cases, the complex function of a herpes break-out can be summarized by the practical impact it has on the patient's physical experience. It prevents sexual intimacy and displays of affection, it satisfies a need for purification through suffering, and it may assist the patient to express anger s/he believes it is not okay to feel.

People who are able to prevent or abort an outbreak acknowledge and appropriately express their emotions, fostering a deeper intimacy with themselves and others. Those who have achieved a cure have been able to change the beliefs that initially made suppression of "unacceptable" feelings seem necessary. As a result, they no longer need to suppress anger, suppress what is true for them, or suppress their sexual needs and sexual pleasure.

QUESTIONS (HSV-1)

Do I feel un-kissable, and if so, why?
What is my truth? Have I left my truth unspoken?
Why do I not want to kiss my intimate partner?
Why do I want to deny my affection?

AGGRAVATING FACTORS (HSV-1)

Guilt/anger around affection and/or kissing/pressure to be affectionate/repressed anger/hostility.

HEALING FACTORS (HSV-1)

Appropriately express anger/appropriately express personal hostile experiences/establish principles around the expression of affection.

QUESTIONS (HSV-2)

Am I angry about sex or my sexual pleasure?
Does it feel acceptable (seem reasonable) to be angry about these things?
Am I angry at my sexual partner?
Does it feel okay to be angry at my sexual partner?
Why do I want to take sex out of my relationship right now?
Who do I want to punish by not being able to have sex right now?
How can I honor my anger or guilt about sex without letting it ruin my sex life?
Can I show love and intimacy in non-sexual ways?

AGGRAVATING FACTORS (HSV-2)

Guilt/anger around sex or the genitals/guilt around perceived sexual performance pressure/repressed anger/hostility about/surrounding sex.

HEALING FACTORS (HSV-2)

Appropriately express anger related to sexuality and sexual performance/establish principles around the expression of sexuality/speak appropriately about negative sexual experiences and angers about sex/identify the beliefs underlying suppressed emotions and replace them with beliefs that produce expansive, loving sexual experiences.

TAKE NOTICE

BASIL • CARDAMOM • CLOVE • COCONUT • TURMERIC

BASIL: Researchers from the island nation of Taiwan have taken a closer look at the possible anti-viral properties of basil extract. Extracts of basil (ocimum basilicum) exhibit a broad spectrum of antiviral activity, including defending against herpes.[5]

CARDAMOM: At the University of Cincinnati College of Medicine, scientists looked at cineole, a major constituent of cardamom, in the context of treating vaginal herpes infections in mice. They determined that sufficient evidence exists to warrant more research using this promising natural treatment modality.[6]

CLOVE: In a series of experiments, Virologists from the Toyama Medical and Pharmaceutical University in Sugitani, Japan determined that eugeniine, a compound purified from the extracts of clove, inhibits viral DNA synthesis in several strains of herpes (I & II), including acyclovir-phosphonoacetic acid-resistant HSV-I.[7]

A Tunesian study determined essential oil of clove extracts has anti-viral properties against herpes.[8]

COCONUT: A crude extract of cocos nucifera L. husk fiber inhibits acyclovir-resistant herpes simplex virus type 1 (HSV-1-ACVr).[9]

TURMERIC: Researchers tested the hypothesis that curcumin, the main active

SUGGESTED BLESSING (HSV 2)

May you see the anger hiding behind your guilt.

May you use your anger like a compass to guide you to the beliefs that need changing so that healing can begin.

SUGGESTED AFFIRMATION (HSV 2)

Sex is natural and sex is fun, and it's done best with harm to no one.

constituent in turmeric, would block viral infection and gene expression of HSV-1 by inhibiting promoters of herpes gene expression. Results showed that curcumin does significantly decrease HSV-1 infectivity and IE gene expression.[10,11]

1   Phan NQ, Siepmann D, Gralow I, Ständer S. *Adjuvant topical therapy with a cannabinoid receptor agonist in facial postherpetic neuralgia.* Competence Center for the Diagnosis and Treatment of Pruritus, Clinic and Polyclinic for Skin Diseases, University Hospital of Münster, Germany. J Dtsch Dermatol Ges. 2010 Feb;8(2):88-91.

2   Maria M Medveczky, Tracy A Sherwood, Thomas W Klein, Herman Friedman, and Peter G Medveczky. *Delta-9 tetrahydrocannabinol (THC) inhibits lytic replication of gamma oncogenic herpesviruses in vitro.* Department of Medical Microbiology and Immunology, MDC Box 10, University of South Florida, and the H. Lee Moffitt Cancer Center, 12901 Bruce B. Downs Blvd, Tampa, FL 33612-4799, USA. BMC Med. 2004; 2: 34.

3   R. Dean Blevins and Michael P. Dumic. T*he Effect of -9-Tetrahydrocannabinol on Herpes Simplex Virus Replication.* Department of Biological Sciences Division of Health Sciences East Tennessee State University, Johnson City, Tenn. 37601, U.S.A. J Gen Virol 49 (1980), 427-431; DOI 10.1099/0022-1317-49-2-427

4   JEROME M. SCHNECK. *The Psychological Component in a Case of Herpes Simplex.* War Department Personnel Center, 1905 SCU Med. Det., Fort MacArthur, California. Psychosomatic Medicine 9:62-64 (1947).

5   Chiang LC, Ng LT, Cheng PW, Chiang W, Lin CC. *Antiviral activities of extracts and selected pure constituents of Ocimum basilicum.* Department of Microbiology, Kaohsiung Medical University, Kaohsiung, Taiwan. Clin Exp Pharmacol Physiol. 2005 Oct;32(10):811-6.

6   Bourne KZ, Bourne N, Reising SF, Stanberry LR. *Plant products as topical microbicide candidates: assessment of in vitro and in vivo activity against herpes simplex virus type 2.* Children's Hospital Research Foundation, Department of Pediatrics, University of Cincinnati College of Medicine, OH 45229-3039, USA. Antiviral Res. 1999 Jul;42(3):219-26.

7   Kurokawa M, Hozumi T, Basnet P, Nakano M, Kadota S, Namba T, Kawana T, Shiraki K. *Purification and characterization of eugeniin as an anti-herpesvirus compound from Geum japonicum and Syzygium aromaticum.* Virology, Toyama Medical and Pharmaceutical University, Sugitani, Toyama 930-01, Japan. J Pharmacol Exp Ther. 1998 Feb;284(2):728-35.

8   Chaieb K, Hajlaoui H, Zmantar T, Kahla-Nakbi AB, Rouabhia M, Mahdouani K, Bakhrouf A. *The chemical composition and biological activity of clove essential oil, Eugenia caryophyllata (Syzigium aromaticum L. Myrtaceae): a short review.* Laboratoire d'Analyses, Traitement et Valorisation des Polluants de l'Environnement et des Produits, Faculté de Pharmacie, rue Avicenne 5000 Monastir, Tunisie. Phytother Res. 2007 Jun;21(6):501-6.

9   Esquenazi D, Wigg MD, Miranda MM, Rodrigues HM, Tostes JB, Rozental S, da Silva AJ, Alviano CS. *Antimicrobial and antiviral activities of polyphenolics from Cocos nucifera Linn. (Palmae) husk fiber extract.* Laboratório de Biologia Celular de Fungos, Instituto de Biofísica Carlos Chagas Filho, Universidade Federal do Rio de Janeiro, 21941-590, Ilha do Fundão, Rio de Janeiro, RJ, Brazil. Res Microbiol. 2002 Dec;153(10):647-52.

10 Kutluay SB, Doroghazi J, Roemer ME, Triezenberg SJ. *Curcumin inhibits herpes simplex virus immediate-early gene expression by a mechanism independent of p300/CBP histone acetyltransferase activity.* Graduate Program in Cell and Molecular Biology, Michigan State University, East Lansing, MI 48824, USA. Virology. 2008 Apr 10;373(2):239-47.

11 Aggarwal BB, Sundaram C, Malani N, Ichikawa H. *Curcumin: the Indian solid gold.* Department of Experimental Therapeutics, The University of Texas M.D. Anderson Cancer Center, Houston, TX 77030, USA. Adv Exp Med Biol. 2007;595:1-75.

Bacterial & Viral Infections
HIV/AIDS

NUMBER OF STUDIES: 1

COMBINED CHI VALUE: 3

The mainstream of orthodox medicine considers acquired immune deficiency syndrome (AIDS) a disease of the immune system that is caused by a human immuno-deficiency virus (HIV) transmitted through sexual or blood contact.

Within a weakened immune system, infectious agents such as parasites, fungi, bacteria, or viruses encounter little resistance from our natural defenses. Regardless of where in the body the infection spreads, the response is fever, sweat, chills, and any other defenses still available. The body's natural filters, such as lymph nodes, liver, and kidneys can become overwhelmed by the invaders, which further increases symptoms of weakness, low energy, and weight loss.

This destructive process can develop into AIDS-related anorexia, cachexia, or wasting syndrome. Common opportunistic infections include lung infections by fungi (pneumocystis) or bacteria (pneumonia, tuberculosis), gastrointestinal infections such as candidiasis (thrush), infection of the nervous systems and the brain by cryptococcal meningitis (fungus), progressive multifocal leukoencephalopathy (virus), or toxoplasmosis (parasite), which can lead to neuropathies (nerve pain) and dementia. Opportunistic diseases may also take the form of cancer (Non-Hodgkin's Lymphoma), affect organs (hepatitis) or the skin (herpes).

Early signs and symptoms may include fatigue, weight loss, shortness of breath, especially during mild exertion, dry coughs, swollen lymph nodes, recurring fevers and chills, frequent episodes of diarrhea, memory loss, skin blemishes (pink, brown, purple, red) of the mucus membranes and/or the skin, candidiasis, frequent colds, coughs or pneumonia. Late-stage symptoms include higher fevers and chills lasting weeks, chronic diarrhea, and continuous weight loss that may develop into wasting, neuropathies (nerve pain), nausea and vomiting. Pneumonia may progress into tuberculosis or pneumocystis. Memory loss may gradually evolve into an altered mental state and AIDS dementia.

No AIDS diagnostic test exists, but depending on what country a person lives in, diagnosis is done by symptoms alone, by testing for HIV, or by a combination of these methods. None of the tests are 100% accurate. Oral tests are available, but produce numerous false positives, indicating HIV infection when none exists. Blood tests include the ELISA and Western blot tests. ELISA tests may yield false positives due to a variety of common pathogens and the body's anti-bodies against them. In the U.S. ELISA positive results must be confirmed by a Western blot test.

The orthodox establishment has no cure for AIDS. Current treatment consists of pharmaceutical anti-viral agents belonging to two classes, namely protease inhibitors and reverse transcriptase inhibitors.

Since the 80's, an AIDS reappraisal movement has emerged that questions many of the orthodox positions. In particular, doubts have been raised about unsubstantiated AIDS epidemic predictions, changing surveillance definitions, unreliable AIDS tests, inconsistent diagnostic methods of AIDS, inconsistent African versus US/EU AIDS presentations, unsafe AIDS pharmaceuticals, curability, the HIV – AIDS hypothesis itself, AIDS and Koch's postulates, the fact that AIDS behaves unlike a contagious disease, and the lack of focus on other possible causative or contributing elements in the development of AIDS.

CANNABIS AND HIV/AIDS (IN GENERAL)

Inspired by courageous early AIDS victims and their caretakers who discovered that cannabis reduces symptoms of AIDS and ameliorates the significant adverse effects of AIDS pharmaceuticals, scientists decided to take a closer look at cannabis in reference to AIDS. Today, a growing body of scientific evidence has elucidated how and why specific cannabinoids benefit patients with AIDS.

In one of the largest of any such studies ever conducted, scientists from Boston collected data from 775 patients living with HIV/AIDS who were suffering from six common symptoms (anxiety, depression, fatigue, diarrhea, nausea, and peripheral neuropathy). Participants came from Kenya, South Africa, Puerto Rico, and 10 different U.S. locations. Results showed that while the differences were relatively small, cannabis was more effective than standard prescription and over-the-counter (OTC) medications for treating 5 of the 6 symptoms studied: anxiety, depression, diarrhea, fatigue and neuropathy. Cannabis was slightly less effective than standard prescriptions and OTC medications for treatment of nausea.[1]

STUDY SUMMARY:

Drugs	Type of Study	Published Year, Place, and Key Results	CHI
Cannabis	775 patients living with HIV/AIDS	2009 – Boston, U.S.: Cannabis is considered effective in treating anxiety and depression, diarrhea, fatigue, and neuropathy.[2]	3

Total CHI Value 3

STRAIN SPECIFIC CONSIDERATIONS

HIV/AIDS patients use both basic strains of cannabis, but often choose a specific strain in response to the severity and presence of their unique symptoms.

EXPLORING MIND–BODY CONSCIOUSNESS

When the "AIDS epidemic" was identified in the late 70's and early 80's, entire groups of people who dared to, or had to, live differently became visible. Social and moral rejection, marginalization, and judgment (often rooted in religious beliefs) rained down on the groups who experienced AIDS first: gays, prostitutes, IV-drug users and Haitians stricken with the ill effects of abject poverty. Some voices in the religious community went so far as to call AIDS "God's punishment for breaking His rules". To many, gays were considered unnatural, prostitutes immoral, IV-drug users worthless, and contemplating sick, poor, third world minorities made people feel uncomfortable, anxious, or guilty.

AIDS was, in many ways, associated with a state of being a victim: a victim of ever-present social rejection, and a victim to a multitude of ever-present pathogens. Some people with HIV or AIDS may have turned these judgments into their bodies where issues of lack of love, hate, rage, punishment, vulnerability, defenselessness, or defensiveness became a deeply personal challenge. This challenge was further amplified by the dire early prediction of physicians and public health experts. They eagerly fanned the fires of fear, warning of a new "plague" brought about by these marginalized groups. As a result, many patients with AIDS say that, through AIDS, they "found out who really loved them" – or not.

AGGRAVATING FACTORS

Defensiveness/defenselessness/love = sex mindset/self-destructive guilt/anger/rage/hatred/self-punishment/testing who loves me/self- loathing.

HEALING FACTORS

Personal power instead of defensiveness; appropriate defenses instead of defenselessness; love is more than sex; constructive release of guilt, anger, hate, and rage; self-forgiveness instead of self-punishment; instead of testing who loves you, find elegant ways of loving and being loved; release self-hatred and loathing, and replace these with self-love and acceptance.

TAKE NOTICE

ACACIA • COCONUT

ACACIA: A study from Mumbai, presented at the 8th International Congress on Drug Therapy in HIV Infection, indicated that the aqueous extract of acacia pods was effective in-vitro against the viral enzyme reverse transcriptase.[3]

COCONUT: The authors of this study from Staten Island, New York write: "Lipids can inactivate enveloped viruses, bacteria, fungi, and protozoa." By adding medium chain fatty acids (MCFA) to HIV-infected blood products researchers learned that they could reduce virus load. Furthermore, the scientists expect that MCFA "…may potentially be used as combination spermicidal and virucidal agents."[4]

---

1 Corless IB, Lindgren T, Holzemer W, Robinson L, Moezzi S, Kirksey K, Coleman C, Tsai YF, Sanzero Eller L, Hamilton MJ, Sefcik EF, Canaval GE, Rivero Mendez M, Kemppainen JK, Bunch EH, Nicholas PK, Nokes KM, Dole P, Reynolds N. *Marijuana Effectiveness as an HIV Self-Care Strategy.* MGH Institute of Health Professions, School of nursing, Boston, Massachusetts 02129, USA. icorless@mghihp.edu Clin Nurs Res. 2009 May;18(2):172-93.

2 Ibid.

SUGGESTED AFFIRMATION (HIV)

I love myself just as I am. I accept myself just as I am.

I can raise my love to a higher octave. Sometimes just letting myself be with hate and rage is a release.

I am powerful, I am creative, and I am able to respond to insult appropriately without harming anyone.

I can respond constructively to judgments, and obtain immunity and protection.

3 Tabassum A Khan, Pratima A Tatke, Satish Y Gabhe. *Evaluation of Aqueous Extract of Babool Pods for in Vitro Anti-HIV Activity. Pharmacy,* C.U. Shah College of Pharmacy, Mumbai, Maharashtra, India. Int Cong Drug Therapy HIV 2006 Nov 12-16;8: Abstract No. P399.

4 Isaacs CE, Kim KS, Thormar H. *Inactivation of enveloped viruses in human bodily fluids by purified lipids.* Department of Developmental Biochemistry, New York State Institute for Basic Research in Developmental Disabilities, Staten Island 10314. Ann N Y Acad Sci. 1994 Jun 6;724:457-64.

Bacterial & Viral Infections
Kaposi's Sarcoma (KS)

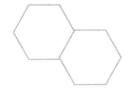

NUMBER OF STUDIES: 2

CHI VALUE: 1

Kaposi's sarcoma is an abnormal connective tissue mass, commonly presenting as multiple lesions on the skin. Moritz Kaposi first described the disease in the late 19th Century. In the early days, it was considered a cancer, a hereditary condition, or a viral infection. The confusion continued at the beginning of the "AIDS epidemic" in the early 1980's, when doctors considered it the signature disease in people diagnosed with AIDS (especially in the gay community). However, by 1994 it was established that KS is a cancer caused by a virus from the herpes family (the eighth human herpes virus), also called HHV-8 or Kaposi's sarcoma-associated herpes virus (KSHV). The allopathic community no longer considers KS to be an indication of AIDS when combined with a positive HIV test.

CANNABIS AND KAPOSI'S SARCOMA

While an Italian laboratory study (2009) discovered that a specific cannabinoid was able to inhibit KS growth, a Los Angeles (2009) experiment focused on a hypothesis proposed by Peter Duesberg that KS development may be influenced by the use of street drugs, particularly amyl nitrite ("poppers"). The results showed that a potential correlation existed between KS and poppers.

STUDY SUMMARY:

Drugs	Type of Study	Published Year, Place, and Key Results	CHI
Synthetic cannabinoid WIN-55,212-2	Laboratory	2009 – Catania, Italy: WIN-55,212-2 reduced viability of human Kaposi's sarcoma cells in vitro.[1]	1
Cannabis vs cocaine or amphetamines and poppers	401 HIV- and HHV-8-coinfected homosexual men	2009 – Los Angeles, California: Patients with a long-term history of using poppers showed a correlation between poppers (amyl nitrite) and KS. Long-term cannabis use was not correlated with an increased risk of developing KS.[2]	0

Total CHI Value   1

STRAIN SPECIFIC SUGGESTIONS

WIN-55,212-2 binds with higher affinity to CB2 receptors than CB1 receptors.

Indicas and indica-dominant strains tend to present a lower THC:CBD ratio, thus relatively favoring CB2 receptor activation.

The lesions formed by KS often develop around the nose and mouth, neck and chest, and thus are very noticeable. Even though the allopathic community was wrong in painting KS as the signature disease of AIDS, to many it retained the highly charged shame and judgment that was born from it.

KS development suggests that a combination of cancer and viral herpes patterns may be activated.

1   Luca T, Di Benedetto G, Scuderi MR, Palumbo M, Clementi S, Bernardini R, Cantarella G. *The CB(1)/CB(2) receptor agonist WIN-55,212-2 reduces viability of human Kaposi's sarcoma cells in vitro.* Department of Experimental and Clinical Pharmacology, University of Catania School of Medicine, 95125 Catania, Italy. Eur J Pharmacol. 2009 Aug 15;616(1-3):16-21.

2   Chao C, Jacobson LP, Jenkins FJ, Tashkin D, Martínez-Maza O, Roth MD, Ng L, Margolick JB, Chmiel JS, Zhang ZF, Detels R. *Recreational Drug Use and Risk of Kaposi's Sarcoma in HIV- and HHV-8-Coinfected Homosexual Men.* Department of Epidemiology and Jonsson Comprehensive Cancer Center, University of California at Los Angeles, 650 Charles E. Young Drive South, Los Angeles, CA 90095, USA. AIDS Res Hum Retroviruses. 2009 Feb;25(2):149-56.

Cancer

COMBINED NUMBER OF STUDIES: 60

COMBINED CHI VALUE: 107

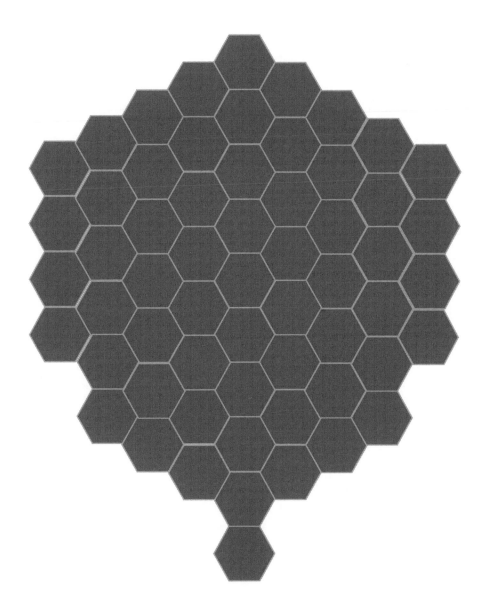

CANCER IN GENERAL

Every year, cancer takes credit for 13% of all deaths worldwide; and, according to the orthodox model of medicine, 30% of all cancers are attributed to known and avoidable risk factors.[1] Cancer-inducing materials, carcinogens, exist almost everywhere, and the list of known carcinogens grows as new information becomes available. A few of those hiding in plain view include: tobacco smoke, industrial poisons in the environment, numerous household products (laundry soap with trisodium nitrilotriacetate), bath and beauty products (containing formaldehyde), pet products (certain flea collars), certain foods (hot dogs with nitrates) and modern medical procedures emitting ionizing radiation (mammograms, CAT scans and any other x-ray devices).[2]

Certain types of infectious agents may also contribute to a cancer's development. Examples include: hepatitis B, an infection of the liver caused by a virus which may lead to liver cancer; human papillomavirus (HPV) may lead to cervical cancer; human herpes virus (HHV-8)—aka Kaposi's sarcoma-associated herpes virus (KSHV)—may produce skin cancer lesions; Helicobacter pylori may facilitate stomach cancer; and a parasite named Schistosoma Mansoni, affecting the urinary tract, may initiate bladder cancer.

Within the orthodox model of medicine, cancer (malignant neoplasm) starts with the corruption of genetic material (a mutation) inside a normally healthy cell. Evidence suggests that cellular cancer may occur quite frequently in everybody, but that normally the body's own proper immune defenses can cure these threats. However, when the body's overall health is weakened, the growth of mutations may overwhelm the capacity of the body to cure them and cancer can take over.

Scientists hypothesize that cellular corruption begins with exposure to a carcinogen (cancer producing toxin). The now-corrupted cell begins to divide, but instead of generating healthy new cells, it begins producing new cancerous cells. Most cancer cells produce tumors but can also destroy adjacent tissue (metastasize) or affect the blood in cases of leukemia. Symptoms vary greatly, depending on where the cancer is located and how far it has progressed. Orthodox treatment is usually limited to chemotherapy, surgery or radiation.

CANNABIS AND CANCER IN GENERAL

As early as 1974, the U.S. Government knew of cannabis' effectiveness against certain types of cancer. While the publication of this particular study became a victim of the war on drugs, an article about the study published by the *Washington Post* survived. The story, written by Victor Cohn, was entitled "Cancer Curb Is Studied: Doctors Eye Drug Found in Marijuana." Cohn reported the active chemical agent in marijuana curbs the growth of three kinds of cancer (lung cancer, breast cancer and viral-induced leukemia) in mice, and may also suppress the immunity reaction that causes rejection of organ transplants, a Medical College of Virginia team has discovered."[3]

Since then the scientific evidence of cannabinoids' ability to counteract certain types of cancer has grown in quantity and detail. Major scientific journals continue to report in great detail about the trial results conducted by an international community of medical researchers and scientists examining the complex impact cannabinoids play in preventing and treating specific cancer formations.

Furthermore, studies also lay claim to cannabinoids' abilities to mitigate common side-effects of chemotherapeutic agents such as cisplatin.[4]

The scientific evidence of therapeutic effects of cannabinoids for patients with specific cancers begin at the end of this section entitled "Cancer in General" (sorted alphabetically for ease of use).

STRAIN AND FORM SPECIFIC CONSIDERATIONS

The review conducted in this chapter examined the results of 60 studies relevant to the use of cannabinoids and the endocannabinoid system in the context of the prevention and treatment of 15 types of cancer. A high overall CHI value of 107 suggests with relative confidence that cannabinoids may prevent, inhibit and destroy cancer cells, as well as exhibit strong therapeutic influences to mitigate nausea, vomiting, pain, night sweats, and improve quality of life.

Research also shows that CB1 and CB2-mediated therapeutic influences may vary depending on the patient's type of cancer or symptoms. In some cases, therapeutic impact occurred via CB1; at other times, via CB2. In all other cases, it was the synergistic effects induced by activation of both CB1 and CB2 receptor sites that was therapeutic.

Sativa and sativa-heavy strains tend to present with a higher THC:CBD/CBN ratio while indicas or indica heavy hybrids tend to contain a lower THC:CBD/CBN ratio. While both strains will activate both CB1 and CB2, in comparison, indicas or indica heavy hybrids tend to activate more CB2 receptors than sativas.

Raw, fresh leaf plant matter, such as cannabis juice, for example, has a significantly higher CBD content in the form of CBD-acid with a greater affinity to activate CB2.

EXPLORING MIND–BODY–CONSCIOUSNESS

Psychotherapists followed 1,353 people over a period of ten years. The researchers discovered that in nine out of ten cases, cancer could be predicted in part on the basis of "an overly rational, anti-emotional attitude."[5] The longest study to date, conducted at John Hopkins, focused on 972 physicians who were followed over a period of 30 years. Results showed that those physicians characterized as "loners," and who were likely to suppress their emotions, were 16 times more likely to develop cancer than their more emotionally expressive peers.[6]

Psychotherapist Lawrence LeShan has worked with cancer patients for the past 50 years. Based on his extensive and numerous successful experiences with even end-stage cancer patients, he published his findings in research papers and books highlighting a common denominator shared by those patients who went into and maintained remission: authenticity, or having learned to "sing their own song in life."[7] In other words, those patients who went into remission had learned to assertively communicate their needs and honestly express their emotions, even those hitherto considered taboo.

> Disease, and especially cancer, is an invitation to find and embrace your other half, hidden in the shadowy recesses of our mind. By the same token, it is also an invitation to dance with the light; to engage whatever brings us joy, aliveness and enthusiasm.

A study conducted at the Veterans Administration Hospital in Houston, Texas, revealed a possible correlation between an individual's body-image and the location of cancer development,[8] thus indicating that psychological constructs such as how we see ourselves may play a part in how and where cancer develops.

J. C. Holland M.D. wrote: "Over the last quarter of the past century, psycho-oncology became a subspecialty of oncology with its own body of knowledge contributing to cancer care. In the new millennium, a significant base of literature,

128

SUGGESTED
BLESSING

May you realize that every feeling retrieved and embraced from the hidden recesses of your mind can serve to reduce the power of cancer.

May you become more conscious of your desire for growth and toward wholeness.

May your journey to the source of all life be the glorious return of a wise wo/man who has become one with the light and with the shadows of your own authentic life.

May you grow in the understanding that the universe offers a lot more to explore than life and death.

May you release all worry and concern about what the world wants of you, and instead be concerned with what brings you aliveness and enthusiasm.

training programs, and a broad research agenda have evolved with applications at all points on the cancer continuum: behavioral research in changing lifestyle and habits to reduce cancer risk; study of behaviors and attitudes to ensure early detection; study of psychological issues related to genetic risk and testing; symptom control (anxiety, depression, delirium, pain, and fatigue) during active treatment; management of psychological sequelae in cancer survivors; and management of the psychological aspects of palliative and end-of-life care. Links between psychological and physiological domains of relevance to cancer risk and survival are being actively explored through psychoneuroimmunology. Research in these areas will occupy the research agenda for the first quarter of the new century."[9]

Today, more than 200 different types of physical cancer classifications exist. And, while the mental/emotional architecture of a particular cancer may be unique to an individual, research suggest some common denominators: negative affect, hostility (overt and covert), lack of emotional authenticity, hopelessness, hopeless anger, and suppresses and repressed emotions foremost among them.

Often, people vulnerable to cancer share low self-esteem early in life. Overly critical authority figures, severe punishments, too much responsibility, a lack of praise or positive feedback - these all can prevent the development of healthy self-esteem. These individuals then seek others' approval to counter their own insecurity. And, while there is nothing wrong with seeking the approval of others, it is not a substitute for self-esteem.

The cancer patient with low self-esteem may attempt to control anything that threatens the social hierarchy they believe in. So they live by the rules. They never rock the boat, do not like to say no, and are nice to everyone around them in order to win their group's appreciation. By the same token, they can be very judgmental of anybody whose values diverge from "normal" within their own social group.

Human emotions against anybody in "the group/family" – emotions such as hatred, hurt, shame, worthlessness, rage or despairing hopelessness - must be hidden at all costs from the self and others. However, where are these feelings to go? Just because we deny them does not mean they don't exist. In cancer these "intolerable emotions", especially hopeless anger, demand to be acknowledged even if it kills us. Interestingly, researchers examining potential psychosomatic causes of breast cancer write: "In some of our patients, we had the feeling that the cancer was being utilized as a form of passive suicide."[10]

Cancer emerges as a living mirror of someone who has the need to demonstrate that s/he is perfect, static, unchanging, and permanent - all qualities that do not exist in life. The first physical symptoms appear. A visit to the physician produces the dreaded diagnosis. The crisis begins to erupt and grow.

Cancer dominates its environment, and stubbornly imposes its will on everything in its path. It's almost as if cancer wants to be God-like, wants to be everywhere, to have power over everything. Cancer cells are theoretically immortal and can be cultured forever. However, cancer is also dumb, as it does not realize that the ultimate destruction of the body leads to its own demise as well.

While the patient previously refused to express thoughts or feelings deemed unacceptable, her body now erupts with these suppressed aspects in a last attempt to find a home for them. The body has no other option. It has harbored these ghosts for too long. To the body, it's either evict them or die. But where can these shadow aspects go?

Now the conscious mind has a unique opportunity to take them into its fold. To own the formerly unacceptable is a step towards authenticity and wholeness that provides support for possible healing.

Constructively used, cancer can serve not only as a way to integrate the shadow self but also to help integrate formerly denied depths of love, intimacy, and passion that were previously feared and similarly hidden away. This produces a real and solid foundation of self-realization where patients fully approve of all aspects of themselves. This can naturally grow into a more solid sense of self-esteem (love I earn from myself), self-respect (comes from feeling all of my feelings), and self-worth (appreciation of my already immortal spiritual nature).

QUESTIONS

Why am I not allowed to fail?
Why is it not okay to make a mistake?
What will happen to me if I stop judging people who have different beliefs?
Why do I have to be perfect?
Why do I have to avoid conflict within my group?
Why do I feel like a nobody on the inside?
Why do I have to project a perfect image to my group?
Why can't I help somebody without making it my problem?
How can I accept a feeling I absolutely hate to feel?
Is it okay for me to feel self-important?
Is it okay for me to feel aggressive, angry or enraged at members of my group?
Can I, at least sometimes, put my needs above those of another?
Is it okay for me to be manipulative?
How can stand up for myself?
What are my needs?
How can I meet my own needs?
How can I give myself the praise I've never gotten before?
What are good ways for me to feel angry?
How can I own and release my aggression?
What happened to my will to live?
Is my desire to live stronger than that of my cancer?
How can I increase my desire to live?
Can I get angry at my cancer?
What do I want to be angry about?
Can I laugh at myself for wanting to be angry?
How can I release the anger I want?

AGGRAVATING FACTORS

Overly rational, anti-emotional attitude/suppressed or repressed anger/hopelessness[11] (hopeless anger)/tendencies for negative affect/seeking approval from other(s)/valuing absolute judgments/self-loathing (repression, or the denial of the existence of anything we hate about ourselves, e.g., self-importance)/refusal to

I am learning the most important word in the universe for me – NO!

There is nothing in my shadow that is not part of the human experience.

I can stand up for myself.

I can meet my own needs.

Sometimes my needs are more important than others.

It is okay to be angry.

I fully embrace my shadow without hurting anyone.

change/little or no self-respect (respect comes from feeling all our feelings)/lack of authenticity.

HEALING FACTORS

Appropriate release of anger/hopeless anger replaced by will, determination, and vision/replacing tendencies for negative affect with those of positive affect/developing self-esteem/values discernment over judgment/self-acceptance (especially what we hate about ourselves, e.g., self-importance)/finding positive ways of changing/developing self-respect (feeling and releasing all our feelings)/developing authenticity.

TAKE NOTICE

ACACIA • BASIL • BUSH TEA • CARAWAY • CARDAMOM • CAYENNE • CLOVE • COCOA • GARLIC • GINGER • MYRRH • NIGELLA • OREGANO • ROSEMARY • TURMERIC

ACACIA: An animal study from India found anti-tumor properties in acacia, suggesting possible cancer preventative abilities.[12]

BASIL: Basil thwarted chemical attempts to produce stomach cancer in rodents.[13]

BUSH TEA: Laboratory studies found that Bush tea possesses DNA-protective and antimutagenic properties.[14] The South African researchers who found that topical application Bush tea inhibits skin tumor formation also confirmed antimutagenic properties of Rooibos.[15]

CARAWAY: Animal research conducted in India suggests that dietary caraway (at a dose of 60mg/kg) can control lipid peroxidation and antioxidant homeostasis, thereby preventing the development of chemically-induced colon cancer lesions.[16] Japanese researchers echoed those results, and asserted that a specific compound from caraway called Ogt-O6-methylguanine-DNA methyltransferase might be responsible for the antimutagenic activity of caraway.[17]

CARDAMOM: Aqueous suspensions of cardamom retain protective effects on experimentally induced colon carcinogenesis.[18]

CAYENNE: After studying cayenne and prostate cancer in the laboratory and in patients, scientists from Madrid, Spain concluded that capsaicin in cayenne "is a promising anti-tumor agent in hormone-refractory prostate cancer, which shows resistance to many chemotherapeutic agents."[19] Injecting capsaicin directly into a tumor resulted in the retardation not just of the injected tumor but also of other similar tumors nearby.[20]

CLOVE: One study from Kolkata, India looked at the properties of aqueous solution of clove and found it to produce apoptosis of lung cancer cells in mice, as well as having other possible cancer protective properties.[21] Another Indian study determined that aqueous solution of clove might also have protective properties against skin papillomas (skin tumors).[22]

COCOA: Researchers at the Georgetown University Medical Center in Washington D.C., examined a cocoa-derived compound called pentameric procyanidin (pentamer) and discovered that it arrested human breast cancer cells in the laboratory.[23]

GARLIC: Using a rodent model, scientists from Hong Kong reported for the first time the high level of success obtained in inhibiting primary tumor formation of the prostrate and a reduction of secondary tumor formation. Another study revealed that garlic possesses potent anti-metastasis (spreading of cancer to other than the primary site) properties, which these scientists believed might also apply to other types of cancer.[24] Population-based case studies conducted in Gdansk, Poland indicated that a relatively high garlic intake reduces the risk of developing certain cancers. It seems that certain compounds contained in garlic prevent and protect against cancer in vivo and in vitro. Researchers attributed the anticancer effect of garlic to its organosulfuric compounds.[25] Diallyl disulfide, a well-known component of garlic, demonstrated repeated ability to induce apoptosis (destruction) of many different cancer cells.[26]

GINGER: Researchers proved that ginger, a spice commonly used in Korean traditional medicine and cuisine, contains the ability to protect and strengthen the heart and liver and function as an anti-inflammatory agent. Scientists are exploring ginger as a potential inhibitor of breast cancer cell growth.[27]

MYRRH: Based on traditional practice and evidence-based discoveries, a researcher from the National Institute of Health, Bethesda, U.S. reported that myrrh's significant antiseptic, anesthetic, and antitumor properties most likely stem from a specific alkene called furanosesquiterpene, present in essential oil of myrrh.[28] Scientists from the University of Texas discovered that naturally-occurring steroids (guggulsterone) from a closely related species called Commiphora mukul could produce apoptosis (destruction of cancer cells) including leukemia, head and neck carcinoma, multiple myeloma, lung carcinoma, melanoma, breast carcinoma, and ovarian carcinoma. Guggulsterone also inhibited the proliferation of drug-resistant cancer cells (e.g., gleevac-resistant leukemia, dexamethasone-resistant multiple myeloma, and doxorubicin-resistant breast cancer cells).[29]

NIGELLA: Scientists at the Henry Ford Hospital in Detroit, U.S. noted that a body of international reports, mostly from the Middle East and Asia, proved nigella possesses an antineoplastic effect (abnormal growth in cells of benign or cancerous tumors) in both the laboratory and actual patients. They isolated a component of nigella called thymoquinone and tested it in a rodent model. They discovered that the nigella-based compound produced apoptosis (the destruction of cancer cells) without notable side effects. These scientists also concluded that thymoquinone might help prevent prostate cancer.[30] A study from Béni-Mellal, Morocco showed that injecting nigella essential oil into the tumor sites significantly reduced solid tumor development, inhibited metastasis, and improved the overall survival of the test mice.[31] In a study from the University of Mississippi Medical Center scientists explored time-proven treatment techniques from the Middle East. They examined the possible therapeutic effects of catechin, found in green tea, and thymoquinone, a major compound from black seed (nigella sativa), on specific colon cancer cells. They compared the effectiveness of both natural products to the current chemotherapeutic drug of choice, 5-fluorouracil, for the treatment of colon cancer cells. Scientists determined that both the green tea catechin and the thymoquinone from nigella sativa "have demonstrated incredible chemotherapeutic responses, thus suggesting that both may have similar chemotherapeutic effects as their pharmacological counterpart 5-fluorouracil, which unlike catechin and thymoquinone has known serious side effects, including cardiac toxicity."[32]

OREGANO: Chemists at the University of Central Florida isolated several compounds from oregano. Studies showed that aristolochic acid I and II possessed cancer-fighting abilities, specifically against leukemia.[33]

ROSEMARY: Scientists from the island nation of Taiwan conducted a series of experiments using a super-critical fluid extraction technique and identified several biologically active constituents from rosemary that can be considered an herbal anti-inflammatory and anti-tumor agent.[34]

TURMERIC: Research during the past five decades, time-proven records from alternative traditions and numerous case studies point toward turmeric's ability to prevent and treat certain forms of cancer. Turmeric has the ability to diminish the creation, production and spread of a wide variety of tumor cells.[35,36]

RADIATION PROTECTION

BUSH TEA • COCOA • GARLIC • NIGELLA • NUTMEG • ROSEMARY

BUSH TEA: Laboratory studies found that Bush tea contains DNA-protective and antimutagenic properties.[37] The South African researchers who determined that topical application of Bush tea inhibits skin tumor formation also confirmed the antimutagenic properties of Rooibos.[38]

COCOA: Researchers from Tokyo, Japan discovered that cacao bean extract, among other compounds, has protective properties against wrinkles causes by excessive UV-light exposure.[39]

GARLIC: In a study from New Delhi, India scientists discovered that giving garlic extract to rodents reduced gamma ray induced damage to their chromosomes in only 5 days. The animals were given doses of 125, 250 and 500 mg of garlic extract per kilogram of body weight.[40]

NIGELLA: Doctors use ionizing radiation to treat many human cancer patients. However, the radiation does not discriminate between cancer cells and healthy cells, and can result in massive tissue damage across the board. A study from Turkey using rodents found that nigella sativa oil ingestion (1ml/kg body weight) and injections of glutathione might minimize radiation damage to healthy tissue. The study reported: "These results clearly show that NS and GSH treatment significantly antagonize the effects of radiation. Therefore, NS and GSH may be a beneficial agent in protection against ionizing radiation-related tissue injury."[41]

NUTMEG: University of Rajasthan scientists evaluated nutmeg's potential to protect mice from the damaging effects of gamma radiation. Gamma radiation resembles x-ray emissions, the major difference being its source. Both are ionizing radiations that penetrate the skin, possibly producing changes in the DNA of each cell. These permutations can result in a variety of cancers and congenital conditions, which may be passed to following generations.[42]

ROSEMARY: In a controlled study from the University of Rajasthan researchers concluded that rosemary can protect laboratory animals from the damage of ionizing radiation.[43]

(E)-β-CARYOPHYLLENE: (E)-β-Caryophyllene or (E)-BCP is a FDA-approved dietary cannabinoid that activates CB2 receptor sites and initiates potent anti-inflammatory actions and protection form oxidative stress,[44,45] both commonly associated with cancer and ill-effects of exposure to ionizing radiation. Spice plants known to contain significant amounts of (E)-BCP in descending order include: BLACK "ASHANTI PEPPER" (PIPER GUINEENSE), WHITE "ASHANTI PEPPER" (PIPER GUINEENSE), INDIAN BAY-LEAF (CINNAMOMUM TAMALA), ALLIGATOR PEPPER (AFRAMOMUM MELEGUETA), BASIL (OCIMUM MICRANTHUM), SRI LANKA CINNAMON (CINNAMOMUM ZEYLANICUM), ROSEMARY (ROSMARINUS OFFICINALIS), BLACK CARAWAY (CARUM NIGRUM), BLACK PEPPER (PIPER NIGRUM), BASIL (OCIMUM GRATISSIMUM), MEXICAN OREGANO (LIPPIA GRAVEOLENS), AND CLOVE (SYZYGIUM AROMATICUM).

1 World Health Organization. *Fact sheet No 297*. Cancer. February 2009.

2 Dr. Gofman, Professor Emeritus in Molecular and Cell Biology at the University of California at Berkeley demonstrated that that past exposure to such ionizing radiation partially caused by medical X-rays' procedures are responsible for more than 50% of all cancers, more than 50% of coronary heart disease cases, and for about 75% of the breast-cancer problem in the United States.

Gofman, John W. *Radiation from Medical Procedures in the Pathogenisis of Cancer and ischemic Heart Disease: Dose Response Studies with Physicians per 100,000 population*. 1999. San Francisco: Committee for Nuclear Responsibility.

Gofman, John W. *Preventing Breast Cancer: The Story of a Major, Proven, Preventable Cause of this Disease*. Committee for Nuclear Responsibility; 2nd edition, February 1996.

3 Victor Cohn (Washington Post Staff Writer). *Cancer Curb Is Studied: Doctors Eye Drug Found In Marijuana*. Washington Post; Aug 18, 1974.

4 Pan H, Mukhopadhyay P, Rajesh M, Patel V, Mukhopadhyay B, Gao B, Haskó G, Pacher P. *Cannabidiol at-*

tenuates cisplatin-induced nephrotoxicity by decreasing oxidative/nitrosative stress, inflammation, and cell death. Department of Urology, The First Affiliated Hospital, College of Medicine, Zhejiang University, Hangzhou, Zhejiang, China. J Pharmacol Exp Ther. 2009 Mar;328(3):708-14.

5 Grossarth-Maticek R, Siegrist J, Vetter H. *Interpersonal repression as a predictor of cancer.* Soc Sci Med. 1982;16(4):493-8.

6 Shaffer JW, Graves PL, Swank RT, Pearson TA. *Clustering of personality traits in youth and the subsequent development of cancer among physicians.* Department of Psychiatry and Behavioral Sciences, Johns Hopkins University School of Medicine, Baltimore, Maryland 21205. J Behav Med. 1987 Oct;10(5):441-7.

7 Lawrence LeShan, PhD *Cancer as a Turning Point: A Handbook for People with Cancer, Their Families, and Health Professionals.* A Plume Book. 1989.

8 SEYMOUR FISHER Ph.D., SIDNEY E. CLEVELAND Ph.D. *Relationship of Body Image to Site of Cancer.* VA Hospital, Houston, Texas. Psychosomatic Medicine 18:304-309 (1956).

9 Jimmie C. Holland, MD. *History of Psycho-Oncology: Overcoming Attitudinal and Conceptual Barriers.* Department of Psychiatry and Behavioral Sciences, Memorial Sloan-Kettering Cancer Center, and Department of Psychiatry, Weill Medical College of Cornell University, New York, NY. Psychosomatic Medicine 64:206-221 (2002).

10 C. Bacon, M.D., R. Rennekerr, M.D., and Max Cutler, M.D. A *Psychosomatic Survey of Cancer of the Breast.* Chicago Tumor Institute. Institute for Psychoanalysis of Chicago. Psychosomatic Medicine November 1, 1952 vol. 14 no. 6 453-460.

11 SA Everson, DE Goldberg, GA Kaplan, RD Cohen, E Pukkala, J Tuomilehto and JT Salonen. *Hopelessness and risk of mortality and incidence of myocardial infarction and cancer.* Human Population Laboratory, Berkeley, CA 94704-1011, USA. Psychosomatic Medicine, Vol 58, Issue 2 113-121, Copyright © 1996 by American Psychosomatic Society.

12 Meena PD, Kaushik P, Shukla S, Soni AK, Kumar M, Kumar A. *Anticancer and Antimutagenic Properties of Acacia nilotica (Linn.) on 7,12-Dimethylbenz(a)anthracene-induced Skin Papillomagenesis in Swiss Albino Mice.* Radiation and Cancer Biology Laboratory,

13 Dasgupta T, Rao AR, Yadava PK. *Chemomodulatory efficacy of basil leaf (Ocimum basilicum) on drug metabolizing and antioxidant enzymes, and on carcinogen-induced skin and forestomach papillomagenesis.* Cancer Biology and Applied Molecular Biology Laboratories, School of Life Sciences, Jawaharlal Nehru University, New Delhi, India. Phytomedicine. 2004 Feb;11(2-3):139-51.

14 Lee EJ, Jang HD. *Antioxidant activity and protective effect on DNA strand scission of Rooibos tea (Aspalathus linearis).* Department of Food and Nutrition, Hannam University, Daejeon, Korea. Biofactors. 2004; 21(1-4-):285-92.

15 Marnewick J, Joubert E, Joseph S, Swanevelder S, Swart P, Gelderblom W. *Inhibition of tumour promotion in mouse skin by extracts of rooibos (Aspalathus linearis) and honeybush (Cyclopia intermedia), unique South African herbal teas.* PROMEC Unit, Medical Research Council, P.O. Box 19070, Tygerberg 7505, South Africa. Cancer Lett. 2005 Jun 28;224(2):193-202.

16 Kamaleeswari M, Nalini N. *Dose-response efficacy of caraway (Carum carvi L.) on tissue lipid peroxidation and antioxidant profile in rat colon carcinogenesis.* Department of Biochemistry, Annamalai University, Annamalainagar, 608 002, Tamilnadu, India. J Pharm Pharmacol. 2006 Aug;58(8):1121-30.

17 Mazaki M, Kataoka K, Kinouchi T, Vinitketkumnuen U, Yamada M, Nohmi T, Kuwahara T, Akimoto S, Ohnishi Y. *Inhibitory effects of caraway (Carum carvi L.) and its component on N-methyl-N'-nitro-N-nitrosoguanidine-induced mutagenicity.* Department of Molecular Bacteriology, Institute of Health Biosciences, The University of Tokushima Graduate School, Japan. J Med Invest. 2006 Feb;53(1-2):123-33.

18 Sengupta A, Ghosh S, Bhattacharjee S. *Dietary cardamom inhibits the formation of azoxymethane-induced*

aberrant crypt foci in mice and reduces COX-2 and iNOS expression in the colon. Department of Cancer Chemoprevention, Chittaranjan National Cancer Institute, Kolkata 700026, India. Asian Pac J Cancer Prev. 2005 Apr-Jun;6(2):118-22.

19 Sánchez AM, Sánchez MG, Malagarie-Cazenave S, Olea N, Díaz-Laviada I. *Induction of apoptosis in prostate tumor PC-3 cells and inhibition of xenograft prostate tumor growth by the vanilloid capsaicin.* Department of Biochemistry and Molecular Biology, School of Medicine, University of Alcalá, Alcalá de Henares, Madrid, 28871, Spain. Apoptosis. 2006 Jan;11(1):89-99.

20 Beltran J, Ghosh AK, Basu S. *Immunotherapy of tumors with neuroimmune ligand capsaicin.* Center for Immunotherapy of Cancer and Infectious Diseases, University of Connecticut School of Medicine, 263 Farmington Avenue, Farmington, CT 06030-1601, USA. J Immunol. 2007 Mar 1;178(5):3260-4.

21 Banerjee S, Panda CK, Das S. *Clove (Syzygium aromaticum L.), a potential chemopreventive agent for lung cancer.* Department of Cancer Chemoprevention, Chittarajan National Cancer Institute, 37, S.P. Mukherjee Road, Kolkata 700026, India. Carcinogenesis. 2006 Aug;27(8):1645-54.

22 Banerjee S, Das S. *Anticarcinogenic effects of an aqueous infusion of cloves on skin carcinogenesis.* Dept. of Cancer Chemoprevention, Chittarajan National Cancer Institute, 37 S.P. Mukherjee Road, Kolkata 700026, West Bengal, India. Asian Pac J Cancer Prev. 2005 Jul-Sep;6(3):304-8.

23 Ramljak D, Romanczyk LJ, Metheny-Barlow LJ, Thompson N, Knezevic V, Galperin M, Ramesh A, Dickson RB. *Pentameric procyanidin from Theobroma cacao selectively inhibits growth of human breast cancer cells.* Department of Oncology, The Research Building, Room W417, Lombardi Comprehensive Cancer Center, Georgetown University Medical Center, 3970 Reservoir Road, NW, Washington, District of Columbia 20057, USA. Mol Cancer Ther. 2005 Apr;4(4):537-46.

24 Howard EW, Ling MT, Chua CW, Cheung HW, Wang X, Wong YC. *Garlic-derived S-allylmercaptocysteine is a novel in vivo antimetastatic agent for androgen-independent prostate cancer.* Cancer Biology Group, Department of Anatomy, Faculty of Medicine, University of Hong Kong, Hong Kong. Clin Cancer Res. 2007 Mar 15;13(6):1847-56.

25 Herman-Antosiewicz A, Powolny AA, Singh SV. *Molecular targets of cancer chemoprevention by garlic-derived organosulfides.* Department of Molecular Biology, University of Gdansk, Kladki 24, 80-822 Gdask, Poland. Acta Pharmacol Sin. 2007 Sep;28(9):1355-1364.

26 Lu HF, Yang JS, Lin YT, Tan TW, Ip SW, Li YC, Tsou MF, Chung JG. *Diallyl Disulfide Induced Signal Transducer and Activatorof Transcription 1 Expression in Human Colon CancerColo 205 Cells using Differential Display RT-PCRy.* Department of Clinical Pathology, Cheng Hsin Rehabilitation Medical Center, Taipei, Taiwan, R.O.C. Cancer Genomics Proteomics. 2007 Mar-Apr;4(2):93-8.

27 Lee HS, Seo EY, Kang NE, Kim WK. *[6]-Gingerol inhibits metastasis of MDA-MB-231 human breast cancer cells.* Department of Sports Sciences, Seoul Sports Graduate University, Seoul 150-034, South Korea. J Nutr Biochem. 2007 Jul 31.

28 Nomicos EY. *Myrrh: medical marvel or myth of the magi?* National Institute of Allergy and Infectious Diseases, National Institute of Health, Bethesda, Maryland. Holist Nurs Pract. 2007 Nov-Dec;21(6):308-23.

29 Shishodia S, Sethi G, Ahn KS, Aggarwal BB. *Guggulsterone inhibits tumor cell proliferation, induces S-phase arrest, and promotes apoptosis through activation of c-Jun N-terminal kinase, suppression of Akt pathway, and downregulation of antiapoptotic gene products.* Cytokine Research Laboratory, Department of Experimental Therapeutics, Unit 143, The University of Texas M. D. Anderson Cancer Center, 1515 Holcombe Boulevard, Houston, TX 77030, United States. Biochem Pharmacol. 2007 Jun 30;74(1):118-30.

30 Kaseb AO, Chinnakannu K, Chen D, Sivanandam A, Tejwani S, Menon M, Dou QP, Reddy GP. *Androgen receptor and E2F-1 targeted thymoquinone therapy for hormone-refractory prostate cancer.* Department of Hematology/Oncology, Henry Ford Hospital, MI 458202, USA. Cancer Res. 2007 Aug 15;67(16):7782-8.

31 Ait Mbarek L, Ait Mouse H, Elabbadi N, Bensalah M, Gamouh A, Aboufatima R, Benharref A, Chait A,

Kamal M, Dalal A, Zyad A. *Anti-tumor properties of blackseed (Nigella sativa L.) extracts.* Laboratory of Immunology, Biochemistry and Molecular Biology, Faculty of Sciences and Technologies, Cadi-Ayyad University, Béni-Mellal, Morocco. Braz J Med Biol Res. 2007 Jun;40(6):839-47.

32 Norwood AA, Tucci M, Benghuzzi H. *A comparison of 5-fluorouracil and natural chemotherapeutic agents, EGCG and thymoquinone, delivered by sustained drug delivery on colon cancer cells.* University of Mississippi Medical Center, 2500 North State Street, Jackson, Mississippi 39216, USA. Biomed Sci Instrum. 2007;43:272-7

33 Goun E, Cunningham G, Solodnikov S, Krasnykch O, Miles H. *Antithrombin activity of some constituents from Origanum vulgare.* Department of Chemistry, University of Central Florida, Orlando, FL 32816, USA. Fitoterapia. 2002 Dec;73(7-8):692-4.

34 Peng CH, Su JD, Chyau CC, Sung TY, Ho SS, Peng CC, Peng RY. *Supercritical fluid extracts of rosemary leaves exhibit potent anti-inflammation and anti-tumor effects.* Division of Basic Medical Science, Hungkuang University, No 34, Chung Chie Rd, Shalu County, Taichung Hsien, 43302, Taiwan. Biosci Biotechnol Biochem. 2007 Sep;71(9):2223-32.

35 Goel A, Kunnumakkara AB, Aggarwal BB. *Curcumin as "Curecumin" From kitchen to clinic.* Gastrointestinal Cancer Research Laboratory, Department of Internal Medicine, Charles A. Sammons Cancer Center and Baylor Research Institute, Baylor University Medical Center, Dallas, TX, United States. Biochem Pharmacol. 2007 Aug 19.

36 Aggarwal BB, Kumar A, Bharti AC. *Anticancer potential of curcumin: preclinical and clinical studies.* Cytokine Research Section, Department of Bioimmunotherapy, University of Texas M. D. Anderson Cancer Center, 1515 Holcombe Boulevard, Box 143, Houston, TX, USA. Anticancer Research. 2003 Jan-Feb;23(1A):363-98.

37 Lee EJ, Jang HD. *Antioxidant activity and protective effect on DNA strand scission of Rooibos tea (Aspalathus linearis).* Department of Food and Nutrition, Hannam University, Daejeon, Korea. Biofactors. 2004; 21(1-4-):285-92.

38 Marnewick J, Joubert E, Joseph S, Swanevelder S, Swart P, Gelderblom W. *Inhibition of tumour promotion in mouse skin by extracts of rooibos (Aspalathus linearis) and honeybush (Cyclopia intermedia), unique South African herbal teas.* PROMEC Unit, Medical Research Council, P.O. Box 19070, Tygerberg 7505, South Africa. Cancer Lett. 2005 Jun 28;224(2):193-202.

39 Mitani H, Ryu A, Suzuki T, Yamashita M, Arakane K, Koide C. *Topical application of plant extracts containing xanthine derivatives can prevent UV-induced wrinkle formation in hairless mice.* Photodermatol Photoimmunol Photomed. 2007 Apr-Jun;23(2-3):86-94.

40 Singh SP, Abraham SK, Kesavan PC. *Radioprotection of mice following garlic pretreatment.* School of Life Sciences, Jawaharlal Nehru Unviersity, New Delhi, India. Br J Cancer Suppl. 1996 Jul;27:S102-4.

41 Cemek M, Enginar H, Karaca T, Unak P. *In vivo radioprotective effects of Nigella sativa L oil and reduced glutathione against irradiation-induced oxidative injury and number of peripheral blood lymphocytes in rats.* Department of Chemistry, Biochemistry Division, Faculty of Science and Arts, Afyon Kocatepe University, Afyon, Turkey. mcemek@yahoo.com Photochem Photobiol. 2006 Nov-Dec;82(6):1691-6.

42 Sharma M, Kumar M. *Radioprotection of Swiss albino mice by Myristica fragrans houtt.* Cell and Molecular Biology Lab, Department of Zoology, University of Rajasthan, Jaipur, India. J Radiat Res (Tokyo). 2007 Mar;48(2):135-41.

43 Soyal D, Jindal A, Singh I, Goyal PK. *Modulation of radiation-induced biochemical alterations in mice by rosemary (Rosemarinus officinalis) extract.* Radiation and Cancer Biology Laboratory, Department of Zoology, University of Rajasthan, Jaipur 302004, India. Phytomedicine. 2007 Oct;14(10):701-5.

44 Béla Horvátha, Partha Mukhopadhyaya, Malek Kechrida, Vivek Patela, Gali Tanchiana, David *A. Winkb, Jürg Gertschc, Pál Pachera. β-Caryophyllene ameliorates cisplatin-induced nephrotoxicity in a cannabinoid 2 receptor-dependent manner.* a Laboratory of Physiologic Studies, National Institute on Alcohol Abuse and Alcoholism, National Institutes of Health, Bethesda, MD 20892, USA. b Radiation Biology Branch, National Cancer

Institute, National Institutes of Health, Bethesda, MD 20892, USA. c Institute of Biochemistry and Molecular Medicine, University of Bern, 3012 Bern, Switzerland. Free Radical Biology and Medicine. Volume 52, Issue 8, 15 April 2012, Pages 1325–133.

45 Gertsch J, Leonti M, Raduner S, Racz I, Chen JZ, Xie XQ, Altmann KH, Karsak M, Zimmer A. *Beta-caryophyllene is a dietary cannabinoid.* Institute of Pharmaceutical Sciences, Department of Chemistry and Applied Biosciences, Eidgenössische Technische Hochschule (ETH) Zurich, 8092 Zürich, Switzerland. Proc Natl Acad Sci U S A. 2008 Jul 1;105(26):9099-104.

Cancer
Bone Cancer

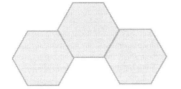

NUMBER OF STUDIES: 3

CHI VALUE: 8

This type of cancer is relatively rare. Here, cancer cells proliferate within the bones' tissues, eventually forming tumors. Orthodox medicine differentiates between bone cancers that originate in the bone, calling these primary, and secondary cancers that develop in the bone tissue after spreading from another place (metastasizing).

Tumors may develop slowly, over time, making their presence known through gradually increasing discomforts, visible deformities, and pain. The tumor often exerts pressure from the inside, which, combined with loss of bone density and strength, may produce fractures of the bones or make them much more vulnerable to breakage.

Orthodox medicinal treatments are limited to chemotherapy, radiation, and surgeries (amputations).

CANNABIS AND BONE CANCER

Patients with bone cancer are often stricken with severe pain. Opiates, while perhaps reducing the pain initially, have been recently associated with further bone destruction, thus contributing to more pain over time. A Tuscon study (2010) treated animals with bone cancer using peripheral synthetic cannabinoids (AM1241) to determine whether the treatment merited any therapeutic potential. Results suggested that daily use (over 7 days) of AM1241 significantly reduced both spontaneous and evoked bone cancer pain. Further, the authors of the study discovered that sustained use of AM1241 significantly reduced bone loss and decreased the incidence of cancer-induced bone fractures. Thus, the CB2 cannabinoid AM1241, achieved reductions in pain, bone cancer induced fractures, and bone loss without the detrimental effects of opiates in animals with bone cancer.[1]

Similarly, researchers from Minnesota (2008) wanted to lean more about the role of endocannabinoids on pain associated with bone cancer. Higher levels of anandamide reduced pains, while lower levels increased pains. The results of this rodent study prompted the authors to write: "the data provides evidence that manipulation of peripheral endocannabinoid signaling is a promising strategy for the management of bone cancer pain."[2]

Lastly, British scientists (2008) conducted a review of the existing literature of cannabinoids and bone disorders which supported the notion that "cannabinoid receptor ligands show a great promise in the treatment of bone diseases associated with accelerated osteoclastic bone resorption, including osteoporosis, rheumatoid arthritis, and bone metastasis."[3]

STUDY SUMMARY:

Drugs	Type of Study	Published Year, Place, and Key Results	CHI
AM1241	Animal study (murine)	2010 – University of Arizona: Reduction in bone cancer pain, bone cancer induced fractures and bone loss without the detrimental effects of opiates.[1]	2
Anandamide (AEA)	Animal study (mice)	2008 – University of Minnesota: Higher levels of anandamide reduced pain.[2]	2
Endocannabinoid system	Review	2008 – University of Edinburgh: Cannabinoid receptors show a great promise in the treatment bone metastasis.[3]	4

Total CHI Value 8

STRAIN SPECIFIC CONSIDERATIONS

The animal study from Tucson, Arizona employed the CB2 stimulating synthetic cannabinoid AM1241. Similarly, CBD has a greater affinity for CB2 receptors than for CB1.

Indica strains have relatively less THC and relatively more CBD/CBN, thus favoring CB2 signaling.

EXPLORING MIND–BODY CONSCIOUSNESS

The human body contains 206 bones.[4] The skeleton protects vital organs and produces a rigid support system which enables the attached flexible counter system of muscles to exert force, allowing the body to contract and expand, thereby producing movement and enabling physical tasks.

Interestingly, a bone's hollowness provides its strength and light weight. The hard outer material is made from collagen and minerals, while the inside is filled with soft and spongy yellow and red bone marrow. Red marrow produces blood cells and yellow marrow stores fat cells as energy reserves.

Thus, the outer shell of bones can be thought of as representing protection and support while the inner parts correlate to blood (family, tribe, joy of life) and energy reserves (passion, intensity). Bone cancer ultimately causes the complete reversal of protection and support where these natural functions are replaced by attack and destruction.

Unexpressed and longstanding resentment or guilt about having to uphold the rules, laws, and regulations of the family or tribe may become the force that ultimately destroys the patient's own protection and support.

Often the internal architecture of guilt is a self-imposed mechanism to force adherence to the perceived rules that 'should' be complied with. Fractures result from built-up pressure exerted by the growing resentments and accumulated guilt for railing against outside authority, the fathers, the rulers, the gods, and their "shoulds" and "shouldn'ts." At this point, patients are unable to move about and are limited in their ability to complete daily tasks.

QUESTIONS

What will you do if I express my hatred for the rules?

What will happen if I let myself rail against my adopted authority?
Will I still be protected, supported, and loved if I do not follow the outside rules?
Can I become my own authority?

1 Lozano-Ondoua AN, Wright C, Vardanyan A, King T, Largent-Milnes TM, Nelson M, Jimenez-Andrade JM, Mantyh PW, Vanderah TW. A cannabinoid 2 receptor agonist attenuates bone cancer-induced pain and bone loss. Department of Pharmacology, College of Medicine, The University of Arizona, Tucson, AZ 85724, United States. Life Sci. 2010 Apr 24;86(17-18):646-53.

2 Khasabova IA, Khasabov SG, Harding-Rose C, Coicou LG, Seybold BA, Lindberg AE, Steevens CD, Simone DA, Seybold VS. A decrease in anandamide signaling contributes to the maintenance of cutaneous mechanical hyperalgesia in a model of bone cancer pain. Department of Diagnostic/Biological Sciences, University of Minnesota, Minneapolis, Minnesota 55455, USA. J Neurosci. 2008 Oct 29;28(44):11141-52.

3 Idris AI. Role of cannabinoid receptors in bone disorders: alternatives for treatment. Bone Research Group, Rheumatic Diseases Unit, University of Edinburgh, General Western Hospital, Edinburgh. Drug News Perspect. 2008 Dec;21(10):533-40.

4 If the sternum is counted as 3 bones, the total number of bones is 208.

SUGGESTED AFFIRMATION

Based on my authentic passion, I choose my own ideals.

I make my own rules as to how to get closer to my ideals.

I am the only enforcer of my rules.

I employ forgiveness, joy, love, and intimacy.

I can express all my feelings with ease and fun, and harm to none.

Cancer
Brain Cancer

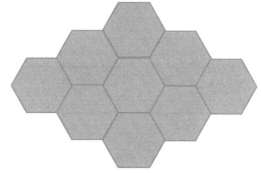

NUMBER OF STUDIES: 9

CHI VALUE: 26

The location and size of cancerous brain tumors largely determines survivability and the various signs and symptoms likely to develop. As tumors grow impairment increases. As a result the whole body as well as the mind may be impacted. Generally speaking, the lower in the brain structurethe tumor is, the poorer the survival outcome. This is because the brain's lower portions control most vital functions such as breathing or heart rate.

Signs and symptoms cover a relatively wide range and can include altered levels of consciousness ranging from mild confusion to epileptic seizures, from odd behavior to full-blown stroke-like handicaps. Additional commonly reported symptoms include headache, visual impairments, and nausea with vomiting.

Orthodox medicine does not know what causes brain cancer. It can neither prevent nor cure it. Its methods of diagnosis include a careful patient history and physical examination, electroencephalography (EEG) measuring the electrical activity of the brain, an extensive eye examination, and the use of imaging techniques such as MRI or CT scans.[1] However, within this model of medicine a definite diagnosis can only be arrived at by using a needle biopsy (a risky procedure of sticking a needle into the affected part of the brain), open brain surgery, or an autopsy. Management consists of the usual three: chemotherapy, radiation, and surgery. Brain cancer progression and treatment may leave the patient with severe impairment, similar to a stroke victim. The five-year survival rate for the most common brain tumors (glioblastomas, astrocytomas, and meningiomas) is 2%, 30% and 70% respectively.[2]

CANNABIS AND BRAIN CANCER

Starting in 2001, an international research team began looking at cannabinoids and brain cancer. The team demonstrated that local injections of the synthetic cannabinoid JWH-133 (a potent CB2 receptor agonist) into mice with brain cancer cells implanted beneath their skin considerably reduced the malignant tumors' sizes.[3] By 2003, two Italian studies expanded our understanding of brain cancer and cannabinoids by suggesting that the non-psychoactive CBD was able to produce a significant anti-brain tumor activity, both in vitro and in vivo,[4] and that CBD selectively produced oxidative stress in brain cancer cells, thus producing apoptosis, leaving normal cells unaffected.[5]

A 2004 Spanish experiment produced another perspective as to why cannabinoids may present a new therapy for patients suffering from brain cancer. Results showed that cannabinoids effectively inhibited a chemical signal needed for the brain tumor to build its blood supply, an essential element for its survival and proliferation. The Spanish researchers considered the blockade of this signal to be one of the most promising antitumoral approaches currently available, and proposed a novel pharmacological target for cannabinoid-based therapies."[6]

To discover whether THC could be injected safely into humans, scientists from Madrid enlisted the cooperation of nine patients with brain cancers which had failed to respond to the standard treatments of either surgery or radiation. The researchers concluded that THC could be safely injected into human brain tumors without causing any overt psychoactive effects.[7]

In 2008, a team of researchers from Israel discovered another way in which cannabinoids may mitigate brain cancer. In this study E2F1 and Cyclin A, two proteins that promote cell cycle progression, were down-regulated and later able to arrest glioblastoma multiforme (brain cancer cells) under the influence of THC.[8]

Several Spanish studies conducted on mice and humans with recurring glioblastoma multiforme brain cancers suggest two more mechanisms by which cannabinoids may counteract cancer. Tissue inhibitors of metalloproteinases (TIMPs) play critical roles in the acquisition of migrating tumor cells and their invasive capacities. TIMP-1 up-regulation is associated with high malignancy and negative prognosis of numerous cancers. Similarly, as matrix metalloproteinase (MMP)-2 up-regulation is associated with high progression and poor prognosis of gliomas (brain cancer), scientists discovered that TIMP-1 down-regulation and MMP down-regulation may be hallmarks of cannabinoid-induced inhibition of glioma progression.[9]

In a more recently published San Francisco study (2010) on brain cancer and cannabinoids, researchers showed in part that two cannabinoids, THC and CBD, acted synergistically to inhibit brain cancer cell growth by inducing reactive oxygen species to produce apoptosis (cancer cell death).[10]

STUDY SUMMARY:

Drugs	Type of Study	Published Year, Place, and Key Results	CHI
CBD and THC	Animal study (rodent)	2010 – California Pacific Medical Center Research Institute, San Francisco, California: Both cannabinoids acted synergistically to inhibit cancer cell growth by inducing reactive oxygen species to produce apoptosis.[11]	2
THC and JWH-133 injected into the tumors of mice	Animal study and 2 human patients with recurrent glioblastoma multiforme (grade IV astrocytoma)	2008 – Complutense University, Madrid, Spain: TIMP-1 down-regulation may be a hallmark of cannabinoid-induced inhibition of glioma progression.[12]	2+3
THC and JWH-133	Animal study and 2 human patients with recurrent glioblastoma multiforme	2008 – Complutense University, Madrid, Spain: MMP-2 down-regulation constitutes a new hallmark of cannabinoid antitumoral activity.[13]	2+3
THC	Laboratory study	2008 – Multi-institutional research team, Israel: THC is shown to significantly affect viability of glioblastoma multiforme (GBM) by downregulation of E2F1 and Cyclin.[14]	1

Drugs	Type of Study	Published Year, Place, and Key Results	CHI
Intracranial injections of THC into the tumor site	Nine end-stage brain cancer patients with recurrent glioblastoma multi forme	2006 – Complutense University, Madrid, Spain: Cannabinoid delivery was safe.[15]	3
THC, WIN-55-,212-2 and anandamide	Laboratory, animal (mice) and human tests	2004 – Multi-institutional research team: Reduced VEGF gene expression, depressed VEGF pathways, decreased production of VEGF, and decreased the activation of VEGF receptors in the brain cancer cells. Corresponding reductions in tumor size in mice.[16]	2+3
Cannabidiol (CBD) e at 0.5mg per mouse	Laboratory and animal tests (mice)	2003 – Multi-institutional research team: Apoptosis of U87 and U373 human glioma cell lines in the laboratory and significant growth inhibition of U87 implanted in mice.[17]	2
Cannabidiol	Laboratory	2003 – University of Milan, Italy: CBD selectively produces oxidative stress in brain cancer cells thus producing apoptosis but not in normal cells.[18]	1
JWH-133 (local injection into tumor 50 µg/day)	Animal tests (mice)	2001 – International & multi-institutional research team: Induced a considerable regression in size of the malignant tumors.[19]	2

Total CHI Value   26

STRAIN AND FORM SPECIFIC CONSIDERATIONS

Both THC and CBD have been found to be potent inhibitors of cancer cell development and to produce apoptosis (cancer cell death). Each works independently in this regard; still greater effect may be produced synergistically when THC and CBD are applied together.

Both basic strains (sativa and indica) deliver the full range of plant cannabinoids. Most patients consider their mental and emotional preferences before determining if a more relaxing or uplifting effect is needed. Indicas are considered generally more relaxing, sedating, or grounding while sativas are more energizing or uplifting. Patients wishing to employ a non-psychoactive form of plant material may take raw juice made from fresh cannabis leaves.

EXPLORING MIND–BODY CONSCIOUSNESS

SUGGESTED BLESSING

May you make it easy for you to trust the process of life.

May you choose authentic beliefs, birthed by your free will and your conscious care.

The brain commonly represents the physical structure associated with the mind; we often use the words mind and brain interchangeably. Both are considered the seat of free will, consciousness, and the authority to govern actions of the body.

Cancer in the brain affects the mind and the whole body, forcing changes of great magnitude. Formerly independent people may become unable to communicate normally, walk, or even complete simple tasks without help. Brain cancer severely disrupts the status quo of free will, consciousness, and the authority to govern actions of the body.

Another consideration centers on the brain's naturally soft and moist environment, consisting of a folded mass of grey matter that thrives on constant changes delivered by the senses. Rigid adherence to mental constructs fueled by fears of change or an unwillingness to change may cause friction in a naturally soft and ever-changing organ.

The mind/brain interprets the continuously incoming sensual data it receives and delivers a response. This is the realm of choices, decisions, thoughts, feelings, attitudes, and beliefs. Cancer in this realm may be reflective of conflicting beliefs, and thereby conflicting thoughts and feelings, making the mind and by association the brain an internal battlefield. The strain of this internal battle against change drains energy, increasing the body's vulnerability.

Change is thrust upon the patient. The body thus becomes the stage to act out the stubborn patterns that may have kept the patient from accepting and working in a healthy way with the inevitable nature of life – change.

It is important to remember that in the context of healing, a particular belief (system) is never right or wrong, but measured by its ability to support health of an individual and the healing process of the patient.

1 CT scans produce a relative high exposure to cancer causing ionizing radiation.

2 Tanya S. Surawicz, Faith Davis, Sally Freels, Edward R. Laws and Herman R. Menck. *Brain tumor survival: Results from the National Cancer Data Base.* Journal of Neuro-Oncology. 1998. Volume 40, Number 2, 151-160.

3 Cristina Sanchez,2 Maria L. de Ceballos,2 Teresa Gomez del Pulgar,2 Daniel Rueda, Cesar Corbacho, Guillermo Velasco, Ismael Galve-Roperh, John W. Huffman, Santiago Ramon y Cajal, and Manuel Guzman.3 *Inhibition of Glioma Growth in Vivo by Selective Activation of the CB2 Cannabinoid Receptor.* Department of Biochemistry and Molecular Biology I, School of Biology, Complutense University, 28040 Madrid, Spain [C. S., T. G. d. P., D. R., G. V., I. G-R., M. G.]; Neurodegeneration Group, Cajal Institute, CSIC, 28002 Madrid, Spain [M. L. d. C.]; Department of Pathology, Clínica Puerta de Hierro, 28035 Madrid, Spain [C. C., S. R. y C.]; and Department of Chemistry, Clemson University, Clemson, South Carolina 29634-1905 [J. W. H.] CANCER RESEARCH 61, 5784 –5789, August 1, 2001.

4 Paola Massi, Angelo Vaccani, Stefania Ceruti, Arianna Colombo, Maria P. Abbracchio and Daniela Parolaro. *Antitumor Effects of Cannabidiol, a Nonpsychoactive Cannabinoid, on Human Glioma Cell Lines.* Department of Pharmacology, Chemotherapy and Toxicology (P.M., A.C.), and Department of Pharmacological Sciences, School of Pharmacy, and Center of Excellence for Neurodegenerative Diseases, University of Milan, Milan, Italy (S.C., M.P.A.); and Department of Structural and Functional Biology, Pharmacology Unit and Center of Neuroscience, University of Insubria, Busto Arsizio (Varese), Italy (A.V., D.P.) JPET March 2004 vol. 308 no. 3 838-845.

5 Massi P, Vaccani A, Bianchessi S, Costa B, Macchi P, Parolaro D. *The non-psychoactive cannabidiol triggers caspase activation and oxidative stress in human glioma cells.* Department of Pharmacology, Chemotherapy and Medical Toxicology, University of Milan, via Vanvitelli 32, 20129 Milan, Italy. Cell Mol Life Sci. 2006 Sep;63(17):2057-66.

6 Cristina Blázquez 1 , Luis González-Feria 4 , Luis Álvarez 2 , Amador Haro 1 , M. Llanos Casanova 3 , and Manuel Guzmán 1 Cannabinoids Inhibit the Vascular Endothelial Growth Factor Pathway in Gliomas. 1Department of Biochemistry and Molecular Biology I, School of Biology, Complutense University; 2 Research Unit, La Paz University Hospital; 3 Project on Cellular and Molecular Biology and Gene Therapy, CIEMAT, Madrid, Spain; and 4 Department of Neurosurgery, University Hospital, Tenerife, Spain. Cancer Res August 15, 2004 64; 5617.

7 Guzman M, Duarte MJ, Blazquez C, Ravina J, Rosa MC, Galve-Roperh I, Sanchez C, Velasco G, Gonzalez-Feria L. *A pilot clinical study of Delta(9)-tetrahydrocannabinol in patients with recurrent glioblastoma multiforme.* Department of Biochemistry and Molecular Biology I, School of Biology, Complutense University, Madrid 28040, Spain. Br J Cancer 2006;95(2):197-203.

8 Gil Galanti1,2, Tamar Fisher2, Iris Kventsel2, Jacob Shoham1, Ruth Gallily3, Raphael Mechoulam4, Gad Lavie5, Ninette Amariglio2, Gideon Rechavi2 and Amos Toren2† *Δ9-Tetrahydrocannabinol inhibits cell cycle pro-*

gression by downregulation of E2F1 in human glioblastoma multiforme cells. 1The Mina and Everard Goodman Faculty of Life Science, Bar-Ilan University, Ramat-Gan, Israel 2Department of Pediatric Hemato-Oncology, Safra Children's Hospital, Sheba Medical Center, Tel Hashomer, Israel 3The Lautenberg Center for General and Tumor Immunology, The Hebrew University Medical Faculty, Ein Kerem Campus, Jerusalem, Israel 4Department of Medicinal Chemistry and Natural Products, Hebrew University Medical Faculty, Jerusalem, Israel 5Blood Center, Sheba Medical Center, Tel-Hashomer, Israel. Acta Oncologica, 2008; 47: 1062

9 Blázquez C, Carracedo A, Salazar M, Lorente M, Egia A, González-Feria L, Haro A, Velasco G, Guzmán M. *Down-regulation of tissue inhibitor of metalloproteinases-1 in gliomas: a new marker of cannabinoid antitumoral activity?* Department of Biochemistry and Molecular Biology I, School of Biology, Complutense University, 28040 Madrid, Spain. Neuropharmacology. 2008 Jan;54(1):235-43.

10 Marcu JP, Christian RT, Lau D, Zielinski AJ, Horowitz MP, Lee J, Pakdel A, Allison J, Limbad C, Moore DH, Yount GL, Desprez PY, McAllister SD. *Cannabidiol Enhances the Inhibitory Effects of {Delta}9-Tetrahydrocannabinol on Human Glioblastoma Cell Proliferation and Survival.* California Pacific Medical Center Research Institute, San Francisco, California 94107, USA. Mol Cancer Ther, 6. Januar 2010.

11 Ibid.

12 Blázquez C, Carracedo A, Salazar M, Lorente M, Egia A, González-Feria L, Haro A, Velasco G, Guzmán M. *Down-regulation of tissue inhibitor of metalloproteinases-1 in gliomas: a new marker of cannabinoid antitumoral activity?* Department of Biochemistry and Molecular Biology I, School of Biology, Complutense University, 28040 Madrid, Spain. Neuropharmacology. 2008 Jan;54(1):235-43.

13 Blázquez C, Salazar M, Carracedo A, Lorente M, Egia A, González-Feria L, Haro A, Velasco G, Guzmán M. *Cannabinoids inhibit glioma cell invasion by down-regulating matrix metalloproteinase-2 expression.* Department of Biochemistry and Molecular Biology I, School of Biology, Complutense University, Madrid, Spain. Cancer Res. 2008 Mar 15;68(6):1945-52.

14 Gil Galanti1,2, Tamar Fisher2, Iris Kventsel2, Jacob Shoham1, Ruth Gallily3, Raphael Mechoulam4, Gad Lavie5, Ninette Amariglio2, Gideon Rechavi2 and Amos Toren2† *Δ9-Tetrahydrocannabinol inhibits cell cycle progression by downregulation of E2F1 in human glioblastoma multiforme cells.* 1The Mina and Everard Goodman Faculty of Life Science, Bar-Ilan University, Ramat-Gan, Israel 2Department of Pediatric Hemato-Oncology, Safra Children's Hospital, Sheba Medical Center, Tel Hashomer, Israel 3The Lautenberg Center for General and Tumor Immunology, The Hebrew University Medical Faculty, Ein Kerem Campus, Jerusalem, Israel 4Department of Medicinal Chemistry and Natural Products, Hebrew University Medical Faculty, Jerusalem, Israel 5Blood Center, Sheba Medical Center, Tel-Hashomer, Israel. †Correspondence: Amos Toren, Department of Pediatric Hemato-Oncology, Safra Children's Hospital, Sheba Medical Center, Tel Hashomer, Israel, 972 3 5303037, 972 3 5303031. Acta Oncologica. 2008, Vol. 47, No. 6, Pages 1062-1070.

15 Guzman M, Duarte MJ, Blazquez C, Ravina J, Rosa MC, Galve-Roperh I, Sanchez C, Velasco G, Gonzalez-Feria L. *A pilot clinical study of Delta(9)-tetrahydrocannabinol in patients with recurrent glioblastoma multiforme.* Department of Biochemistry and Molecular Biology I, School of Biology, Complutense University, Madrid 28040, Spain. Br J Cancer 2006;95(2):197-203.

16 Cristina Blázquez 1 , Luis González-Feria 4 , Luis Álvarez 2 , Amador Haro 1 , M. Llanos Casanova 3 , and Manuel Guzmán 1 *Cannabinoids Inhibit the Vascular Endothelial Growth Factor Pathway in Gliomas.* 1Department of Biochemistry and Molecular Biology I, School of Biology, Complutense University; 2 Research Unit, La Paz University Hospital; 3 Project on Cellular and Molecular Biology and Gene Therapy, CIEMAT, Madrid, Spain; and 4 Department of Neurosurgery, University Hospital, Tenerife, Spain. Cancer Res August 15, 2004 64; 5617

17 Massi P, Vaccani A, Bianchessi S, Costa B, Macchi P, Parolaro D. *The non-psychoactive cannabidiol triggers caspase activation and oxidative stress in human glioma cells.* Department of Pharmacology, Chemotherapy and Medical Toxicology, University of Milan, via Vanvitelli 32, 20129 Milan, Italy. Cell Mol Life Sci. 2006 Sep;63(17):2057-66.

18 Paola Massi, Angelo Vaccani, Stefania Ceruti, Arianna Colombo, Maria P. Abbracchio and Daniela Parolaro. *Antitumor Effects of Cannabidiol, a Nonpsychoactive Cannabinoid, on Human Glioma Cell Lines.* Department of Pharmacology, Chemotherapy and Toxicology (P.M., A.C.), and Department of Pharmacological Sciences,

School of Pharmacy, and Center of Excellence for Neurodegenerative Diseases, University of Milan, Milan, Italy (S.C., M.P.A.); and Department of Structural and Functional Biology, Pharmacology Unit and Center of Neuroscience, University of Insubria, Busto Arsizio (Varese), Italy (A.V., D.P.) JPET March 2004 vol. 308 no. 3 838-845.

19   Cristina Sanchez,2 Marıa L. de Ceballos,2 Teresa Gomez del Pulgar,2 Daniel Rueda, Cesar Corbacho, Guillermo Velasco, Ismael Galve-Roperh, John W. Huffman, Santiago Ramon y Cajal, and Manuel Guzman.3 *Inhibition of Glioma Growth in Vivo by Selective Activation of the CB2 Cannabinoid Receptor.* Department of Biochemistry and Molecular Biology I, School of Biology, Complutense University, 28040 Madrid, Spain [C. S., T. G. d. P., D. R., G. V., I. G-R., M. G.]; Neurodegeneration Group, Cajal Institute, CSIC, 28002 Madrid, Spain [M. L. d. C.]; Department of Pathology, Clınica Puerta de Hierro, 28035 Madrid, Spain [C. C., S. R. y C.]; and Department of Chemistry, Clemson University, Clemson, South Carolina 29634-1905 [J. W. H.] CANCER RE-SEARCH 61, 5784 –5789, August 1, 2001.

Cancer
Breast Cancer

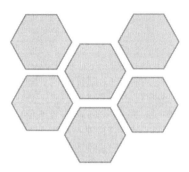

NUMBER OF STUDIES: 6

CHI VALUE: 11

By 2004, reported global estimates of breast cancer deaths exceeded 500,000 victims.[1] The vast majority were women. This type of cancer most commonly originates in the milk ducts from a corrupted breast cell(s), which left unchecked can invade surrounding breast tissue with devastating results.

While benign in origin, a dreaded lump in the breast can develop into a cancerous growth. Chronically swollen lymph nodes around the breast or in the armpit may also be signs of cancer. Other symptoms include single nipple discharge, pain in the area, inverted nipple, discoloration, heat, redness, and swelling to the affected tissue, or a change in breast tissue texture. Orthodox treatment is usually limited to surgery, pharmaceuticals (chemotherapy), or radiation.

Although a multitude of possible known factors contribute to the genesis of cancers (see Cancer in General), one controllable risk factor for breast cancer is high levels of estrogen. In fact, the development of breast cancer remains a serious effect of hormone replacement therapy. Body fat is another source of high levels of estrogen. In addition, women's fat cells store excess estrogen after menopause.

Exposure to ionizing radiation is another known risk factor.[2] Mammograms, CAT (or CT) scans, and any other x-rays produce ionizing radiation. Dr. Gofman, Professor Emeritus from UC Berkeley, demonstrated that past exposure to ionizing radiation - primarily medical x-rays - is responsible for about 75% of breast-cancer cases in the United States. He also reported some good news. Since the radiation dosage given today by medical procedures can be significantly reduced without interfering with a single useful procedure, numerous future cases of breast-cancer can be prevented.[3]

In the case of mothers, women who breast-feed longer tend to form greater protection against breast cancer.[4]

CANNABIS AND BREAST CANCER

In 1998, a team of researchers from Naples, Italy, discovered that the endogenous cannabinoid anandamide blocks human breast cancer cell growth in vitro.[5] By

2000, researchers discovered a potential mechanism by which anandamide might inhibit breast cancer cell growth. Cannabinoids suppressed certain growth factors and prolactin receptors, which lead to an inhibition of certain types of breast cancer cell lines.[6]

By 2006, another Italian team had formulated more interesting insights. Researchers compared the specific anti-tumor properties of five individual cannabinoids to a whole cannabis extract. Of the five individual cannabinoids (cannabidiol, cannabigerol, cannabichromene, cannabidiol acid, THC acid, and cannabis extract), cannabidiol emerged as the most potent anti-breast cancer substance, on par with the cannabidiol-rich whole plant extract. The authors wrote: "our experiments indicate that the cannabidiol effect is due to its capability of inducing apoptosis via[…]elevation of intracellular Ca2+ and reactive oxygen species."[7]

In the same year, a team of Spanish scientists found that cannabinoids are involved in the process of breast cell proliferation, differentiation, and survival. The authors of this study suggested several specific mechanisms, one of which proved "that Δ9-tetrahydrocannabinol (THC), through activation of CB2 cannabinoid receptors, reduces human breast cancer cell proliferation by blocking the progression of the cell cycle, and by inducing apoptosis."[8] The Spanish researchers wrote: "Taken together, these data might set the bases for a cannabinoid therapy for the management of breast cancer."

In 2007, a team from San Francisco examined cannabinoids in the context of cases involving a rapid spread of aggressive breast cancer cells. To date, oncologists have a very limited supply of options, each with their own set of toxic or dangerous adverse effects. In this experiment, scientists wrote about a key finding: "Here, we report that cannabidiol (CBD), a cannabinoid with a low-toxicity profile, could down-regulate Id-1 expression in aggressive human breast cancer cells. […]In conclusion, CBD represents the first nontoxic exogenous agent that can significantly decrease Id-1 expression in metastatic breast cancer cells leading to the down-regulation of tumor aggressiveness."[9]

Perhaps the most exciting research comes from Spain, where scientists discovered for the first time that cannabinoids therapeutically influence a genetic component involved in breast cancer progression. The authors wrote: "In summary, this is the first report showing not only that cannabinoids regulate a protein called transcription factor jun-D, which in humans is encoded in a JUND gene but, more generally, that jun-D activation reduces the proliferation of cancer cells, which points to a new target to inhibit breast cancer progression."[10]

STUDY SUMMARY:

Drugs	Type of Study	Published Year, Place, and Key Results	CHI
THC	Laboratory and animal study (mice)	2008 – Complutense University, Madrid, Spain: Discovery of a mechanism by which THC reduces proliferation of human breast cancer cells.[10]	1+2
CBD	Laboratory and animal study (mice)	2007 – California Pacific Medical Center, San Francisco, U.S.: CBD represents the first nontoxic agent that can significantly decrease breast cancer aggressiveness.[9]	1+2
THC	Laboratory	2006 – Multi-institutional research team Madrid, Spain: THC reduces human breast cancer cell proliferation.[8]	1

Drugs	Type of Study	Published Year, Place, and Key Results	CHI
Cannabidiol, cannabigerol, cannabichromene, cannabidiol acid and THC acid v. whole plant extract	Animal study (mice)	2006 – Multi-institutional research team, Italy: Cannabidiol was the most potent anti-breast cancer substance, on par with the cannabidiol rich whole plant extract.[7]	2
Anandamide	Laboratory	2000 – Multi-institutional research team Naples, Italy: Inhibiting prolactin-responsive human breast cancer cells was achieved by down-regulating of the long form of the prolactin receptors.[6]	1
Anandamide	Laboratory	1998 – Multi-institutional research team Naples, Italy: Anandamide blocks human breast cancer cell growth.[5]	1

Total CHI Value 11

STRAIN SPECIFIC CONSIDERATIONS

Pre-clinical animal trials demonstrated that anandamide, the body's own endocannabinoid, and numerous plant cannabinoids such as THC but especially CBD have the abilities to limit breast cancer cell proliferation and produce apoptosis (death of cancer cells). Current research results also suggest that therapeutic mechanisms begin at CB2 receptor sites.

Indica strains, or indica-heavy hybrids tend to have a higher CBD profile. A CBD profile of more than 3-4% is considered potent.

EXPLORING MIND–BODY CONSCIOUSNESS

As early as the 1950s, physicians examined possible correlations between the psyche and cancer. Researchers enrolled 40 breast cancer patients in a study to evaluate the prevalence of common behavioral characteristics. Results exposed unresolved conflicts with their mothers. These included: competition and guilt; sexual inhibition; inhibited motherhood; masochistic character structures; denial; self-sacrifice; an inability to discharge or deal appropriately with anger, aggressiveness, or hostility, and a tendency to hide these emotions behind a façade of pleasantness.[11]

More recently, London scientists examining a possible link between emotional expressions and breast cancer discovered that "…IgA levels[12] were found to be significantly higher in patients who habitually suppressed anger than in those who were able to express anger."[13]

Another study, from the University of Arizona, similarly confirmed that acceptance of emotions and emotional processing decreased overall mortality from breast cancer. Furthermore, research results also showed that close relationships which included confiding and dependable support, were protective against breast cancer progression.[14] In addition, psychiatrists trying to understand the impact of emotional states on patients' personalities prior to the clinical manifestation of breast cancer suggested that a depressive reaction decreased host immunity, especially disturbances in the person, sex, and maternal drive.[15]

Contrary to these above-mentioned study results, a large-scale research project from Australia found no significant correlation between anger management or negative affect and risk of breast cancer (and only weak links between anger management and prostate, lung and colorectal cancer).[16]

For mothers and the infant, breasts are a source of love, pleasure, life, and nourishment. Breastfeeding after birth releases oxytocin, a hormone that induces uterine contractions and thereby stops post partum bleeding (a great benefit to the health and survival of the mother).[17] Oxytocin also relaxes the mother and increases her feelings of love and bonding for the child. Breast milk provides the mother with easy access to all the food, immune protection, and nourishment the infant needs. Breastfeeding also supplies the mother with a host of health benefits. It is interesting to note that mothers who breastfeed lower their risk for developing breast cancer and a host of other diseases.[18,19,20]

Breasts also represent nurturing and the pleasure of nurturing in general. In a healthy situation, offering the breasts to another human being brings pleasure to the child or the lover, as well as the woman herself. Taking pleasure in a woman's breast can be a beautiful part of the human experience. The breast tissue, especially the areolas and nipples, are very sensitive, and sucking produces intensely pleasurable experiences for the happy infant, the aroused lover, and the woman alike. However, sometimes there is trouble in paradise.

Feeling arousal in the nipples during sex is considered normal, but arousal during breastfeeding is often discomforting. To women who consider motherhood holy and sex dirty, this sensation does not fit into the mental construct of what life should be like. Here we have a source of possible guilt and conflicting emotions involving the breasts. Many of these feelings can never be communicated, and may even have to be hidden from her. But where can they go?

Most kids take mom's love for granted. "A face only a mother could love." "No matter what I do mother loves me." It is assumed that her love is unconditional. But what about the many times when a mother doesn't feel that way? She is a human being, capable of feeling emotions not normally associated with the impossible and idealized version of motherhood; arousal, anger, rage, self-importance, envy, or jealousy of those in her care, be they child, husband, mother, father, or God. Yet she is a mother now, or a wife, or a loving daughter, or a God-fearing woman, and she likes to see herself and others as being only loving. Her soft bosoms, which should provide loving, nurturing hugs, may become a repository for all those distasteful and unwanted emotional experiences that are part of anybody's life.

When it comes to sex, the breasts are everywhere. No other organ induces such primary urges in males as the mammary glands of women. No other organ is as used and abused in social power plays by entire industries, as well as by both genders, as the breast. Unexpressed hurt, anger, and silent rage born of this use and abuse may find the breast a perfect stage and repository to force attention on the core issues, thus presenting a serious demand for change.

While the intense focus on the importance of breasts is virtually everywhere, it is also reflected in medical statistics. In 2008, more than 300,000 women in the U.S. received voluntary cosmetic breast augmentations[21] while, in 2010, another 200,000 women were diagnosed with dreaded breast cancer.[22] Inside this soft place of pleasure, love, nurturing, and nourishment, now looms an aggressive, hurtful threat, not just to the perceived front of womanhood, but also to life itself.

Women who give and give might feel that their breasts exist solely for the pleasure of others. In such cases, women may forget to take pleasure in their own breasts, and by extension in the capacities they represent. Here, these capacities for life, love, pleasure and nourishment are not applied to herself. Over time, a woman may feel chronically stressed by this costly one-way giving and lack of replenishment. She might even blame her lot (gender) in life for the stress that she feels.

Her stress can soon form into feeling unappreciated, fueling a righteous control of those in her care. When left unchecked, this disintegrating process may even turn love or her loving bosoms into a form of smothering. It is as if her pattern of suppressing anything not in line with her ideal of what a good mother, woman, daughter, or member of her church should be soon superimposes itself onto those who behave differently than she thinks they should. She can become disrespectful, hard, and invasive, using righteous indignation as justification for dominating others into behaving according to her values and beliefs. She may treat others as she treats herself.

QUESTIONS

What does it mean to me to be a woman?
Is it okay for me to enjoy my breasts as a celebration of my sensuality?
How do I feel about wearing clothes that reveal my cleavage?
How do I feel about women who prominently display their breasts?
How do I feel about women who have larger or smaller breasts than mine?
What beliefs underlie those feelings?
Do these beliefs and the feelings they engender serve me well?

What does it mean to be a mother?
Is it okay for a mother to be aroused?
Is it okay to be aroused by breastfeeding my child?

What does it mean to be a daughter?
What does it mean to be a good daughter?

What does it mean to be a lover/wife?
What does it mean to be a good wife?

Do I have to 'put out' to be a good wife?
What does it mean to be a God-fearing woman?
Is motherhood/martyrdom for me, if I must suffer for the noble cause?
If I did not have breasts, how would I define being a woman?

Does nurturing necessarily entail sacrifice?
What do I get from nurturing others?
What does nurturing mean to me?
Do I make time to nurture myself?
How do I feel if I make time to nurture myself?
Can I trust myself to find my authentic self?
Can I support others in their attempt to become their ideal selves?

AGGRAVATING FACTORS

Suppressed anger / depressive reaction/decreased immunity / unresolved conflicts with the mother, such as competition and guilt, sexual inhibitio, inhibited motherhood / masochistic character structures / denial / self-sacrifice / and an inability to discharge or deal appropriately with anger, aggressiveness, or hostility / the desire to hide behind a façade of pleasantness.

HEALING FACTORS

Acceptance of emotions / willingness to process emotions / close relationships, particularly those which included confiding and dependable support.

TAKE NOTICE

ANISE • COCOA • GINGER • MYRRH

ANISE: Greek herbalists have used anise and fennel to promote menstruation, increase breast milk production, facilitate birth, and enhance libido. University of Athens' scientists have taken a closer look at anise in the context of finding a safe alternative to estrogen replacement therapies to prevent osteoporosis. Anise exhibited estrogen receptor modulator-like properties that produce bone-cell formation without causing breast and cervical cancer cells to proliferate.[23]

COCOA: Researchers at the Georgetown University Medical Center in Washington, D.C., examined a cocoa-derived compound called pentameric procyanidin (pentamer) and discovered that it arrested human breast cancer cells.[24]

GINGER: Researchers from Seoul proved that ginger, a spice commonly used in Korean traditional medicine and cuisine, has the ability to protect and strengthen the heart and liver and function as an anti-inflammatory agent. Scientists are exploring ginger as am inhibitor of breast cancer cells.[25]

MYRRH: Based on traditional practice and evidence-based discoveries, this author reported that myrrh's significant antiseptic, anesthetic, and antitumor properties most likely stem from a specific alkene called furanosesquiterpene, which is present in essential oil of myrrh.[26] Scientists from the University of Texas discovered that naturally occurring steroids (guggulsterone) from a closely related species called *Commiphora mukul* could produce apoptosis (destruction of cancer cells) "including leukemia, head and neck carcinoma, multiple myeloma, lung carcinoma, melanoma, breast carcinoma, and ovarian carcinoma. Guggulsterone also inhibited the proliferation of drug-resistant cancer cells (e.g., gleevac-resistant leukemia, dexamethasone-resistant multiple myeloma, and doxorubicin-resistant breast cancer cells)."[27]

1 World Health Organization. *Fact sheet No 297*. Cancer. February 2009.

2 U.S. National Institute of Health. National Cancer institute. Breast Cancer Prevention (PDQ®). *Factors Associated With Increased Risk of Breast Cancer. Ionizing radiation*. July 23, 2010. http://www.cancer.gov/cancertopics/pdq/prevention/breast/healthprofessional#Section_178

3 John W. Gofman, M.D., Ph.D. *Preventing Breast Cancer: The story of a Major, Proven, Preventable Cause of This Disease*. Committee for Nuclear Responsibility; Second Edition: 1996.

4 Collaborative Group on Hormonal Factors in Breast Cancer. *Breast cancer and breastfeeding: collaborative reanalysis of individual data from 47 epidemiological studies in 30 countries, including 50302 women with breast cancer and 96973 women without the disease*. Lancet 360 (9328): 187-95, 2002.

5 Luciano De Petrocellis * , †, Dominique Melck * , ‡, Antonella Palmisano §, Tiziana Bisogno ‡, Chiara Laezza ¶, Maurizio Bifulco ¶, and Vincenzo Di Marzo ‡ , ⊠. *The endogenous cannabinoid anandamide inhibits human breast cancer cell proliferation*. †Istituto di Cibernetica and ‡Istituto per la Chimica di Molecole di Interesse Biologico (affiliated with the National Institute for the Chemistry of Biological Systems, Consiglio Nazionale delle Ricerche), Consiglio Nazionale delle Ricerche, Via Toiano 6, 80072 Arco Felice, Naples, Italy; § Istituto di Ricerche sull'Adattamento dei Bovini e dei Bufali all'Ambiente del Mezzogiorno, Consiglio Nazionale delle Ricerche, Ponticelli, 80147 Naples, Italy; and ¶Centro di Studio der l'Endocrinologia e l'Oncologia Sperimentale, Consiglio Nazionale Delle Richerche and Dipartimento di Biologia e Patologia Cellulare e Molecolare, Università di Napoli 'Federico II', 80131 Naples, Italy. PNAS July 7, 1998 vol. 95 no. 14 8375-8380

6 Dominique Melck, Luciano De Petrocellis, Pierangelo Orlando, Tiziana Bisogno, Chiara Laezza, Maurizio Bifulco and Vincenzo Di Marzo. *Suppression of Nerve Growth Factor Trk Receptors and Prolactin Receptors by Endocannabinoids Leads to Inhibition of Human Breast and Prostate Cancer Cell Proliferation*. stituto per la Chimica di Molecole di Interesse Biologico (D.M., T.B., V.D.M.), Istituto di Cibernetica (L.D.P.), and Istituto di Biochimica delle Proteine ed Enzimologia (P.O.), Consiglio Nazionale delle Ricerche, 80072 Arco Felice (NA); and Centro di Endocrinologia e Oncologia Sperimentale, Consiglio Nazionale delle Ricerche, and Dipartimento di Biologia e Patologia Cellulare e Molecolare, Università di Napoli Federico II (C.L., M.B.), 80131 Naples, Italy. Endocrinology 2000. Vol. 141, No. 1 118-126.

7 Alessia Ligresti, Aniello Schiano Moriello, Katarzyna Starowicz, Isabel Matias, Simona Pisanti, Luciano De Petrocellis, Chiara Laezza, Giuseppe Portella, Maurizio Bifulco and Vincenzo Di Marzo. *Antitumor Activity of Plant Cannabinoids with Emphasis on the Effect of Cannabidiol on Human Breast Carcinoma*. Endocannabinoid Research Group, Istituto di Chimica Biomolecolare (A.L., A.S.M., K.S., I.M., V.D.M.), and Istituto di Cibernetica (A.S.M., L.D.P.), Consiglio Nazionale delle Ricerche Pozzuoli, Italy; Dipartimento di Biologia e Patologia Cellulare e Molecolare "L. Califano", Università di Napoli "Federico II", Napoli, Italy (S.P., C.L., G.P., M.B.); and Dipartimento di Scienze Farmaceutiche, Università degli Studi di Salerno, Fisciano, Italy (S.P., M.B.). JPET September 2006 vol. 318 no. 3 1375-1387.

8 María M. Caffarel1, David Sarrió2, José Palacios2, Manuel Guzmán1, and Cristina Sánchez1. *Δ9-Tetrahydrocannabinol Inhibits Cell Cycle Progression in Human Breast Cancer Cells through Cdc2 Regulation*. 1Department of Biochemistry and Molecular Biology I, School of Biology, Complutense University and 2Breast and Gynecological Cancer Group, Molecular Pathology Programme, Centro Nacional de Investigaciones Oncológicas, Madrid, Spain. Cancer Res July 1, 2006 66; 6615.

9 McAllister SD, Christian RT, Horowitz MP, Garcia A, Desprez PY. *Cannabidiol as a novel inhibitor of Id-1 gene expression in aggressive breast cancer cells*. California Pacific Medical Center, Research Institute, 475 Brannan Street, San Francisco, CA 94107, USA. Mol Cancer Ther. 2007 Nov;6(11):2921-7.

10 Caffarel MM, Moreno-Bueno G, Cerutti C, Palacios J, Guzman M, Mechta-Grigoriou F, Sanchez C. *JunD is involved in the antiproliferative effect of Delta9-tetrahydrocannabinol on human breast cancer cells*. Department of Biochemistry and Molecular Biology I, School of Biology, Complutense University, Madrid, Spain. Oncogene. 2008 Aug 28;27(37):5033-44.

11 C. Bacon, M.D., R. Rennekerr, M.D., and Max Cutler, M.D. *A Psychosomatic survey of Cancer of the Breast*. Chicago Tumor Institute. Institute for Psychoanalysis of Chicago. Psychosomatic Medicine November 1, 1952 vol. 14 no. 6 453-460.

12 Immunoglobulin A (IgA): antibodies made by the body's immune system in response to an invasion such as from cancer.

13 Pettingale KW, Greer S, Tee DEH. *Serum IgA and emotional expression in breast cancer patients.* Faith Courtauld Unit for Human Studies in Cancer, King's College Hospital Medical School, Denmark Hill, London S.E.5., England. J Psychosom Med 1977; 21: 395–9.

14 Karen L. Weihs, MD, Timothy M. Enright, PhD and Samuel J. Simmens, PhD. Close Relationships and Emotional Processing Predict Decreased Mortality in Women with Breast Cancer: Preliminary Evidence. Department of Psychiatry (K.L.W.) and the Arizona Cancer Center, University of Arizona, Tucson, Arizona; Department of Psychiatry and Behavioral Sciences (T.M.E.), The George Washington University, Washington, DC; and the Departments of Epidemiology and Biostatistics (S.J.S.), The George Washington University, Washington, DC. Psychosomatic Medicine January 1, 2008 vol. 70 no. 1 117-124.

15 RICHARD E. RENNEKER M.D., ROBERT CUTLER M.D., JEROME HORA M.D., CATHERINE BACON M.D., GARNET BRADLEY M.D., JOHN KEARNEY M.D., and MAX CUTLER M.D. Psychoanalytical Explorations of Emotional Correlates of Cancer of the Breast. Psychosomatic Medicine 25:106-123 (1963).

16 Victoria M. White, PhD, Dallas R. English, PhD, Hamish Coates, PhD, Magdalena Lagerlund, PhD, Ron Borland, PhD and Graham G. Giles, PhD. *Is Cancer Risk Associated With Anger Control and Negative Affect? Findings from a Prospective Cohort Study.* Centre for Behavioural Research in Cancer (V.M.W.), The Cancer Council Victoria, Australia; Cancer Epidemiology Centre (D.R.E., G.G.G.), The Cancer Council Victoria, Australia; School of Population Health (D.R.E., G.G.G.), University of Melbourne, Australia; Department of Epidemiology and Preventive Medicine (D.R.E., G.G.G.), Monash University, Australia; Centre for the Study of Higher Education (H.C.), University of Melbourne, Australia; Department of Epidemiology and Biostatistics (M.L.), University of Western Ontario, Canada; VicHealth Centre for Tobacco Control (R.B.), The Cancer Council Victoria, Australia. Psychosomatic Medicine 69:667-674 (2007).

17 Chua S, Arulkumaran S, Lim I, Selamat N, Ratnam SS. *Influence of breastfeeding and nipple stimulation on postpartum uterine activity.* Br J Obstet Gynaecol. 1994;101 :804 –805.

18 Newcomb PA, Storer BE, Longnecker MP, et al. *Lactation and a reduced risk of premenopausal breast cancer.* N Engl J Med. 1994;330 :81 –87.

19 Collaborative Group on Hormonal Factors in Breast Cancer. *Breast cancer and breastfeeding: collaborative reanalysis of individual data from 47 epidemiological studies in 30 countries, including 50302 women with breast cancer and 96973 women without the disease.* Lancet. 2002;360 :187 –195.

20 Tryggvadottir L, Tulinius H, Eyfjord JE, Sigurvinsson T. *Breastfeeding and reduced risk of breast cancer in an Icelandic cohort study.* Am J Epidemiol. 2001;154 :37 –42.

21 American Society of Plastic Surgeons (ASPS). *2000/2007/2008 National Plastic Surgery Statistics.*

22 *Cancer Facts and Figures 2010.* Atlanta, Ga: American Cancer Society, 2010.

23 Kassi E, Papoutsi Z, Fokialakis N, Messari I, Mitakou S, Moutsatsou P. *Greek plant extracts exhibit selective estrogen receptor modulator (SERM)-like properties.* Department of Biological Chemistry, Medical School, University of Athens, 115 27 Athens, Greece. J Agric Food Chem. 2004 Nov 17;52(23):6956-61.

24 Ramljak D, Romanczyk LJ, Metheny-Barlow LJ, Thompson N, Knezevic V, Galperin M, Ramesh A, Dickson RB. *Pentameric procyanidin from Theobroma cacao selectively inhibits growth of human breast cancer cells.* Department of Oncology, The Research Building, Room W417, Lombardi Comprehensive Cancer Center, Georgetown University Medical Center, 3970 Reservoir Road, NW, Washington, District of Columbia 20057, USA. Mol Cancer Ther. 2005 Apr;4(4):537-46.

25 Lee HS, Seo EY, Kang NE, Kim WK. *[6]-Gingerol inhibits metastasis of MDA-MB-231 human breast cancer cells.* Department of Sports Sciences, Seoul Sports Graduate University, Seoul 150-034, South Korea. J Nutr Biochem. 2007 Jul 31.

26 Nomicos EY. *Myrrh: medical marvel or myth of the magi?* National Institute of Allergy and Infectious Diseases, National Institute of Health, Bethesda, Maryland. Holist Nurs Pract. 2007 Nov-Dec;21(6):308-23.

27 Shishodia S, Sethi G, Ahn KS, Aggarwal BB. *Guggulsterone inhibits tumor cell proliferation, induces S-phase arrest, and promotes apoptosis through activation of c-Jun N-terminal kinase, suppression of Akt pathway, and downregulation of antiapoptotic gene products.* Cytokine Research Laboratory, Department of Experimental Therapeutics, Unit 143, The University of Texas M. D. Anderson Cancer Center, 1515 Holcombe Boulevard, Houston, TX 77030, United States. Biochem Pharmacol. 2007 Jun 30;74(1):118-30.

Cancer Caused by Cannabis?

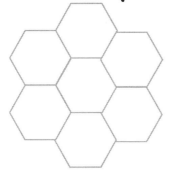

NUMBER OF STUDIES: 7

CHI VALUE: -1

Plant and animal products, such as those used in smoking or barbequing, are known to produce carcinogenic substances. Additionally, smoking tobacco has been clearly implicated in the genesis of lung cancer.

However, studies examining whether cannabis smoke leads to lung cancer have been confounded by test subjects who also smoked tobacco. No study examined risk of lung cancer when cannabis is smoked without tobacco. No study examined the possible risk of lung cancer associated with smoking cannabis using various vaporizers, which produce no or very little smoke.

Two studies using interviews and statistical mathematics indicate a possible link between frequent cannabis smoke and the more rare of two forms of testicular cancer.

A large Los Angeles study perhaps yields the most reliable current scientific indicator. It concluded: "the association of these cancers with marijuana, even long-term or heavy use, is not strong and may be below practically detectable limits."

STUDY SUMMARY:

Drugs	Type of Study	Published Year, Place, and Key Results	CHI
Cannabis smoke, tobacco smoke, alcohol	Human case study (interview-based)	2011 – National Institutes of Health: Results suggested that cannabis might be associated with one of two types of testicular cancers.[1]	-3
Cannabis smoke	Laboratory	2009 – University of Leicester, United Kingdom: Cannabis smoke can damage DNA.[2]	-1
Cannabis smoke, tobacco smoke, alcohol	Human case study (interview-based)	2009 – Division of Public Health Sciences, F. Hutchinson Cancer Research Center, Seattle: Results suggested that cannabis might be associated with one of two types of testicular cancers.[3]	-3
Cannabis/Tobacco smoke	Human subjects	2008 – International Agency for Research on Cancer, Lyon, France: Cannabis smoking may be a risk factor for lung cancer.[4]	0
Cannabis/Tobacco smoke	76 patients with lung cancer and 324 people without	2008 – Medical Research Institute of New Zealand, Wellington, New Zealand: Long-term cannabis with tobacco smoke increases the risk of lung cancer in young adults.[5]	-3
Cannabis	2,252 human subjects	2006 – International Agency for Research on Cancer Lyon, France: Cannabis, even long-term or heavy use, is unlikely to cause oral cancer or throat cancer.[6]	5

Drugs	Type of Study	Published Year, Place, and Key Results	CHI
Cannabis smoke	Meta-analysis	2005 – International Agency for Research on Cancer, Lyon, France: In general, increased risk of lung cancer was not observed.[7]	4

Total CHI Value   -1

1 Trabert B, Sigurdson AJ, Sweeney AM, Strom SS, McGlynn KA. *Marijuana use and testicular germ cell tumors.* Hormonal and Reproductive Epidemiology Branch, Division of Cancer Epidemiology and Genetics, National Cancer Institute, National Institutes of Health, Department of Health and Human Services, Rockville, Maryland, USA. Cancer. 2011 Feb 15;117(4):848-53.

2 Singh R, Sandhu J, Kaur B, Juren T, Steward WP, Segerbäck D, Farmer PB. *Evaluation of the DNA damaging potential of cannabis cigarette smoke by the determination of acetaldehyde derived N2-ethyl-2'-deoxyguanosine adducts.* Cancer Biomarkers and Prevention Group, Biocentre, Department of Cancer Studies and Molecular Medicine, University of Leicester, University Road, Leicester LE1 7RH, United Kingdom. rs25@le.ac.uk Chem Res Toxicol. 2009 Jun;22(6):1181-8.

3 Daling, J.R., et al. *Association of marijuana use and the incidence of testicular germ cell tumors.* Cancer 115(6):1215–1223, 2009.

4 Berthiller J, Straif K, Boniol M, Voirin N, Benhaïm-Luzon V, Ayoub WB, Dari I, Laouamri S, Hamdi-Cherif M, Bartal M, Ayed FB, Sasco AJ. *Cannabis smoking and risk of lung cancer in men: a pooled analysis of three studies in Maghreb.* International Agency for Research on Cancer, Lyon, France.

5 Aldington S, Harwood M, Cox B, Weatherall M, Beckert L, Hansell A, Pritchard A, Robinson G, Beasley R; Cannabis and Respiratory Disease Research Group. *Cannabis use and risk of lung cancer: a case-control study.* Medical Research Institute of New Zealand, Wellington, New Zealand. Eur Respir J. 2008 Feb;31(2):280-6.

6 Hashibe M, Morgenstern H, Cui Y, Tashkin DP, Zhang ZF, Cozen W, Mack TM, Greenland S. *Marijuana use and the risk of lung and upper aerodigestive tract cancers: results of a population-based case-control study.* IARC, Lyon, France. Cancer Epidemiol Biomarkers Prev. 2006 Oct;15(10):1829-34.

7 Hashibe M, Straif K, Tashkin DP, Morgenstern H, Greenland S, Zhang ZF. *Epidemiologic review of marijuana use and cancer risk.* International Agency for Research on Cancer, 69008 Lyon, France. Alcohol. 2005 Apr;35(3):265-75.

Cancer
Cancer Induced Night Sweats

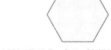

NUMBER OF STUDIES: 1

CHI VALUE: 3

Night sweats, relatively common in end stage cancer patients, are partly responsible for disrupted sleep patterns. This factor directly and indirectly further reduces the patient's overall quality of life. The orthodox medical system believes the sympathetic nervous system controls sweating via the hypothalamus. This almond sized, centrally located portion of the brain releases hormones to control numerous autonomic functions, such as temperature, circadian cycles, sleep, hunger and thirst. Environmental signals such as light, stress, smell, or pheromones can activate the hypothalamus. It responds quickly to these indicators and other changes in heart rate, respiratory rate, blood, shifts in hormonal profiles, and to the presence of pathogens.

Perspiration also functions as a balancing mechanism by releasing excess water, dumping toxic material, and introducing molecules such as pheromones into the immediate environment. Sweat is excreted through sweat glands (apocrine and eccrine glands) strategically located throughout the skin.

CANNABIS AND NIGHT SWEATS

A 2007 study from Fukuoka, Japan challenges the orthodox hypothesis of temperature controlled solely by the hypothalamus. Researchers hypothesized that the endocannabinoid system, especially CB1, may regulate body temperature independent of the hypothalamus.[1]

Cannabis, used within the appropriate therapeutic range, is well-known for its ability to induce relaxation and, by extension, improve sleep. Now scientists (2008) have tested this age-old knowledge in the context of cancer–induced night sweats. A synthetic orally administered cannabinoid, nabilone (similar to THC), was effectively used in treating night sweats. Cancer patients who suffered the ill-effects of interrupted sleep experienced an improved quality of life during nabilone treatment. Further, the cannabinoid positively affected pains, anorexia, and nausea.[2]

STUDY SUMMARY:

Drugs	Type of Study	Published Year, Place, and Key Results	CHI
Nabilone 1mg 1 x daily; and patients with more severe pains 1mg 2 x daily	Case study	2008 – University of Toronto: Significant reduction of night sweats.[3]	3

STRAIN SPECIFIC CONSIDERATIONS

CB1 receptors are located primarily in the brain and central nervous system, including the sympathetic nervous system and the hypothalamus, which are both involved in perspiration. The synthetic cannabinoid nabilone, similar to THC, has been shown to therapeutically influence perspiration patterns in humans. Here, the logic of the available science would suggest a sativa with higher THC:CBD ratios. However, an indica or indica-heavy strain is advised in order to access a balanced and synergistic approach with the body and the mind. Indicas still provide the CB1 activation involved in the mechanism of night sweats, yet also activate CB2 receptors involved in inducing an overall calming and restful state.

EXPLORING MIND–BODY CONSCIOUSNESS

SUGGESTED BLESSING

May you relax and release all fears.

May you find your antidote to fear.

Anxiety, intense fears, dread, or guilt are common emotional states that keep the mind in an endless attempt to control what cannot be controlled. This continuous process can drain every bit of energy and at the same time prevent release, relaxation, and sleep. Even when sleep arrives, these intense emotions may find their expression in the dream world. The body reacts to the dreams with physiological responses. Intense dreams, struggling with uncomfortable topics or nightmares, are commonly associated with night sweats.

SUGGESTED AFFIRMATION

There is a place in me where I am completely safe.

1 Hayakawa K, Mishima K, Nozako M, Hazekawa M, Ogata A, Fujioka M, Harada K, Mishima S, Orito K, Egashira N, Iwasaki K, Fujiwara M. *Delta9-tetrahydrocannabinol (Delta9-THC) prevents cerebral infarction via hypothalamic-independent hypothermia.* Department of Neuropharmacology, Faculty of Pharmaceutical Sciences, Fukuoka University, Nanakuma 8-19-1, Fukuoka City, Fukuoka, Japan. Life Sci 2007 Mar 27; 80(16):1466-71.

2 Maida V. *Nabilone for the treatment of paraneoplastic night sweats: a report of four cases.* Division of Palliative Medicine, William Osler Health Centre, University of Toronto, Toronto, Canada. vincent.maida@utoronto.ca J Palliat Med. 2008 Jul;11(6):929-34.

3 Ibid.

Cancer
Cervical Cancer

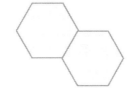

NUMBER OF STUDIES: 2

CHI VALUE: 2

Cervix is Latin for neck. Cancer of the cervix uteri is the development of cancerous cells at the narrow neck of the uterus. The uterus begins at the end of the vagina and together with the fallopian tubes and ovaries comprises the female reproductive system.

Initial symptoms of cervical cancer may include vaginal bleeding, discharge, and painful intercourse. Symptoms of more advanced cancerous development may include lower abdominal pains, pelvic pain, lower back pain, groin pain and persistent vaginal bleeding. Other general signs often associated with cancer may also be present such as loss of appetite, weight loss, and low energy.

Orthodox medicine hypothesizes numerous possible causes and co-factors for the development of cervical cancer among higher risk females. Higher risk is defined by the presence of statistically significant co-factors, such as a family history of cervical cancer, poverty, substance abuse, human papillomavirus (HPV), HIV/AIDS, herpes simplex, use of pharmaceutical birth control, multiple prior pregnancies, dietary factors, and a high number of sex partners.

Allopathic prevention methods of cervical cancer may include the use of HPV vaccine. Diagnosis involves progressive tests, including pap smears, colposcopies (visual inspection of the cervix using acetic acid), or biopsies. Treatment comprises surgery, chemotherapy, or radiation.

Some alternative leaning physicians may also recommend a diet high in vegetable consumption, especially fruits and vegetables containing lycopene. Recent studies have shown that lycopene may be protective against HPV persistence.[1] The fruit containing by far the highest amout of lycopene is a Southeast Asian native called gac (Spiny bitter gourd, lat. Momordica cochinchinensis). Other sources of lycopene include tomatoes, water melon, papaya, pink guava, rosehip or pink grapefruit.

CANNABIS AND CERVICAL CANCER

A Geneva study (2004) demonstrated that anandamide, the body's own cannabinoid, possesses the ability to protect healthy cervical cells from developing cancer via both CB1 and CB2 receptor sites. Beyond protective abilities, anandamide was found to induce suicide (apoptosis) in cervical cells which had mutated into cancerous forms.[2] By 2008, the Rostock experiment continued to add to our scientific knowledge by confirming anandamide's abilities, as well as that of THC, to significantly decrease cell tumor invasiveness, even at very low dosages.[3]

STUDY SUMMARY:

Drugs	Type of Study	Published Year, Place, and Key Results	CHI
Anandamide analog, meth-anandamide and THC	Laboratory test performed on human cervical cancer cells	2008 – University of Rostock, Germany: Cannabinoid-elicits decrease in tumor cell invasiveness.[3]	1
Anandamide	Laboratory test performed on human cervical cancer cells	2004 – University Hospital, Geneva, Switzerland: Anandamide produces apoptosis in cancer cells and exhibits a protective effect via CB1 and CB2.[2]	1

Total CHI Value   2

STRAIN SPECIFIC CONSIDERATIONS

Pre-clinical experiments suggest a potential mechanism involving both CB1 and CB2 in the destruction of human cervical cancer cells, at least in laboratory tests. Both the body's own anandamide and the plant cannabinoid THC bind with CB1 and CB2. In addition, sativas and indicas contain THC.

EXPLORING MIND–BODY CONSCIOUSNESS

The uterus is where the fertilized egg nests and develops from an embryo to a fetus. It is a cradle of physical life. The neck of the uterus is narrow, but flexible enough to be able to contain and eventually release the fully-grown fetus. The mucosal lining of the uterus sheds monthly in an ancient embodied rhythm of life, death, and rebirth.

See also OBGYN and CANCER IN GENERAL

TAKE NOTICE

SAFFRON

SAFFRON: Crocus sativus L. or saffron may poccess anti-cancer activity including against ovarian cancer.[4]

1 Sedjo RL, Roe DJ, Abrahamsen M, Harris RB, Craft N, Baldwin S, Giuliano AR. *Vitamin A, carotenoids, and risk of persistent oncogenic human papillomavirus infection.* Arizona Cancer Center, University of Arizona, Tucson, Arizona 85724, USA. Cancer Epidemiol Biomarkers Prev. 2002 Sep;11(9):876-84.

2 Contassot E, Tenan M, Schnüriger V, Pelte MF, Dietrich PY. *Arachidonyl ethanolamide induces apoptosis of uterine cervix cancer cells via aberrantly expressed vanilloid receptor-1.* Gynecol Oncol. 2004 Apr;93(1):182-8. Oncology Division, Laboratory of Tumor Immunology, University Hospital, Geneva, Switzerland.

3 Ramer R, Hinz B. *Inhibition of cancer cell invasion by cannabinoids via increased expression of tissue inhibitor of matrix metalloproteinases-1.* Institute of Toxicology and Pharmacology, University of Rostock, Schillingallee 70, Rostock D-18057, Germany. J Natl Cancer Inst. 2008 Jan 2;100(1):59-69.

4 Deng Y, Guo ZG, Zeng ZL, Wang Z. *Studies on the pharmacological effects of saffron(Crocus sativus L.)--a review.* Dept. of Chemical Engineering, Tsinghua University, Beijing 100084, China. Zhongguo Zhong Yao Za Zhi. 2002 Aug;27(8):565-8.

Cancer
Colon Cancer

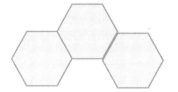

NUMBER OF STUDIES: 3

CHI VALUE: 4

The large intestines (colon) - basically absorb water and salts (electrolytes) from digested matter prior to elimination. In contrast, the small intestins primarily digest and absord nutrients. The majority of nutrients have been absorbed by the time the remaining matter reaches the colon. The large intestines consist of the ascending, transverse and descending colon, followed by the sigmoid colon, closest to the rectum. The colon is lined with a mucus membrane, facilitating the movement of waste and essential gut flora (symbiotic bacteria) involved in the production of vitamins and healthy immune function.

Colon cancer develops in the epithelial cells (lining), which may be found as high up as the junction between the large and small intestine or anywhere following its pathway to the anus. Signs and symptoms depend on location and the spread of the cancer but may include abdominal pain, nausea, vomiting, narrow stools, and unexplained changes in bowel movement, waste color or texture. However, numerous other bowel diseases exhibit similar symptoms.

Hypothesized causes include cellular mutations by inheritance or dietary exposure to carcinogens. Other known aspects that increase the risk of developing colon cancer are the presence of colon polyps, IBS, and ulcerative colitis. Additional risk factors include: smoking tobacco, use of alcohol alcohol, aged 50 or over, male gender, obesity, a sedentary lifestyle, the presence of other environmental carcinogens, African American heritage, and receiving radiation therapy for cancer.

In 2010, the National Cancer Institute at the National Institute for Health estimated the U.S. had over 100,000 new colon cancer patients and more than 50,000 fatalities from rectal and colon cancer combined.[1] Within allopathic medicine, colon cancer is diagnosed by colonoscopies, biopsies, or using imaging technology utilizing ionizing radiation, such as contrast x-rays and CT-scans. Treatments include chemotherapy, radiation, or surgery.

CANNABIS AND COLON CANCER

While other cancer-related studies have shown how cannabinoids can induce cancer cell death through apoptosis, both the Uppsala(2011)[2] and Bristol(2005)[3] experiment indicated another possible mechanism involving the inhibition of the enzyme cyclooxygenase 2 (COX-2). The genetic and pharmacologic studies from Nashville (2008) demonstrated in part that activation of CB1 reduced intestinal tumor growth in mice. It suggests endogenous cannabinoid receptors (CB1) as a possible target of novel mechanism for prevention and treatment of colon cancer using the body's own anandamide.[4]

STUDY SUMMARY:

Drugs/Study Focus	Type of Study	Published Year, Place, and Key Results	CHI
Tetrahydrocannabinol (Δ^9-THC), tetrahydrocannabinolic acid (Δ^9-THC-A), cannabidiol (CBD), cannabidiolic acid (CBDA), cannabigerol (CBG) and cannabigerolic acid (CBGA)	Laboratory	2011 – Uppsala University, Uppsala, Sweden: Cannabinoids inhibited cyclooxygenase enzyme.[2]	1
Endogenous cannabinoid receptor (CB1)	Animal study (mice)	2008 – Vanderbilt University Medical Center, Nashville, Tennessee: CB1 expression may reduce intestinal tumor growth.[4]	2
Anandamide	Laboratory	2005 – University of Bristol, Bristol, UK: Anandamide-induced colorectal carcinoma cell death produced by neither apoptosis nor necrosis.[3]	1

Total CHI Value   4

STRAIN AND FORM SPECIFIC CONSIDERATIONS

THC, THC-acid, CBD, CBD-acid, CBG and CBG-acid and endogenous (body's own) anandamide inhibited colon caner cell proliferation in the laboratory. CB1 activation has been shown to reduce colon cancer in mice.

Anandamide and THC activate both CB1 and CB2, while CBD has a greater affinity for CB2. Sativa strains with a higher THC:CBD ratio tend to activate CB1 in greater proportions than indica strains with a generally lower THC:CBD ratio.

Juice obtained from fresh leaves of both indica and sativa strains contain non-psychoactive forms of plant cannabinoids, THC-acid, CBD-acid, and CBG-acid. Sativa strains with a higher THC-acid:CBD-acid ratio tend to activate CB1 in greater proportions than indica strains with a generally lower THC-acid:CBD-acid ratio.

Isolated synthetic cannabinoid prescription medications containing THC, such as sativex, dronabinol, marinol, or nabilone activate both CB1 and CB2.

EXPLORING MIND–BODY CONSCIOUSNESS

SUGGESTED BLESSING

May you find a way to replace any beliefs that suppress or inhibit your emotions.

A study conducted by Australian psychiatrists on more than 637 newly-confirmed colon cancer patients showed a psychological framework unique to the participants when compared to healthy people of similar age and social situation. They included: "…denial and repression of anger, and of other negative emotions, a commitment to prevailing social norms resulting in the external appearance of a 'nice' or 'good' person, and a suppression of reactions which may offend others and the avoidance of conflict."[5]

QUESTIONS

What are the beliefs, thoughts and feelings that I cannot digest, absorb, and eliminate?

AGGRAVATING FACTORS

Suppressed emotions / repression of anger / seeking approval from other(s) / suppression of reactions.

HEALING FACTORS

Appropriate release of emotions / raising self-esteem / adhering to one's own ideals and standards rather than those of others.

TAKE NOTICE

BASIL • CARAWAY • CARDAMOM • CUMIN • NIGELLA • SAFFRON • TURMERIC

BASIL: Basil thwarted chemical attempts to produce stomach cancer in rodents.[6]

CARAWAY: Caraway has been used in an experimental model on rats to determine if the spice, commonly used in Ayurvedic medicine for gastro-intestinal difficulties, has any impact on the development of chemically-induced colon cancer. The researchers determined that dietary caraway (at a dose of 60mg/kg) indeed has properties that are able to control lipid peroxidation and antioxidant homeostasis, thereby preventing the development of chemically-induced colon cancer lesions.[7] Another rodent-based study confirmed these results and further determined that the most optimal dose was 60mg/kg.[8]

CARDAMOM: Nearby, in the city of Kolkata, researchers at the Chittaranjan National Cancer Institute published results of cardamom study: "These results suggest that aqueous suspensions of cardamom have protective effects on experimentally induced colon carcinogenesis."[9] These findings echo the time-proven Unani and Ayurvedic application of cardamom as a treatment in certain gastrointestinal diseases.

CUMIN: Traditional healers in India have been using cumin to treat various gastro-intestinal complaints for hundreds of years. To test the potential therapeutic benefits of cumin, a chemical known to produce colon cancer called 1,2-dimethylhydrazine (DMH) was given to rats to produce colon cancer tumors. For the following 32 weeks, the rats with colon cancer were fed cumin seeds as part of their standard pellet diet.[10] Results showed that dietary cumin significantly suppressesed colon carcinogensis in the test animals.

Another report, this time from New Delhi, suggests similar anti-colon cancer properties of cumin. In a study published in the Journal of Nutrition and Cancer, the researchers state: "The results strongly suggest the cancer chemopreventive potentials of cumin seed could be attributed to its ability to modulate carcinogen metabolism."[11]

NIGELLA: In a University of Mississippi Medical Center study, Mississippi scientists explored a time-proven technique from the Middle East. They examined the possible therapeutic effects of catechin, found in green tea, and thymoquinone, a major compound from black seed (nigella sativa), on specific colon cancer cells. They compared both natural products with the effectiveness of the current chemotherapeutic drug of choice - 5-fluorouracil - against colon cancer cell lines. Scientists determined that both the green tea – catechin - and the thymoquinone from nigella sativa "have demonstrated incredible chemotherapeutic responses,[12] thus suggesting that both may have similar chemotherapeutic effects as their pharmacological counterpart 5-fluorouracil, which has known serious side effects, including cardiac toxicity."

SAFFRON: Crocus sativus L. or saffron may poccess anti-cancer activity including against colon adenocarcinoma.[13]

TURMERIC: In this meta-analysis, scientists provided an overview of decades of scientific studies on turmeric. They summarized a long list of turmeric's potential therapeutic properties: cancer and diabetic prevention, cancer treatment, promoter of wound-healing, and a therapeutic agent in Alzheimer's, Parkinson's, cardio-vascular, and pulmonary diseases, arthritis, adenomatous polyposis (multiple polyps in the large intestines – precursor to colon cancer), inflammatory bowel disease (IBS), ulcerative colitis (colon inflammation with ulcers), atherosclerosis, pancreatitis, psoriasis, chronic anterior and uveitis (inflammation of the middle layer of the eye).[14]

1 National Cancer Institute at the National Institute for Health. *Colon and Rectal Cancer. Estimated new cases and deaths from colon and rectal cancer in the United States in 2010*: http://www.cancer.gov/cancertopics/types/colon-and-rectal

2 Ruhaak LR, Felth J, Karlsson PC, Rafter JJ, Verpoorte R, Bohlin L. *Evaluation of the cyclooxygenase inhibiting effects of six major cannabinoids isolated from Cannabis sativa.* Division of Pharmacognosy, Department of Medicinal Chemistry, Biomedical Centre, Uppsala University, Uppsala, Sweden. Biol Pharm Bull. 2011;34(5):774-8.

3 H A Patsos1, D J Hicks1, R R H Dobson1, A Greenhough1, N Woodman1, J D Lane2, A C Williams1, C Paraskeva1 *The endogenous cannabinoid, anandamide, induces cell death in colorectal carcinoma cells: a possible role for cyclooxygenase 2.* 1Cancer Research UK Colorectal Tumour Biology Group, Department of Pathology and Microbiology, School of Medical Sciences, University of Bristol, Bristol, UK. 2Department of Biochemistry, School of Medical Sciences, University of Bristol, Bristol, UK Correspondence to: Professor C Paraskeva Cancer Research UK Colorectal Tumour Biology Group, Department of Pathology and Microbiology, School of Medical Sciences, University Walk, University of Bristol, Bristol BS8 1TD, UK. Gut 2005;54:1741-1750.

4 Wang D, Wang H, Ning W, Backlund MG, Dey SK, Dubois RN. *Loss of cannabinoid receptor 1 accelerates intestinal tumor growth.* Departments of Medicine, Vanderbilt University Medical Center, Nashville, Tenessee, USA. Cancer Res. 2008 Aug 1;68(15):6468-76.

5 Gabriel A. Kunea1, Susan Kunea1, Lyndsey F. Watsona1 and Claus Bahne Bahnsona1 *Personality as a risk factor in large bowel cancer: data from the Melbourne Colorectal Cancer Study.* 1 Department of Surgery, University of Melbourne, Australia; Departments of Family Medicine and Psychiatry, University of California, San Francisco, Fresno Campus, USA. Psychological Medicine (1991), 21: 29-41.

6 Dasgupta T, Rao AR, Yadava PK. *Chemomodulatory efficacy of basil leaf (Ocimum basilicum) on drug metabolizing and antioxidant enzymes, and on carcinogen-induced skin and forestomach papillomagenesis.* Cancer Biology and Applied Molecular Biology Laboratories, School of Life Sciences, Jawaharlal Nehru University, New Delhi, India. Phytomedicine. 2004 Feb;11(2-3):139-51.

7   Kamaleeswari M, Nalini N. *Dose-response efficacy of caraway (Carum carvi L.) on tissue lipid peroxidation and antioxidant profile in rat colon carcinogenesis.* Department of Biochemistry, Annamalai University, Annamalainagar, 608 002, Tamilnadu, India. J Pharm Pharmacol. 2006 Aug;58(8):1121-30.

8   Deeptha K, Kamaleeswari M, Sengottuvelan M, Nalini N. *Dose dependent inhibitory effect of dietary caraway on 1,2-dimethylhydrazine induced colonic aberrant crypt foci and bacterial enzyme activity in rats.* Department of Biochemistry and Biotechnology, Annamalai University, Annamalainagar 608 002, Tamilnadu, India. Invest New Drugs. 2006 Nov;24(6):479-88.

9   Sengupta A, Ghosh S, Bhattacharjee S. *Dietary cardamom inhibits the formation of azoxymethane-induced aberrant crypt foci in mice and reduces COX-2 and iNOS expression in the colon.* Department of Cancer Chemoprevention, Chittaranjan National Cancer Institute, Kolkata 700026, India. Asian Pac J Cancer Prev. 2005 Apr-Jun;6(2):118-22.

10   Nalini N, Manju V, Menon VP. *Effect of spices on lipid metabolism in 1,2-dimethylhydrazine-induced rat colon carcinogenesis.* Department of Biochemistry, Annamalai University, Annamalainagar, Tamilnadu, India. J Med Food. 2006 Summer;9(2):237-45.

11   Gagandeep, Dhanalakshmi S, Méndiz E, Rao AR, Kale RK. *Chemopreventive effects of Cuminum cyminum in chemically induced forestomach and uterine cervix tumors in murine model systems.* Radiation and Cancer Biology Laboratory, School of Life Sciences, Jawaharlal Nehru University, New Delhi-110067, India. Nutr Cancer. 2003;47(2):171-80.

12   Norwood AA, Tucci M, Benghuzzi H. *A comparison of 5-fluorouracil and natural chemotherapeutic agents, EGCG and thymoquinone, delivered by sustained drug delivery on colon cancer cells.* University of Mississippi Medical Center, 2500 North State Street, Jackson, Mississippi 39216, USA. Biomed Sci Instrum. 2007;43:272-7.

13   Deng Y, Guo ZG, Zeng ZL, Wang Z. *Studies on the pharmacological effects of saffron(Crocus sativus L.)--a review.* Dept. of Chemical Engineering, Tsinghua University, Beijing 100084, China. Zhongguo Zhong Yao Za Zhi. 2002 Aug;27(8):565-8.

14   Goel A, Kunnumakkara AB, Aggarwal BB. *Curcumin as "Curecumin": From kitchen to clinic.* Gastrointestinal Cancer Research Laboratory, Department of Internal Medicine, Charles A. Sammons Cancer Center and Baylor Research Institute, Baylor University Medical Center, Dallas, TX, United States. Biochem Pharmacol. 2007 Aug 19.

Cancer
Leukemia and Lymphoma

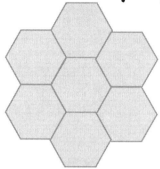

COMBINED NUMBER OF STUDIES: 7

COMBINED CHI VALUE: 9

Leukemia is a type of blood cancer which usually begins in the bone marrow. Here, under normal circumstances, production takes place for red and white blood cells and platelets. Cancerous mutations of blood cells at their point of genesis can lead to serious impairment of the functions associated with each type of blood cell.

Lymphomas are cancers which typically form tumors inside lymph nodes. Both white blood cells (natural killer cells, T-cells, B-cells) and lymph nodes, which filter waste and toxins, are important parts of the body's immune system. Therefore, leukemia and lymphoma are closely related and can be considered cancers of the immune system.

A common observation in leukemia is the production of too many poorly functioning white blood cells, which severely reduces natural immunity and increase the risk of infections. Further, this glut of malformed white blood cells can displace red blood cells and platelets, which carry oxygen and are responsible for blood clotting, respectively.

As one would suspect, signs and symptoms of leukemia include a high white blood cell count, anemia, clotting problems leading to opportunistic infections, easy bruising, and spontaneous pinprick bleeds. Depending on severity, anemia symptoms may progress from feelings of weakness to shortness of breath. Other symptoms may mimic the disease, such as malaria or flu, with nausea, vomiting, fever, chills, diaphoresis, bone and joint aches, muscular weakness or pain, and enlarged liver, spleen, and lymph nodes.

Lymphomas are basically classified as Hodgkin's and non-Hodgkin's lymphomas, with dozens of sub-classifications depending on the country or system used. Lymphoma's symptoms are similar to leukemia, but more commonly include swollen lymph nodes resulting from the backup of unmoved waste materials and tumors inside the nodes.

Depending on the speed of disease development and specific tissues affected, leukemia is generally classified into acute and chronic forms and further broken down as either acute or chronic myeloid or lymphoblastic leukemia. Leukemia can develop in the very young and adults alike. "It is estimated that 43,050 men and women (24,690 men and 18,360 women) will be diagnosed with, and 21,840 men and women will die of, leukemia in 2010."[1] However, of all children suffering from cancers, roughly 1 out of 3 suffers from leukemia.

Within the orthodox medical community, the exact causes of the various leukemia types are only partially known, but several risk factors have been identified. Causative relations are found between prior chemotherapies for cancer, ionizing radiation and exposure to benzene, formaldehyde and other chemical toxins. Risk factors may include genetic pre-disposition, smoking, viral influences, Down syndrome, and extremely low frequencies (ELF) commonly associated with high voltage electrical power lines.[2]

Depending on the presence of symptoms, diagnosis occurs by physical examination, lymph node biopsies, or tests of blood and bone marrow. In some cases, doctors perform imaging techniques, such as ultra sound, magnetic resonance imaging (MRI), or ionizing radiation via X-rays or CT scan. Allopathic treatments include chemotherapy, bone marrow transplants, and radiation.

1 Howlader N, Noone AM, Krapcho M, Neyman N, Aminou R, Waldron W, Altekruse SF, Kosary CL, Ruhl J, Tatalovich Z, Cho H, Mariotto A, Eisner MP, Lewis DR, Chen HS, Feuer EJ, Cronin KA, Edwards BK (eds). *SEER Cancer Statistics Review, 1975-2008*, National Cancer Institute. Bethesda, MD, http://seer.cancer.gov/csr/1975_2008/, based on November 2010 SEER data submission, posted to the SEER web site, 2011.

2 World Health Organization (WHO). *IARC Monographs on the Evaluation of Carcinogenic Risks to Humans. Non-Ionizing Radiation, Part 1: Static and Extremely Low-Frequency (ELF) Electric and Magnetic Fields.* Volume 80 (2002).

Abdominal section of a healthy lymphatic system

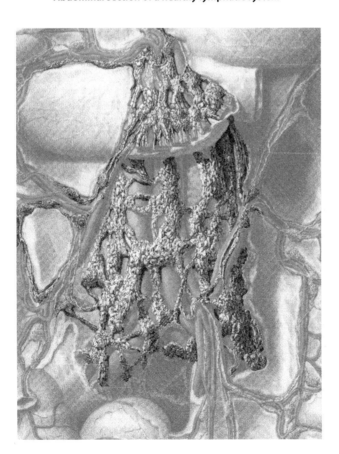

Cancer
Leukemia

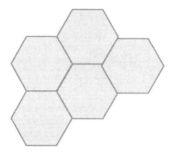

NUMBER OF STUDIES: 5

CHI VALUE: 7

The Lymphoma Foundation of America has acknowledged the medical and therapeutic benefits of marijuana and supports its legal use for patients with serious medical conditions.

While a 2004 London study suggested that THC does not work synergistically with chemotherapy agents, a 2008 analysis concluded that THC does in fact enhance the effectiveness of anti-cancer drugs to induce death in leukemia cells.

During this same period (2006), a Columbia team discovered that CBD, via CB2 pathways, produced apoptosis of leukemia cells, reduced tumor burden, and increased tumor apoptosis, suggesting that CBD may be a novel and highly selective treatment for leukemia.

A couple of years later, the London studies and the Colombia/Virginia experiments confirmed THC's ability to induce apoptosis in leukemia cancer cells and that therapeutic modulation was likely to involve CB1 and CB2 receptors. In addition, Swedish researchers demonstrated the potential of CB1 and CB2-mediated reduction in size and spread of lymphomas.

CANNABIS AND LEUKEMIA STUDY SUMMARY:

Drugs/Study Focus	Type of Study	Published Year, Place, and Key Results	CHI
Anandamide analog R(+)-methanand-amide (R(+)-MA)	Laboratory and 'in vivo' studies on mice	2008 - Karolinska University Hospital Huddinge, Stockholm, Sweden:Anandamide analog R(+)-methanandamide (R(+)-MA) halts the spread and growth of cancerous tumors in animals with non-Hodgkin lymphoma.[3]	1+2
THC	Laboratory study on Leukemia cell lines	2008 - Department of Oncology, St George's University of London, London, UK: "Clear synergistic interactions between THC and the cytotoxic agents in leukemic cells."[4]	1
CBD	Laboratory and 'in vivo' studies	2006 – University of South Carolina School of Medicine, Columbia, SC: CBD, via CB2 pathways, produced apoptosis of leukemia cells, reduced tumor burden and increased tumor apoptosis.[5]	1
THC	Laboratory	2006 – Multi-institutional, Columbia, SC: Raf-1/MEK/ERK/RSK-mediated translocation played a critical role in THC-induced apoptosis in Jurkat cells (Leukemia cells).[6]	1

Drugs	Type of Study	Published Year, Place, and Key Results	CHI
THC	Laboratory	2004 – Multi-institutional, London, UK: THC induces apoptosis in leukemia cancer cells in 'test tube.'[7]	1

Total CHI Value 7

TAKE NOTICE

TURMERIC • SAFFRON

TURMERIC: The rate for childhood leukemia in Asia is significant lower and researchers increasingly consider environmental factor such as diet a major factor. Scientist increasingly focus on turmeric. Over a dozen studies have examined turmeric an leukemia. For instance, studies from Singapore, Chengdu, China and Bethesda, MD have demonstrated that curcumin, the compound that gives turmeric its bright yellow color, was able to arrest the growth of leukemia in the laboratory.[8,9,10] Physicians have treated a total of 50 patients with chronic lymphocytic leukemia and concluded that curcumin may be contributing to a more effective therapy for leukemia patients.[11]

SAFFRON: Crocus sativus L. or Saffron may poccess anti cancer activity including against leukemia.[12]

3 Gustafsson K, Wang X, Severa D, Eriksson M, Kimby E, Merup M, Christensson B, Flygare J, Sander B. *Expression of cannabinoid receptors type 1 and type 2 in non-Hodgkin lymphoma: growth inhibition by receptor activation.* Department of Laboratory Medicine, Division of Pathology, Karolinska Institutet and Karolinska University Hospital Huddinge, F-46, SE-14186 Stockholm, Sweden. Int J Cancer. 2008 Sep 1;123(5):1025-33.

4 Liu WM, Scott KA, Shamash J, Joel S, Powles TB. *Enhancing the in vitro cytotoxic activity of Delta(9)-tetrahydrocannabinol in leukemic cells through a combinatorial approach.* Department of Oncology, St George's University of London, Jenner Wing, London, UK. w.liu@sgul.ac.uk Leuk Lymphoma. 2008 Sep;49(9):1800-9.

5 Robert J. McKallip, Wentao Jia, Jerome Schlomer, James W. Warren, Prakash S. Nagarkatti and Mitzi Nagarkatti. *Cannabidiol-Induced Apoptosis in Human Leukemia Cells: A Novel Role of Cannabidiol in the Regulation of p22phox and Nox4 Expression.* Department of Pathology, Microbiology, and Immunology, University of South Carolina School of Medicine, 6439 Garner's Ferry Road, Columbia, SC 29209, USA. Mol Pharmacol. 2006 Sep;70(3):897-908.

6 Wentao Jia2, Venkatesh L. Hegde1, Narendra P. Singh1, Daniel Sisco1, Steven Grant3, Mitzi Nagarkatti1 and Prakash S. Nagarkatti1. *Δ9-Tetrahydrocannabinol-Induced Apoptosis in Jurkat Leukemia T Cells Is Regulated by Translocation of Bad to Mitochondria.* 1Department of Pathology, Microbiology, and Immunology, University of South Carolina School of Medicine, Columbia, South Carolina and Departments of 2Pharmacology and Toxicology and 3Medicine, Medical College of Virginia Campus, Virginia Commonwealth University, Richmond, Virginia. Mol Cancer Res 2006;4(8):549–62.

7 Thomas Powles, Robert te Poele, Jonathan Shamash, Tracy Chaplin, David Propper, Simon Joel, Tim Oliver, and Wai Man Liu. *Cannabis-induced cytotoxicity in leukemic cell lines: the role of the cannabinoid receptors and the MAPK pathway.* From the New Drug Study Group, St Bartholomew's Hospital (SBH), London, United Kingdom; the Department of Medical Oncology, SBH, London, United Kingdom; the Centre for Cancer Therapeutics, Institute of Cancer Research, Surrey, United Kingdom; the Department of Medical Oncology, Charterhouse Square, London, United Kingdom; and the Barry Reed Oncology Laboratory, SBH, London, United Kingdom. Blood February 1, 2005 vol. 105 no. 3 1214-1221.

8 Tan KL, Koh SB, Ee RP, Khan M, Go ML. *Curcumin analogues with potent and selective anti-proliferative activity on acute promyelocytic leukemia: involvement of accumulated misfolded nuclear receptor co-repressor (N-CoR) protein as a basis for selective activity.* Department of Pharmacy, National University of Singapore, 18 Science Drive 4, Singapore 117543, Singapore. ChemMedChem. 2012 Sep;7(9):1567-79.

9 Shan QQ, Gong YP, Guo Y, Lin J, Zhou RQ, Yang X. *Anti-tumor effect of tanshinone II A, tetrandrine, honokiol, curcumin, oridonin and paeonol on leukemia cell lines.* Department of Hematology, State Key Laboratory of Biotherapy, West China Hospital, Sichuan University, Chengdu 610041, China. Sichuan Da Xue Xue Bao Yi Xue Ban. 2012 May;43(3):362-6.

10 Kim YS, Farrar W, Colburn NH, Milner JA. *Cancer stem cells: potential target for bioactive food components.* Nutritional Science Research Group, Division of Cancer Prevention, National Cancer Institute, Bethesda, MD 20892, USA. J Nutr Biochem. 2012 Jul;23(7):691-8

11 Guenova ML, Michova A, Balatzenko GN, Yosifov DY, Stoyanov N, Taskov H, Berger MR, Konstantinov SM. *A particular expression pattern of CD13 epitope 7H5 in chronic lymphocytic leukaemia - a possible new therapeutic target.* Laboratory of Haematopathology and Immunology, National Specialised Hospital for Active Treatment of Haematological Diseases, Sofia, Bulgaria. Hematology. 2012 May;17(3):132-9.

12 Deng Y, Guo ZG, Zeng ZL, Wang Z. *Studies on the pharmacological effects of saffron(Crocus sativus L.)--a review.* Dept. of Chemical Engineering, Tsinghua University, Beijing 100084, China. Zhongguo Zhong Yao Za Zhi. 2002 Aug;27(8):565-8.

Cancer
Lymphoma

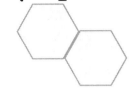

NUMBER OF STUDIES: 2

CHI VALUE: 2

A Swedish study (2009) revealed that the anti-cancer properties of cannabinoids increased synergistically with the rise of ceramide, a naturally-occurring lipid (fat) commonly found in cell membranes. This followed an Italian team's confirmation (2000) that the endocannabinoid anandamide induces apoptosis in lymphoma cancer cells.

CANNABIS AND LYMPHOMA STUDY SUMMARY:

Drugs	Type of Study	Published Year, Place, and Key Results	CHI
Endocannabinoid analogue R(+)-meth-anandamide (R-MA)	Laboratory	2009 – Karolinska University Hospital Huddinge, Stockholm, Sweden: The cannabinoid R-MA produces MCL cell death & the cytotoxic effect of R-MA is enhanced by modulation of ceramide metabolism.[12]	1
Anandamide	Laboratory	2000 - Ministero dell'Università e della Ricerca Scientifica e Tecnologica, Rome, Italy: Andndamide produced apoptosis in human cancer cells (neuroblastoma CHP100 and lymphoma U937 cells).[13]	1

Total CHI Value 2

STRAIN SPECIFIC CONSIDERATIONS

These pre-clinical laboratory studies and animal experiments highlight the endocannabinoid system in the destruction (apoptosis) of both leukemia and lymphoma cell lines. The body's own anandamide, as well as THC and CBD, have proven to be toxic to these types of cancers, at least in the laboratory. The majority of these studies have been conducted on anandamide and THC, which bind to both CB1 and CB2 receptors. However, one experiment also demonstrated that CBD exhibited the ability to produce apoptosis via CB2 mechanisms.

Sativas or sativa-heavy strains tend to have a higher THC:CBD ratio, binding to both CB1 and CB2, while indicas or indica-heavy strains tend to have a lower THC:CBD ratio, binding to CB1 with a greater affinity.

EXPLORING MIND–BODY CONSCIOUSNESS

My flesh and blood. Blood bother. Blood is thicker than water. These idioms, similar in many cultures, suggest issues related to family. A study conducted on several patients diagnosed with leukemia reported that symptoms occurred while trying to handle multiple stressors from varying sources. Seventeen out of the twenty patients participating in this study claimed significant stress from a common source; the separation of a significant other (father, mother, wife, or other mother-figure) mainly due to death or from separation due to sibling and offspring conflict. Compounding stressors included quick and sudden changes related to work, infection, injury, or surgery.[14]

A study examining potential psychological risk factors for the genesis of acute leukemia discovered that family conflict involving inabilities to express feelings and emotions (alexithymia) due to guilt, repression and denial were among the significant risk factors common in those who developed the disease.[15]

See also EXPLORING MIND–BODY–CONSCIOUSNESS for CANCER IN GENERAL, and SICKLE CELL DISEASE.

TAKE NOTICE

MYRRH • OREGANO

MYRRH: Based on traditional practice and evidence-based discoveries, this researcher reported that myrrh's significant antiseptic, anesthetic, and antitumor properties are most likely attributed to a specific alkene called furanosesquiterpene, present in essential oil of myrrh.[16] University of Texas scientists discovered that naturally-occurring steroids (guggulsterone) from a closely related species called Commiphora mukul could produce apoptosis (destruction of cancer cells); "…including leukemia, head and neck carcinoma, multiple myeloma, lung carcinoma, melanoma, breast carcinoma, and ovarian carcinoma. Guggulsterone also inhibited the proliferation of drug-resistant cancer cells (e.g., gleevac-resistant leukemia, dexamethasone-resistant multiple myeloma, and doxorubicin-resistant breast cancer cells)."[17]

OREGANO: Chemists at the University of Central Florida isolated several compounds from oregano. Studies showed that aristolochic acid I and II possessed cancer-fighting abilities targeted at leukemia.[18]

12 Gustafsson K, Sander B, Bielawski J, Hannun YA, Flygare J. *Potentiation of cannabinoid-induced cytotoxicity in mantle cell lymphoma through modulation of ceramide metabolism.* Department of Laboratory Medicine, Division of Pathology, Karolinska Institutet and Karolinska University Hospital Huddinge, Stockholm, Sweden. Mol Cancer Res 2009;7(7):1086-98.

13 Mauro Maccarrone, Tatiana Lorenzon, Monica Bari, Gerry Melino and Alessandro Finazzi-Agrò. *Anandamide Induces Apoptosis in Human Cells via Vanilloid Receptors EVIDENCE FOR A PROTECTIVE ROLE OF CANNABINOID RECEPTORS.* Istituto Superiore di Sanità (III AIDS Program), by Ministero dell'Università e della Ricerca Scientifica e Tecnologica, Rome October 13, 2000 The Journal of Biological Chemistry, 275, 31938-31945.

14 William A. Greene Jr. M.D.1 Psychological Factors and Reticuloendothelial Disease. I. *Preliminary Observations on a Group of Males with Lymphomas and Leukemias.* 1Departments of Psychiatry and Medicine, University of Rochester School of Medicine and Dentistry, and Strong Memorial Hospital and Rochester Municipal Hospital Rochester, New York. Psychosomatic Medicine 16:220-230 (1954).

15 Gouva M., Damigos D., Kaltsouda A., Bouranta P., Tsabouri S., Mavreas V., Bourantas K.L. *Psychological Risk Factors in Acute Leukemia.* 1 University of Ioannina - Medical School, Ioannina, 2 Department of Nursing, TEI of Epirus, Greece. Interscientific Health Care (2009) 1, 16-20.

16 Nomicos EY. *Myrrh: medical marvel or myth of the magi?* National Institute of Allergy and Infectious Diseases, National Institute of Health, Bethesda, Maryland. Holist Nurs Pract. 2007 Nov-Dec;21(6):308-23.

17 Shishodia S, Sethi G, Ahn KS, Aggarwal BB. *Guggulsterone inhibits tumor cell proliferation, induces S-phase arrest, and promotes apoptosis through activation of c-Jun N-terminal kinase, suppression of Akt pathway, and downregulation of antiapoptotic gene products.* Cytokine Research Laboratory, Department of Experimental Therapeutics, Unit 143, The University of Texas M. D. Anderson Cancer Center, 1515 Holcombe Boulevard, Houston, TX 77030, United States. Biochem Pharmacol. 2007 Jun 30;74(1):118-30.

18 Goun E, Cunningham G, Solodnikov S, Krasnykch O, Miles H. *Antithrombin activity of some constituents from Origanum vulgare.* Department of Chemistry, University of Central Florida, Orlando, FL 32816, USA. Fitoterapia. 2002 Dec;73(7-8):692-4.

Cancer
Liver Cancer

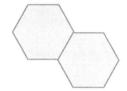

NUMBER OF STUDIES: 2

CHI VALUE: 4

Hepatocellular carcinoma (HCC) is the third leading cause of cancer-related death worldwide.[1] While numerous types of liver cancers exist, HCC is by far the most common form. Signs and symptoms may include: right upper abdominal distention, tenderness, pain (may be radiating), jaundice (yellow skin, sclera), brown urine, weight loss, nausea, and vomiting.

The allopathic community cannot pinpoint the exact cause of liver cancer. Statistically significant risk factors in the development of liver cancer may include: gender (more common in males), history of chronic hepatitis B or C, cirrhosis, fatty liver, diabetes, toxins, alcoholism, L-carnitine deficiencies, or obesity.

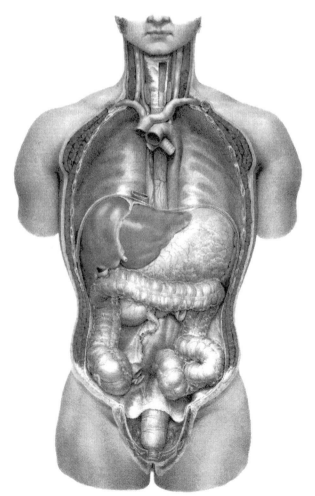

Orthodox diagnosis is conducted via blood tests (examining liver values), imaging tests (X-ray, ultrasound, MRI) or biopsy. Traditional treatment consists of chemotherapy, radiation, surgery (tumor removal or transplant), cold applications (cryoprobe), heat (radiofrequency ablation), and injections of pure alcohol into the tumor sites.

CANNABIS AND LIVER CANCER

In 2009, researchers from Palermo, Italy, wrote: "It has recently been shown that cannabinoids induce growth inhibition and apoptosis in different tumor cell lines." The results confirmed that WIN produced liver cancer cell death or apoptosis (programmed cell death) in a fashion that was determined to be both dose-and time-dependent. The authors wrote: "…the results seem to indicate a potential therapeutic role of WIN, a synthetic cannabinoid, in hepatic cancer treatment."[2]

Two years later, in another experiment from Madrid, Spain, researchers looking for novel treatment options in cases of liver cancers investigated the effects of the cannabinoids THC and JWH-015 (synthetic cannabinoid) on various liver cancer cell lines. Results showed that both cannabinoids were able to inhibit liver cancer tumor growth in animal models.[3]

STUDY SUMMARY:

Drugs	Type of Study	Published Year, Place, and Key Results	CHI
THC and JWH-015	Animal and laboratory tests	2011 – Alcalá University, Madrid, Spain: Both cannabinoids inhibit liver cancer tumors growth.	1+2
WIN 55,212-2 (Synthetic cannabinoid receptor agonist)	Laboratory	2009 – Università di Palermo, Palermo, Italy: "…potential therapeutic role of WIN in hepatic cancer treatment."	1

Total CHI Value   4

STRAIN SPECIFIC CONSIDERATIONS

The two experiments reviewed here used THC and the synthetic cannabinoids WIN 55,212-2 and JWH-015. Each displayed the ability to inhibit liver cancer cell lines or to induce apoptosis (programmed cancer cell death), at least in the laboratory and in animal tests.

THC binds with both CB1 and CB2. WIN 55,212-2 binds with higher affinity to CB2 than the CB1 receptor. Similarly, JWH-015 has higher affinities for CB2 than CB1.

Both sativa, sativa-heavy strains, indicas and indica-heavy strains bind to CB1 and CB2 but indicas and indica heavy strains tend to have a lower THC:CBD ratio, which may favor CB2 activation.

EXPLORING MIND–BODY CONSCIOUSNESS

See EXPLORING MIND–BODY CONSCIOUSNESS for HEPATITIS and CANCER IN GENERAL.

QUESTIONS

What feeling(s) am I unable to let go of?
What feeling(s) am I unable to filter through?

1 Vara D, Salazar M, Olea-Herrero N, Guzmán M, Velasco G, Díaz-Laviada I. *Anti-tumoral action of cannabinoids on hepatocellular carcinoma: role of AMPK-dependent activation of autophagy.* Department of Biochemistry and Molecular Biology, School of Medicine, Alcalá University, Madrid, Spain. Cell Death Differ. 2011 Apr 8.

2 Giuliano M, Pellerito O, Portanova P, Calvaruso G, Santulli A, De Blasio A, Vento R, Tesoriere G. *Apoptosis induced in HepG2 cells by the synthetic cannabinoid WIN: Involvement of the transcription factor PPARgamma.* Dipartimento di Scienze Biochimiche, Università di Palermo, Via del Vespro 129, 90127 Palermo, Italy. Biochimie. 2009 Apr;91(4):457-65.

3 Ibid.

4 Felder CC, Joyce KE, Briley EM, Mansouri J, Mackie K, Blond O, Lai Y, Ma AL, Mitchell RL. *Comparison of the pharmacology and signal transduction of the human cannabinoid CB1 and CB2 receptors.* Laboratory of Cell Biology, National Institute of Mental Health, Bethesda, Maryland 20892, USA. Mol Pharmacol. 1995 Sep;48(3):443-50.

Cancer
Lung Cancer

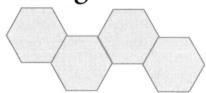

NUMBER OF STUDIES: 4

CHI VALUE: 7

Historically, Lung cancer was a rare diagnosis until it emerged as a major killer with the advent of the industrial revolution, the introduction of cigarettes (tobacco smoke and second hand smoke are recognized as the major cause for developing lung cancer), increasing levels of air pollution (e.g. exhaust, asbestos, coal dust, soot), and the cumulative damage of ionizing radiation (x-rays).[1] Lung cancer is now the number one cancer and leading fatal cancer in the world; some types are highly aggressive and resistant to allopathic treatments. Diagnosis consists of chest x-rays and biopsies, and treatment is limited to chemotherapy, radiation, or surgery.

CANNABIS AND LUNG CANCER

While inhaling any burned substance is generally bad for the lungs, the cannabinoid THC may prevent lung cancer. As early as 1975, the U.S. Government discovered that cannabis plant cannabinoids were able to inhibit lung cancer growth, reduce tumor size, and increase survival rates in animal test subjects. The later studies from Lyon (2006),[2] Rostock (2006)[3] and Harvard (2008)[4] elucidated potential mechanisms: signaling via CB1 and CB2 receptor sites, inducing protection against lung cancer, and inducing cancer-infected cells to self-destruct (apoptosis).

STUDY SUMMARY:

Drugs	Type of Study	Published Year, Place, and Key Results	CHI
THC	Animal studies (mice) and laboratory tests	2008 – Harvard Medical School, Boston, MA: Tested lung cancer cells contained CB1 and CB2 sites. Significant inhibition of the subcutaneous tumor growth and lung metastasis were found.[4]	1+2
Anandamide analog, meth-anandamide and delta9-tetrahydrocannabinol (THC)	Laboratory test performed on human lung cancer cells	2008 – University of Rostock, Germany: Cannabinoid-elicits decrease in tumor cell invasiveness.[3]	1
Cannabis	2,252 human subjects	2006 – International Agency for Research on Cancer, Lyon, France: Population study found no association between lung cancer and long-term cannabis use.[2]	N/A
Delta-9-tetrahydrocannabinol, delta-8-tetrahydrocannabinol, and cannabinol (CBN), and cannabidiol (CBD)	Animal (mice) and laboratory tests	1975 – Virginia Commonwealth University. Richmond, VA: THC, CBN but not CBD retarded lung cancer cell growth, reduction in tumor size, increased survival rates.[5]	1+2

STRAIN-SPECIFIC CONSIDERATIONS

Lung cancer cells have been shown to contain both CB1 and CB2 receptor sites. The reviewed pre-clinical experiments conducted in the laboratory and on animals revealed that the body's own anandamide and plant cannabinoids THC and CBN produced anti-lung cancer cell activity ranging from inhibition of growth to initiation of apoptosis (cancer cell self destruction).

CBN has a higher affinity for CB2, while THC and anandamide bind relatively equally to both CB1 and CB2.

Both sativa, sativa-heavy strains, indicas, and indica-heavy strains bind to CB1 and CB2, but indicas and indica-heavy strains tend to have a lower THC:CBN ratio, which may favor CB2 activation.

EXPLORING MIND–BODY CONSCIOUSNESS

All types of lung cancers affect males significantly more than females. In 1961, scientists explored a hypothesized link between personality constructs and the development of lung cancer. The authors of the study wrote: "The available evidence suggests that lung cancer patients have personality features distinct from the general cigarette smoking population."[6] By 1984 scientists trying to learn more about the differences between organic and psychological predictors in the development of lung cancer discovered that: "Some psychosocial variables, like rationality and anti-emotionality, or long-lasting hopelessness, were about as relevant as the strongest organic predictors..."[7] In another study, published in 1991, researchers discovered possible predictable psychological conditions in the development of lung cancer that included "...low expression of anxiety, and unfulfilled need for closeness ...."[8]

Breathing in and breathing out. Taking life in and letting it go again can become a difficult and often painful process, depending on the disease's progression. More often than not, the feelings and emotions we have around the symptoms of lung cancer are often a clue to judged emotions and stifled expressions.

See also EXPLORING MIND–BODY–CONSCIOUSNESS for CANCER IN GENERAL and COUGHING.

QUESTIONS

Do you value feelings or emotions? If not, why not?
What are logic, fact, and reason protecting you from?
What thoughts and feeling(s) are always in the air that must not be allowed in?
What would happen if you were to breathe them in?
What feeling(s) are you hopeless or helpless about?

AGGRAVATING FACTORS

Rationality, anti-emotionality, or long-lasting hopelessness, low expression of anxiety, and unfulfilled need for closeness.

> **SUGGESTED BLESSING**
>
> *May your breath and your emotions flow as easy as one, two, three. May you find the seeds of new vision in the depths of hopelessness.*

> **SUGGESTED AFFIRMATION**
>
> *I allow all my feelings and emotions to come and go in fullness, and I express them with intensity, appropriately, and with harm to none.*
>
> *I express and fulfill my need for closeness in healthy ways.*

Learning to value feelings and emotions, express and release emotions, define your feelings and emotions, and feel close with your emotions fosters in self-respect.

TAKE NOTICE

CLOVE • MYRRH

CLOVE: A study from Kolkata looked at the properties of aqueous solution of clove. It found the spice could produce apoptosis of lung cancer cells in mice and held other possible cancer-protective properties.[9]

MYRRH: Based on traditional practice and evidence-based discoveries, this researcher reported that myrrh's significant antiseptic, anesthetic, and antitumor properties are most likely attributed to a specific alkene called furanosesquiterpene, present in essential oil of myrrh.[10]

Scientists from the University of Texas discovered that naturally-occurring steroids (guggulsterone) from a closely related species called Commiphora mukul was able to produce apoptosis (destruction of cancer cells). This included: "…leukemia, head and neck carcinoma, multiple myeloma, lung carcinoma, melanoma, breast carcinoma, and ovarian carcinoma. Guggulsterone also inhibited the proliferation of drug-resistant cancer cells (e.g., gleevac-resistant leukemia, dexamethasone-resistant multiple myeloma, and doxorubicin-resistant breast cancer cells)."[11]

1 John Gofman M.D., Ph.D. Professor emeritus of molecular and cell biology at the UC. Berkeley. *Radiation from Medical Procedures in the Pathogenisis of Cancer and Ischemic Heart Disease*. First Edition 1999. Center for Nuclear Responsibility, Inc. P.O.Box 421993 San Francisco, CA 94142.

2 Hashibe M, Morgenstern H, Cui Y, Tashkin DP, Zhang ZF, Cozen W, Mack TM, Greenland S. *Marijuana use and the risk of lung and upper aerodigestive tract cancers: results of a population-based case-control study*. IARC, Lyon, France. Cancer Epidemiol Biomarkers Prev. 2006 Oct;15(10):1829-34.

3 Ramer R, Hinz B. *Inhibition of cancer cell invasion by cannabinoids via increased expression of tissue inhibitor of matrix metalloproteinases-1*. Institute of Toxicology and Pharmacology, University of Rostock, Schillingallee 70, Rostock D-18057, Germany. J Natl Cancer Inst. 2008 Jan 2;100(1):59-69.

4 Preet A, Ganju RK, Groopman JE. *Delta9-Tetrahydrocannabinol inhibits epithelial growth factor-induced lung cancer cell migration in vitro as well as its growth and metastasis in vivo*. Division of Experimental Medicine, Department of Medicine, Beth Israel Deaconess Medical Center, Harvard Medical School, Boston, MA, USA. Oncogene. 2008 Jan 10;27(3):339-46.

5 A.E. Munson, L.S. Harris, M.A. Friedman, W.L. Dewey, and R.A. Carchman. *Antineoplastic activity of cannabinoids*. Journal of the National Cancer Institute, Vol. 55, No. 3, September 1975. Supported by Public Health Service grant DA00490 from the National Institute on Drug Abuse, Health Services & Mental Health Administration; by a grant from the Alexander and Margaret Stewart Trust Fund; and by an institutional grant from the American Cancer Society. Department of Pharmacology and the MCV/VCU Cancer Center, Medical College of Virginia, Virginia Commonwealth University. Richmond, Va. 23298. Journal of the National Cancer Institute, Vol. 55, No. 3, September 1975.

6 David M. Kissen and H. J. Eysenck. *Personality in male lung cancer patients*. Journal of Psychosomatic Re-

search. From the Department of Psychological Medicine (Southern General Hospital), University of Glasgow, and the Department of Psychology, the Institute of Psychiatry, London. Volume 6, Issue 2, April-June 1962, Pages 123-127.

7 Ronald Grossarth-Maticek, Dusan T. Kanazir, Peter Schmidt and Hermann Vetter. Psychosocial and organic variables as predictors of lung cancer, cardiac infarct and apoplexy: *Some differential predictors. Social Scientific Oncology*, Prospective Epidemiology and Experimental Behavioral Medicine, 6900 Heidelberg, Schloss-Wolfsbrunnenweg 16, F.R.G. University of Belgrade, Studentski trg I, Belgrade, Yugoslavia. Justus-Liebig University Giessen, Ludwigstrasse 23, 6300 Giessen, F.R.G. Personality and Individual Differences. Volume 6, Issue 3, 1985, Pages 313-321.

8 Jutta Quander-Blaznik. P*ersonality as a predictor of lung cancer: A replication.* Institut für Psychologie, Freie Universität, Berlin, F.R.G. Personality and Individual Differences. Volume 12, Issue 2, 1991, Pages 125-130.

9 Banerjee S, Panda CK, Das S. Clove (Syzygium aromaticum L.), a potential chemopreventive agent for lung cancer. Department of Cancer Chemoprevention, Chittarajan National Cancer Institute, 37, S.P. Mukherjee Road, Kolkata 700026, India. Carcinogenesis. 2006 Aug;27(8):1645-54.

10 Nomicos EY. *Myrrh: medical marvel or myth of the magi?* National Institute of Allergy and Infectious Diseases, National Institute of Health, Bethesda, Maryland. Holist Nurs Pract. 2007 Nov-Dec;21(6):308-23.

11 Shishodia S, Sethi G, Ahn KS, Aggarwal BB. *Guggulsterone inhibits tumor cell proliferation, induces S-phase arrest, and promotes apoptosis through activation of c-Jun N-terminal kinase, suppression of Akt pathway, and downregulation of antiapoptotic gene products.* Cytokine Research Laboratory, Department of Experimental Therapeutics, Unit 143, The University of Texas M. D. Anderson Cancer Center, 1515 Holcombe Boulevard, Houston, TX 77030, United States. Biochem Pharmacol. 2007 Jun 30;74(1):118-30.

Cancer
Melanoma

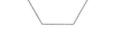

NUMBER OF STUDIES: 1

CHI VALUE: 1

Melanin, produced by specialized skin cells (melanocytes), is the brownish pigment responsible for skin tone variants as well as for the coloring that occurs in tanning, freckles and moles. Exposure to UV light increases melanin production as a protective mechanism from excessive harmful rays. Melanin converts the majority of UV light to harmless heat preventing cellular mutation, thus protecting the skin from damage. The darker your skin means the greater your body's protective ability. The majority of melanocytes lay in the base of the epidermis (outer skin layer).

While the majority of skin cancers are non-melanomas, melanomas make up the majorities of deaths. Melanoma affects more Caucasians than other ethnicities. While direct sun exposure is healthy, natural and excessive sun exposure can contribute to mutation of DNA in melanocytes. The highest incidence of melanoma occurs in whites living in Australia.

Diagnosis begins with the examination of suspicious tissue, moles or lesions. Practitioners carefully look at the A, B, C, D, and E's of affected skin. A stands for asymmetry; B for borders (irregularly shaped); C for uneven color(s) presentation (white, pink, red, blue, brown, black); D for diameter (moles larger than 6mm are more suspicious); and E for evolving or rapid development of shape, color and size (weeks or months, rather than years). Other signs include pain, itching, scar-like tissue development, a pink growth, a reddish patch, or ulceration with discharge or bleeding.

Allopathic treatment includes surgical removal, chemotherapy or radiation.

It's interesting to note that the majority of sunscreens contain ingredients which are considered carcinogenic, or can become carcinogenic in reaction with UV light. Furthermore, using sun block prevents UVB light-induced vitamin D synthesis, which may protect against certain cancers.[1] This last discovery is especially important to dark-skinned people. Thus, a careful balance between the need for healthy sun exposure and a reduction in excessive sun exposure and associated cancer risk should be maintained.

Ten to fifteen minutes of unclothed exposure to the sun before 10AM or after 3PM about three times per week is optimal. This stimulates a gentle and gradual production in melanin for photo protection and supports a healthy immune response mediated in part by the conversion of cholesterol into vitamin D. Dark-skinned people, women who wear veils, and people rarely exposed to the sun may want to consider vitamin D supplementation.

CANNABIS AND MELANOMA

Several studies have confirmed the antiemetic benefits of cannabinoids on melanoma patients undergoing radiation treatment[2] and chemotherapy.[3] Indeed, case study reports of successful applications of extracted cannabis oil against melanoma exist, notably from the citizen experiments of Rick Simpson and reports by Cannabis Science, Inc.[4] Still, scientific studies examining the efficacy of cannabis on melanoma are mostly wanting with the exception of the study conducted by the National Institute of Oncology in Budapest where researchers proved that CB1 modulation induces apoptosis of human melanoma cells.

STUDY SUMMARY:

Drugs/Study Focus	Type of Study	Published Year, Place, and Key Results	CHI
CB1 receptor agonist, Met-F-AEA, CB1 antagonist, AM251	Laboratory study on human melanoma cell lines	2008 – National Inst. of Oncology, Budapest, Hungary: CB1 modulation induces apoptosis of human melanoma cells.[5]	1

Total CHI Value 1

STRAIN SPECIFIC CONSIDERATIONS

A Hungarian laboratory experiment highlights a potential pathway involving CB1 receptor activation in the destruction of human melanoma cells. The synthetic cannabinoid Met-F-AEA is similar to naturally-occurring anandamide, which binds relatively equally to CB1 and CB2.

Sativas and sativa-heavy strains tend to have a higher THC:CBN ratio, which may increase CB1 activation when compared to indicas and indica-heavy strains with lower THC:CBD ratios that may increase CB2 activation.

EXPLORING MIND–BODY CONSCIOUSNESS

See SKIN CANCER (NON-MELANOMA) and CANCER IN GENERAL.

TAKE NOTICE

BUSH TEA • CLOVE • MYRRH

Numerous marijuana patients and advocates alike have reported cases of successful melanoma treatments using highly concentrated solvent extracts of flowers of cannabis.[6]

BUSH TEA: Laboratory studies have found that Bush tea contains DNA-protective and antimutagenic properties.[7] South African researchers who discovered that topical Bush tea application inhibits skin tumor formation have confirmed the antimutagenic properties of Rooibos as well.[8]

CLOVE: An Indian study determined that aqueous solutions of clove might also have protective properties against skin papillomas (skin tumor).[9]

MYRRH: Based on traditional practice and evidence-based discoveries, this researcher reported that myrrh's significant antiseptic, anesthetic, and antitumor properties are most likely attributed to a specific alkene called furanosesquiterpene, present in essential oil of myrrh.[10] University of Texas scientists discovered that naturally-occurring steroids (guggulsterone) from a closely related species called Commiphora mukul produced apoptosis (destruction of cancer cells), "... including leukemia, head and neck carcinoma, multiple myeloma, lung carcinoma, melanoma, breast carcinoma, and ovarian carcinoma. Guggulsterone also inhibited the proliferation of drug-resistant cancer cells (e.g., gleevac-resistant leukemia, dexamethasone-resistant multiple myeloma, and doxorubicin-resistant breast cancer cells)."[11]

1 Grant WB. *An estimate of premature cancer mortality in the U.S. due to inadequate doses of solar ultraviolet-B radiation.* Cancer. 2002 Mar 15;94(6):1867-75.

2 Gonzalez-Rosales F, Walsh D. *Intractable nausea and vomiting due to gastrointestinal mucosal metastases relieved by tetrahydrocannabinol (dronabinol).* Department of Hematology/Oncology, Cleveland Clinic Cancer Center, Cleveland Clinic Foundation, Ohio 44195, USA. Journal of Pain and Symptom Management 1997;14(5):311-314.

3 Zutt M, Hanssle H, Emmert S, Neumann C, Kretschmer L. *Dronabinol for supportive therapy in patients with malignant melanoma and liver metastases.* Hautklinik und Poliklinik der Georg-August-Universitat Gottingen, Germany. Hautarzt 2006;57(5):423-7.

4 Med Knowledge Base. *CBIS Rockford cannabis extract kills melanoma cells.* DENVER, Mar 09, 2011 (BUSINESS WIRE) -- Cannabis Science, Inc. (CBIS) a pioneering U.S. biotech company developing pharmaceutical cannabis (marijuana derivative) products, is pleased to announce that we have now received verbal confirmation that the sites of the former cancerous lesions are free of cancer cells, and we are now awaiting official physician documentation of the patient's history and biopsy reports. Dr. Robert J. Melamede, the CEO and President of Cannabis Science Inc., stated, "The photographic documentation in our last press release demonstrated that cannabis extracts appeared to be effective against what seems to be the patient's third incidence of basal cell carcinoma. For accuracy, it should be noted that a before-treatment biopsy of the lesion on the nose had not been performed. It is obvious that there was a lesion-centered response to the application of the cannabis extract. This patient had a previous surgically-removed lesion, as well as a biopsied basal cell carcinoma on the right cheek. The lesion on the cheek was also self-treated and resolved with cannabis extracts over a half year ago."

5 Jozsef Timar, Balazs Bani, Norbert Varga and Istvan Kenessey. *Cannabinoid receptor-1 modulation induces apoptosis of human melanoma cells.* National Inst. of Oncology, Budapest, Hungary. 99th American Association for Cancer Research (AACR) Annual Meeting-- Apr 12-16, 2008; San Diego, CA.

6 A simple search for 'Phoenix Tears,' or that of its advocate, Rick Simpson, will yield numerous results on any server or media sites, such as YouTube. You can also go directly to: Phoenix Tears Foundation (http://www.phoenixtearsfoundation.com), which was founded to pursue Cannabinoid research and treatment, or visit Rick Simpson's home site (http://phoenixtears.ca/) or 'Patients out of Time' an all-volunteer non-profit 501c3 educational charity (http://www.medicalcannabis.com/)

7 Lee EJ, Jang HD. *Antioxidant activity and protective effect on DNA strand scission of Rooibos tea (Aspalathus linearis).* Department of Food and Nutrition, Hannam University, Daejeon, Korea. Biofactors. 2004; 21(1-4-):285-92.

8 Marnewick J, Joubert E, Joseph S, Swanevelder S, Swart P, Gelderblom W. *Inhibition of tumour promotion in mouse skin by extracts of rooibos (Aspalathus linearis) and honeybush (Cyclopia intermedia), unique South*

African herbal teas. PROMEC Unit, Medical Research Council, P.O. Box 19070, Tygerberg 7505, South Africa. Cancer Lett. 2005 Jun 28;224(2):193-202.

9 Banerjee S, Das S. *Anticarcinogenic effects of an aqueous infusion of cloves on skin carcinogenesis.* Dept. of Cancer Chemoprevention, Chittarajan National Cancer Institute, 37 S.P. Mukherjee Road, Kolkata 700026, West Bengal, India. Asian Pac J Cancer Prev. 2005 Jul-Sep;6(3):304-8.

10 Nomicos EY. *Myrrh: medical marvel or myth of the magi?* National Institute of Allergy and Infectious Diseases, National Institute of Health, Bethesda, Maryland. Holist Nurs Pract. 2007 Nov-Dec;21(6):308-23.

11 Shishodia S, Sethi G, Ahn KS, Aggarwal BB. *Guggulsterone inhibits tumor cell proliferation, induces S-phase arrest, and promotes apoptosis through activation of c-Jun N-terminal kinase, suppression of Akt pathway, and downregulation of antiapoptotic gene products.* Cytokine Research Laboratory, Department of Experimental Therapeutics, Unit 143, The University of Texas M. D. Anderson Cancer Center, 1515 Holcombe Boulevard, Houston, TX 77030, United States. Biochem Pharmacol. 2007 Jun 30;74(1):118-30.

Cancer
Pancreatic Cancer

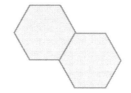

NUMBER OF STUDIES: 2

CHI VALUE: 4

One of the most malignant forms of cancer, pancreatic cancer usually has poor outcomes. Onset symptoms may include gastrointestinal difficulties, such as abdominal pain (often radiating to the back), lack of appetite, nausea and vomiting, diarrhea, weight loss, jaundice, or diabetes. Traditional allopathic treatments of surgery and chemotherapy offer meager success rates. "Pancreatic cancer prognosis remains very poor with a 5-year survival rate of less than 5% in most reports."[1]

CANNABIS AND PANCREATIC CANCER

The urgency of this particularly aggressive cancer, and the lack of effective treatments, has generated a demand for research into new and more successful care. Madrid took the first steps in 2006 after discovering an increased presence of cannabinoid receptors in pancreatic cancer cells.[2] Experiments in the laboratory and in animals confirmed the potential; cannabinoids effectively induced apoptosis in cancerous cells, leaving normal cells unaffected.[3] That same year, scientists in Pisa, Italy, discovered that a novel endocannabinoid mechanism which was not regulated via typical CB1 or CB2 receptors possessed properties to destroy pancreatic cancer lines in the laboratory.[4]

STUDY SUMMARY:

Drugs	Type of Study	Published Year, Place, and Key Results	CHI
THC and other cannabinoids	Laboratory and in vivo animal studies	2006 – Complutense University, Madrid, Spain: Anti pancreatic tumor effect via CB2 receptors.	1+2
AM251 (potent CB1 antagonist)	Laboratory	2006 – University of Pisa, Italy: Endocannabinoids produce a significant cytotoxic effect via a receptor-independent mechanism.	1

Total CHI Value 4

STRAIN SPECIFIC CONSIDERATIONS

The results of these pre-clinical trials suggests a CB2-initiated mechanism by which cannabinoids produce toxic effects on pancreatic cancer cell lines.

Indicas and indica-heavy hybrids usually present with a lower THC:CBD/CBN ratio typically promoting an increased CB2 activation.

EXPLORING MIND–BODY CONSCIOUSNESS

If the heart is metaphorically where we feel our feelings, then the liver is where we process them. The pancreas is where we store these feelings until we put them in proper perspective, "making sense" of them in the larger context of our lives. The latter may be echoed in the pancreatic production of insulin where it is needed to utilize sugar. Without it, sugar remains in the blood unused, causing many of the symptoms associated with hyperglycemia (diabetes). Similarly, in emotional terms, feelings flow in the stream of our emotional reality until we transcend them, just like sugar is converted to life sustaining energy.

See also chapters on DIABETES, CANCER IN GENERAL and INFLAMMATORY DIS-EASES - PANCREATITIS.

TAKE NOTICE

TURMERIC • NIGELLA

TURMERIC: A study from Detroit, Michigan showed that diflourinated-curcumin (CDF), a novel analogue of the turmeric spice component curcumin was able to inhibit pancreatic cancer tumor growth and aggressiveness in the laboratory.[5]

NIGELLA: Researchers form Wenzhou, China report that thymoquinone (TQ), a component derived from the medicinal spice Nigella sativa, exhibited inhibitory effects on cell proliferation of pancreatic cell lines in the laboratory and in animal experiments. "Consequently, these results provide important insights into thymoquinone as an antimetastatic agent for the treatment of human pancreatic cancer."[6]

1 World Health Organization (WHO) 2011. http://www.who.int/tobacco/research/cancer/en/

2 Carracedo A, Gironella M, Lorente M, Garcia S, Guzmán M, Velasco G, Iovanna JL. *Cannabinoids Induce Apoptosis of Pancreatic Tumor Cells via Endoplasmic Reticulum Stress–Related Genes.* Department of Biochemistry and Molecular Biology I, School of Biology, Complutense University, c/ José Antonio Novais s/n, 28040 Madrid, Spain. Cancer Res July 1, 2006 66; 6748-55.

3 Ibid.

4 Fogli S, Nieri P, Chicca A, Adinolfi B, Mariotti V, Iacopetti P, Breschi MC, Pellegrini S. *Cannabinoid derivatives induce cell death in pancreatic MIA PaCa-2 cells via a receptor-independent mechanism.* Department of Psychiatry, University of Pisa, Via Bonanno, 6, 56126 Pisa, PI, Italy. FEBS Lett. 2006 Mar 20;580(7):1733-9.

5 Bao B, Ali S, Banerjee S, Wang Z, Logna F, Azmi AS, Kong D, Ahmad A, Li Y, Padhye S, Sarkar FH. *Curcumin analogue CDF inhibits pancreatic tumor growth by switching on suppressor microRNAs and attenuating EZH2 expression.* Department of Pathology, Karmanos Cancer Institute, Wayne State University, Detroit, Michigan 48201, USA. Cancer Res. 2012 Jan 1;72(1):335-45.

6 Wu ZH, Chen Z, Shen Y, Huang LL, Jiang P. *Anti-metastasis effect of thymoquinone on human pancreatic cancer.* Second Affiliated Hospital of Wenzhou Medical College, Wenzhou 325027, China. Yao Xue Xue Bao. 2011 Aug;46(8):910-4.

SUGGESTED BLESSING

May I learn to provide space for my feelings without letting them control my life.

SUGGESTED AFFIRMATION

I store my feelings only as long as it takes to put them in proper perspective.

Cancer
Prostate Cancer

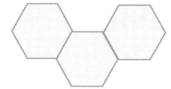

NUMBER OF STUDIES: 3

CHI VALUE: 3

The prostate gland is part of the male reproductive system. Located at the outlet of the urinary bladder, the prostate is about the size of a walnut in its healthy state. The urethra, the opening from the bladder, leads through the prostate to the tip of the penis. The gland produces and stores seminal fluids in which sperm originating in the testes move about during ejaculation.

Similarly, females have a glandular tissue called Skene's glands or periurethral glands that produce fluid almost identical to the male version which may be ejaculated during orgasm. However, the 'female prostate' is not usually subject to cancerous proliferation.

Prostate cancer is one of the most common cancers in elderly males yet is generally very slow growing. While many patients never have any particular symptoms, an enlargement of the prostate commonly underlies cancer pathologies. The enlargement exerts pressure on the urethra making urinating and fully emptying the bladder difficult. Other possible symptoms of prostate cancer may include sexual dysfunction, bloody urine, painful urination or pain in that general region.

In days past, a prostate problem was called "priests disease", due to the hypothesis that lack of sexual activity may be related to the development of prostate cancer. A significant study conducted over a period of eight years aincluding almost 30,000 males confirmed this association. Results revealed that increased sexual activity (more than 21 ejaculation per month) correlated to a 30% decreased risk of developing prostate cancer over a lifetime when compared to males who only ejaculate four to seven times per month.[1]

More specific causes of prostate cancer remain a mystery to the scientific community. Traditional treatment includes chemotherapy, radiation, and surgery.

CANNABIS AND PROSTATE CANCER

In 2000, a laboratory experiment conducted in Naples, Italy, demonstrated to researchers that the body's own cannabinoid, anandamide, was able to inhibit the growth of both breast cancer and prostate cancer cells.[2] A 2004 US study followed, led by scientists from Wisconsin who found that prostate cancer cells contained significantly higher expressions of both CB1 and CB2 receptors. This in turn led them to suggest a possible novel approach to treating prostrate cancer.[3] More insights came in 2009, from Debrecen, Hungary. For the first time, CB1 was identified in epithelial and smooth muscle cells of the healthy human prostate. Researchers confirmed the study results, and strongly argued that CB1 possessed a promising future role in the treatment of prostate cancer.[4]

STUDY SUMMARY:

Drugs/Study Focus	Type of Study	Published Year, Place, and Key Results	CHI
Drug receptor CB1	Labratory study on healthy and cancerous prostate cells	2009 – University of Debrecen, Hungary: CB1 found in healthy prostate cells.	1
WIN-55,212-2 and SR141716 (CB1) and SR144528 (CB2)	Labratory study on prostate cancer cells	2004 – University of Wisconsin: Prostate cancer cells contained significantly higher expressions of both CB1 and CB2 receptors.	1
Anandamide, HU-210, BML-190, SR141716A, SR144528	Labratory study on prostate and breast cancer cells	2000 – Multi-institutional: Anandamide inhibits the growth of breast cancer and prostate cancer cells.	1

Total CHI Value 3

STRAIN SPECIFIC CONSIDERATION

Prostate cancer cells contain significantly higher expressions of both CB1 and CB2 receptors, which has prompted researchers to suggest a possible novel approach in treating prostrate cancer. Further, anandamide inhibits the growth of prostate cancer cells in the laboratory. Anandamide and THC bind relatively equally with CB1 and CB2.

While both sativas and indicas as well as hybrids bind with CB1 and CB2, sativas and sativa dominant strains contain a higher THC:CBD ratio, thus providing an increased similarity to the cannabinoid profile of anandamide.

EXPLORING MIND–BODY CONSCIOUSNESS

Researchers have discovered a link between psychological stress and healthy prostate function. Results of a study conducted on 83 men diagnosed with benign prostatic hyperplasia (BPH) reveal that stress and hostility influence prostate volume and residual urine volume.[5] Researchers hypothesize that the effect is mediated via the sympathetic nervous system and hypothalamic–pituitary–gonadal axis.

A large-scale and long-term study of 19,730 adults over a period of nine years somewhat confirmed these results. Researchers discovered that anger control and negative affect have a small role in the risk of prostate cancer.[6]

An enlarged male gland applies pressure and strangles the urethra thus producing the most commonly observed symptom: a struggle to release urine.

Derived from the ancient Greek word for "protector or "guardian," the prostate represents survival, safety and security. An impaired flow of urine is associated with being 'pissed off.' 'Have I made enough money to live on?' 'Do I have enough for those I love?' 'Am I a good enough provider?'

Other issues include pressure from suppressed anger at old age in connection with male energy, image, or virility ('Am I still hard, strong, tough, or fast enough?'). Additionally, pressure from self-judgments about goals never

SUGGESTED BLESSING

May you find a way to forgive and release any pressure(s) surrounding your masculinity.

SUGGESTED AFFIRMATION

I can generate youthful spiritual energy, no matter what age I am.

reached or achieved, or pressure from negative self-image or self-talk that says 'old is useless, weak and decrepit' may be present and in need of healing.

Sexual performance pressure is another issue commonly found in patients dealing with prostate enlargement or cancer. Many males deal with performance pressure by denial, or by looking at outside causes and cures rather than taking an inward look. Blaming a partner, or using oral or injectable erectile enhancements does not resolve the underpinning psychology. Sexual conflict due to guilt, anxiety, fear, shame, betrayal, or humiliation and past traumatic events all can produce performance pressure, and may require attention to produce permanent change.

QUESTIONS

Have I made enough money to live on?
Do I have enough for those I love?
Am I a good enough provider?
Am I still hard, strong, tough or fast enough?
Where do I feel useless, weak or decrepit?
What do I think of having feelings?
What feelings or emotions do I hold in?
What do I think of "the feminine" in me?
What am I holding in?
What blocks a complete release?
Where do I struggle to let go?

AGGRAVATING FACTORS

Chronic life-long stress / acute stress / hostility / negative affect / male pressure to be anti-emotional / performance pressure / male guilt / suppressed male anger / negative older male self-image.

HEALING FACTORS

Stress reduction or management define and release feelings and emotions around male image, age, and sex / transforming tendencies for negative affect by re-evaluating emotionally limiting beliefs and attitudes.

TAKE NOTICE

CAYENNE • GARLIC

CAYENNE: After studying cayenne and prostate cancer in the laboratory and in patients, scientists concluded that capsaicin in cayenne "is a promising anti-tumor agent in hormone-refractory prostate cancer, which shows resistance to many chemotherapeutic agents."[7]

GARLIC: Applying garlic to rodents, Hong Kong scientists reported significant success in inhibiting primary tumor formation of the prostrate, and a reduction of secondary tumor formation. Another study concluded that garlic possesses potent anti-metastasis properties (preventing cancer from spreading), which may also apply to other types of cancer.[8]

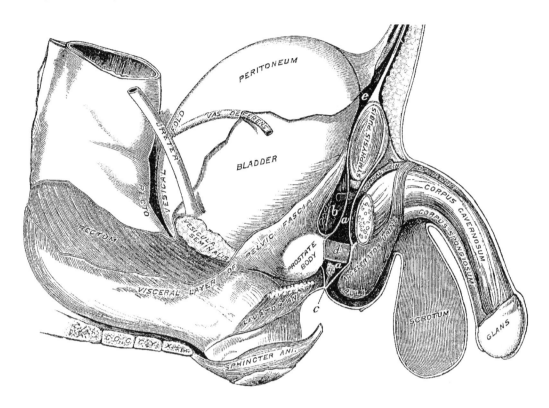

1 Leitzmann MF, Platz EA, Stampfer MJ, Willett WC, Giovannucci E. *Ejaculation frequency and subsequent risk of prostate cancer.* Division of Cancer Epidemiology and Genetics, National Cancer Institute, National Institutes of Health, Department of Health and Human Services, Bethesda, Md 20892, USA. JAMA. 2004 Apr 7;291(13):1578-86.

2 Dominique Melck, Luciano De Petrocellis, Pierangelo Orlando, Tiziana Bisogno, Chiara Laezza, Maurizio Bifulco and Vincenzo Di Marzo. *Suppression of Nerve Growth Factor Trk Receptors and Prolactin Receptors by Endocannabinoids Leads to Inhibition of Human Breast and Prostate Cancer Cell Proliferation.* Istituto per la Chimica di Molecole di Interesse Biologico (D.M., T.B., V.D.M.), Istituto di Cibernetica (L.D.P.), and Istituto di Biochimica delle Proteine ed Enzimologia (P.O.), Consiglio Nazionale delle Ricerche, 80072 Arco Felice (NA); and Centro di Endocrinologia e Oncologia Sperimentale, Consiglio Nazionale delle Ricerche, and Dipartimento di Biologia e Patologia Cellulare e Molecolare, Università di Napoli Federico II (C.L., M.B.), 80131 Naples, Italy. Endocrinology, 2000. Vol. 141, No. 1 118-126.

3 Sami Sarfaraz, Farrukh Afaq, Vaqar M. Adhami, and Hasan Mukhtar. *Cannabinoid Receptor as a Novel Target for the Treatment of Prostate Cancer.* Department of Dermatology, University of Wisconsin, Medical Sciences Center, Room B-25, 1300 University Avenue, Madison, WI 53706. Cancer Res March 1, 2005 65; 1635.

4 Czifra G, Varga A, Nyeste K, Marincsák R, Tóth BI, Kovács I, Kovács L, Bíró T. *Increased expressions of cannabinoid receptor-1 and transient receptor potential vanilloid-1 in human prostate carcinoma.* Department of Physiology, Medical and Health Science Center, Research Center for Molecular Medicine, University of Debrecen, Debrecen, Hungary. J Cancer Res Clin Oncol. 2009 Apr;135(4):507-14.

5 Philip M. Ullrich, PhD, Susan K. Lutgendorf, PhD, Jane Leserman, PhD, Derek G. Turesky, BA and Karl J. Kreder, MD. Stress, *Hostility, and Disease Parameters of Benign Prostatic Hyperplasia.* Department of Rehabilitation Medicine, University of Washington, Seattle, WA (P.M.U.); the Departments of Psychology and Obstetrics and Gynecology (S.K.L., D.G.T.) and Urology (K.J.K.), University of Iowa, Iowa City, IA; and the Department of

Psychiatry, University of North Carolina, Chapel Hill, NC (J.L.). Psychosomatic Medicine 67:476-482 (2005).

6 Victoria M. White, PhD, Dallas R. English, PhD, Hamish Coates, PhD, Magdalena Lagerlund, PhD, Ron Borland, PhD and Graham G. Giles, PhD. *Is Cancer Risk Associated With Anger Control and Negative Affect? Findings from a Prospective Cohort Study*. Centre for Behavioural Research in Cancer (V.M.W.), The Cancer Council Victoria, Australia; Cancer Epidemiology Centre (D.R.E., G.G.G.), The Cancer Council Victoria, Australia; School of Population Health (D.R.E., G.G.G.), University of Melbourne, Australia; Department of Epidemiology and Preventive Medicine (D.R.E., G.G.G.), Monash University, Australia; Centre for the Study of Higher Education (H.C.), University of Melbourne, Australia; Department of Epidemiology and Biostatistics (M.L.), University of Western Ontario, Canada; VicHealth Centre for Tobacco Control (R.B.), The Cancer Council Victoria, Australia. Psychosomatic Medicine 69:667-674 (2007).

7 Sánchez AM, Sánchez MG, Malagarie-Cazenave S, Olea N, Díaz-Laviada I. *Induction of apoptosis in prostate tumor PC-3 cells and inhibition of xenograft prostate tumor growth by the vanilloid capsaicin*. Department of Biochemistry and Molecular Biology, School of Medicine, University of Alcalá, Alcalá de Henares, Madrid, 28871, Spain. Apoptosis. 2006 Jan;11(1):89-99.

8 Howard EW, Ling MT, Chua CW, Cheung HW, Wang X, Wong YC. *Garlic-derived S-allylmercaptocysteine is a novel in vivo antimetastatic agent for androgen-independent prostate cancer*. Cancer Biology Group, Department of Anatomy, Faculty of Medicine, University of Hong Kong, Hong Kong. Clin Cancer Res. 2007 Mar 15;13(6):1847-56.

Cancer
Rhabdomyosarcoma

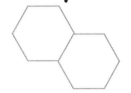

NUMBER OF STUDIES: 2

CHI VALUE: 1

This type of cancer is typically a fast-growing and highly malignant tumor found most often in children. It affects the connective tissue and is believed to begin in progenitor cells (similar to stem cells), which later differentiate into muscle cells. The most common location of rhabdomyosarcoma development is the head and neck, followed by the genitourinary tract. Allopaths traditionally suspect hereditary causes, and treatment is limited to chemotherapy, surgery, and radiation. The survival rate in the late 1960s was a mere 10-15%, but by 2000 it had risen to over 70%.[1]

CANNABIS AND RHABDOMYOSARCOMA

A 1993 Pittsburgh survey found a possible correlation between a child's development of rhabdomyosarcoma when their birth parent used cocaine and marijuana in the year preceding the child's birth. Cannabis use was one potential co-factor, in conjunction with cocaine, in the development of the cancer.[2] To date, no studies have explored whether use of cannabis alone increases the risk of rhabdomyosarcoma.

In fact, 16 years later, Swiss researchers were able to kill rhabdomyosarcoma cells in a laboratory test using a synthetic cannabinoid. The scientists confirmed the test results in vivo by xenografting rhabdomyosarcoma cancer cells treated with the cannabinoid, which led to a significant suppression of the tumor growth. The Swiss study provides a basis for considering cannabinoids as a new treatment approach for rhabdomyosarcoma.[3]

STUDY SUMMARY:

Drugs	Type of Study	Published Year, Place, and Key Results	CHI
HU210 and THC	Laboratory and animal studies	2009 – University Children's Hospital, Zurich, Switzerland: HU210 and THC produced cancer cell death.[3]	1
Cocaine and marijuana		1993 – University of Pittsburgh School of Medicine: Survey of parents of 322 patients with rhabdomyosarcoma. Parental use of cocaine and marijuana in the year before conception may increase the risk of rhabdomyosarcoma by two to fivefold.[2]	0

Total CHI Value   1

STRAIN SPECIFIC CONSIDERATIONS

To date, two cannabinoids have been tested against rhabdomyosarcoma: HU210, a synthetic cannabinoid with a higher affinity for the CB1 receptors, and THC, which binds relatively equally to CB1 and CB2.

Sativas and sativa-heavy strains tend to present with a higher THC:CBD ratio, thus activating CB1 and CB2 in relative equal proportions.

EXPLORING MIND–BODY CONSCIOUSNESS

Applying the paradigm of co-creation to the dreadful events of often fatal infant and childhood diseases or accidents remains a very challenging task. What belief(s) in punishment, what guilt, how much harbored anger, and what responsibility can a baby have?

If we were privy to the intention and choices made, beyond the veil of conception, or after death's final curtain falls, it would perhaps be easier to understand the elusive why(s). However, discovery may take place in the experiences of present moments, and in the process of finding the most effective road to healing.

TAKE NOTICE

SAFFRON

SAFFRON: Crocus sativus L. or Saffron may poccess anti cancer activity including against rhabdomyosarcoma.[4]

1 M.Kaefer, RC Rink. *Genitourinary Rhabdomyosarcoma.* Treatment Options. Department of Pediatric Urology, James Whitcomb Riley Hospital for Children, Indiana University Medical Center, Indianapolis, USA. Urologic Clinics of North America, Volume 27, Issue 3, Pages 471-487.

2 Grufferman S, Schwartz AG, Ruymann FB, Maurer HM. *Parents' use of cocaine and marijuana and increased risk of rhabdomyosarcoma in their children.* Intergroup Rhabdomyosarcoma Study, Department of Clinical Epidemiology and Family Medicine, University of Pittsburgh School of Medicine, PA. Cancer Causes Control. 1993 May;4(3):217-24.

3 Oesch S, Walter D, Wachtel M, Pretre K, Salazar M, Guzmán M, Velasco G, Schäfer BW. *Cannabinoid receptor 1 is a potential drug target for treatment of translocation-positive rhabdomyosarcoma.* Department of Oncology, University Children's Hospital, Zurich, Switzerland. Mol Cancer Ther, 9. Juni 2009.

4 Deng Y, Guo ZG, Zeng ZL, Wang Z. *Studies on the pharmacological effects of saffron(Crocus sativus L.)--a review.* Dept. of Chemical Engineering, Tsinghua University, Beijing 100084, China. Zhongguo Zhong Yao Za Zhi. 2002 Aug;27(8):565-8.

Cancer
Skin Cancer

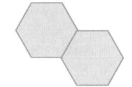

NUMBER OF STUDIES: 2

CHI VALUE: 11

The skin is the largest organ of the body. It transmits sensations to the brain, provides temperature regulation, and protects us from environmental toxins and pathogens. Our skin has three basic layers: the outer layer (epidermis), the middle layer (dermis), and lower subcutaneous tissue.

There are two types of non-melanoma skin cancer (NMSC). Squamous cell carcinoma originates in the outermost layer of the epidermis (which is comprised of squamous cells). Basal cell carcinoma originates in the lowest layer, (comprised of basal cells).

Non-melanoma skin cancers are one of the most common cancers diagnosed to date. With a relatively easy diagnosis and treatment, most non-melanoma skin cancers favor a positive outcome.

During initial stages, a cancerous growh may have a mole-like appearance. To distinguish possible skin cancers from normal moles, practitioners look at the A, B, C, D, and E's of cancerous lesions: A stands for asymmetry; B for borders (irregularly shaped); C for uneven color(s) presentation (white, pink, red, blue, brown, black); D for diameter (melanoma is typically ¼ inch); and E for evolving or rapid development of shape, color and size (weeks or months rather than years). Other warning signs include pain, itching, scar-like tissue development, a pink growth, a reddish patch, or ulceration with discharge or bleeding.

Allopathic treatment includes forms of surgical removal using type-appropriate tools to shave off the cancerous tissue. The actual slicing may involve using a topical electrical current to stop bleeding and, ideally, to zap the remaining cancer cells. Surgeons may use lasers to vaporize tissue, a wire brush to sand off skin, or freeze the affected tissue (cryosurgery). Depending on the breadth and depth of the cancer, physicians may also use chemotherapies or radiation.

Mohs micrographic surgery is another commonly used method for the removal of non-melanoma skin cancer, especially when found on the nose, ears, or eyelids where it is extremely important to shave off as little tissue as possible. A local anesthetic is injected, and very thin layers of skin are sliced off and immediately examined under a microscope to determine if the last layer removed is free of cancerous cells.

CANNABIS AND SKIN CANCER (NON-MELANOMA)

Most Materia Medicas of both the Eastern and the Western healing traditions reference historical applications of whole-plant cannabis topicals for the treatment of skin cancer.

In 2003, a team of researchers from Madrid, Spain, and Clemons, South Carolina, investigated cannabinoids' effectiveness as a non-melanoma skin cancer therapy. The team showed that CB1 and CB2 receptors exist in both healthy and cancerous skin tissue of humans and mice, and that both CB1 and CB2 receptors play a role in the induction of apoptosis of skin tumor cells and the regression of skin carcinomas. Further, they compared the effects of cannabinoids on cell cultures containing normal skin cells and cultures containing cancerous skin cells. Results revealed the destruction of cancerous cells, while normal cells remained unaffected. The authors concluded that: "These results support a new therapeutic approach for the treatment of skin tumors."[1]

Six years later, in 2009, another team of international researchers concluded that the main function of the presence of an endocannabinoid system (ECS) in the skin is to control and balance growth, differentiation, and survival of skin cells, as well as to produce proper immune responses. The team believed that manipulation of the ECS might be beneficial in a multitude of human skin diseases, including acne, dermatitis, dry skin, hair loss (alopecia, effluvium), hirsutism (excessive hair growth), itching, seborrhea, skin tumors, pain, and psoriasis. The authors of the study hypothesized that, in the case of skin cancers, an up-regulation of both ECS receptors CB1 and CB2 would suppress cancerous growths, angiogenesis (blood supply to the tumor), and metastasis (rapid spread of cancer), and even induce apoptosis (cancer cell death).[2]

STUDY SUMMARY:

Drugs/Study Focus	Type of Study	Published Year, Place, and Key Results	CHI
Endocannabinoid system (ECS) and cannabinoids	Meta-analysis	2009 – Multi-center international study from Germany, Hungary, United Kingdom, and the United States: "…targeted manipulation of the ECS (…) might be beneficial in a multitude of human skin diseases."[2]	**4**
JWH-133 (CB2 agonist), WIN-55,212-2 (CB1&CB2 agonist), SR141716 (CB1 antagonist) and SR144528 (CB2 antagonist)	Laboratory cultures, mice and human study	2003 – Multi-center international study from Spain and the United States: CB1 and CB2 are present in normal skin and skin tumors of mice and humans. Cannabinoid receptor activation induces skin tumor cell apoptosis.[1]	**1+2+4**

Total CHI Value   11

STRAIN SPECIFIC CONSIDERATIONS

In this review, JWH-133, a CB2 agonist, and WIN-55,212-2, a CB1 and CB2 agonist, were tested successfully against non-melanoma skin cancer cells in vitro (cell cultures) and in vivo (animal tested).

Both sativa and indica strains contain cannabinoids that activate CB1 and CB2 receptors. THC binds with both CB1 and CB2 receptors relatively equally, while CBD has a greater affinity for CB2.

EXPLORING MIND–BODY CONSCIOUSNESS

The skin is a boundary that lets us know precisely where we end and the outside world begins. It is also the image we present to the world.

Since doctors diagnose the majority of skin cancers on the face, neck, back of hands, upper arms and upper torso, the potential for subjective meaning and understanding varies accordingly. For example, the face communicates emotional states through obvious and subtle micro-expressions. Perhaps more than any other physicality, the face represents the image we present to the world, and the nose leads the way. Scent is processed differently from other senses, in that it quickly and directly targets the more ancient part of the brain (limbic system), where emotions such as fear or arousal, rapid hormonal changes, long-term memory, and related behavior are rapidly initiated.

Idioms related to the nose reveal self-controlling judgments and an underlying need for perfection. *Brown nosing. Nose to the Grindstone. Cut off your nose to spite your face. Hard nosed. Don't stick your nose where it does not belong. Nosy. Pay through the nose. Rub his nose in it. Nose up in the air.*

The fairytale archetype of the evil witch with the pronounced mole on her nose also springs to mind.

See also SKIN DISEASE and CANCER IN GENERAL.

SUGGESTED BLESSING

May you feel safe and secure inside your skin.

SUGGESTED AFFIRMATION

I love and value my boundaries. I love the constant sensual dance between my skin and the world.

QUESTIONS

Am I comfortable in my own skin?
Do I like my skin?
Which part don't I like?
How do I feel about it, and why?
What part of my skin don't I want anybody to see, and why?
What does that part represent?
What has gotten under my skin that is eating me up?

AGGRAVATING FACTORS

Negative self-image / belief in visible punishment.

HEALING FACTORS

Release the negative / build a positive self-image and a belief in self-forgiveness.

TAKE NOTICE

BUSH TEA • CLOVE

BUSH TEA: Laboratory studies found that Bush tea contains DNA-protective and antimutagenic properties.[3] South African researchers who learned that topical Bush tea application inhibits skin tumor formation have confirmed the antimutagenic properties of Rooibos as well.[4]

CLOVE: One study from Kolkata looked at the properties of aqueous solution of clove and found it to produce apoptosis of lung cancer cells in mice as well as having other possible cancer protective properties.[5] Another Indian study determined that aqueous solution of clove might also have protective properties against skin papillomas (skin tumors).[6]

RADIATION PROTECTION: See CANCER IN GENERAL under TAKE NOTICE - RADIATION PROTECTION.

1 M. Llanos Casanova1, Cristina Blázquez2, Jesús Martínez-Palacio1, Concepción Villanueva3, M. Jesús Fernández-Aceñero3, John W. Huffman4, José L. Jorcano1 and Manuel Guzmán2 *Inhibition of skin tumor growth and angiogenesis in vivo by activation of cannabinoid receptors.* 1Project on Cellular and Molecular Biology and Gene Therapy, Centro de Investigaciones Energéticas, Medioambientales y Tecnológicas, Madrid, Spain 2 Department of Biochemistry and Molecular Biology I, School of Biology, Complutense University, Madrid, Spain 3 Department of Pathology, Hospital General de Móstoles, Madrid, Spain 4 Department of Chemistry, Clemson University, Clemson, South Carolina, USA. J Clin Invest. 2003;111(1):43–50.

2 Tamás Bíró,1 Balázs I. Tóth,1 György Haskó,2 Ralf Paus,3,4 and Pál Pacher5 *The endocannabinoid system of the skin in health and disease: novel perspectives and therapeutic opportunities.* 1Department of Physiology, University of Debrecen, Research Center for Molecular Medicine, Debrecen 4032, Hungary. 2University of Medicine and Dentistry, Department of Surgery, New Jersey Medical School, Newark, NJ 07103, USA. 3Department of Dermatology, University Hospital Schleswig-Holstein, University of Lübeck, Lübeck 23538, Germany. 4School of Translational Medicine, University of Manchester, Manchester, M13 9PL, UK. 5Section on Oxidative Stress Tissue Injury, Laboratory of Physiological Studies, National Institutes of Health/NIAAA, Rockville, MD 20892-9413, USA. Trends Pharmacol Sci. 2009 August; 30(8): 411–420.

3 Lee EJ, Jang HD. *Antioxidant activity and protective effect on DNA strand scission of Rooibos tea (Aspalathus linearis).* Department of Food and Nutrition, Hannam University, Daejeon, Korea. Biofactors. 2004; 21(1-4-):285-92.

4 Marnewick J, Joubert E, Joseph S, Swanevelder S, Swart P, Gelderblom W. *Inhibition of tumour promotion in mouse skin by extracts of rooibos (Aspalathus linearis) and honeybush (Cyclopia intermedia), unique South African herbal teas.* PROMEC Unit, Medical Research Council, P.O. Box 19070, Tygerberg 7505, South Africa. Cancer Lett. 2005 Jun 28;224(2):193-202.

5 Banerjee S, Panda CK, Das S. *Clove (Syzygium aromaticum L.), a potential chemopreventive agent for lung cancer.* Department of Cancer Chemoprevention, Chittarajan National Cancer Institute, 37, S.P. Mukherjee Road, Kolkata 700026, India. Carcinogenesis. 2006 Aug;27(8):1645-54.

6 Banerjee S, Das S. *Anticarcinogenic effects of an aqueous infusion of cloves on skin carcinogenesis. Dept. of Cancer Chemoprevention,* Chittarajan National Cancer Institute, 37 S.P. Mukherjee Road, Kolkata 700026, West Bengal, India. Asian Pac J Cancer Prev. 2005 Jul-Sep;6(3):304-8.

Cancer
Thyroid Cancer

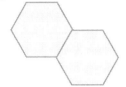

NUMBER OF STUDIES: 2

CHI VALUE: 3

Guided by hormones from the pituitary and hypothalamus glands, the thyroid (Greek for shield) is an integral part of the human endocrine system. Its butterfly-like shape appears to shield or embrace the front of the Adam's apple in males and females alike. It produces thyroid hormones, mainly triiodothyronine (T3) and thyroxine (T4), which are intricately involved in physiological development, growth, and cellular metabolism. In addition, the thyroid enhances and extends the catecholamine effects of adrenaline (increases alertness, and "fight or flight" responses).

Minor thyroid diseases fall into two basic categories: hypothyroidism (underproduction of T3 and T4), or hyperthyroidism (overproduction of T3 and T4). The thyroid produces both T3 and T4 by utilizing dietary iodine.

In previous decades, a major cause of thyroid cancer stemmed from orthodox medical procedures involving ionizing radiation. From 1940 to 1960, orthodox medicine used radiation on the necks and heads of many young children to treat relatively mild diseases.[1] Ten to thirty years later, many of those children developed thyroid cancer, which affects women at twice the rate as males. Thyroid's affinity for the element iodine also makes it vulnerable to the ill-affects of numerous iodine isotopes, such as iodine 131, released by nuclear accidents and explosions.

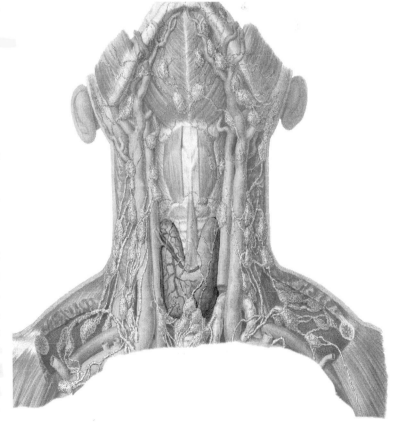

Signs and symptoms may include a feeling of pressure in the throat that will not go away, the physical presence of lumps or nodules, a change in voice, swollen lymph nodes beneath the jaw and neck, or difficulty swallowing. These symptoms may also co-exist or be preceded by hyperthyroidism or hypothyroidism, both of which may lead to autoimmune difficulties. The chart below lists some common signs and symptoms.

Hyperthyroidism (symptoms)	Hypothyroidism (symptoms)
Weight loss with increased appetite	Weight gain with poor appetite
Feeling hot	Feeling cold
Rapid heart beats (tachycardia)	Slow heart beats (bradycardia)
	Dry, coarse hair and/or hair loss, dry skin, brittle fingernails
Toxic goiter (swelling of the lower neck)	Non-toxic goiter (less common)
Protruding eyes	Puffy appearance of face
Diaphoresis (sweating) increased	Diaphoresis (sweating) decreased
Diarrhea	Constipation
Nervousness, anxiety, restlessness	Depression
Tremors (hands and fingers)	Joint and muscle pains/cramps
Feeling weak or easily fatigued	Feeling weak or easily fatigued
Difficulty sleeping	
Mood swings	Slower thinking
Light menses	Heavy menses

Diagnosis involves a blood test (balance of thyroid hormones), imaging techniques and a needle biopsy of suspect tissue. Allopathic treatment includes surgery, radiation with iodine 131, and chemotherapy.

CANNABIS AND THYROID CANCER

Laboratory tests revealed that thyroid cancer cells are inhibited by cannabinoids. In 2006, Italian scientists from Pozzuoli examined the effects of isolated cannabinoids and cannabis extracts on thyroid cancer cell lines implanted in rodents. Of the five natural compounds tested, scientists discovered cannabidiol and cannabidiol-acid to be the most potent inhibitors of thyroid cancer cells.[2] Test results also revealed that while cannabinoids are toxic to cancer cells, they exert less potent effects on normal cells.

Another laboratory study from Naples, Italy, (2010) confirmed these initial findings when researchers exposed cancerous thyroid cells to an analog of anandamide. The exposure inhibited the growth of the cancer cells and led to an increase of apoptosis (death of cancer cells). The scientists also discovered elevated levels of cannabinoid receptor 1 (CB1) expression, thus suggesting that the toxic effect to the mutated cells likely occurred from interaction with the CB1 receptors.[3]

STUDY SUMMARY:

Drugs	Type of Study	Published Year, Place, and Key Results	CHI
2-methyl-2'-F-anandamide (Met-F-AEA), a metabolically stable analogue of anandamide	Laboratory	2010 – University of Naples Federico II, Naples, Italy: Growth inhibition found in cell lines derived from thyroid carcinoma.[3]	1
Cannabidiol (CBD), cannabigerol (CBG), cannabichromene, cannabidiol acid (CBD-A) and THC acid (THC-A)	Laboratory and animal (rat) study	2006 – Istituto di Chimica Biomolecolare, Consiglio Nazionale delle Ricerche Pozzuoli, Italy: Both cannabidiol and the cannabidiol-rich extract inhibited the growth of injected thyroid tumor cells.[2]	2

Total CHI Value 3

STRAIN AND FORM-SPECIFIC CONSIDERATIONS

Scientists tested six cannabinoids against thyroid cancer cells. Significant among them were anandamide, the body's own cannabinoid, which binds relatively equally to CB1 and CB2, the plant cannabinoids cannabidiol (CBD), and cannabidiol acid (CBD-A). These elements possess a greater affinity for the CB2 receptor than for the CB1.

Indica or indica-heavy hybrids tend to have a lower THC:CBD ratio, thus increasing the probability of enhanced CB2 activation. Further, CBD-acid is present at higher concentration in fresh, raw leaf. Cannabis-using patients often consume it in juice form.

EXPLORING MIND–BODY CONSCIOUSNESS

Hyperthyroidism can cause excess production of thyroid hormones. This excess, also referred to as thyrotoxicosis, can lead to the development of Grave's Disease, an autoimmune disorder due to an overactive thyroid.

Nineteenth Century observers noticed a correlation between combat stress from the Bohr War and WWI and the development of Grave's Disease. Later, psychosomatic studies described the thyroid as "the gland of the emotions," and thyrotoxicosis as "crystallized fright."[5]

More specifically, early researchers found that thyrotoxicosis was significantly more likely to develop when, a patient's emotional stability rested on a particular person in the family. Further, they observed that a threat to or from that person appeared to induce thyrotoxicosis. Participating patients proved to be unduly vulnerable because "…their development had led to overdependence upon parental love and shelter; or fear of repudiation by parents; or excessively high ideals of parenthood, of social and moral duties…"[6]

Another psychiatric study enrolled two hundred patients at the Presbyterian Hospital in New York and found that female hyperthyroid patients "…make a desperate and life-long struggle to win their mother's approval, and to achieve likeness to her, at the same time that they fear her pain. … The men also show fear of deprivation of their mother's comfort, but the fear of loss of approval is less specific, appearing as fear of public disgrace."[7]

The thyroid is centered in the throat, the seat of expression and communication. When individual needs, desires, or feelings are not appropriately expressed and communicated, but rather are repressed or harbored, throat problems may provide a vehicle to draw attention to these issues of self-expression.

Although lung cancer rates are significantly higher in males, thyroid cancer affects many more women than men. And while researchers point to correlations between lung cancer and rationality and anti-emotionality, a similar case involving thyroid cancer could be made; for instance, women not speaking up for themselves, especially relative to authority or parental figures.

See also COLDS AND FLU, COUGHING and CANCER IN GENERAL.

SUGGESTED BLESSING

May you realize that it is okay to be who you are right now, no matter what others might think.

May you realize that every feeling retrieved and embraced from the hidden recesses of your mind can serve to reduce the power of cancer.

May you experience the self-respect gained from feeling and releasing all your feelings.

QUESTIONS

When do I fail to speak up for myself?
How long has this been going on?
When did it start?
How do I feel about it?
What does "not standing up for myself" mean about me?
How important is what my mother/father thinks of me?
How important is what I think of me?

AGGRAVATING FACTORS

Fear (acute or chronic) / fear of loss of parental approval / fear of loss of shelter / overdependence upon parental love and shelter / fear of repudiation by parents / excessively high ideals of parenthood or of social and moral duties / Female hyperthyroid patients "…make a desperate and life-long struggle to win their mother's approval and to achieve likeness to her, at the same time that they fear her pain. … The men also show fear of deprivation of their mother's comfort, but the fear of loss of approval is less specific, appearing as fear of public disgrace."[7]

HEALING FACTORS

Build self-esteem / reduce fear, worry, and stress / release the need for perfection / let mother and father be mere humans with all their quirks and foibles / love is letting go of fear.

1 Erika Masuda Alford, MD1, Mimi I. Hu, MD1, Peter Ahn , MD2, Jeffrey P. Lamont, MD3. *Thyroid and Parathyroid Cancers.* 1 Department of Endocrine Neoplasia and Hormonal Disorders, M. D. Anderson Cancer Center. 2 Department of Radiation Oncology, Thomas Jefferson University. 3 Division of Surgery, Baylor University Medical Center. Cancer Management: A Multidisciplinary Approach. 13th Edition. CMPMedica, 2011.

2 Ligresti A, Moriello AS, Starowicz K, Matias I, Pisanti S, De Petrocellis L, Laezza C, Portella G, Bifulco M, Di Marzo V. *Antitumor activity of plant cannabinoids with emphasis on the effect of cannabidiol on human breast carcinoma.* Istituto di Chimica Biomolecolare, Consiglio Nazionale delle Ricerche Pozzuoli, Italy. J Pharmacol Exp Ther. 2006 Sep;318(3):1375-87.

3 Cozzolino R, Calì G, Bifulco M, Laccetti P. *A metabolically stable analogue of anandamide, Met-F-AEA, inhibits human thyroid carcinoma cell lines by activation of apoptosis.* Department of Structural and Functional Biology, University of Naples Federico II, 80126 Naples, Italy. cozzolino1@interfree.it Invest New Drugs. 2010 Apr;28(2):115-23.

4 Harland, W.H. *Notes on two cases of exophthalmic goiter appearing suddenly in men who have been in action.* Brit. M. J. 2:584, 1900.

5 Theodore Lidz, M.D. *Emotional Factors in the Etiology of Hyperthyroidism.* Psychiatric Medical Department. School of Medicine. John Hopkins University. Psychosomatic Medicine January 1, 1949 vol. 11 no. 1 2-8.

6 Mittelman B. *Psychogenic factors and psychotherapy in hyperthyreosis and rapid heart imbalance.* J. Nerv. and Ment. Dis. 77:465, 1933.

7 Conrad Agnes. *A psychiatric study of hyperthyroid patients.* J. Nerv. & Ment. Dis. 79:505, 1934.

Cardiovascular Health

Heart Disease

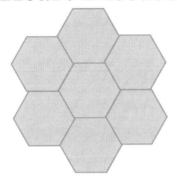

NUMBER OF STUDIES: 7

CHI VALUE: 16

The human heart is about the size of a fist. It has four chambers, which it uses in a particular sequence to move blood throughout the entire body. It beats an average of 70 times per minute, or over 100,000 times a day for the duration of a lifetime. It keeps blood flowing constantly, thus taking care of the basic needs of the trillion or so cells that make up our bodies.

The heart is a unique muscle that gets its own nourishment from three main vessels called the coronary arteries. In western medicine's model, when one or more of these coronary arteries is slowly or suddenly blocked (as in the case of a blood clot) or gradually narrows (as in the case of atherosclerosis a build-up of plaque), the heart muscle begins to ache. If not corrected, this 'ache' can progress to tissue death called a myocardial infarction or heart attack. The size of the infarct determines survivability. In 2007, the Center for Disease Control publicized a report identifying heart disease as the leading cause of death in the U.S. with over 600,000 victims that year.[1]

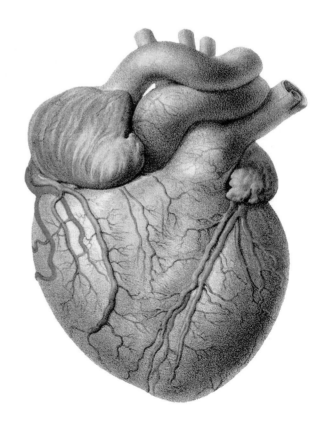

Other common causes of damaged hearts or contributing factors include: high blood pressure, metabolic syndrome (insulin resistance), excess weight, drug use (especially "uppers" such as cocaine, crack, methamphetamines), stress (especially chronic stress), mineral imbalances, pharmaceutical drugs including those designed to prevent irregular heartbeats, surgical procedures such as bypass or angioplasty, build-up of toxins (such as lead, mercury, etc.) and degeneration from chronic overexposure to free radicals. Whatever the underlying sudden or chronic cause for acute heartaches, in orthodox medicine it boils down to a lack of oxygen. Allopathic treatments include supplemental oxygen, pharmaceuticals, emergency interventions and surgery.

In 2004, researchers from Fukuoka City, Japan, reported that the cannabinoids CBN and THC significantly reduced heart attack size in mice. Interpretation of the study data indicated that the neuroprotective effects of THC were medicated via CB1 receptors.[2]

Researchers in Ramat-Gan, Israel (2006) developed a laboratory experiment, in part, to learn more about THC's mechanism for producing this cardioprotective effect. Results suggested, in a sense, that THC protects heart cells against damage from hypoxia by induction of nitric oxide. THC prepares the heart cells to better withstand hypoxia.[3] The Israeli scientists confirmed that THC has a beneficial effect on the cardiovascular system during stress conditions.

Discoveries in the same year from Montreal further established the groundwork for a better scientific understanding of the role cannabinoids play in protecting the heart from damage. First, endocannabinoid receptors CB1 and CB2 naturally reside in heart tissue. Second, "This endogenous cardiac cannabinoid system is involved in several phenomena associated with cardioprotective effects." These phenomena include a reduction of infarct (heart attack) size after induced ischemia (restriction of blood flow and oxygen). Thirdly, cannabinoids exert direct cardioprotective effects, which were confirmed both in vivo and in vitro. The Canadian authors concluded that: "Thus, the endogenous cardiac cannabinoid system, through activation of CB2-receptors, appears to be an important mechanism of protection against myocardial (heart muscle) ischemia."[4]

News from Jerusalem (2007) suggested that cannabidiol (CBD) could have significant cardioprotective effects from ischemia and infarct in rats.[5] The authors wrote: "Inasmuch as CBD has previously been administered to humans without causing side effects, it may represent a promising novel treatment for myocardial ischemia."

In 2007 researchers from the island nation of New Zealand conducted a meta-analysis (a review of studies on a topic) on the influence of cannabinoid drugs on the heart. The study revealed that cannabinoids positively influence "...vasodilation, cardiac protection, modulation of the baroreceptor reflex in the control of systolic blood pressure, and inhibition of endothelial inflammation and the progress of atherosclerosis..."[6]

The Brazilian research team discovered (2009) that the cannabidiol (CBD) calms autonomic responses to stress, such as rapid heart rates, by engaging receptors that select serotonin to achieve such down regulation (calming effect).[7]

A Geneva study (2009) of trauma or chronic illness in brain and nervous system tissues showed that CB2 activation might also protect ischemic (oxygen starved) heart cells during angina pectoris or myocardial infarctions (heart attack).[8]

STUDY SUMMARY:

Drugs	Type of Study	Published Year, Place, and Key Results	CHI
Injection of CB2 agonist JWH-133	Animal study (mice)	2009 – Geneva, Switzerland. Reduction of infarct size and oxidative stress.	2
Injected cannabidiol (CBD)	Animal study (rats)	2009 – São Paulo, Brazil. Cannabidiol (CBD) reduced all stress responses such as anxiety, high blood pressure and rapid heart rate.	2
Cannabinoid drugs	Meta-analysis	2007 – New Zealand, Dunedin. Endocannabinoid receptors are involved in vasodilation, cardiac protection, control of systolic blood pressure, inhibition of endothelial inflammation and the progress of atherosclerosis.	4
Cannabidiol (CBD)	Animal (rats) and laboratory	2007 – Jerusalem, Israel. CBD induces a substantial in vivo cardioprotective effect from ischemia.	2+1
Endocannabinoids and synthetic cannabinoids	Animal study (rats and mice)	2006 – Montreal, Canada. Synthetic cannabinoids exert direct cardioprotective effects.	2
THC	Laboratory study	2006 – Ramat-Gan, Israel. THC protects cardiac cells against hypoxia.	1
CBD and THC	Animal study (mice)	2004 – Fukuoka City, Japan . CBD and THC significantly reduced heart attack size.	2

Total CHI Valu   16

STRAIN AND FORM SPECIFIC CONSIDERATIONS

Preclinical trials proved that cannabinoids (whether plant, synthetic or endogeneous) have cardio protective properties. Additionally, research highlighted a yet unknown mechanism for the delivery of CBD's protection.[9]

Sativas and indicas activate CB1 and CB2 receptors; however, the non-psychoactive CBD in indicas or indica heavy hybrids tends to possess higher CBD content than sativas. Raw, fresh leaf or leaf juice contains significantly higher amounts of CBD-acid than heated or processed plant matter.

Another way to stimulate CB2 receptors, which has no psychoactive effects, is to ingest plants known to contain significant amounts of the dietary cannabinoid (E)-BCP (see TAKE NOTICE).

EXPLORING MIND–BODY CONSCIOUSNESS

"From the beginning of our understanding of coronary heart disease, psychological variables have been thought to play an important etiological (causative) role."[10] Researchers who hoped to learn more about this interplay of emotion and heart disease devised a two-fold approach. One involved a meta-analysis of studies correlating emotions with heart disease; the other enrolled 255 medical students, measured their hostility scores and followed them over a period of 25 years.

Results of the medical student study indicated that those inidividuals prone to hostility, competitiveness and impatience were likely to experience "… an attitude which would tend to make one distrustful of and isolated from others."[11] And the higher their hostility scores, the higher their incidence of

206

SUGGESTED

BLESSING

May you learn to love the natural function, of your heart: to feel

May you erase your fear of emotion.

May all hard-heartedness melt away as you feel your feeling.

May you experience the joy of the emotional ebb and flow of life.

developing coronary heart disease later in life. The first meta-analysis study also confirmed these conclusions.

Ann Arbor researchers followed 696 men and women between the ages of 30 and 69. During a 17-year period, they examined the relationship between anger-coping responses (suppressive or expressive) and mortality. Results showed that both men and women who suppressed their anger had significantly higher blood pressure, higher rates of cardiovascular disease and a lower life expectancy.[12]

Two other significant studies examined the effects of suppressed and harbored anger on the development of heart disease. Significant co-factors in coronary mortality included both proneness to anger[13] and suppressed anger.[14]

Besides the tangible connection of unexpressed emotions or propensity to constricting feelings, researchers discovered one other significant emotional connection. In a 1996 study from Berkeley, California, hopelessness emerged as a predictor in developing ailments such as heart disease and cancer.[15]

A study titled "Is the Glass Half Empty or Half Full?" presented another emotional aspect in the context of developing heart disease. Studying 1,306 males during a 10-year period, researchers discovered that optimism might protect against the risk of coronary heart disease in older men.[16]

While scientifically a heart attack is measured in the size of the infarct, mentally/emotionally it might be measured by a person's reservoir of suppressed emotions and their frequency to respond with negative affect.

QUESTIONS

SUGGESTED

AFFIRMATION

The rhythm of my heart is calm, yet strong bold and beautiful.

I embrace all my human emotions.

I release all fears.

I feel connected with all humans through the knowledge that we share a capacity for any and all emotions.

What do I think of feelings period?
What feeling(s) do I tend to avoid?
Which feeling do I have to avoid at all cost?
Where am I afraid to love?
What story or definition of belief is my fear of love connected to?
Where do I believe in punishment?
Where am I hard-hearted with myself?
Where am I hard-hearted with others?
What is unforgivable?
If I cannot forgive the what, can I forgive the why?
How else do I block the flow of my love?

AGGRAVATING FACTORS

Negative affect / hostility / competitiveness / impatience / distrust / isolation / suppressed anger / proneness to anger / pessimism and hopelessness.

HEALING FACTORS

Optimism / tendency for positive affect / emotional release work / feeling all feelings / a sense of humor / love / trusting life / trusting those who are trustworthy / transcending hopelessness / will or determination.

WARNING: IF YOU OR A LOVED ONE EXPERIENCES ANY OF THESE SIGNS AND SYMPTOMS, ESPECIALLY IN COMBINATION, CALL 911 RIGHT AWAY.

Chest pains
Nausea, sometimes with vomiting
Weakness
Sweating
Pale skin
Shortness of breath
Dizziness
Palpitations (feeling of skipped beats)
Fainting

TAKE NOTICE

ACACIA • CARDAMOM • COCOA • COCONUT • GARLIC • GINGER • NIGELLA • ROSEMARY • SAFFRON • TURMERIC AND (E)-β-CARYOPHYLLENE CONTAINING SPICES.

ACACIA: A study from Riyadh, Saudi Arabia, suggests that gum Arabic/acacia contains cardio-protective properties superoxide scavengers - potent anti-oxidants.[17]

CARDAMON: Scientists from the city of Mysore, India, discovered that cardamom extract protects platelets (blood particles) from aggregation (clotting) and lipid peroxidation (breakdown of fat-like molecules); both may play a part in the development of cardio-vascular disease.[18]

COCOA: Scientists at the McGill University School of Dietetics and Human Nutrition, Quebec, Canada, cautiously suggest that the consumption of dark chocolate may have a protective impact on heart and vascular illness, and protect against bad cholesterol (LDL).[19]

COCONUT: Researcher Hans Kaunitz correlated data from several laboratory animal studies with the findings from the United Nations. He reported that death from ischemic heart disease is lowest where coconut fat intake is highest.[20]

GARLIC: Garlic is one of Cuba's most versatile herbs. It is used for the treatment of peripheral signs and symptoms relevant to heart disease such as water retention, spasms, thrombophlebitis, inflammations, viral infections and hypertension, and can be used as an overall tonic and to promote healthy veins.[21]

German Commission E approved garlic as a treatment supportive to dietary measures at elevated levels of lipids in blood and as a preventative measure for age-dependent vascular changes.[22]

For the first time, Japanese researchers have scientifically proven what many traditional practitioners have suspected: garlic, or specifically allicin, contains potent antioxidant properties.[23]

Another Japanese study suggested that odorless garlic powder might play a beneficial role in preventing destructive thrombus (clod) formation such as in heart attacks. Apparently it suppresses the formation of clots by destroying fibrin, a protein involved in the clotting of blood.[24]

A Singapore study determined that S-allylcysteine (SAC), an organosulphur-containing compound produced from garlic, offers protection in myocardial infarction (heart attacks).[25]

GINGER: Scientists from Jinan, China, reported that components of ginger protect the epithelium (tissue lining inside the arteries) when exposed to an environment of high fat diets. This rodent-based study confirmed that ginger reduced the thickening of the arterial wall as measured by intima-media thickness of the aorta.[26]

NIGELLA: Two kinds of cardiac hypertrophy exist. One is pathological and produces a variety of heart problems; the other is physiological, usually brought on by regular exercise, and enhancing overall heart functions. King Faisal University scientists from Dammam, Saudi Arabia, discovered that rats, when fed 800mg/kg black seed during a two-month period, developed physiological cardiac hypertrophy. This is the first such study to date that examined nigella's potential for overall heart function and health.[27]

ROSEMARY: In another experiment from Taichung Hsien, Taiwan, scientists concluded that: "…rosemary is an excellent multifunctional therapeutic herb; by looking at its potentially potent antiglycative bioactivity, it may become a good adjuvant medicine for the prevention and treatment of diabetic, cardiovascular, and other neurodegenerative diseases."[28]

SAFFRON: Crocus sativus L. or Saffron may poccess anti cancer activity including against rhabdomyosarcoma.[29]

TURMERIC: In this meta-study scientists provide an overview of decade-long scientific studies on turmeric. They summarize a long list of turmeric's potential therapeutic properties: cancer and diabetic preventative, a cancer treatment, promoter of wound-healing, therapeutic agent in Alzheimer's, Parkinson's, cardio-vascular and pulmonary diseases, arthritis, adenomatous polyposis (multiple polyps in the large intestines – a precursor to colon cancer), inflammatory bowel disease (IBS), ulcerative colitis (colon inflammation with ulcers), atherosclerosis, pancreatitis, psoriasis, chronic anterior and uveitis (inflammation of the middle layer of the eye).[30]

(E)-β-CARYOPHYLLENE: Orally administed β-caryophyllene produced strong anti-inflammatory and analgesic effects in animal studies. (E)-β-Caryophyllene or (E)-BCP is a FDA-approved dietary plant-cannabinoid that activates CB2 receptor sites and initiates potent anti-inflammatory actions and protection form oxidative stress, both potential underlying factors in heart disease.

Spice plants known to contain significant amounts of (E)-BCP in descending order include: BLACK "ASHANTI PEPPER" (PIPER GUINEENSE), WHITE "ASHANTI PEPPER" (PIPER GUINEENSE), INDIAN BAY-LEAF (CINNAMOMUM TAMALA), ALLIGATOR PEPPER (AFRAMOMUM MELEGUETA), BASIL (OCIMUM MICRANTHUM), SRI LANKA CINNAMON (CINNAMOMUM ZEYLANICUM),

ROSEMARY (ROSMARINUS OFFICINALIS), BLACK CARAWAY (CARUM NIGRUM), BLACK PEPPER (PIPER NIGRUM), BASIL (OCIMUM GRATISSIMUM), MEXICAN OREGANO (LIPPIA GRAVEOLENS), AND CLOVE (SYZYGIUM AROMATICUM).

1 Xu JQ, Kochanek KD, Murphy SL, Tejada-Vera B. Deaths: Final data for 2007. *National vital statistics reports* web release; vol 58 no 19. Hyattsville, Maryland: National Center for Health Statistics. Released May, 2010.

2 Hayakawa K, Mishima K, Abe K, Hasebe N, Takamatsu F, Yasuda H, Ikeda T, Inui K, Egashira N, Iwasaki K, Fujiwara M. *Cannabidiol prevents infarction via the non-CB1 cannabinoid receptor mechanism.* Department of Neuropharmacology, Faculty of Pharmaceutical Sciences, Fukuoka University, Nanakuma 8-19-1, Fukuoka City, Fukuoka, 814-0180, Japan. Neuroreport. 2004 Oct 25;15(15):2381-5.

3 Shmist YA, Goncharov I, Eichler M, Shneyvays V, Isaac A, Vogel Z, Shainberg A. *Delta-9-tetrahydrocannabinol protects cardiac cells from hypoxia via CB2 receptor activation and nitric oxide production.* Faculty of Life Sciences, Bar-Ilan University, Ramat-Gan, Israel. Mol Cell Biochem. 2006 Feb;283(1-2):75-83.

4 Lamontagne D, Lépicier P, Lagneux C, Bouchard JF. *The endogenous cardiac cannabinoid system: a new protective mechanism against myocardial ischemia.* Faculté de pharmacie, Université de Montréal, QC, Canada. daniel.lamontagne@umontreal.ca Arch Mal Coeur Vaiss. 2006 Mar;99(3):242-6.

5 Ronen Durst,1 Haim Danenberg,1 Ruth Gallily,2 Raphael Mechoulam,3 Keren Meir,4 Etty Grad,1 Ronen Beeri,1 Thea Pugatsch,1 Elizabet Tarsish,1 and Chaim Lotan1 *Cannabidiol, a nonpsychoactive Cannabis constituent, protects against myocardial ischemic reperfusion injury.* 1Cardiology Department and 4Pathology Department, Hadassah Hebrew University Medical Center, 2Lautenberg Center for General and Tumor Immunology, and 3Department of Medicinal Chemistry and Natural Products, Pharmacy School, Hebrew University Medical School, Jerusalem, Israel. Am J Physiol Heart Circ Physiol 293: H3602-H3607, 2007.

6 Ashton JC, Smith PF. *Cannabinoids and cardiovascular disease: the outlook for clinical treatments.* Department of Pharmacology and Toxicology, University of Otago, Dunedin, New Zealand. john.ashton@stonebow.otago.ac.nz Curr Vasc Pharmacol. 2007 Jul;5(3):175-85.

7 Resstel LB, Tavares RF, Lisboa SF, Joca SR, Corrêa FM, Guimarães FS. *5-HT receptors are involved in the cannabidiol-induced attenuation of behavioural and cardiovascular responses to acute restraint stress in rats.* Department of Pharmacology, School of Medicine of Ribeirão Preto, University of São Paulo, Ribeirão Preto, SP, Brazil. leoresstel@yahoo.com.br Br J Pharmacol. 2009 Jan;156(1):181-8.

8 Montecucco F, Lenglet S, Braunersreuther V, Burger F, Pelli G, Bertolotto M, Mach F, Steffens S. *CB(2) cannabinoid receptor activation is cardioprotective in a mouse model of ischemia/reperfusion.* Division of Cardiology, Foundation for Medical Researches, Department of Internal Medicine, University Hospital, Geneva, Switzerland. J Mol Cell Cardiol. 2009 May;46(5):612-20.

9 Hayakawa K, Mishima K, Abe K, Hasebe N, Takamatsu F, Yasuda H, Ikeda T, Inui K, Egashira N, Iwasaki K, Fujiwara M. *Cannabidiol prevents infarction via the non-CB1 cannabinoid receptor mechanism.* Department of Neuropharmacology, Faculty of Pharmaceutical Sciences, Fukuoka University, Nanakuma 8-19-1, Fukuoka City, Fukuoka, 814-0180, Japan. Neuroreport. 2004 Oct 25;15(15):2381-5.

10 Barefoot JC, Dahlstrom WG, Williams RB Jr. *Hostility, CHD incidence, and total mortality: a 25-year follow-up study of 255 physicians.* Department of Biostatistics and Psychology, University of North Carolina and Department of Psychiatry and Internal Medicine, Duke University, Durham North Carolina. Psychosom Med. 1983 Mar;45(1):59-63.

11 Ibid.

12 Ernest Harburg, PhD, Mara Julius, ScD, Niko Kaciroti, PhD, Lillian Gleiberman, PhD and M. Anthony Schork, PhD. *Expressive/Suppressive Anger-Coping Responses, Gender, and Types of Mortality: a 17-Year Follow-Up (Tecumseh, Michigan, 1971–1988).* Department of Epidemiology, School of Public Health (E.H., M.J.),

Biostatistics, School of Public Health (M.A.S.), Psychology (E.H.), Internal Medicine (L.G.), and the Center for Human Growth and Development (N.K.), University of Michigan, Ann Arbor, Michigan. Psychosomatic Medicine 65:588-597 (2003).

13 Janice E. Williams, PhD, MPH; Catherine C. Paton, MSPH; Ilene C. Siegler, PhD, MPH; Marsha L. Eigenbrodt, MD, MPH; F. Javier Nieto, MD, PhD; Herman A. Tyroler, MD. *Anger Proneness Predicts Coronary Heart Disease Risk.* University of North Carolina (J.E.W., C.C.P., M.L.E., H.A.T.), Chapel Hill, NC; Duke University Medical Center (I.C.S.), Durham, NC; and Johns Hopkins University, Baltimore, Md (F.J.N.). Circulation. 2000;101:2034-2039. Copyright © 2011 by American Heart Association, Inc.

14 Ernest Harburg, PhD, Mara Julius, ScD, Niko Kaciroti, PhD, Lillian Gleiberman, PhD and M. Anthony Schork, PhD. *Expressive/Suppressive Anger-Coping Responses, Gender, and Types of Mortality: a 17-Year Follow-Up (Tecumseh, Michigan, 1971–1988).* Department of Epidemiology, School of Public Health (E.H., M.J.), Biostatistics, School of Public Health (M.A.S.), Psychology (E.H.), Internal Medicine (L.G.), and the Center for Human Growth and Development (N.K.), University of Michigan, Ann Arbor, Michigan. Psychosomatic Medicine 65:588-597 (2003).

15 SA Everson, DE Goldberg, GA Kaplan, RD Cohen, E Pukkala, J Tuomilehto and JT Salonen. *Hopelessness and risk of mortality and incidence of myocardial infarction and cancer.* Human Population Laboratory, Berkeley, CA 94704-1011, USA. Psychosomatic Medicine, Vol 58, Issue 2 113-121, Copyright © 1996 by American Psychosomatic Society.

16 Laura D. Kubzansky, PhD, David Sparrow, DSc, Pantel Vokonas, MD and Ichiro Kawachi, MD. *Is the Glass Half Empty or Half Full? A Prospective Study of Optimism and Coronary Heart Disease in the Normative Aging Study.* Department of Health and Social Behavior, Harvard School of Public Health (L.K., I.K.), and Channing Laboratory, Harvard Medical School (I.K., D.S.), Boston; Normative Aging Study, Department of Veterans Affairs Outpatient Clinic, and Department of Medicine, Boston University School of Medicine (D.S., P.V.), Boston, MA. Psychosomatic Medicine 63:910-916 (2001).

17 Abd-Allah AR, Al-Majed AA, Mostafa AM, Al-Shabanah OA, Din AG, Nagi MN. *Protective effect of arabic gum against cardiotoxicity induced by doxorubicin in mice: a possible mechanism of protection.* Department of Pharmacology, College of Pharmacy, King Saud University, P O Box 2457, Riyadh 11451, Saudi Arabia. J Biochem Mol Toxicol. 2002;16(5):254-9.

18 Suneetha WJ, Krishnakantha TP. *Cardamom extract as inhibitor of human platelet aggregation.* Department of Biochemistry and Nutrition, Central Food Technological Research Institute, Mysore 570 020, India. Phytother Res. 2005 May;19(5):437-40.

19 Rudkowska I, Jones PJ. *Functional foods for the prevention and treatment of cardiovascular diseases: cholesterol and beyond.* School of Dietetics and Human Nutrition McGill University, St-Anne-de-Bellevue, Quebec, Canada. Expert Rev Cardiovasc Ther. 2007 May;5(3):477-90.

20 Kaunitz H. *Medium chain triglycerides (MCT) in aging and arteriosclerosis.* J Environ Pathol Toxicol Oncol. 1986 Mar-Apr;6(3-4):115-21.

21 *Therapeutic Guide to Plant Pharmaceuticals and Honey Pharmaceuticals (Guia Terapeutica Dispensarial de Fitofarmacos y Apifarmacos* - Ministerio de Salud Publica, Ciudad de La Habana - Republica de Cuba 1992). Cuban Ministry of Public Health, Havana.

22 *Monographien der E-Kommission* (Phyto-Therapie) (380 monographs). A therapeutic guide to herbal medicine evaluating the safety and efficacy of herbs for licensed medical prescribing in Germany. Published between 1984 and 1994 in the Bundesanzeiger (official publication by the Federal Republic of Germany). Copies of the monographs are available at the Heilpflanzen-Welt Bibliothek: http://buecher.heilpflanzen-welt.de/BGA-Commission-E-Monographs/

23 Okada Y, Tanaka K, Sato E, Okajima H. *Kinetic and mechanistic studies of allicin as an antioxidant.* Department of Analytical Chemistry, Faculty of Health Sciences, Kyorin University, 476 Miyasita-cho, Hachioji, Tokyo, 192-8508, Japan. Org Biomol Chem. 2006 Nov 21;4(22):4113-7.

24 6 Fukao H, Yoshida H, Tazawa Y, Hada T. *Antithrombotic effects of odorless garlic powder both in vitro and in vivo*. Department of Nutritional Sciences, Faculty of Food Culture, Kurashiki Sakuyo University, Japan. Biosci Biotechnol Biochem. 2007 Jan;71(1):84-90.

25 Chuah SC, Moore PK, Zhu YZ. S-allylcysteine mediates cardioprotection in an acute myocardial infarction rat model via a hydrogen sulphide mediated pathway. Dept. of Pharmacology, National University of Singapore, Singapore, Singapore. Am J Physiol Heart Circ Physiol. August 31, 2007.

26 Wu CX, Wei XB, Ding H, Sun X, Cheng XM. *Protective effect of effective parts of Zingiber Offecinal on vascular endothelium of the experimental hyperlipidemic rats*. Department of Pharmacology, School of Medicine Shandong University, Jinan 250012, China. wcxzzl@eyou.com Zhong Yao Cai. 2006 Aug;29(8):810-3.

27 El-Bahai MN, Al-Hariri MT, Yar T, Bamosa AO. *Cardiac inotropic and hypertrophic effects of Nigella sativa supplementation in rats*. Department of Physiology, College of Medicine, King Faisal University, PO Box 2114, Dammam, 31451, Saudi Arabia. Int J Cardiol. 2007 Oct 9.

28 Hsieh CL, Peng CH, Chyau CC, Lin YC, Wang HE, Peng RY. *Low-density lipoprotein, collagen, and thrombin models reveal that Rosemarinus officinalis L. exhibits potent antiglycative effects*. Department of Food and Nutrition, Research Institute of Biotechnology, and Division of Basic Medical Sciences, Hung-Kuang University, No. 34 Chung-Chie Road, Shalu County, Taichung Hsien, Taiwan. J Agric Food Chem. 2007 Apr 18;55(8):2884-91.

29 Deng Y, Guo ZG, Zeng ZL, Wang Z. *Studies on the pharmacological effects of saffron(Crocus sativus L.)--a review*. Dept. of Chemical Engineering, Tsinghua University, Beijing 100084, China. Zhongguo Zhong Yao Za Zhi. 2002 Aug;27(8):565-8.

30 Goel A, Kunnumakkara AB, Aggarwal BB. *Curcumin as "Curecumin": From kitchen to clinic*. Gastrointestinal Cancer Research Laboratory, Department of Internal Medicine, Charles A. Sammons Cancer Center and Baylor Research Institute, Baylor University Medical Center, Dallas, TX, United States. Biochem Pharmacol. 2007 Aug 19.

Cardiovascular Health
Hypertension

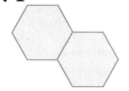

NUMBER OF STUDIES: 2

CHI VALUE: 5

Approximately 24% of US adults have hypertension."[1] The allopathic system of medicine considers high blood pressure or hypertension to be a chronic condition that can develop into an acute expression. Both chronic and acute hypertension can contribute to a host of other serious medical conditions, such as heart attacks, strokes, kidney failure, eye problems, atherosclerosis (arterial plaque deposits) or aneurisms (bulging blood vessels).

Two factors determine blood pressure: the amount of blood inside the body and the size of the blood vessels. Smooth muscles, which line the larger blood vessels, regulate blood pressure by expansion or contraction. Blood pressure naturally changes many times during the day in response to different stimuli such as emotions, temperature or level of physical activity.

Orthodox medicine has no cure for hypertension and has not yet discovered a direct cause. However, it has identified several co-factors. These include age, family history, obesity, poor diet, smoking, alcohol abuse, physical inactivity, arteriosclerosis (hardening of the arteries), depression, anxiety, insulin resistance, and diabetes.

Within this system of medicine, "normal" pressure is 120/80. However, optimal pressure is not clearly defined. Some people are happy and healthy with either lower or slightly higher numbers. However, The Seventh Report of the Joint National Committee on Prevention, Detection, Evaluation, and Treatment of High Blood Pressure suggests that: "The risk of coronary vascular disease, beginning at 115/75 mm Hg, doubles with each increment of 20/10 mm Hg."[2]

The two numbers reflect the pressure that blood exerts against the walls of the arteries as the heart contracts and relaxes, respectively. The more blood the heart moves and the tighter your arteries, the higher your blood pressure rises.

Many patients with chronic but mild or even moderate hypertension demonstrate no signs or symptoms until many years later. When symptoms do appear, they may include dizziness, headaches, blurred vision, nausea or vomiting.

Orthodox treatment is limited to life-long pharmaceutical management and intervention during acute phases.

CANNABIS AND HYPERTENSION

Researchers from Washington, DC, wanted to learn more about the relationship between simultaneous changes in heart rate, blood pressure and intraocular pressure in people with normal blood pressure, high blood pressure and open-angle glaucoma patients after inhalation of tetrahydrocannabinol (THC). The results revealed that patients responded to the inhalation of 2.8% THC with an increase in heart rate (when compared to the control group) followed by a substantial drop in blood pressure (both systolic and diastolic) as well as a drop in intraocular pressure. Scientists also noted that the increase in heart rate allowed the body to maintain adequate perfusion (cardiac output) while lowering both blood and intraocular pressures in a parallel fashion.[3]

In the Nottingham animal trial (2009) conducted on rats, researchers artificially induced hypertension, then intravenously administered the endocannabinoid anandamide and the synthetic cannabinoids WIN55,212-2 to study their effects on high blood pressure. The naturally occurring endocannabinoid anandamide lowered blood pressure in hypertension but did not affect rats with normal blood pressure. The synthetic cannabinoids WIN55,212-2 also reduced blood pressure in hypertensive rats but also raised blood pressure in rats with normal blood pressures. Both cannabinoids achieved the pressure lowering effects through increased vasodilatation.[4]

Both the Nottingham and the Washington, DC, studies indicated that the plant based cannabinoid THC and the endocannabinoid anandamide mutually lowered blood pressure without compromising overall perfusion and the commonly associated side effects - an effect not completely reproducible by the synthetic version WIN55,212-2.

STUDY SUMMARY:

Drugs	Type of Study	Published Year, Place, and Key Results	CHI
Intra-veinous endocannabinoid anandamide & synthetic cannabinoids WIN55,212-2	Animal study (rats)	2009 – Nottingham, UK. Endocannabinoid anandamide and the synthetic cannabinoid WIN55,212-2 lowered high blood pressure through vasodilatation.	2
2.8% THC inhalation	Human clinical trial	1976 –Washington, DC. Reduction in blood pressure and intraocular pressure while maintaining adequate perfusion.	3

Total CHI Value   5

STRAIN AND FORM SPECIFIC CONSIDERATIONS

The body's own cannabinoid, anandamide, the synthetic cannabinoid WIN55,212-2 and the plant based cannabinoid THC have been tested in the context of hypertension. Study results showed that each of the cannabinoids achieved a drop in blood pressure via vasodilation.

Anandamide and THC bind with CB1 and CB2 relatively equally, while synthetic WIN 55212-2 has a higher affinity for CB2 than the CB1 receptors. Cannabinoid research supports the implication of both CB1 and CB2 in activating vasodilation.[5]

Sativas and indicas contain cannabinoids that bind with CB1 and CB2. Indicas and indica-heavy strains present with a lower THC:CBD ratio, thus favoring CB2 expression.

Raw, fresh leaf or juice contains non-psychoactive CBD acid also favoring CB2 activation.

For those wishing to further stimulate non-psychoactive CB2 activation, consider plants known to contain significant amounts of the dietary cannabinoid (E)-BCP (see TAKE NOTICE).

EXPLORING MIND–BODY CONSCIOUSNESS

The physicians Grace and Graham discovered a link between attitude and hypertension. They wrote: "Arterial hypertension occurred when an individual felt that he must constantly be prepared to meet all possible threats." Typical statements were: " I had to ready for anything. … Nobody is ever going to beat me, I'm ready for everything. … It was up to me to take care of all the worries."[6]

Atlanta scientists conducted a long-term experiment on 3,310 initially normotensive and chronic disease-free persons. During a period of 22 years, doctors measured and recorded participants' blood pressure. Each participant cooperated in evaluations using two basic emotional scales, the 'Relaxed vs. Anxious' scale (GWB-A),[7] which assesses nervousness, stress, strain, pressure, anxiety, worry, and tension and the 'Cheerful vs. Depressed' scale (GWB-D), which assesses unhappiness, sadness, discouragement, hopelessness, and lack of cheerfulness. After adjusting for cofactors, the analysis revealed that those participants rating high on depression and anxiety developed hypertension at an increased rate greater than those who rated high on the relaxed and cheerfulness ends of the scales.[8] These results confirmed anxiety and depression as predictive signs for the future development of hypertension.[9]

Another large population study conducted on 3,308 adults between the ages of 18 and 30 shared similar findings at 15-year follow-ups. These researchers concluded that tendencies for impatience and hostility suggested a future risk for developing hypertension.[10]

Another study from Texas enrolled 2,564 cross-sectional Mexican Americans aged 65 and older and evaluated possible correlations between primary measures of blood pressure values and a positive emotion score. Results suggested that subjects were less likely to be hypertensive if they identified with the feeling that 'I was just as good as other people', felt happy, felt hopeful about the future, and enjoyed life.[11] Echoing these results, a Harvard study entitled *Positive Emotion and Health: Going Beyond the Negative*, discovered an association between higher levels of curiosity and hope with the decreased likelihood of hypertension.[12]

The orthodox medical tradition acknowledges effects of certain emotional stressors such as fear, anxiety and depression. These emotions trigger the release of adrenaline, which in turn speeds up the heart and signals the smooth muscles in the arteries to constrict thus increasing blood pressure.

Furthermore, in the chronically stressed state, the same adrenal glands that discharge adrenaline also release corticosteroids. Unchecked release of corticosteroids weakens the immune system, making the patient more vulnerable to other diseases. The increased hormonal (adrenaline) and steroidal impact on the body can lead to a host of other problems including sexual dysfunction, muscle spasms or hair loss. Each of these consequences can develop into reasons for more stress, fueling the vicious cycle.

Preventive measures such as dietary changes, stress reduction (meditation, noise reduction, dimming of lights, breathing techniques, watching an aquarium), appropriate exercise, quitting smoking and reducing heavy alcohol use have all proven to significantly assist in reducing hypertension.

However, release from chronically constricting emotions such as fears, anxieties, worries, stress, strain, impatience, hostility and harbored or suppressed anger may be more lasting when root causes are identified and transcended.

QUESTIONS

What family related pressure am I aware of?
Which fears are my constant companions?
How long have I had them?
Where did they come from?
Why am I maintaining them?
What definitions or beliefs are they rooted to?
Why won't I release these roots?
What positive effects do I derive from these roots?
Can I replace these effects with something else so I can let go of the root?
What am I going to plant instead?

AGGRAVATING FACTORS

Anxiety / nervousness / stress / strain / pressure / anxiety / worry / unhappiness / sadness / discouragement / hopelessness / lack of cheerfulness / impatience / hostility and constant threat perceptions

HEALING FACTORS

Feeling OK about self / feeling happy / feeling joyful / feeling hopeful about the future / hope and curiosity

ANECDOTE

Of course not every case of hypertension can be connected to measurable propensity for negative affect. An additional perspective is demonstrated by the case of a 43 year-old African American woman who suffered from chronic and severe hypertension with complications that could not be controlled, even with aggressive pharmaceutical interventions.[13] There was no reported stress or distress other than that associated with her blood pressure. Despite employing multiple blood pressure medications for about a decade, her hypertension remained dangerously uncontrollable.

Then, after an apparently normal conversation with her nephew, she began experiencing recurring nightmares. she dreamt a man was approaching

her from behind and grabbing her, which caused her to wake up screaming. She was terrified to go to bed. Her physician asked if she had ever been attacked? Hesitant, the patient reported that since the nightmares' onset, she had started to recall fragmented memories of rape by her uncle. She remembered ever telling only her father, who promised, "I'll take care of it, baby". He never did. The rapist had long since left the family. She had suppressed the episode for 30 years until her now grown nephew, who resembled her uncle, triggered the emergence of the event. In the past she had remembered bits and pieces of the rape but felt only numb and detached.

Now, however, she was very agitated recalling the event, and kept repeating: "He hurt me, he hurt me." She agreed to counseling, and after several sessions also revealed that her abusive ex-husband attempted to strangle her while her father, whom she adored, was present but did nothing to protect her. In subsequent sessions, the emotional intensity of her memories strengthened. For the first time, the patient reported feeling powerlessness, betrayal and rage at her uncle and her father. By processing her emotions, she started to identify first as a victim, and than as a survivor. By ending her own silence about the abuse she had suffered she took back some of her own power. With new energy and insight, she was than able to explore how best to protect herself as a self-aware adult.

These changes were followed by a dramatic and sustained improvement in her blood pressure. Over a period of 18 months, her blood pressure returned to normal, and there was no recurrence of nightmares despite a gradual reduction of pharmaceuticals.

TAKE NOTICE

BUSH TEA • CARAWAY • COCOA • GARLIC • (E)-β-CARYOPHYLLENE CONTAINING SPICES.

BUSH TEA: A recent study from Karachi, Pakistan, determined why Bush tea is effective in treating hyperactive gastrointestinal problems, respiratory difficulty and high blood pressure. Bush tea is a bronchodilator and antispasmodic with blood pressure-lowering properties. It apparently achieves this by portassium (ATP) channel activation with a selective bronchodilatory effect.[14]

CARAWAY: North African traditional healers from FEZ, Morocco, use caraway as a diuretic for patients experiencing water retention, passing urine and, in some cases, high blood pressure need attention. Through an animal study, Moroccan scientists determined that caraway does possess strong diuretic properties,[15] which apparently work similarly to the commonly used anti-hypertensive pharmacological drugs Lasix and Hydrochlorthiazide (HCTZ).

COCOA: Scientists at the McGill University School of Dietetics and Human Nutrition in Quebec, Canada, cautiously suggest that the consumption of dark chocolate may have protective impact on heart and vascular illnesses and their connections to oxidized bad cholesterol (LDL).[16]

A meta-analysis of similar studies from Köln, Germany, looking at dietary intake of cocoa and the reduction in blood pressure suggest that food rich in cocoa may contribute to a reduction of high blood pressure.[17]

GARLIC: Garlic is one of Cuba's most versatile herbs. It is used for the treatment of peripheral signs and symptoms relevant to heart disease, such as decreased water retention, spasms, thrombophlebitis, inflammations, viral infections and hypertension. It is used as an overall tonic and promoter of healthy veins.[18]

German Commission E: Approved as a treatment for: "Supportive to dietary measures at elevated levels of lipids in blood. Preventative measures for age-dependent vascular changes."[19]

For the first time, Japanese scientists have been able to scientifically prove what many traditional practitioners have suspected - garlic, or specifically allicin, contains potent antioxidant properties.[20] Another study from Japan suggests that odorless garlic powder can play a beneficial role in preventing destructive thrombus (clod) formation, such as in heart attacks. Apparently it suppresses the formation of clots by destroying fibrin, a protein involved in blood clotting.[21]

(E)-β-CARYOPHYLLENE: (E)-β-Caryophyllene or (E)-BCP is a FDA-approved dietary plant-cannabinoid that activates CB2 receptor sites which have been shown to be involved in the modulation of blood pressure, inflammation and oxidative stress common in patients with hypertension. Spice plants known to contain significant amounts of (E)-BCP in descending order include: BLACK "ASHANTI PEPPER" (PIPER GUINEENSE), WHITE "ASHANTI PEPPER" (PIPER GUINEENSE), INDIAN BAY-LEAF (CINNAMOMUM TAMALA), ALLIGATOR PEPPER (AFRAMOMUM MELEGUETA), BASIL (OCIMUM MICRANTHUM), SRI LANKA CINNAMON (CINNAMOMUM ZEYLANICUM), ROSEMARY (ROSMARINUS OFFICINALIS), BLACK CARAWAY (CARUM NIGRUM), BLACK PEPPER (PIPER NIGRUM), BASIL (OCIMUM GRATISSIMUM), MEXICAN OREGANO (LIPPIA GRAVEOLENS), AND CLOVE (SYZYGIUM AROMATICUM).

1 He J, Whelton PK. *Epidemiology and prevention of hypertension*. Department of Biostatistics and Epidemiology, Tulane University School of Public Health and Tropical Medicine, New Orleans, Louisiana, USA. Med Clin North Am. 1997 Sep;81(5):1077-97.

2 Chobanian AV, Bakris GL, Black HR, Cushman WC, Green LA, Izzo JL Jr, Jones DW, Materson BJ, Oparil S, Wright JT Jr, Roccella EJ; *The Seventh Report of the Joint National Committee on Prevention, Detection, Evaluation, and Treatment of High Blood Pressure: the JNC 7 report*. National Heart, Lung, and Blood Institute Joint National Committee on Prevention, Detection, Evaluation, and Treatment of High Blood Pressure; National High Blood Pressure Education Program Coordinating Committee. JAMA 2003;289:2560–72.

3 Crawford WJ, Merritt JC. *Effects of tetrahydrocannabinol on arterial and intraocular hypertension*. Glaucoma Clinic at Howard University Hospital, Washington, DC. Int J Clin Pharmacol Biopharm. 1979 May;17(5):191-6.

4 Ho WS, Gardiner SM. *Acute hypertension reveals depressor and vasodilator effects of cannabinoids in conscious rats*. School of Biomedical Sciences, University of Nottingham Medical School, Queen's Medical Centre, Nottingham, UK. 2009 Jan;156(1):94-104.

5 Ashton JC, Smith PF. *Cannabinoids and cardiovascular disease: the outlook for clinical treatments.* Department of Pharmacology and Toxicology, University of Otago, Dunedin, New Zealand. john.ashton@stonebow.otago.ac.nz Curr Vasc Pharmacol. 2007 Jul;5(3):175-85.

6 William J. Grace, M.D. and David T. Graham, M.D. *Relationship of Specific Attitudes and Emotions to Certain Bodily Diseases.* Dept. of Medicine, of the New York Hospital-Cornell Medical Center. Psychosomatic Medicine July 1, 1952 vol. 14 no. 4 243-251.

7 GWB-A & GWB-D taken from the General Well-being Schedule.

8 Bruce S. Jonas, ScM, PhD and James F. Lando, MD, MPH. *Negative Affect as a Prospective Risk Factor for Hypertension.* Office of Analysis (B.S.J.), Epidemiology and Health Promotion, National Center for Health Statistics, US Centers for Disease Control and Prevention, Hyattsville, MD; and Epidemiology Program Office (J.F.L.), US Centers for Disease Control and Prevention, Atlanta, GA. Psychosomatic Medicine 62:188-196 (2000).

9 Bruce S. Jonas, PhD; Peter Franks, MD; Deborah D. Ingram, PhD. *Are Symptoms of Anxiety and Depression Risk Factors for Hypertension?* Longitudinal Evidence From the National Health and Nutrition Examination Survey I Epidemiologic Follow-up Study. National Center for Health Statistics, Centers for Disease Control and Prevention, Hyattsville, Md (Drs Jonas and Ingram); and the Primary Care Institute, Highland Hospital, and the Department of Family Medicine, University of Rochester, Rochester, NY (Dr Franks). Arch Fam Med. 1997;6(1):43-49.

10 Lijing L. Yan, PhD, MPH; Kiang Liu, PhD; Karen A. Matthews, PhD; Martha L. Daviglus, MD, PhD; T. Freeman Ferguson, MPH, MSPH; Catarina I. Kiefe, MD, PhD. *Psychosocial Factors and Risk of Hypertension: The Coronary Artery Risk Development in Young Adults (CARDIA) Study.* Department of Preventive Medicine, Feinberg School of Medicine, Northwestern University, Chicago, Ill (Drs Yan, Liu, and Daviglus); Department of Psychiatry, University of Pittsburgh, Pittsburgh, Pa (Dr Matthews); and Division of Preventive Medicine, University of Alabama at Birmingham, Birmingham (Ms Ferguson and Dr Kiefe) and Birmingham Veterans Affairs Medical Center (Dr Kiefe). JAMA. 2003;290(16):2138-2148.

11 Glenn V. Ostir, PhD, Ivonne M. Berges, PhD, Kyriakos S. Markides, PhD and Kenneth J. Ottenbacher, PhD. *Hypertension in Older Adults and the Role of Positive Emotions.* Sealy Center on Aging (G.V.O., I.M.B., K.J.O.), the Division of Geriatrics, Department of Medicine (G.V.O., K.S.M.), the Department of Preventive Medicine and Community Health (G.V.O., K.S.M.), and the Division of Rehabilitation Sciences (K.J.O.), University of Texas Medical Branch, Galveston, Texas. Psychosomatic Medicine 68:727-733 (2006).

12 Richman LS, Kubzansky L, Maselko J, Kawachi I, Choo P, Bauer M. *Positive emotion and health: going beyond the negative.* Department of Society, Human Development, and Health, Harvard School of Public Health, Cambridge, MA, USA. Health Psychol. 2005 Jul;24(4):422-9.

13 SJ Mann and M Delon. *Improved hypertension control after disclosure of decades-old trauma.* Cardiovascular Center, New York Hospital--Cornell Medical Center, New York 10021, USA. Psychosomatic Medicine, Vol 57, Issue 5 501-505

14 Khan AU, Gilani AH. *Selective bronchodilatory effect of Rooibos tea (Aspalathus linearis) and its flavonoid, chrysoeriol.* Dept. of Biological and Biomedical Sciences, The Aga Khan University Medical College, Karachi, 74800, Pakistan. Eur J Nutr. 2006 Dec; 45(8):463-9.

15 Lahlou S, Tahraoui A, Israili Z, Lyoussi B. *Diuretic activity of the aqueous extracts of Carum carvi and Tanacetum vulgare in normal rats.* UFR Physiology-Pharmacology, Laboratory of Animal Physiology, Department of Biology, Fez, Morocco. J Ethnopharmacol. 2007 Apr 4;110(3):458-63.

16 Rudkowska I, Jones PJ. *Functional foods for the prevention and treatment of cardiovascular diseases: cholesterol and beyond.* School of Dietetics and Human Nutrition McGill University, St-Anne-de-Bellevue, Quebec, Canada. Expert Rev Cardiovasc Ther. 2007 May;5(3):477-90.

17 Taubert D, Roesen R, Schomig E. *Effect of cocoa and tea intake on blood pressure: a meta-analysis.* Department of Pharmacology, University Hospital of Cologne, Gleueler Strasse 24, D-50931 Cologne, Germany. Arch Intern Med. 2007 Apr 9;167(7):626-34.

18 *Therapeutic Guide to Plant Pharmaceuticals and Honey Pharmaceuticals (Guia Terapeutica Dispensarial de Fitofarmacos y Apifarmacos* - Ministerio de Salud Publica, Ciudad de La Habana - Republica de Cuba 1992). Cuban Ministry of Public Health, Havana.

19 *Monographien der E-Kommission* (Phyto-Therapie) (380 monographs). A therapeutic guide to herbal medicine evaluating the safety and efficacy of herbs for licensed medical prescriptions in Germany. Published between 1984 and 1994 in the Bundesanzeiger (official publication by the Federal Republic of Germany). Copies of the monographs are available at the Heilpflanzen-Welt Bibliothek: http://buecher.heilpflanzen-welt.de/BGA-Commission-E-Monographs/

20 Okada Y, Tanaka K, Sato E, Okajima H. *Kinetic and mechanistic studies of allicin as an antioxidant.* Department of Analytical Chemistry, Faculty of Health Sciences, Kyorin University, 476 Miyasita-cho, Hachioji, Tokyo, 192-8508, Japan. Org Biomol Chem. 2006 Nov 21;4(22):4113-7.

21 Fukao H, Yoshida H, Tazawa Y, Hada T. *Antithrombotic effects of odorless garlic powder both in vitro and in vivo.* Department of Nutritional Sciences, Faculty of Food Culture, Kurashiki Sakuyo University, Japan. Biosci Biotechnol Biochem. 2007 Jan;71(1):84-90.

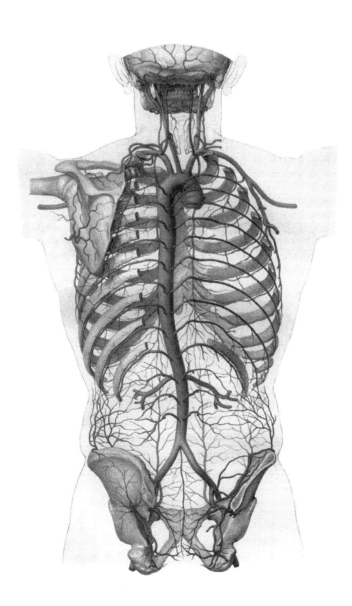

Cardiovascular Health
Stroke

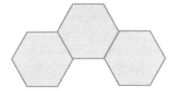

NUMBER OF STUDIES: 3

CHI VALUE: 8

A stroke (cerebrovascular accident or CVA) is a loss of brain function. There are two types of strokes: ischemic and hemorrhagic. In an ischemic stroke, an obstruction (thrombosis, embolism) prevents blood from reaching the brain cells on the other side of the obstruction; thus, it blocks oxygen and may cause tissue damage or death. A hemorrhagic stroke, which results from a ruptured blood vessel causing blood leaks, produces the same consequences.

Epidemiological and clinical studies have identified common modifiable and non-modifiable predictors or co-factors in the development of stroke. Modifiable co-factors include alcohol abuse, smoking, inactivity, diabetes, obesity and hypertension, while non-modifiable co-factors include age, race, and hereditary factors.

Depending on the size of the stroke and where it occurs, the loss of certain brain function may be limited and self-correcting as in transient ischemic attacks (TIA), or it can be massive (CVA) involving loss of major motor function. A massive stroke may cause complete flaccidity in one half of the body. High blood pressure is considered the main contributing factor in stroke. A stroke in the lower parts of the brain, which regulate heartbeat and breathing, can rapidly lead to death. Therefore, time is of great importance. The sooner an effective treatment begins, the fewer brain cells will die.

Allopathic treatment of an ischemic stroke includes either thrombolysis, where doctors use pharmaceuticals (anticoagulants and thrombolytics) to break the clod apart or a thrombectomy, a mechanical means to remove the clod. Hemorrhagic stroke cannot be treated by anticoagulants and thrombolytics as they might exascerbate the bleed. Instead, doctors may opt for surgery to relieve pressure caused by the leaking blood. The majority of fatal strokes are hemorrhagic strokes, and presently there is no way to fix a leaking blood vessel in the brain. However, since the symptoms of both types of strokes are basically the same, perhaps the biggest challenge for the treating physician is determining which type of stroke occured.

Signs and symptoms may come and go especially in TIA's. However, in a massive stroke, they are usually sudden and noticeable. Symptoms in massive stokes include: headache, nausea, vomiting, slurred speech, expressive aphasia (not finding proper words), dizziness, blurred vision, unequal grips or facial expressions, weakness on one side of the body, numbness, ataxia (inability to walk), high blood pressure (or history of hypertension) altered mental status, (confusion, irritability, aggression), loss of consciousness, incontinence or drooling.

If you notice symptoms of stroke, call 911 or visit the nearest Emergency Room. Clearly, the first hour following the onset of symptoms is crucial. To get the most out of the limited allopathic treatment options currently available, it helps to immediately start the process of differentiating the underlying type of stroke followed by the appropriate treatment.

CANNABIS AND STROKE

In 2003, the U.S. Federal Government issued itself a patent on a newly found property of cannabis making it "…useful in the treatment and prophylaxis of a wide variety of oxidation associated diseases, such as ischemic, age-related, inflammatory and autoimmune diseases. The cannabinoids are found to have particular application as neuroprotectants, for example in limiting neurological damage following ischemic insults, such as stroke and trauma, or in the treatment of neurodegenerative diseases, such as Alzheimer's disease, Parkinson's disease and HIV dementia."[1]

Researchers from Fukuoka, Japan, further enlightened the U.S. Government's patented findings on the plant's neuroprotective properties. Examining strokes in animals, scientists compared the effects of two cannabinoids (THC and CBD). The discoveries offered promise. THC treatment administered prior to a stroke in mice reduced the resulting infarction, which was measured at intervals up to 3 days. Even more promising, cannabidiol treatment offered before and after resulted in potent and long-lasting neuroprotection. Scientists concluded that: "Cannabidiol provides potent and long-lasting neuroprotection through an anti-inflammatory CB(1) receptor-independent mechanism, suggesting that cannabidiol will have a palliative action and open new therapeutic possibilities for treating cerebrovascular disorders."[2]

The same team of scientists from Fukuoka also concluded that 24 hours after the induced stroke in mice, THC significantly increased the expression of CB1 receptor in both the striatum and cortex but not in the hypothalamus (responsible for body temperature regulation). These and other observations led the team to conclude that THC prevents stroke by producing a lower body temperature independent of the hypothalamus.[3] These findings describe a new mechanism of body temperature control.

The U.S. Government's patent on the neuroprotective properties of cannabinoids presents a scientific foundation for the use of cannabinoids in patients with stroke. If the Japanese results can be confirmed in humans, cannabinoids, especially cannabidiol, may one day be used as neuroprotective agents in patients prone to stroke as well as a first line drug treatment in patients with an acute stroke.

STUDY SUMMARY:

Drugs	Type of Study	Published Year, Place, and Key Results	CHI
THC and CBD	Animal study (mice)	2007 – Fukuoka, Japan. Increased CB1 receptors in striatum and cortex, but not in hypothalamus. THC is neuroprotective when given before CVA. Cannabidiol is neuroprotective when given before and after CVA.	2

Drugs	Type of Study	Published Year, Place, and Key Results	CHI
THC and CBD	Animal study (mice)	2007 – Fukuoka, Japan. THC prevents stroke by reducing body temperature not mediated via hypothalamus; Cannabidiol provides potent and long-lasting neuroprotection through an anti-inflammatory CB(1) receptor-independent mechanism.	2
Cannabinoids	Meta-analysis	2004 – United States Government. Cannabinoids neuroprotective in stroke.	4

Total CHI Value   8

STRAIN AND FORM SPECIFIC CONSIDERATION

The results of these pre-clinical-studies may suggest the possibility that THC is neuroprotective before a stroke; that CBD is neuroprotective when used before and after a stroke; that CBD may provide neuroprotection independent of the currently known cannabinoids receptor system. CBD has a higher affinity for CB2, while THC binds relatively equally to CB1 and CB2. Clinical trials conducted on humans will ultimately prove whether or not the pre-clinical results translate directly to the human condition.

Both basic strains provide biologically active full spectrum cannabinoid and non-cannabinoid plant materials. Indicas and indica heavy hybrids contain a lower THC:CBD ratio favoring CB2 expression when compared to sativas or sativa heavy strains.

Raw, fresh leaf or juice contains non-psychoactive CBD-acid at higher concentrations, thereby increasing CB2 activation.

EXPLORING MIND–BODY CONSCIOUSNESS

SUGGESTED BLESSING

May you ease the pressure in your body and your mind.

May you relax and release all that is stubborn and inflexible.

May you in protect both halves of your brain.

May you integrate your previously hidden or oppressed half and emerge more balanced and anew.

This multi-institutional study from Texas involved 2,478 elderly participants studied during a period of six years. Participants were asked to fill out questionnaires asking yes or no questions leading to indicative feelings or symptoms during the last week. High scores on the 16 following CES-D scale[4] items made up the negative affect measure and were significantly associated with an increase in stroke.[5]

"I felt that I could not shake off the blues even with help from my family and friends."
"I felt depressed."
"I thought my life had been a failure."
"I felt fearful."
"I felt lonely."
"I had crying spells."
"I felt sad."
"I was bothered by things that usually don't bother me."
"I did not feel like eating; my appetite was poor."
"I had trouble keeping my mind on what I was doing."
"I felt everything I did was an effort."
"My sleep was restless."
"It seemed that I talked less than usual."
"People were unfriendly."
"I felt that people disliked me."

"I could not get going."

The remaining items made up the positive affect measure. A high score on this scale indicated positive affect. Researchers concluded that positive affect seems to play a role in protecting against stroke in older adults.[6]

"I felt that I was just as good as other people."
"I felt hopeful about the future."
"I was happy."
"I enjoyed life."

QUESTIONS

What is my blood pressure trying to tell me?
Where am I hard and inflexible?
Where do I resist change?
Where am I consistently or deadly stubborn?
What belief or definition fuels my stress?

The brain is divided into two hemispheres (halves). While both halves can generally complete all tasks, each side varies in its strengths. The right half of the brain governs the left side of the body associated with intuition, art, focus on the big picture, creativity and emotion (considered female characteristics). The left half of the brain governs the right side of the body associated with logic, language, reason, focus on detail and analytical thinking (considered male characteristics). In cases of one-sided loss of function, patients are helpless. Patients are confined to bed because their other half is gone. The affected half is lifeless, simply being lugged along by the healthy side. In such instances, it appears that the body is a mirror for the mind's routine of numbing or ignoring the male or female side.

Which side was taken from me?
What is my relationship to my male/female characteristics?
Did I judge, hate or ignore those characteristics?
Where am I a one-sided person?
Can I make peace with my lost side and breathe new life into it?
What am I going to use to build my new other half?

Stroke survivors face many developmental tasks. They must re-learn how to speak, do, and think. They will be different than their former selves.

AGGRAVATING FACTORS

Negative affect / depression

HEALING FACTORS

Positive affect / emotional release work / especially with hurt and anger

TAKE NOTICE

BUSH TEA • COCOA • GARLIC • GINGER •

(E)-β-CARYOPHYLLENE CONTAINING SPICES.

BUSH TEA: A recent study from Karachi, Pakistan determined why Bush tea is effective in treating hyperactive gastrointestinal problems, respiratory difficulty and high blood pressure. Bush tea is a bronchodilator, antispasmodic and has blood pressure-lowering properties. It operates by potassium (ATP) channel activation with a selective bronchodilatory effect.[7]

COCOA: Scientists at the McGill University School of Dietetics and Human Nutrition, Quebec, Canada, cautiously suggest that the consumption of dark chocolate may have protective impact on heart and vascular illness and their connection to oxidized bad cholesterol (LDL).[8]

GARLIC: Garlic is one of Cuba's most versatile herbs. It is used for the treatment of peripheral signs and symptoms relevant to heart disease such as water retention, spasms, thrombophlebitis, inflammations, viral infections and hypertension. It is also considered an overall tonic and promoter of healthy veins.[9]

German Commission E: Approved as a treatment for: "Supportive to dietary measures at elevated levels of lipids in blood. Preventative measures for age-dependent vascular changes."[10]

For the first time, Japanese scientists have been able to scientifically prove what many traditional practitioners have suspected, that garlic, or specifically allicin, has potent antioxidant properties.[11]

Another study from Japan suggests that odorless garlic powder can play a beneficial role in preventing destructive thrombus (clod) formation such as in heart attacks. Apparently it suppresses the formation of clots and destroys fibrin, a protein involved in the clotting of blood.[12]

GINGER: Scientists from Jinan, China, have shown that components of ginger protect the epithelium (tissue lining inside the arteries) when exposed to an environment of high fat diets. This rodent-based study confirmed that ginger reduced the thickening of the artery wall as measured by intima-media thickness of the aorta.[13]

(E)-β-CARYOPHYLLENE: (E)-β-Caryophyllene or (E)-BCP is a FDA-approved dietary plant-cannabinoid that activates CB2 receptor sites which have been shown to be involved in the modulation of blood pressure, inflammation and oxidative stress common in patients with hypertension. Spice plants known to contain significant amounts of (E)-BCP in descending order include: BLACK "ASHANTI PEPPER" (PIPER GUINEENSE), WHITE "ASHANTI PEPPER" (PIPER GUINEENSE), INDIAN BAY-LEAF (CINNAMOMUM TAMALA), ALLIGATOR PEPPER (AFRAMOMUM MELEGUETA), BASIL (OCIMUM MICRANTHUM), SRI LANKA CINNAMON (CINNAMOMUM ZEYLANICUM), ROSEMARY (ROSMARINUS OFFICINALIS), BLACK CARAWAY (CARUM NIGRUM), BLACK PEPPER (PIPER NIGRUM), BASIL (OCI-

MUM GRATISSIMUM), MEXICAN OREGANO (LIPPIA GRAVEOLENS), AND CLOVE (SYZYGIUM AROMATICUM).

See also HYPERTENSION, HEART DISEASES, and INFLAMMATORY DISEASES.

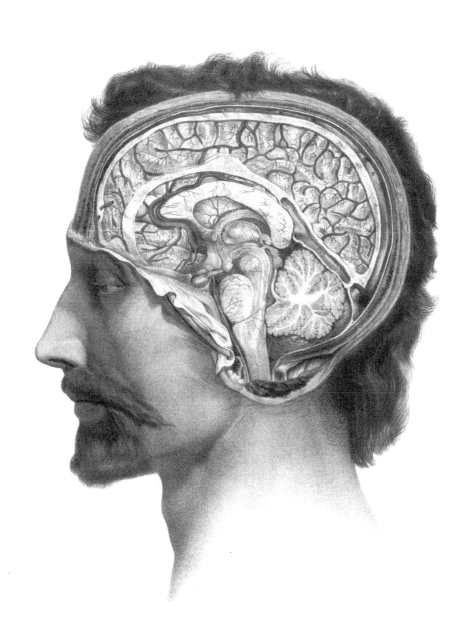

1 The United States of America as represented by the Department of Health and Human Services. (Aidan J. Hampson, Julius Axelrod and Maurizio Grimaldi) Patent No. 09/674028 filed on 02/02/2001. Patent 6630507 issued on October 7, 2003. Estimated expiration date: 2021. Cannabinoids as antioxidants and neuroprotectants. http://www.patentstorm.us/patents/6630507.html

2 Hayakawa K, Mishima K, Nozako M, Hazekawa M, Irie K, Fujioka M, Orito K, Abe K, Hasebe N, Egashira N, Iwasaki K, Fujiwara M. *Delayed treatment with cannabidiol has a cerebroprotective action via a cannabinoid receptor-independent myeloperoxidase-inhibiting mechanism.* Department of Neuropharmacology, Faculty of Pharmaceutical Sciences, Fukuoka University, Fukuoka, Japan. J Neurochem 2007 Sep; 102(5):1488-96.

3 Hayakawa K, Mishima K, Nozako M, Hazekawa M, Ogata A, Fujioka M, Harada K, Mishima S, Orito K, Egashira N, Iwasaki K, Fujiwara M. *Delta9-tetrahydrocannabinol (Delta9-THC) prevents cerebral infarction via hypothalamic-independent hypothermia.* Department of Neuropharmacology, Faculty of Pharmaceutical Sciences, Fukuoka University, Nanakuma 8-19-1, Fukuoka City, Fukuoka, Japan. Life Sci 2007 Mar 27; 80(16):1466-71.

4 CES-D = Center for Epidemiological Studies Depression Scale.

5 Glenn V. Ostir, PhD, Kyriakos S. Markides, PhD, M. Kristen Peek, PhD and James S. Goodwin, MD. *The Association Between Emotional Well-Being and the Incidence of Stroke in Older Adults.* Department of Preventive Medicine and Community Health (G.V.O., K.S.M., J.S.G.), Sealy Center on Aging (G.V.O., K.S.M., M.K.P., J.S.G.), Department of Internal Medicine (J.S.G.), and Department of Health Promotion and Gerontology (M.K.P.), University of Texas Medical Branch, Galveston, Texas. Psychosomatic Medicine 63:210-215 (2001).

6 Ibid.

7 Khan AU, Gilani AH. *Selective bronchodilatory effect of Rooibos tea (Aspalathus linearis) and its flavonoid, chrysoeriol.* Dept. of Biological and Biomedical Sciences, The Aga Khan University Medical College, Karachi, 74800, Pakistan. Eur J Nutr. 2006 Dec; 45(8):463-9.

8 Rudkowska I, Jones PJ. *Functional foods for the prevention and treatment of cardiovascular diseases: cholesterol and beyond.* School of Dietetics and Human Nutrition McGill University, St-Anne-de-Bellevue, Quebec, Canada. Expert Rev Cardiovasc Ther. 2007 May;5(3):477-90.

9 *Therapeutic Guide to Plant Pharmaceuticals and Honey Pharmaceuticals (Guia Terapeutica Dispensarial de Fitofarmacos y Apifarmacos* - Ministerio de Salud Publica, Ciudad de La Habana - Republica de Cuba 1992). Cuban Ministry of Public Health, Havana.

10 *Monographien der E-Kommission* (Phyto-Therapie) (380 monographs). A therapeutic guide to herbal medicine evaluating the safety and efficacy of herbs for licensed medical prescribing in Germany. Published between 1984 and 1994 in the Bundesanzeiger (official publication by the Federal Republic of Germany). Copies of the monographs are available at the Heilpflanzen-Welt Bibliothek: http://buecher.heilpflanzen-welt.de/BGA-Commission-E-Monographs/

11 Okada Y, Tanaka K, Sato E, Okajima H. *Kinetic and mechanistic studies of allicin as an antioxidant.* Department of Analytical Chemistry, Faculty of Health Sciences, Kyorin University, 476 Miyasita-cho, Hachioji, Tokyo, 192-8508, Japan. Org Biomol Chem. 2006 Nov 21;4(22):4113-7.

12 Fukao H, Yoshida H, Tazawa Y, Hada T. *Antithrombotic effects of odorless garlic powder both in vitro and in vivo.* Department of Nutritional Sciences, Faculty of Food Culture, Kurashiki Sakuyo University, Japan. Biosci Biotechnol Biochem. 2007 Jan;71(1):84-90.

13 Wu CX, Wei XB, Ding H, Sun X, Cheng XM. *Protective effect of effective parts of Zingiber Offecinal on vascular endothelium of the experimental hyperlipidemic rats.* Department of Pharmacology, School of Medicine Shandong University, Jinan 250012, China. wcxzzl@eyou.com Zhong Yao Cai. 2006 Aug;29(8):810-3.

Diabetes Mellitus

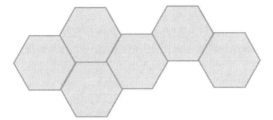

NUMBER OF STUDIES: 6

CHI VALUE: 11

Ancient physicians used the Greek word diabetes, which translates as fountain, due to their observation of frequent urination in diabetic patients (the body's natural means to rid itself of excess sugar). They also noticed that their urine tasted quite sweet, as evidenced by the many ants collecting about it. Mellitus derives from the Greek word honey; thus, *diabetes mellitus.*

Diabetes is a disease related to the pancreas, a relatively small gland located behind the stomach and in front of the spine that opens into the duodenum (small intestines). Of all the glands in the endocrine system, the pancreas, along with the adrenals, sits directly in the body's center. The pancreas produces hormones such as insulin and glucagon as well as digestive enzymes that break down food into basic sugar molecules usable as food/energy by each cell of the human body.

Between the years 1958 and 1993, the number of diabetic patients in the U.S. increased five-fold.[1] Therefore, diabetes emerged as a major public-health concern of the 21st century. Still, the number of insulin-controlled diabetic patients varies greatly between different countries. "On average, less than one per 100,000 people in Shanghai, China, have diabetes; while for, example, whites in Allegheny County, Pennsylvania, have been diagnosed with diabetes at a rate 26 times higher. Populations in Finland fare even worse with a more than 50 times greater incidence of the disease."[2]

Orthodox medicine lacks a cure and has not yet located the exact origins of the illness. However, mainstream science considers a likely cause to be genetic predisposition in conjunction with some form of environmental trigger(s) or life stressor(s). One primary environmental cause considered includes the emergence of industrial food production with its decline in nutrient densities and the widespread use of pesticides and hormones, and/or modern food processing and storage methods that contain endocrine disruptors. Other potential causes include certain pharmaceutical drugs, infectious pathogens, life-style factors (poor diet, lack of exercise, chronic stress) or an overzealous immune system that turns on itself. Higher maternal age at birth or the lack or duration of breastfeeding are also cited as possible causes, particularly in cases of pedeatric diabetes.

Alternatively, some researchers consider diabetes a metabolic disease involving cellular resistance to two specific hormones: insulin, which is produced by the pancreas and leptin, which is made by adipose tissue (fat cells). Leptin signals the brain to reduce hunger. Leptin sensitive people will feel satiated sooner and convert fat faster while leptin resistant individuals will eat longer and keep energy stored in fat.

Insulin tells individual cells when to turn fat or sugar into energy. Insulin sensitive people easily convert fat and sugar into energy. In insulin resistant people, cells do not get the message and the sugar remains poorly used, thus fat accumulates.

Other recent scientific discoveries suggest still another cause for the early genesis of diabetes - fatty livers. Here, scientists propose that eating excessive or unhealthy sugar induces the liver to convert the sugar into unhealthy types of fats, which are deposited in the liver, among other places. Fatty livers produce insulin resistance (metabolic syndrome) in both obese and healthy people alike, increasing the risk of cancer and heart disease. Evidence suggests that avoiding sugar and eating low glycemic foods quickly rids the body of liver/abdominal fat, and insulin resistance disappears.

Traditionally, orthodox medicine categorizes diabetes into three kinds: Type I, Type II and gestational diabetes. Type I diabetes was once called juvenile diabetes because it occurred mostly in children or adolescents. In Type I, the pancreas stops producing the hormone insulin. Without insulin the body cannot use the food life depends on, cellular sugar. Treatment in the orthodox paradigm consists of daily insulin injections normally administered by the patients themselves.

Type II diabetes, or adult onset diabetes, is the most common form of the disease. In Type II the pancreas does not produce enough insulin or the body's cells are insensitive to the presence of insulin and ignore it. This prevents the body from converting sugar into energy. Early Type II usually does not require the use of insulin; modern medical practitioners generally prescribes oral pharmaceuticals instead.

Diabetes, especially Type I or advanced Type II, is potentially life-threatening. Complications diminish one's life expectancy and quality of life.

Gestational diabetes (diabetes that occurs during some pregnancies), most often self-corrects after delivery. While not very well understood, it is hypothesized that hormonal changes during pregnancy may produce a temporary resistance to insulin, thereby producing higher than normal blood sugar levels.

Early signs and symptoms of diabetes include: frequent urination, sweet smelling urine, and increased thirst and hunger. Over long periods of time, symptoms may progress to cold, pale and clammy skin, altered levels of consciousness, unconsciousness, neuropathies, skin ulcers, peripheral vascular diseases, kidney problems, acute metabolic problems (diabetic ketoacidosis, hypoglycemia, diabetic coma, lactic acidosis), loss of vision, heart disease, stroke, infections, sepsis and periodontal disease.

Diagnostic tools include a simple blood test used to measure sugar content. Measurements between 80 and 120 are considered normal. Orthodox disease management is limited to pharmaceutical treatments (oral or injections), nutritional and dietary recommendations and lifestyle changes.

CANNABIS AND DIABETES

While cannabis oil has been used historically in the treatment of diabetes, and while many diabetic patients claim that cannabis lowers high blood sugar levels, stabilizes mood changes and mental irritability, to date, no human studies have been conducted to examine the general effects of cannabinoids on diabetic patients. However, the known anti-inflammatory and immunomodulating properties of the plant have prompted the following experiments relevant in the context of diabetes.

Israeli scientists demonstrated a potential link between endocannabinoid receptor sites and diabetes. The Jerusalem studies (2006 & 2008) suggest that the cannabinoid cannabidiol (CBD) might possibly be a novel therapeutic agent for treatment of Type I diabetes. An Edinburgh laboratory study (2009) discovered a synthetic cannabinoid's ability to grow nerve extensions in a glucose rich environment, thus providing a basis for potentially novel neuroprotective drugs for diabetic patients. Two US studies from Augusta, GA (2006) and East Lansing, MI (2001) conducted on rodents demonstrated that the cannabinoids THC and CBD could reduce diabetic neuropathies. Scientists observed a reduction in retinal oxidative stress with an additional attenuation of autoimmune diabetes in the mice. A Polish research team (2008) learned more about the mechanism by which cannabinoids ease diabetic neuropathies (nerve pain). This team discovered that certain pharmaceutical medications (COX-1 inhibitors such as indomethacin) work synergistically to further ease such pains.[3]

STUDY SUMMARY:

Drugs	Type of Study	Published Year, Place, and Key Results	CHI
Synthetic cannabinoid HU210	Laboratory	2009 – School of Life Sciences, Edinburgh Napier University, Scotland, UK. Neurite growth may play a therapeutic role in reversing neuropathies.[4]	1
CB-1 and CB-2 receptor agonists WIN 55,212-2; Met-F-AEA; and AM1241	Animals study (mice)	2008 – Department of Pharma-codynamics, Medical University of Warsaw, Warsaw, Poland. CB1 & CB2 agonists reduce sensitivity to pain in a dose dependent fashion and COX-1 inhibitors e.g. (indomethacin) and may increase these cannabinoid properties at low dosages.[5]	2
Cannabidiol (CBD)	Animals study (mice)	2008 – Department of Bone Marrow Transplantation and Cancer Immunotherapy, Hadassah Hebrew University Hospital, Jerusalem, Israel. CBD reduced the manifestations of diabetes and exhibited more intact islets of Langerhans than a control group.[6]	2
Cannabidiol (CBD)	Animals study (mice)	2006 – Hadassah University Hospital, Department of Bone Marrow Transplantation & Cancer Immunotherapy, Jerusalem, Israel. CBD treatment significantly reduced the incidence of diabetes in non-obese diabetic mice.[7]	2
Cannabidiol (CBD)	Animals study (rats)	2006 – Multi-institutional Research Team Augusta, Georgia. Rats treated with cannabidiol (CBD) experienced significant protection from developing diabetic retinopathy.[8]	2
Delta9-THC administered orally in corn oil at 150 mg/kg for 11 days	Animals study (mice)	2001 – Michigan State University, East Lansing. Mice with induced autoimmune diabetes. Delta9-THC is capable of attenuating the severity of the autoimmune diabetes in mice.[9]	2

Total CHI Value   11

STRAIN SPECIFIC CONSIDERATIONS

In these studies, the synthetic cannabinoids (WIN 55,212-2; AM1241, HU210) and the plant cannabinoids THC but especially CBD underwent testing relevant to diabetes.

WIN 55,212-2 and AM 1241 bind with higher affinity to CB2 while HU210 has a higher affinity for the CB1 receptors. THC binds relatively equally to CB1 and CB2 while CBD has a greater affinity for CB2.

Indicas and indica heavy strains contain lower THC:CBD ratios, which tends to result in activation of both CB1 and CB2; but it initiates more CB2 than sativa strains.

Results from a Harvard study entitled Positive Emotion and Health: Going Beyond the Negative, alluded to the role that emotions play in the genesis of diabetes. Scientists discovered an association of higher levels of curiosity and hope with a lower incidence of diabetes.[10]

Becoming an insulin dependent diabetic poses a serious demand for change and forces a significant shift in lifestyle with a focus on attention to details. The individual must now seriously monitor sugar levels, carefully determine when and how to nurture the body and understand when and how to exercise. Depending on the progression of the disease, the patient must become sensitive to the early signals, subtle sensations and internal experiences that indicate hypoglycemia if s/he wants to avert an acute event. The body plays out the core issues of diabetes. The patient appears locked into a constant struggle to gain access to the energy that fuels and sustains physical life.

In the diabetic patient, sugar is not converted into cellular energy, thus keeping individual cells from operating efficiently. As a result, a wide variety of diabetic symptoms ensue. In hyperglycemia, sugar remains suspended in blood, available but not utilized. In other words, there is plenty of food in the pantry but the key to the locked door - insulin - is missing. In severe cases of hyperglycemia, the patient initially presents with thirst and frequent urination, which when left untreated can progress to lethargy and confusion until s/he slips into a silent diabetic coma.

In the self-treating insulin dependent diabetic patient, a delicate daily balance between insulin dose and measured blood sugar levels are essential to maintain healthy bodily functions. A simple error can quickly lead to too much insulin in the bloodstream causing hypoglycemia where sugar absorbs at such a rapid pace that too little remains for sustained cellular function. The hypoglycemic symptoms, including expressions of irritability, anger, confusion, pale and very moist skin, often lead to a variety of expressions. These range from a quiet fury or rage to physical combativeness when approached by caregivers such as paramedics.

Thus, paradoxically, a diabetic person may be physically either too sweet or not sweet enough but at its cellular core in both cases, exists a struggle to convert sugar or fat into life-sustaining energy or power. The central emotion observed in both hypoglycemia and hyperglycemia appears as a rage turned inward. This rage, focused on the center organ of the body, the pancreas, effectively renders the whole body useless in activating available power.

In the context of diabetes, rage is not simply louder anger. Rage is a complex and paradoxical emotion that can be empowering or disempowering; it can be destructive or instructive; it can be imprisoning or liberating. Rage can be a vicious enemy or a protective ally, and in the context of diabetes, it finds association with the inappropriate use of powers or unwillingness to be truly powerful.

In juvenile diabetes, the source of disempowering rage can often be traced to family power dynamics; while in adult onset diabetes, this disempowering rage is often connected to societal issues.

"Many patients believe that their diabetes has been caused by stress or an adverse life event."[11] When thinking back to the first appearance of diabetes, patients might recall experiencing 'trigger events' such as: the violation of deeply valued ideals, a defiling of one's sense of worth, the removal of power or crushing of one's spirit. There may have been a single event of great intensity or an onslaught of repeated events that caused damage over time.

In addition to the notion of trigger events, researchers noted that interventions aimed at reducing family conflict and caregiver involvement garnered positive results in improving diabetes' outcome.[12] These beliefs and findings indicate that psychosomatic origins of diabetes likely occur in power dynamics involving conflict, anger, fury, resentment and rage where the person feels hopeless and resigned or unable to change anything.

POWER–RAGE DYNAMICS: Lacking the will to be powerful or perceiving oneself as powerless may be a psychosomatic link to diabetes.

When a child is to assume responsibilities that require adult powers childhood ends prematurely. Intense longing for this stolen childhood and rage about having to be the grown up in the family may result for the child or juvenile. Diabetes may emerge as an unconscious strategy to reclaim childhood. While it may work to shift the power-responsibility dynamic of the family, the well-intentioned and initially helpful strategy, left unhealed, can ultimately evolve into a serious liability.

Alternatively, a caregiver may be over-reaching or actively suppress growth, age-appropriated responsibility and emerging power of the developing child/person in an attempt to retain control, driven by fear of loosing them. Sick and unable to attend school or have diabetes may be a childs attempt to provide a troubled parent with the control they seek.

Nature automatically takes the body from infancy through adolescence and into adulthood. However, the maturing of the mind is a process involving conscious growth, engagement and work. Rage at having to do this work is a rage directed at the source of life itself. The refusal to be responsible and the implicit entitlement in "I should not have to do this work" emerges in the diabetic expression of not wanting to utilize the energy or power to be responsible for one's own growth and well-being.

When a person in a position of power demands blind loyalty from others or when a subordinate provides blind loyalty to an unprincipled or scrupulous leader, a fertile and vast breeding ground for abusive behavior or the condoning of abuse unfolds. While both will have a reason or justification for such a misuse of power, neither will truly be able to utilize the available powers, strengths or talents inherent in every human.

Somewhere hidden in this depth of rage, patients can discover root belief(s), from which such rage was born. Examples may include: power cannot be trusted; power corrupts; I am safe when I am powerless; I cannot be trusted with power; I am resigned to letting others have power; others cannot be trusted with power.

See also PAIN – NEUROPATHIES.

QUESTIONS

Think back: what was going on when you first started to have symptoms?
Was there a feeling of loss for a private treasure (self, power, value, self-worth)?
Which treasures does my rage hold for me?

What have I given to my rage?

Where am I too sweet with an abusive person?

Where can I not speak truth to power?

In what situation am I a "yes" wo/man?

How can I respond consciously and constructively to the power in my family?

How can I express my rage (fury, resentment, anger) constructively but without hurting anyone?

What are my feelings about receiving nourishment from others?

How do I feel about nourishing myself?

Do I want to nurture myself?

Does this power/rage apply to me?

If so, how can I answer the power/rage dynamic?

How do I feel about nurturing myself with constant attention to details?

AGGRAVATING FACTORS

Hypoglycemia – not sweet enough (being hard on self, lack of deservability) / Hyperglycemia – being too sweet (over caring, helping others but suffering to do so)

HEALING FACTORS

Develop a caring that does not involve personal suffering. For example, gratitude makes it difficult to be hard on oneself, feel undeserving, over-care or help others while suffering / Embrace hope and curiosity

TAKE NOTICE

β-CARYOPHYLLENE CONTAINING SPICES: BLACK AND WHITE ASHANTI (WEST AFRICAN) PEPPERS, INDIAN BAY-LEAF, ALLIGATOR PEPPER, BASIL, CINNAMON, ROSEMARY, CARAWAY, BLACK PEPPER, MEXICAN OREGANO AND CLOVE.

CAYENNE • COCOA • CUMIN • GARLIC • GINGER • NUTMEG • TURMERIC

β-CARYOPHYLLENE CONTAINING SPICES: Researchers suggest that activation of CB2 receptors via β-caryophyllene containing spices may present a new and additional therapeutic strategy in the treatment of a multitude of diseases associated with inflammation and oxidative stress; both are underlying factors in diabetes.[13,14]

This dietary cannabinoid is approved by the U.S. Government with the FDA's seal of approval and key β-caryophyllene containing organic spices, which are relatively easy to obtain. Spices that contain β-caryophyllene include: BLACK AND WHITE ASHANTI (WEST AFRICAN) PEPPERS, INDIAN BAY-LEAF, ALLIGATOR PEPPER, BASIL, CINNAMON, ROSEMARY, CARAWAY, BLACK PEPPER, MEXICAN OREGANO AND CLOVE. For more information on these specific spices go the chapter "Cannabinoid Research."

CARAWAY: Moroccan scientists from the city of Errachidia determined in animal-based studies that caraway could lower blood sugar levels without increasing the body's production of insulin.[15]

CAYENNE: Fat and sugar balancing effects of cayenne (among other herbs) have been documented at the Johann Wolfgang Goethe University in Frankfurt, Germany. Results of this study suggest a rationale for the use of cayenne in diabetic treatment.[16]

Doctors from Bangkok, Thailand, noted an increase in metabolic rates and a slowing of sugar (glucose) uptake after giving 5gm of fresh cayenne to a group of women. This, in turn, may provide scientists with an appreciation for traditional healers worldwide who use cayenne as a means to treat certain forms of diabetes.[17]

CINNAMON: Canadian researchers have determined that cinnamon may be a valuable candidate for new anti-diabetic medications.[18]

The spice is widely used in Ayurvedic medicine in the treatment of diabetes. Studies from Tamil Nadu indicate that cinnamon contains hypoglycemic and hypolipidemic properties[19] and improves glucose metabolism.[20]

CLOVE: Scientists at Vanderbilt University School of Medicine, in Nashville, explored clove because it has insulin-like effects, which may prove beneficial in the treatment of diabetes.[21] The data revealed that clove, much like insulin, stimulates a certain gene sequence expression and thereby sets in motion chemical reactions important in effective sugar metabolism.

COCOA: Although traditional practitioners used cocoa to work with diabetic patients, cocoa's exact working mechanism remains a mystery. However, University Putra scientists in Selangor, Malaysia, have confirmed that cocoa extract may indeed possess dose-dependent hypoglycemic and hypocholestrolemic properties.[22]

CUMIN: A meta-analysis from Mysore, India, conducted animal and clinical trials to determine that cumin, among other select spices, contains beneficial antidiabetic food adjuncts.[23]

> **Improve Cellular Fat and Sugar Metabolism Naturally by:**
>
> 1. Eating foods with a low glycemic index.
>
> 2. Avoiding toxic sugars:
> Aspartame (NutraSweet®), Sucralose (Splenda®) and Splenda® essentials (a new form of Splenda® dressed up as a health food with added vitamins, fiber or minerals), Saccharin (Sweet'n Low®), and high fructose corn syrup. Agave nectar is *not* a traditional, natural, low glycemic sugar, despite being marketed as such. It is a highly processed chemical product to be avoided.
>
> 3. Using healthy sugars such as:
> Xylitol, Fructoligosaccharides (FOS) and Stevia.

GARLIC: Scientists at the Russian Academy of Medical Sciences conducted a live double-blind placebo-controlled study on 60 Type II diabetic patients.[24] They used time controlled garlic powder tablets and found that garlic produced improved metabolic control in patients due to lowered blood glucose and triglyceride levels. These scientists now recommend garlic in conjunction with dietary control and other measures in the treatment of adult onset diabetes. Scientists believe garlic helps make glucose and fat metabolism more efficient, thereby contributing to the prevention of long-term complications such as heart attacks.

GINGER: Scientists in Safat, Kuwat, examined the effectiveness of ginger to alleviate diabetic rats' incapacity to breakdown sugar and convert it to usable energy. They discovered that ginger dosed at 500mg/kg could lower blood glucose, cholesterol and triacylglycerol levels when compared to the control group of rats not receiving the treatment.[25]

A researcher from Durban, South Africa supports the time-proven use of ginger by traditional African healers as an effective means to treat painful and chronic arthritic inflammatory conditions and to achieve better metabolic control in patients with Type II adult-onset diabetes.[26]

NUTMEG: Korean scientists from Yusong-gu explored the use of an isolated nutmeg extract in the treatment of Type II diabetes and obesity. They discovered that the extract inhibited a certain protein expression, thereby enhancing insulin signals inside the cells.[27]

OREGANO: Endocrinologists in Errachidia, Morocco, examined the potential of a water-based extract of oregano as a therapeutic agent in treating hyperglycemia. They found, in an animal model, that the extract could reduce sugar levels without increasing blood insulin concentrations.[28]

ROSEMARY: University scientists from Taichung Hsien, Taiwan, concluded that, "… rosemary is an excellent multifunctional therapeutic herb; by looking at its potentially potent antiglycative bioactivity, it may become a good adjuvant medicine for the prevention and treatment of diabetic, cardiovascular, and other neurodegenerative diseases."[29]

TURMERIC: In this meta-study, scientists from Dallas, Texas, provided an overview of decades of scientific studies on turmeric. Researchers summarized a long list of turmeric's potential therapeutic properties, including as a diabetic and pancreatitis preventative.[30]

1 Ronald Aubert. *Diabetes in America*. 2nd Edition. Published by the National Institute of Health No. 95-1468. 1995. Page 3.

2 Ibid.

3 Bujalska M. *Effect of Cannabinoid Receptor Agonists on Streptozotocin-Induced Hyperalgesia in Diabetic Neuropathy*. Department of Pharmacodynamics, Medical University of Warsaw, Warsaw, Poland. mbujalska@gmail.com Pharmacology. 2008;82(3):193-200.

4 Zhang F, Challapalli SC, Smith PJ. *Cannabinoid CB(1) receptor activation stimulates neurite outgrowth and inhibits capsaicin-induced Ca(2+) influx in an in vitro model of diabetic neuropathy*. School of Life Sciences, Edinburgh Napier University, Scotland, UK. Neuropharmacology. 2009 Aug;57(2):88-96.

5 Bujalska M. *Effect of Cannabinoid Receptor Agonists on Streptozotocin-Induced Hyperalgesia in Diabetic Neuropathy*. Department of Pharmacodynamics, Medical University of Warsaw, Warsaw, Poland. mbujalska@gmail.com Pharmacology. 2008;82(3):193-200.

6 Weiss L, Zeira M, Reich S, Slavin S, Raz I, Mechoulam R, Gallily R. *Cannabidiol arrests onset of autoimmune diabetes in NOD mice*. Department of Bone Marrow Transplantation and Cancer Immunotherapy, Hadassah Hebrew University Hospital, Jerusalem 91120, Israel. lolaw@hadassa.org.il Neuropharmacology. 2008 Jan;54(1):244-9.

7 Weiss L, Zeira M, Reich S, Har-Noy M, Mechoulam R, Slavin S, Gallily R. *Cannabidiol lowers incidence of diabetes in non-obese diabetic mice*. Hadassah University Hospital, Department of Bone Marrow Transplantation &

Cancer Immunotherapy, POB 12000, Jerusalem, 91120, Israel. Autoimmunity. 2006 Mar;39(2):143-51.

8 Azza B. El-Remessy*, Mohamed Al-Shabrawey, Yousuf Khalifa, Nai-Tse Tsai, Ruth B. Caldwell and Gregory I. Liou. *Neuroprotective and Blood-Retinal Barrier-Preserving Effects of Cannabidiol in Experimental Diabetes.* From the Departments of Pharmacology and Toxicology* and Ophthalmology, the Vascular Biology Center, Cellular Biology and Anatomy, and the Medical College of Georgia; and the Veterans Affairs Medical Center, Augusta, Georgia. American Journal of Pathology. 2006;168:235-244.

9 Li X, Kaminski NE, Fischer LJ. *Examination of the immunosuppressive effect of delta9-tetrahydrocannabinol in streptozotocin-induced autoimmune diabetes.* Department of Pharmacology and Toxicology, Michigan State University, East Lansing 48824, USA. Int Immunopharmacol. 2001 Apr;1(4):699-712.

10 Richman LS, Kubzansky L, Maselko J, Kawachi I, Choo P, Bauer M. *Positive emotion and health: going beyond the negative.* Department of Society, Human Development, and Health, Harvard School of Public Health, Cambridge, MA, USA. Health Psychol. 2005 Jul;24(4):422-9.

11 Wales JK. *Does psychological stress cause diabetes?* Division of Medicine, University of Leeds, UK. Diabet Med. 1995 Feb;12(2):109-12.

12 Ingerski LM, Anderson BJ, Dolan LM, Hood KK. *Blood glucose monitoring and glycemic control in adolescence: contribution of diabetes-specific responsibility and family conflict.* Division of Behavioral Medicine and Clinical Psychology, Center for Treatment Adherence, Cincinnati Children's Hospital Medical Center, Cincinnati, Ohio 45229-3039, USA. J Adolesc Health. 2010 Aug;47(2):191-7.

13 Gertsch J, Leonti M, Raduner S, Racz I, Chen JZ, Xie XQ, Altmann KH, Karsak M, Zimmer A. *Beta-caryophyllene is a dietary cannabinoid.* Institute of Pharmaceutical Sciences, Department of Chemistry and Applied Biosciences, Eidgenössische Technische Hochschule (ETH) Zurich, 8092 Zürich, Switzerland. Proc Natl Acad Sci U S A. 2008 Jul 1;105(26):9099-104.

14 Béla Horvátha, Partha Mukhopadhyaya, Malek Kechrida, Vivek Patela, Gali Tanchiana, David A. Winkb, Jürg Gertschc, Pál Pachera. *β-Caryophyllene ameliorates cisplatin-induced nephrotoxicity in a cannabinoid 2 receptor-dependent manner.* a Laboratory of Physiologic Studies, National Institute on Alcohol Abuse and Alcoholism, National Institutes of Health, Bethesda, MD 20892, USA. b Radiation Biology Branch, National Cancer Institute, National Institutes of Health, Bethesda, MD 20892, USA. c Institute of Biochemistry and Molecular Medicine, University of Bern, 3012 Bern, Switzerland. Free Radical Biology and Medicine. Volume 52, Issue 8, 15 April 2012, Pages 1325–133.

15 Eddouks M, Lemhadri A, Michel JB. *Caraway and caper: potential anti-hyperglycaemic plants in diabetic rats.* Laboratory of Endocrinian Physiology, FSTE Boutalamine and Pharmacology, EDDOUKS, UFR PNPE, BP 21, Errachidia 52000, Morocco. J Ethnopharmacol. 2004 Sep;94(1):143-8.

16 Rau O, Wurglics M, Dingermann T, Abdel-Tawab M, Schubert-Zsilavecz M. *Screening of herbal extracts for activation of the human peroxisome proliferator-activated receptor.* Johann Wolfgang Goethe University Frankfurt, Institute of Pharmaceutical Chemistry/ZAFES, Frankfurt/Main, Germany. Pharmazie. 2006 Nov;61(11):952-6.

17 Chaiyata P, Puttadechakum S, Komindr S. *Effect of chili pepper (Capsicum frutescens) ingestion on plasma glucose response and metabolic rate in Thai women.* Research Center, Ramathibodi Hospital, Mahidol University, Bangkok 10400, Thailand. J Med Assoc Thai. 2003 Sep;86(9):854-60.

18 Kim W, Khil LY, Clark R, Bok SH, Kim EE, Lee S, Jun HS, Yoon JW. *Naphthalenemethyl ester derivative of dihydroxyhydrocinnamic acid, a component of cinnamon, increases glucose disposal by enhancing translocation of glucose transporter.* Julia McFarlane Diabetes Research Centre and Department of Microbiology and Infectious Diseases, Faculty of Medicine, University of Calgary, Calgary, AB, Canada. Diabetologia. 2006 Oct;49(10):2437-48.

19 Subash Babu P, Prabuseenivasan S, Ignacimuthu S. Phytomedicine. *Cinnamaldehyde-A potential antidiabetic agent.* Division of Ethnopharmacology, Entomology Research Institute, Loyola College, Chennai 600 034, Tamil Nadu, India. 2007 Jan;14(1):15-22. Phytomedicine. 2007 Jan;14(1):15-22

20 Kannappan S, Jayaraman T, Rajasekar P, Ravichandran MK, Anuradha CV. *Cinnamon bark extract improves glucose metabolism and lipid profile in the fructose-fed rat.* Department of Biochemistry, Annamalai University, Annamalai Nagar, Tamil Nadu 608002, India. Singapore Med J. 2006 Oct;47(10):858-63.

21 Prasad RC, Herzog B, Boone B, Sims L, Waltner-Law M. *An extract of Syzygium aromaticum represses genes encoding hepatic gluconeogenic enzymes.* Department of Molecular Physiology and Biophysics, Vanderbilt University School of Medicine, Nashville, TN 37232, USA. J Ethnopharmacol. 2005 Jan 4;96(1-2):295-301.

22 Ruzaidi A, Amin I, Nawalyah AG, Hamid M, Faizul HA. *The effect of Malaysian cocoa extract on glucose levels and lipid profiles in diabetic rats.* Department of Nutrition and Health Sciences, Faculty of Medicine and Health Sciences, University Putra Malaysia, 43400 Serdang, Selangor, Malaysia. J Ethnopharmacol. 2005 Apr 8;98(1-2):55-60.

23 Srinivasan K. *Plant foods in the management of diabetes mellitus: spices as beneficial antidiabetic food adjuncts.* Department of Biochemistry & Nutrition, Central Food Technological Research Institute, Mysore-570013, India. Int J Food Sci Nutr. 2005 Sep;56(6):399-414.

24 Sobenin IA, Nedosugova LV, Filatova LV, Balabolkin MI, Gorchakova TV, Orekhov AN. *Metabolic effects of time-released garlic powder tablets in type 2 diabetes mellitus: the results of double-blinded placebo-controlled study.* Institute of General Pathology and Pathophysiology, Russian Academy of Medical Sciences, Moscow, Russia. Acta Diabetol. September 6, 2007.

25 Al-Amin ZM, Thomson M, Al-Qattan KK, Peltonen-Shalaby R, Ali M. *Anti-diabetic and hypolipidaemic properties of ginger (Zingiber officinale) in streptozotocin-induced diabetic rats.* Department of Biological Sciences, Faculty of Science, Kuwait University, 13060-Safat, Kuwait. Br J Nutr. 2006 Oct;96(4):660-6.

26 Ojewole JA. *Analgesic, antiinflammatory and hypoglycaemic effects of ethanol extract of Zingiber officinale (Roscoe) rhizomes (Zingiberaceae) in mice and rats.* Department of Pharmacology, Faculty of Health Sciences, University of KwaZulu-Natal, Private Bag X54001, Durban, South Africa. ojewolej@ukzn.ac.za Phytother Res. 2006 Sep;20(9):764-72.

27 Yang S, Na MK, Jang JP, Kim KA, Kim BY, Sung NJ, Oh WK, Ahn JS. *Inhibition of protein tyrosine phosphatase 1B by lignans from Myristica fragrans.* Korea Research Institute of Bioscience and Biotechnology (KRIBB), 52 Eoeun-dong, Yusong-gu, Daejeon 305-333, Korea. Phytother Res. 2006 Aug;20(8):680-2.

28 Lemhadri A, Zeggwagh NA, Maghrani M, Jouad H, Eddouks M. *Anti-hyperglycaemic activity of the aqueous extract of Origanum vulgare growing wild in Tafilalet region.* Laboratory of Endocrinian Physiology, F.S.T.E. Boutalamine and Pharmacology, UFR PNPE, BP 21, Errachidia 52000, Morocco. J Ethnopharmacol. 2004 Jun;92(2-3):251-6.

29 Hsieh CL, Peng CH, Chyau CC, Lin YC, Wang HE, Peng RY. *Low-density lipoprotein, collagen, and thrombin models reveal that Rosemarinus officinalis L. exhibits potent antiglycative effects.* Department of Food and Nutrition, Research Institute of Biotechnology, and Division of Basic Medical Sciences, Hung-Kuang University, No. 34 Chung-Chie Road, Shalu County, Taichung Hsien, Taiwan. J Agric Food Chem. 2007 Apr 18;55(8):2884-91.

30 Goel A, Kunnumakkara AB, Aggarwal BB. *Curcumin as "Curecumin": From kitchen to clinic.* Gastrointestinal Cancer Research Laboratory, Department of Internal Medicine, Charles A. Sammons Cancer Center and Baylor Research Institute, Baylor University Medical Center, Dallas, TX, United States. Biochem Pharmacol. 2007 Aug 19.

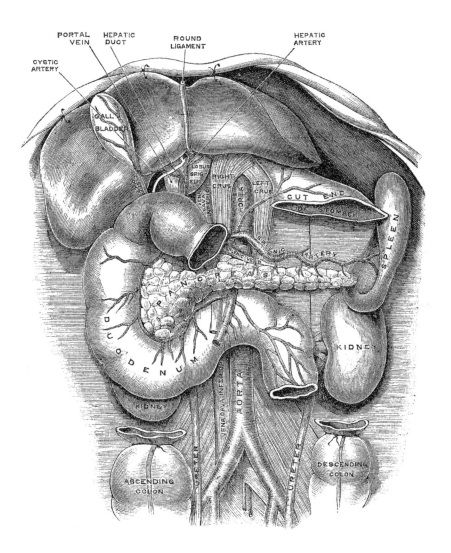

Eye Disease and Eye Function
Age Related Macular Degeneration

NUMBER OF STUDIES: 1

CHI VALUE: 1

This painless eye disease is characterized by loss of accurate vision in the center of the field of vision. Most common in seniors, age related macular degeneration (ARMD) is due to damage of the retina (the tissue lining the inner surface of the eye). It exists in wet or dry forms. Orthodox medicine has no cure and does not know the exact mechanism causing the disease's development. Possible causes include: aging, family history, plaque build up, high glycemic index food consumption, high blood pressure, smoking and damage from oxidative stress.

Signs and symptoms may include but are not limited to drusen (tissue build-up on the eye), sudden loss of visual accuracy, blurred vision and loss of central vision. The disease will not cause blindness and many people learn to function with peripheral vision alone. However, patients might lose the ability to drive or see faces. Various treatments exist. The more orthodox of these involves injections of pharmaceutical agents directly into the eye. Presently, scientists are testing experimental treatments using stem cells. In addition, natural treatments currently practiced include dietary changes and nutritional supplements such as lutein, carotenoids and omega-3 fatty acids.

CANNABIS AND ARMD

Researchers widely agree that cannabinoid receptors are present in nerve cells. The endocannabinoid system plays an important role as a potential therapeutic agents in neurodegenerative diseases. However, until 2009, it remained uncertain whether receptors existed in human retinal pigment epithelial (RPE) cells and, more importantly, what role they might play in ARMD.

Results from a study in Shanghai, China (2009) showed that RPE cells indeed contain cannabinoid receptors CB1 and CB2. In fact, they note that the presence of cannabinoids triggers a cellular response in RPE cells in such a way as to significantly protect them from oxidative damage, considered one of the possible causes of ARMD.[1]

STUDY SUMMARY:

Drugs	Type of Study	Published Year, Place, and Key Results	CHI
Cannabinoid receptors and one enzyme responsible for endocannabinoid hydrolysis, fatty acid amide hydrolase (FAAH)	Laboratory test	2009 – Department of Ophthalmology, Ruijin Hospital, Shanghai Jiaotong University School of Medicine, Shanghai, People's Republic of China. RPE cells contain CB1 & CB2. Cannabinoids may protect the retina from oxidative stress - one of the causes of ARMD.	1

Total CHI Value 1

STRAIN SPECIFIC CONSIDERATIONS

RPE cells contain CB1 and CB2 receptors. Sativas and indicas, as well as their varied hybrids, contain cannabinoids that will activate CB1 and CB2.

QUESTIONS

What is at the center of my life that I do not want to see?
Why do I want to focus only on the periphery of my world?
Why do I not want to see your face?
What is going to happen if I see clearly?
What don't I what to see?
Might I have difficulty facing you on an emotional level?

TAKE NOTICE

OXIDATIVE STRESS REDUCTION: ACACIA • CINNAMON • CLOVE • COCOA • CUMIN • FENNEL • GINGER • OREGANO • TURMERIC

ACACIA: Gum Arabic/acacia protects from oxidative stress by means of super-oxide scavengers (potent anti-oxidants).[2]

CINNAMON: This Indian study from Mysore revealed that a cinnamon fruit powder water extract contains potent antioxidant properties.[3]

CLOVE: Scientists from Vienna discovered more about the mechanism of how the essential oil of clove's potent anti-oxidant properties work.[4]

COCOA: University Hospital doctors from Zürich highlight the antioxidant properties of cocoa among other therapeutic effects.[5]

CUMIN: This study from Andhra Pradesh, India, looked at the antioxidant activity of aqueous extract of cumin when compared to that of ascorbic acid (vitamin C). Researchers determined that cumin actually scavenges super-oxide radicals while inhibiting lipid peroxide and hydroxyl radicals to perform the same tasks.[6]

FENNEL: Researchers examined the anti-oxidant properties of fennel in an animal experiment from Afyon, Turkey.[7]

GINGER: Indian scientists from Mysore determined that ginger protects the body by multiple means including to scavenging free radicals (strong anti-oxidants).[8]

OREGANO: Scientists from the Department of Pharmacology and Biochemistry at the University of Medicine, Varna, Bulgaria, conducted studies following the model of traditional Bulgarian herbalists. Using a tea preparation of oregano, they discovered it has a high phenolic content as well as significant anti-oxidant properties.[9]

SUGGESTED BLESSING

May a pristine focus and crisp clarity inform everything you see.

SUGGESTED AFFIRMATION

I can create a life that is wondrous to see no matter what perspective I choose.

TURMERIC: Based on the evidence of numerous laboratory and animal trials, these scientists from Vandoeuvre-Lès-Nancy, France, contend, "…that curcumin plays a protective role in numerous diseases; its therapeutic action being on the prevention or modulation of inflammation and oxidative stress."[10]

In this meta-study from Dallas, Texas, scientists give an overview of decades of scientific studies on turmeric. They summarize a long list of turmeric's potential therapeutic properties including protection from chronic anterior uveitis (inflammation of the middle layer of the eye).[11]

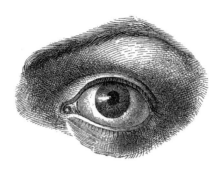

1 Wei Y, Wang X, Wang L. *Presence and regulation of cannabinoid receptors in human retinal pigment epithelial cells.* Department of Ophthalmology, Ruijin Hospital, Shanghai Jiaotong University School of Medicine, Shanghai, People's Republic of China. Mol Vis. 2009 Jun 14;15:1243-51.

2 Abd-Allah AR, Al-Majed AA, Mostafa AM, Al-Shabanah OA, Din AG, Nagi MN. *Protective effect of Arabic gum against cardiotoxicity induced by doxorubicin in mice: a possible mechanism of protection.* Department of Pharmacology, College of Pharmacy, King Saud University, P O Box 2457, Riyadh 11451, Saudi Arabia. J Biochem Mol Toxicol. 2002;16(5):254-9.

3 Jayaprakasha GK, Ohnishi-Kameyama M, Ono H, Yoshida M, Jaganmohan Rao L. *Phenolic constituents in the fruits of Cinnamomum zeylanicum and their antioxidant activity.* Central Food Technological Research Institute, Mysore, India. J Agric Food Chem. 2006 Mar 8;54(5):1672-9.

4 Jirovetz L, Buchbauer G, Stoilova I, Stoyanova A, Krastanov A, Schmidt E. *Chemical composition and antioxidant properties of clove leaf essential oil.* Department of Clinical Pharmacy and Diagnostics, University of Vienna, Althanstrasse 14, A-1090 Vienna, Austria. J Agric Food Chem. 2006 Aug 23;54(17):6303-7.

5 Hermann F, Ruschitzka F, Spieker L, Sudano I, Noll G, Corti R. *The sweet secret of dark chocolate.* HerzKreislaufzentrum, Kardiologie, Universitätsspital Zürich. Ther Umsch. 2005 Sep;62(9):635-7.

6 Satyanarayana S, Sushruta K, Sarma GS, Srinivas N, Subba Raju GV. *Antioxidant activity of the aqueous extracts of spicy food additives--evaluation and comparison with ascorbic acid in in-vitro systems.* Pharmacology Division, Department of Pharmaceutical Services, Andhra University, Visakhapatnam, Andhra Pradesh 530-003, India. J Herb Pharmacother. 2004;4(2):1-10.

7 Birdane FM, Cemek M, Birdane YO, Gülçin I, Büyükokurolu ME. B*eneficial effects of Foeniculum vulgare on ethanol-induced acute gastric mucosal injury in rats.* Department of Pharmacology, Faculty of Veterinary Medicine, Afyon Kocatepe University, Afyon, Turkey. World J Gastroenterol. 2007 Jan 28;13(4):607-11.

8 Siddaraju MN, Dharmesh SM. *Inhibition of gastric H+, K+-ATPase and Helicobacter pylori growth by phenolic antioxidants of Zingiber officinale.* Department of Biochemistry and Nutrition, Central Food Technological Research Institute, Mysore 570-020, Karnataka, India. Mol Nutr Food Res. 2007 Mar;51(3):324-32.

9 Ivanova D, Gerova D, Chervenkov T, Yankova T. *Polyphenols and antioxidant capacity of Bulgarian medicinal plants.* Department of Pharmacology and Biochemistry, University of Medicine Varna, 55 Marin Drinov Street, 9002 Varna, Bulgaria. J Ethnopharmacol. 2005 Jan 4;96(1-2):145-50.

10 Venkatesan N, Punithavathi D, Babu M. Protection from acute and chronic lung diseases by curcumin. Faculte de Medecine, UMR-7561, CNRS UHP, Vandoeuvre lès Nancy, France. vnar12@yahoo.com Adv Exp Med Biol. 2007;595:379-405.

11 Goel A, Kunnumakkara AB, Aggarwal BB. *Curcumin as "Curecumin": From kitchen to clinic.* Gastrointestinal Cancer Research Laboratory, Department of Internal Medicine, Charles A. Sammons Cancer Center and Baylor Research Institute, Baylor University Medical Center, Dallas, TX, United States. Biochem Pharmacol. 2007 Aug 19.

Eye Disease and Eye Function
Glaucoma

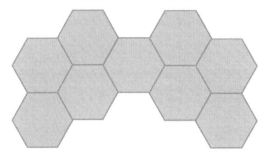

NUMBER OF STUDIES: 9

CHI VALUE: 19

Glaucoma can be classified as a group of eye diseases in which vision can be partially or completely lost, sometimes without warning. Early glaucoma patients may not even be aware of the disease's progress. Ultimately, glaucoma causes the optic nerve leading from the eye to the brain to become damaged, resulting in partial or complete blindness. While other factors may play a role in the disease's development chronic or acute increased intraocular pressure (IOP) is commonly present, allthough some glaucoma patients maintain normal IOP. Normally aqueous humor (fluid inside the eye) flows through channels to maintain eye health and function. In glaucoma patients this fluid becomes blocked.

Allopathic medicine has neither a cure for glaucoma nor the ability to restore lost vision due to glaucoma. Instead, doctors focus on surgery and prescription medications to slow the disease's progression. While glaucoma is commonly observed in the senior population, it may develop at any age.

Statistically, people over 40, those with a family history of glaucoma or vision problems, diabetic patients, and people taking corticosteroid prescription medications are at increased risk for glaucoma. In addition, the following ethnic groups are at increased risk: African-American, Hispanic, Inuit, Irish, Japanese, Russian, and people of Scandinavian descent.

Symptoms may include: loss of peripheral vision, red sclera (white of eye), loss of visual acuity, eye aches, tunnel vision or, in some cases, nausea and vomiting.

To diagnose glaucoma, an ophthalmologist (eye doctor) will test vision and then examine the eyes after administering a medicated eye drop, which dilates the pupil.

CANNABIS AND GLAUCOMA

Cannabis has been part of traditional medicine's treatment of eye disease for millennia. Most historical Materia Medicas include cannabis prescriptions for the treatment of eye problems. Of late, the discovery of ocular cannabinoid receptors has stimulated a new round of ophthalmic cannabinoid research. Potential areas of investigation include the neuroprotective properties of cannabinoids, the stimulation of neural microcirculation, and the suppression of both apoptosis (cell death) and damaging free radical reactions.

Modern scientists showed renewed interest in cannabis in 1971 when it was first noted in scientific literature that smoking marijuana lowered intraocular pressure. In this first study, modern researchers enlisted eleven healthy youths to smoke 2 gm of cannabis with a 0.9% THC content provided by the National Institute for Mental Health. Prior to and one hour following smoking cannabis, complete ocular examinations were performed, and a substantial decrease in intraocular pressure was observed in 9 of 11 subjects.[1]

A 1976 Washington, DC study further examined the impact of THC. It revealed that patients responded to the inhalation of 2.8% THC with an increase in heart rate (when compared to a control group), followed by a substantial drop in blood pressure (both systolic and diastolic), and a drop in intraocular pressure. Scientists also noted that increased heart rate allowed the body to maintain adequate perfusion (cardiac output) while lowering both blood and intraocular pressures in parallel fashion.[2] Risk versus benefit analyses were conducted between 1977 and 1998. These studies concluded that IOP follows a parallel course to that of arterial blood pressure. While some scientists considered an increased heart rate an adverse effect, other researchers considered it a balancing mechanism protecting the patient from the effects of hypotension (low blood pressure).

New insights emerged from an animal study in Louisville, KY (2000). Results indicated that the reduction of IOP is mediated by CB1 cannabinoid receptors in the eye itself, and that the synthetic cannabinoid WIN55212-2 (like natural cannabinoids) can also reduce IOP.[3] Scientists at Oxford followed this work in 2006 with a randomized, double-blind, placebo-controlled, 4-way crossover human study on patients with increased intraocular pressure (ocular hypertension). Subjects either received a single dose of 5 mg Delta-9-THC, 20 mg CBD, 40 mg CBD, or a placebo. The authors wrote: "A single 5 mg sublingual dose of Delta-9-THC reduced the IOP temporarily and was well tolerated by most patients. Sublingual administration of 20 mg CBD did not reduce IOP, whereas 40 mg CBD produced a transient increase IOP rise."[4] The apparent differing effects of isolated cannabinoids may point to the complex yet synergistic mechanisms by which these cannabinoids naturally combine to achieve therapeutic effects.

Recently, in Aachen, Germany, scientists gave THC in the form of marinol to healthy physicians to test its impact on blood circulation of the eye, as well as its effect on intraocular pressure (IOP). Two hours after ingestion, the drug reduced IOP and retinal arteriovenous passage time. The authors concluded that this effect may be beneficial in ocular circulatory disorders, including glaucoma.[5]

STUDY SUMMARY:

Drugs	Study Subjects	Published Year, Place, and Key Results	CHI
THC as Marinol (7.5mg)	8 healthy physicians	2007 – RWTH Aachen University, Department of Ophthalmology, Aachen, Germany. THC reduced intraocular pressure and improved blood circulation of the eye.[6]	4
Single daily dose of either 5 mg Delta-9-THC, 20 mg CBD, 40 mg CBD, or placebo	6 patients with increased intraocular pressure	2006 – Department of Ophthalmology, Aberdeen Royal Infirmary, School of Medical Sciences, Institute of Medical Sciences, University of Aberdeen, UK. Dose specific therapeutic effect (5mg THC by mouth).[7]	5

Drugs	Study Subjects	Published Year, Place, and Key Results	CHI
Synthetic cannabinoid WIN55212-2	Animal study (rabbits)	2000 – Department of Pharmacology and Toxicology, University of Louisville School of Medicine, Louisville, US. WIN55212-2 also reduces intraocular pressure an IOP reduction is mediated by CB1 cannabinoid receptors in the eye.[8]	1
Smoked cannabis v. cannabinoids	Discussion/analysis	1998 – Department of Ophthalmology, Medical College of Georgia, Augusta, US. Benefits do not outweigh adverse effects.[9]	0
Topical solution of 0.05% and 0.1% THC in light mineral oil	6 glaucoma patients	1981 -Smoked THC lowers occular and systolic pressur. Topical treatment ineffective.[10]	3
Smoked cannabis	18 glaucoma patients	1980 - Increased heart rate, decreased blood pressure and IOP with side effects.[11]	0
2.8% THC inhalation	Human clinical trial	1979 – Glaucoma Clinic at Howard University Hospital, Washington, D.C. Reduction in blood pressure, intraocular pressure while maintaining adequate perfusion.[12]	3
THC intravenously. Two strengths were used--0.022 mg/ kg of body weight and 0.044 mg/kg of body weight.	10 people with normal IOP	1977 - Increased heart rate (22% to 65%), decreased IOP (average 37%).[13]	0
2 gm inhaled cannabis (THC 0.9%)	A group of 11 healthy youthful subjects	1971 – Substantial decrease in intraocular pressure observed in a large percentage of subjects.[14]	3

Total CHI Value **19**

STRAIN SPECIFIC CONSIDERATIONS

The majority of clinical studies have examined the impact of cannabinoids, primarily in the form of THC, on glaucoma. THC binds relatively equally with both CB1 and CB2. Both sativas and indicas contain CB1 and CB2 binding cannabinoids.

EXPLORING MIND–BODY CONSCIOUSNESS

A Yale University School of Medicine study conducted on seven glaucoma patients and a healthy control group concluded that hypnosis could be an important tool in reducing objective and subjective symptoms of glaucoma. All patients showed a significant reduction in intraocular pressure. Subjective improvements were reported as follows: fewer headaches, less tearing, feeling generally more relaxed, and sleeping better. The authors suggested also that: "these findings serve to emphasize the significant role of the emotions in glaucoma, although the mechanisms involved remain obscure."[15]

In glaucoma, the fluid of the eye is under too much pressure with no release in sight.

THE POWER OF QUESTIONS

What tears have I refused to shed?
What past hurt is still in need of healing?

What am I refusing to release?
Where can I apply forgiveness to bring about release?

AGGRAVATING FACTORS

Emotional pressure building up over long periods of time.

HEALING FACTORS

Forgiving oneself for the iron-willed determination to hold on to emotional baggage.

TAKE NOTICE

Consider TAKE NOTICE section in chapter on HYPERTENSION and ARMD.

1 Hepler RS, Frank IR. *Marihuana smoking and intraocular pressure.* Journal of the American Medical Association 1971;217(10):1392.

2 Crawford WJ, Merritt JC. *Effects of tetrahydrocannabinol on arterial and intraocular hypertension.* Glaucoma Clinic at Howard University Hospital, Washington, DC. Int J Clin Pharmacol Biopharm. 1979 May;17(5):191-6.

3 Song ZH, Slowey CA. *Involvement of cannabinoid receptors in the intraocular pressure-lowering effects of WIN55212-2.* Department of Pharmacology and Toxicology, University of Louisville School of Medicine, Louisville, KY 40292, USA. zhsong@louisville.edu J Pharmacol Exp Ther. 2000 Jan;292(1):136-9.

4 Tomida I, Azuara-Blanco A, House H, Flint M, Pertwee RG, Robson PJ. *Effect of Sublingual Application of Cannabinoids on Intraocular Pressure: A Pilot Study.* Department of Ophthalmology, Aberdeen Royal Infirmary, School of Medical Sciences, Institute of Medical Sciences, University of Aberdeen, UK, Cannabinoid Research Institute, Magdalen Centre, Oxford Science Park, Oxford OX4 4GA. J Glaucoma 2006 15(5):349-353.

5 Plange N, Arend KO, Kaup M, Doehmen B, Adams H, Hendricks S, Cordes A, Huth J, Sponsel WE, Remky A. *Dronabinol and retinal hemodynamics in humans.* Department of Ophthalmology, RWTH Aachen University, Pauwelstrasse 30, 52057 Aachen, Germany. nplange@ukaachen.de Am J Ophthalmol. 2007 Jan;143(1):173-4.

6 Plange N, Arend KO, Kaup M, Doehmen B, Adams H, Hendricks S, Cordes A, Huth J, Sponsel WE, Remky A. *Dronabinol and retinal hemodynamics in humans.* Department of Ophthalmology, RWTH Aachen University, Pauwelstrasse 30, 52057 Aachen, Germany. nplange@ukaachen.de Am J Ophthalmol. 2007 Jan;143(1):173-4.

7 Tomida I, Azuara-Blanco A, House H, Flint M, Pertwee RG, Robson PJ. *Effect of Sublingual Application of Cannabinoids on Intraocular Pressure: A Pilot Study.* Department of Ophthalmology, Aberdeen Royal Infirmary, School of Medical Sciences, Institute of Medical Sciences, University of Aberdeen, UK, Cannabinoid Research Institute, Magdalen Centre, Oxford Science Park, Oxford OX4 4GA. J Glaucoma 2006 15(5):349-353.

8 Song ZH, Slowey CA. *Involvement of cannabinoid receptors in the intraocular pressure-lowering effects of WIN55212-2.* Department of Pharmacology and Toxicology, University of Louisville School of Medicine, Louisville, KY 40292, USA. zhsong@louisville.edu J Pharmacol Exp Ther. 2000 Jan;292(1):136-9.

9 Green K. *Marijuana smoking vs cannabinoids for glaucoma therapy.* Department of Ophthalmology, Medical College of Georgia, Augusta, USA. kgreen@mail.mcg.edu Arch Ophthalmol. 1998 Nov;116(11):1433-7.

10 Merritt JC, Perry DD, Russell DN, Jones BF. Topical delta 9-tetrahydrocannabinol and aqueous dynamics in glaucoma. J Clin Pharmacol. 1981 Aug-Sep;21(8-9 Suppl):467S-471S.

11 Merritt JC, Crawford WJ, Alexander PC, Anduze AL, Gelbart SS. *Effect of marihuana on intraocular and blood pressure in glaucoma.* Ophthalmology 1980;87(3):222-8.

12 Crawford WJ, Merritt JC. *Effects of tetrahydrocannabinol on arterial and intraocular hypertension.* Glaucoma Clinic at Howard University Hospital, Washington, DC. Int J Clin Pharmacol Biopharm. 1979 May;17(5):191-6.

13 Cooler P, Gregg JM. *Effect of delta-9-tetrahydrocannabinol on intraocular pressure in humans.* South Med J. 1977 Aug;70(8):951-4.

14 Hepler RS, Frank IR. *Marihuana smoking and intraocular pressure.* Journal of the American Medical Association 1971;217(10):1392.

15 ALLAN S. BERGER M.D.1 and PAUL J. SIMEL M.D.1 *Effect of Hypnosis on Intraocular Pressure in Normal and Glaucomatous Subjects.* 1 Department of Psychiatry, Yale University School of Medicine, and the Department of Surgery, Section of Ophthalmology, Grace-New Haven Community Hospital, New Haven, Conn. Psychosomatic Medicine 20:321-327 (1958).

Eye Disease and Eye Function
Improved Night Vision

NUMBER OF STUDIES: 1

CHI VALUE: 3

A team of international researchers from the United States, Spain and Morocco "… have documented (2004) an improvement in night vision among Jamaican fishermen after ingestion of a crude tincture of herbal cannabis, while two members of this group noted that Moroccan fishermen and mountain dwellers observe an analogous improvement after smoking kif, sifted Cannabis sativa mixed with tobacco (Nicotiana rustica)." To field test these anecdotal reports researchers devised a placebo-controlled double-blind trial using volunteers. Volunteers were given either placebo or oral THC in the form of marinol or smoking kif. Improvements in night vision were noted after the ingestion of THC and after the smoking of kif. The authors write: "It is believed that this effect is dose-dependent and cannabinoid-mediated at the retinal level. Further testing may assess possible clinical application of these results in retinitis pigmentosa or other conditions."[1]

STUDY SUMMARY:

Drugs	Study Subjects	Published Year, Place, and Key Results	CHI
Marinol (THC) 20mg and smoked kif	4 healthy subjects	2004 – International research team. Improved night vision	3

Total CHI Value   3

1 E. B. Russo, , a, A. Merzoukib, c, J. Molero Mesab, K. A. Freyd and P. J. Bach.e *Cannabis improves night vision: a case study of dark adaptometry and scotopic sensitivity in kif smokers of the Rif mountains of northern Morocco.* a 2235 Wylie Avenue, Missoula, MT 59802, USA. b Department of Botany, Faculty of Pharmacy, University of Granada, Granada 18071, Spain. c Laboratory of Ethnobotany, Faculty of Sciences, University Abdelmalek Essaadi, Tétouan, Morocco. d Montana State University School of Nursing, 236 Corbin Hall, University of Montana, Missoula, MT 59812, USA. e Montana Neurobehavioral Specialists, 900 North Orange St., Missoula, MT 59802, USA. J Ethnopharmacol. 2004 Jul;93(1):99-104.

Fever/Temperature Regulation
Fever

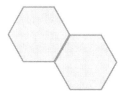

NUMBER OF STUDIES: 2

CHI VALUE: 4

The body's temperature changes all the time. Things like clothing, exertion and exercise, environmental conditions, and hormonal changes (for example, during menstruation) can all affect the body's temperature.

A normal body temperature is generally considered about 37C° or 98.5F°; a mild fever between 99F° to 101F°; and a high fever above 103F°. Body temperatures above 42C°/108F° are potentially fatal.

The body's immune system induces fever in an attempt to rid itself of an invader. This invader could be as simple as a cold virus or as exotic as a malarial parasite. The body's rise in temperature is designed to destroy much of these invading armies of microbes while simultaneously recruiting production of the body's police force, the white blood cells. Therefore, fever is actually a good thing when it remains low and lasts only for a short time.

Most fevers tend to lessen in a day or two. If you have a fever for more than two days or higher than 101 degrees, consult a physician to find the underlying causes and to discuss an appropriate treatment plan. Remember, mild short fever can help in healing the body, but high fevers, especially long-term high fevers, can kill.

WARNING

Aspirin is a common medication people use quite effectively to treat minor pains and fevers. Salicin, the active ingredient in aspirin, was originally isolated from willow bark but is now produced synthetically. Long ago, willow bark was used as effectively and in the same way that we use aspirin today.

However, use caution when considering aspirin for young children and young adults (younger than 19 years). It is recommended to never give a child or adolescent aspirin or other medication containing salicin if they may have a viral infection such as a cold, flu, or other common childhood disease like chickenpox together with a fever. Why? Under those conditions salicin can be fatal to a child/young adult. It is called Reye's Syndrome.

REYE'S SYNDROME

While the exact cause of Reye's Syndrome remains unknown, it has been noted that a very high percentage of youngsters who develop the condition previously had taken aspirin (or other medications containing salicin) during a viral infection. Reye's syndrome is a potentially deadly condition which affects the liver and the brain. Those who survive Reye's syndrome are often left physically and mentally handicapped.

Signs and symptoms of Reye's syndrome include: nausea and vomiting, increased generalized weakness, bizarre behavior, altered mental status, acting as if drunk, loss of consciousness, and seizures.

Western medicine has no cure. Treatment is usually performed in intensive care units, and is focused primarily on reducing swelling of the brain, or preventing liver damage or a score of other potentially severe complications.

FEBRILE SEIZURES

A seizure may occur while a child of three months to four years has a fever.

The precise reasons for febrile seizures are not known. One hypothesis: When a child is born, the brain is not finished growing. During the subsequent months and even years, the brain and nervous system continue to expand and develop. However, the part of the brain responsible for temperature regulation in the body sometimes develops at a slower pace. Therefore, it is argued that during times of fever, an 'overload' to the neurological system occurs producing a seizure. Once the temperature regulating part of the brain is fully developed, seizures during fevers cease.

What should you do when you have a child between three months and five years who suddenly has a seizure? Put the child on a bed or clean flat surface. Roll the child onto his side so as to avoid any mucus (spit) or vomit from entering the lungs. Protect the child from hitting his head against the floor or other standing objects. Have someone call 911 immediately. In most places in the US, a paramedic should arrive within a few minutes. Most febrile seizures will stop by themselves in a few seconds or a few minutes.

An emergency room definition for status epilepticus (SE) is continuous seizure activity lasting longer than 5 minutes or multiple seizures without regaining consciousness between seizures. This is considered a true emergency. SE is a potentially life-threatening condition in which the brain and by extension the entire nervous system enter into excessive nerve cell activity.

CANNABIS AND SEIZURES

To date, two studies exist examining the potential properties of cannabinoids relevant to fever genesis and pediatric fever-induced seizures. In 2006, Philadelphia scientists attempted to induce fevers by injecting rats with lipopolysaccharide, a component of the outer membrane of Gram-negative bacteria. Results showed that: "…cannabinoids interact with systemic bacterial lipopolysaccharide injections and indicate a role of the CB1 receptor subtype in the pathogenesis of lipopolysaccharide fever."[1]

A 2007 study in Fukuoka, Japan, concluded that the endocannabinoid system, especially CB1, may regulate body temperature, independent of the hypothalamus previously assumed to be solely responsible for body temperature regulation.[2]

See also NEUROLOGICAL DISEASES – EPILEPTIC SEIZURES

STUDY SUMMARY:

Drugs	Study Subjects	Published Year, Place, and Key Results	CHI
THC and cannabidiol	Animal study (mice)	2007 – Department of Neuropharmacology, Faculty of Pharmaceutical Sciences, Fukuoka University, Fukuoka, Japan. Increased CB1 receptors in striatum and cortex, but not in hypothalamus. Indicate CB1 may play a role in fever.	2
WIN 55,212-2	Animal study (rats)	2006 – Multi-institutional research team. CB1 may play a role in fever.	2

Total CHI Value   4

STRAIN SPECIFIC CONSIDERATIONS

THC binds with CB1 and CB2 relatively equally. CBD and WIN 55212-2 have a higher affinity to CB2.

Sativas or sativa dominant strains tend to present with a higher THC:CBD ratio.

EXPLORING MIND–BODY CONSCIOUSNESS

The body commonly responds to an invasion of pathogens with a fever to 'boil off' pathogens. In cases of a mild invasion, a low-grade fever will suffice to regain health and well-being. If the threat is more serious, the body will try to meet the challenge by raising the temperature and extending the length of the fever.

However, in some cases a high fever may begin to depress the level of consciousness of the patient, produce hallucinations, seizures, loss of consciousness, and sometimes results in death.

It is as if a door to the unconscious has opened and unleashed a series of uncontrollable experiences. For more information go to the chapter on NEUROLOGICAL DISEASES – EPILEPTIC SEIZURES or the chapter on CANCER – CANCER INDUCED NIGHTSWEATS.

1 Khalid Benamar, Menachem Yondorf, Joseph J. Meissler, Ellen B. Geller, Ronald J. Tallarida, Toby K. Eisenstein and Martin W. Adler. *A Novel Role of Cannabinoids: Implication in the Fever Induced by Bacterial Lipopolysaccharide.* Center for Substance Abuse Research (K.B., M.Y., E.B.G., M.W.A.) and Departments of Microbiology and Immunology (J.J.M., T.K.E.) and Pharmacology (R.J.T.), Temple University School of Medicine, Philadelphia, Pennsylvania. JPET March 2007 vol. 320 no. 3 1127-1133

2 Hayakawa K, Mishima K, Nozako M, Hazekawa M, Ogata A, Fujioka M, Harada K, Mishima S, Orito K, Egashira N, Iwasaki K, Fujiwara M. *Delta9-tetrahydrocannabinol (Delta9-THC) prevents cerebral infarction via hypothalamic-independent hypothermia.* Department of Neuropharmacology, Faculty of Pharmaceutical Sciences, Fukuoka University, Nanakuma 8-19-1, Fukuoka City, Fukuoka, Japan. Life Sci 2007 Mar 27; 80(16):1466-71.

Fibromyalgia

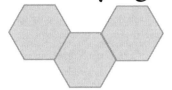

NUMBER OF STUDIES: 3

CHI VALUE: 14

Fibromyalgia, an illness characterized by chronic pain combined with some form of psychiatric diagnosis, remains absent of an observable underlying pathology. The disease picture of fibromyalgia usually includes widespread chronic pains in muscles and connective tissue, joint stiffness, general weakness, exhaustion, depression, anxiety and insomnia. "Nearly 2 percent of the general population in the United States suffers from fibromyalgia, the majority of them being middle-aged females."[1]

No specific test exists to determine an exact diagnosis. Symptoms are often similar to those of rheumatism, osteoporosis or arthritis. Physicians try to diagnose by process of elimination. Diagnostic criteria established by the American College of Rheumatology list the following criteria: 1. A history of diffused and chronic pains for more than three months and present in all four quadrants of the body. 2. The presence of pain in at least 11 of 18 specific trigger points.

Orthodox pharmaceutical treatment includes muscle relaxants, pain medication (opiods), anti-depressants, anti-seizure medication, dopamine agonists, and cannabinoids.

CANNABIS AND FIBROMYALGIA

In 2007, researchers in Winnipeg, Canada, enrolled 40 fibromyalgia patients to measure the effects of nabilone, a synthetic cannabinoid, on pain and quality of life. The results of this randomized, double-blind, placebo-controlled trial showed that: "Nabilone appears to be a beneficial, well-tolerated treatment option for fibromyalgia patients, with significant benefits in pain relief and functional improvement."[2]

While most studies have focused on using cannabis for the treatment of fibromyalgia pains, another randomized, double-blind, placebo-controlled, crossover clinical trial from Montreal, Cananda (2008) examined the effects of this

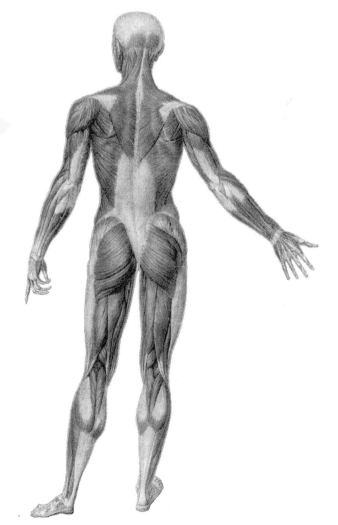

synthetic cannabinoid on insomnia. Twenty-nine patients with the disease completed a course in which they either received nabilone or the tricyclic antidepressant amitriptyline, commonly prescribed for insomnia with fibromyalgia. Each patient received a course of nabilone (0.5-1.0 mg before bedtime) or amitriptyline (10-20 mg before bedtime) for a period of two weeks with a two-week period of no medication in between. The results showed that while both medications significantly improved people's sleep, nabilone was superior.[3]

In 2009, Scientists from Worcester, Massachusetts conducted a meta-analysis of recent and relevant studies and found that "...all classes of cannabinoids, including the endogenous cannabinoid such as anandamide, related compounds such as the elmiric acids (EMAs), and noncannabinoid components (200-250 constituents) of cannabis show anti-inflammatory action."[4] The analysis demonstrated that all types of cannabinoids as well as noncannabinoid parts of the plant are effective in reducing pain from inflammation as in post-surgery patients, rheumatism, rheumatoid arthritis, chronic neuropathic pain and fibromyalgia.

STUDY SUMMARY:

Drugs	Type of Study	Published Year, Place, and Key Results	CHI
All types of cannabinoids (endogeneous, plant-based and synthetic)	Meta-analysis (2004-2009)	2009 – University of Massachusetts Medical School - Cannabinoids effective in pain from post-surgery patients, rheumatism, rheumatoid arthritis, chronic neuropathic pain and fibromyalgia.	4
Synthetic cannabinoid nabilone 0.5-1.0mg at night	29 patients with fibromyalgia	2008 – Pain Clinic, McGill University Health Centre, Montreal, Quebec, Canada - Improved sleep.	5
Synthetic cannabinoid nabilone 2mg orally	40 patients with fibromyalgia	2007 – Section of Physical Medicine and Rehabilitation, University of Manitoba, Rehabilitation Hospital, Health Sciences Centre, Winnipeg, Manitoba, Canada - Significant reduction of pain and improvement of quality of life.	5

Total CHI Value   14

STRAIN SPECIFIC CONSIDERATIONS

Two of the studies reviewed used primarily the synthetic cannabinoid nabilone (similar to THC), which binds relatively equally to CB1 and CB2.

Both sativa and indica strains contain cannabinoids that activate CB1 and CB2. However, sativas or sativa-heavy strains tend to produce higher THC:CBD ratios than indica strains.

EXPLORING MIND–BODY CONSCIOUSNESS

While examining the differences of fibromyalgia patients and healthy people using functional brain imaging studies, neurotransmitter studies, and brain anatomy studies, researchers discovered "...that fibromyalgia patients have alterations in central nervous system (CNS) anatomy, physiology, and chemistry that potentially contribute to the symptoms experienced by these patients."[5] Furthermore, the authors of these studies write: "The frequent comorbidity of fibromyalgia with stress-related disorders, such as chronic fatigue, post-traumatic stress disorder, irritable bowel syndrome, and depression, as well as the similarity of many CNS abnormalities, suggests at least a partial common substrate for these disorders." The authors further conclude: "Despite the numerous cerebral alterations, fibromyalgia might not be a primary disorder of the brain but may be a consequence of early life stress or prolonged or severe stress, affecting brain modulatory circuitry of pain and emotions in genetically susceptible individuals."

Arizona researchers studying fibromyalgia patients discovered that low positive affect, especially during stressful weeks, was a key component in fibromyalgia. This insight provided a new direction away from the commonly held notion that negative affect was a significant factor. Interventions that focus on improving positive affective resources, especially during times of stress, could thus provide a more positive therapeutic experience.[6]

Research also revealed that fibromyalgia patients experienced improved psychological well-being and a reduction in pain and fatigue through emotional expression of personal traumatic experiences simply by writing about them for 20 minutes, three times a week.[7]

Another study conducted by researchers from the University of Washington concluded that: "Fibromyalgia seems to be associated with increased risk of victimization, particularly adult physical abuse. Sexual, physical, and emotional trauma may be important factors in the development and maintenance of this disorder and its associated disability in many patients."[8]

AGGRAVATING FACTORS

Early life stress / prolonged severe stress / low levels of positive emotions (affect) especially during times of stress / increased risk of victimization / particularly adult physical abuse / sexual, physical, and emotional trauma.

HEALING FACTORS

Expressing personal traumatic experiences increases positive affect during times of stress.

QUESTIONS

Why does it hurt to move in life?
What age-old pains are still stressing me?
What does the pain remind me of?
What purposes do my aches and pains serve?
How do I release pain?
Are there other ways to release pain?
What is keeping me from reaching my potential?
Can I employ forgiveness?

TAKE NOTICE

TAI CHI

Researchers conducted a single-blind, randomized trial of classic Yang-style tai chi comparing stretching exercises to wellness education as put forth by the American College of Rheumatology 1990 criteria. Results showed that of the 66 enrolled patients with fibromyalgia those 33 who were included in the tai chi group showed measurable clinical improvement and a general increase in quality of life. The investigators of the study noticed that the benefits of tai chi were still present after six months and no adverse effects were observed.[9] So it would appear with a little effort and gentle daily practice symptoms will diminish and life will improve with no worries about side effects.

1 Chakrabarty S, Zoorob R. *Fibromyalgia*. Department of Family and Community Medicine, Meharry Medical College, Nashville, TN 37208, USA. schakrabarty@mmc.edu Am Fam Physician. 2007 Jul 15;76(2):247-54.

2 Skrabek RQ, Galimova L, Ethansand Daryl K. *Nabilone for the treatment of pain in fibromyalgia*. Section of Physical Medicine and Rehabilitation, University of Manitoba, Rehabilitation Hospital, Health Sciences Centre, Winnipeg, Manitoba, Canada, rskrabek@hotmail.com 31: J Pain. 2007 Oct 30.

3 Ware MA, Fitzcharles MA, Joseph L, Shir Y. *The Effects of Nabilone on Sleep in Fibromyalgia: Results of a Randomized Controlled Trial*. Pain Clinic, McGill University Health Centre, Montreal, Quebec, Canada. mark.ware@muhc.mcgill.c Anesth Analg, 2010.

4 Sumner H. Burstein1,2 and Robert B. Zurier2. *Cannabinoids, Endocannabinoids, and Related Analogs in Inflammation*. 1Department of Biochemistry & Molecular Pharmacology, University of Massachusetts Medical School, 364 Plantation St., Worcester, Massachusetts 01605 USA. 2Department of Medicine, University of Massachusetts Medical School, 364 Plantation St., Worcester, Massachusetts 01605 USA. AAPS J. 2009 March; 11(1): 109–119.

5 Schweinhardt P, Sauro KM, Bushnell MC. *Fibromyalgia: a disorder of the brain?* Alan Edwards Centre for Research on Pain, Faculty of Dentistry, McGill University, Canada. Neuroscientist. 2008 Oct;14(5):415-21.

6 Alex J. Zautra, PhD, Robert Fasman, MA, John W. Reich, PhD, Peter Harakas, MSc, Lisa M. Johnson, MA, Maureen E. Olmsted, PhD and Mary C. Davis, PhD. *Fibromyalgia: Evidence for Deficits in Positive Affect Regulation*. Department of Psychology, Arizona State University, Tempe, Arizona. Psychosomatic Medicine 67:147-155 (2005).

7 Joan E. Broderick, PhD, Doerte U. Junghaenel, MA and Joseph E. Schwartz, PhD. *Written Emotional Expression Produces Health Benefits in Fibromyalgia Patients*. Department of Psychiatry and Behavioral Sciences, Stony Brook University, Stony Brook, NY (J.E.B., J.E.S.); and the Department of Psychology, Stony Brook University, Stony Brook, NY (D.U.J.). Psychosomatic Medicine 67:326-334 (2005).

8 EA Walker, D Keegan, G Gardner, M Sullivan, D Bernstein and WJ Katon. Psychosocial factors in fibromyalgia compared with rheumatoid arthritis: II. Sexual, physical, and emotional abuse and neglect. Department of Psychiatry and Behavioral Sciences, University of Washington, Seattle 98195, USA. Psychosomatic Medicine, Vol 59, Issue 6 572-577, Copyright © 1997.

9 Chenchen Wang, M.D., M.P.H., Christopher H. Schmid, Ph.D., Ramel Rones, B.S., Robert Kalish, M.D., Janeth Yinh, M.D., Don L. Goldenberg, M.D., Yoojin Lee, M.S. and Timothy McAlindon, M.D., M.P.H. *A Randomized Trial of Tai Chi for Fibromyalgia*. Division of Rheumatology (C.W., R.K., J.Y., T.M.) and the Institute for Clinical Research and Health Policy Studies (C.H.S., Y.L.), Tufts Medical Center, Tufts University School of Medicine; and Mind–Body Therapies (R.R.) — both in Boston; and Newton–Wellesley Hospital, Newton, MA (D.L.G.). N Engl J Med 2010; 363:743-75

Hemorrhoids

NO MODERN CANNABIS STUDIES AVAILABLE

The structures of the anus contain channels or hemorrhoids, which are comprised of connective tissue filled with small arterial and venous blood vessels that function to make the passing of stool easier. Only when they become inflamed, swollen or begin to bleed are they cause for concern. In the western world, about half of the population has had some form of symptomatic hemorrhoidal issue. Symptoms include: itching, pain, bleeding, external and internal protrusion of hemorrhoids, minor anal leakage and painful bowel movements.

Hemorrhoidal swelling and inflammation occurs after pressure in the anal region through pregnancy, chronic constipation or diarrhea, long periods of sitting in the same position, or severe straining during bowel movements.

Allopathic medicine uses pharmaceutical and surgical procedures in the treatment of hemorrhoids. Medicated creams, oils, ointments, and suppositories aim to relieve pain, inflammation, or itching and to produce easier elimination. Minor procedures include rubber band ligation, injections or coagulation using a laser. Surgical procedures include stapling and hemorrhoidectomies.

CANNABIS AND HEMORRHOIDS

In 1845, European historical medical literature described hemp leaf oil as effective at reducing inflammation and managing neuralgic pains in cases of hemorrhoids.[1] A paste of cannabis leaves was reportedly used for treatment in India.[2] More than a century later (1972), the Canadian Government issued a report on its examination of the medical use of cannabis as past treatment for hemorrhoids.[3]

Case reports from patients suffering from hemorrhoids suggest potential benefits of cannabis-infused oils such as hemp or almond oil in the care of inflamed hemorrhoidal tissues. The lubricating and tissue-soothing properties of basic food-grade hemp oil infused with cannabis flowers potentially combines anti-inflammatory, antiseptic and analgesic properties.

EXPLORING MIND–BODY CONSCIOUSNESS

Grace and Graham write: "Constipation occurs when an individual was grimly determined to carry on even though faced with a problem he could not solve." Typical statements were (17 patients with constipation): "I have to keep on with this, but I know I'm not going to like it." "It's a lousy job but it's the best I can do." "This marriage is never going to get any better but I won't quit." "I'll have to keep on with this but I'm not going to like it." "I'll stick with it even though nothing good will come of it."[4] The authors concluded: "Constipation is a phenomenon of holding on without change." This corresponds to the patients' attitude of trying to continue with things as they are, without hope of immediate improvement despite definite desire to do something different.

One of the main functions of the colon is to retrieve water from chyme (waste). The element water is commonly associated with feelings and emotions. The dryer the stool, the harder it is to release. Chronic or acute constipation often result in inflamed and protruding hemorrhoids. Dry paper worsens inflammation and moist towelettes ease the pain. While holding onto every bit of water may be the body's signal of dehydration, for some it may also mirror a psychological structure indicative of a lack of emotional ownership. Others have described it as being stingy with one's feeling or emotional release. Hemorrhoids may also represent fear of letting go or the fear of getting hurt when letting go.

Emotionally speaking, constant irritation, inflammation and associated pains may be messages to pay attention throughout the day and relax rectal sphincter muscles. Until the pain sets in, many hemorrhoid sufferers are simply unaware that they carry a lot of tension in the form of anxiety (often undefined fears or aggression) in the rectal region, thus contributing to constant strain of the tissue affected. Becoming more conscious of the tension and choosing instead to gently relax the region can bring relief.

QUESTIONS

Do I hold tension in my buttocks or rectum?
What is the feeling or emotion associated with the tension?
Can I gently release these feelings?
Can I choose to relax the region whenever I become aware of tension?
Where do I believe I have to hold back on feeling?
Do I have to ration my emotions?
Why does it hurt to let go?
Why is it a struggle to let go?
Do I believe that it hurts to let go?

AGGRAVATING FACTORS

Holding on to something we don't like, while lacking desire or ability to change it; fear of letting go or the fear of getting hurt when letting go / chronic irritation or inflamed thinking around the topics of safety and security.

HEALING FACTORS

Emotional release work that gently addresses issues around safety and security / think of impossible, as: I am possible.

ANECDOTE

Johnny used to have hemorrhoid flare-ups with different intensities. Sometimes it was just a painless bleed after a bowel movement. Other times his hemorrhoids were excruciatingly painful while bearing down. In such cases the pain would last for hours. He tried the usual herbal and pharmaceuticals to ease his pain and discomfort without much success. After a bit of research on the adverse effects of a surgical procedure, Johnny opted against it.

He tried cannabis oil topically before and after a bowel movement. This provided significant relief by reducing the inflammation and the time it took to feel better after strain-induced flare-ups. However, while the oil reduced symptoms, his hemorrhoidal condition remained a chronic issue until he began noticing the same emotional state every time he decided to go to the bathroom.

Johnny used some of the oil internally and allowed his emotions to come to the forefront of his awareness. He felt anxious, dreading a bowel movement, anticipating the struggle and the burning pains. He allowed the feeling to take him deeper and noticed that he was feeling the same way about his financial situation.

Johnny bought whatever he wanted in the moment, even if it meant falling deeper into credit card debt. For years he spent today, not thinking about tomorrow. Soon he was in over his head, and used one credit card to pay the monthly debt on another. He was late more and more often. He dreaded the debt collector's calls, feeling anxious with each ring of the telephone. He realized his poor financial choices and poor dietary choices led to the same emotional states.

Johnny started to make better food choices, taking into account the delayed effect of his food choices. However, while drinking more water and eating more fiber helped to ease his symptoms, his hemorrhoids did not cease to be an issue until he began making serious changes in his financial life as well.

He designed a budget and stuck to it. He stopped using his cards and began the process of digging himself out of debt. He made purchasing choices with tomorrow in mind. And it was here that Johnny noticed his anxieties had lifted and his hemorrhoids stopped being an issue for him.

For Johnny, the message of the hemorrhoids was to start caring more for himself by considering the long-term emotional impact of his financial and dietary choices. Once he understood the message of the disease and answered it, his hemorrhoids ceased to be an issue at all.

TAKE NOTICE

ACACIA • CLOVE • GARLIC

ACACIA: Acacia improves stool consistency and reduces the occurrence of fecal incontinence in adults.[5] Some alternative practitioners in the U.S. have begun to use this highly soluble fiber to ease symptoms of irritable bowel syndrome (IBS). Further studies are under way to determine the mechanism whereby acacia appears to reduce sugar-induced weight gain.

CLOVE: Patients suffering from chronic anal fissures were given a clove oil 1% cream preparation. Healing occurred in five times as many patients as in the control group. The 1% clove cream patients also had a greater reduction in resting anal pressure than those in the control group.[6]

GARLIC: One of Cuba's most versatile herbs, garlic is used for the treatment of asthma to bring up phlegm, to prevent and treat infections caused by bacteria, and to decrease water retention, spasms and thrombophlebitis. Used to treat fungal infections, garlic also works as a tonic, promotes healthy veins, and prevents parasites, inflammation, hemorrhoids, bacterial infections, viral infections, hypertension, muscular pains, back pains, synovitis (inflammation of a membrane in the knee joint) and varicose veins.[7]

HEMORRHOIDS MAY DEMAND NEW EATING HABITS

Animal products contain no fiber while all vegetable matter is essentially fiber, soluble or non-soluble. Consider leaning more and more toward a vegan diet.

Increase water intake. If the body does not receive enough water it will take its needed portions from chyme, causing harder stool, forcing us to struggle with elimination.

Stop using dry tissue paper. Instead, use moist towelettes without any irritating additives, or simply use water to clean the rectum (bidet or shower). Use cold water to ease the inflammation and burning sensation. Use a topical astringent (which contracts swollen tissue) such as witch hazel. Use continuous proper hygiene.

In cases of constipation, use a bulb syringe filled with warm organic coconut oil to lubricate the anal passage. This allows for easy stool passage and reduces strain.

Avoid long periods of sitting. Get the body moving frequently.

After each cleansing, use a couple of drops of cannabis-infused hemp or coconut oil to keep the area slightly lubricated.

Rapid eating and poor food choices ought to be replaced by relaxed eating and a healthy diet with plenty of fiber. Relax your bottom when eating. Try to check for aggression and anxieties before eating. If they are present, try to let it be OK that they are there, or relax in spite of them.

1 M. Donovan. *On the physical and medicinal qualities of Indian hemp (Cannabis Indica); with observations on the best mode of administration, and cases illustrative of its powers.* Dublin Journal of Medical Science (1836-1845), Vol. 26, No. 3. (1 January 1845), pp. 368-402.

2 Shah, N.C. & Joshi, *An ethnobotanical study of the Kumaon region of India.* M.G. 1971. Economic Botany VoL 25(4):414-422.

3 Canadian Government Commission of Inquiry into the Non-Medical Use of Drugs. 2.Cannabis and Its Effects. Medical Use. Published by Information Canada, Ottawa, Canada, 1972.

4 William J. Grace, M.D. and David T. Graham, M.D. *Relationship of Specific Attitudes and Emotions to Certain Bodily Diseases.* Dept. of Medicine, of the New York Hospital-Cornell Medical Center. Psychosomatic Medicine July 1, 1952 vol. 14 no. 4 243-251.

5 Bliss DZ, Jung HJ, Savik K, Lowry A, LeMoine M, Jensen L, Werner C, Schaffer K. *Supplementation with dietary fiber improves fecal incontinence.* School of Nursing, University of Minnesota, Minneapolis 55455, USA. Nurs Res. 2001 Jul-Aug;50(4):203-13.

6 Elwakeel HA, Moneim HA, Farid M, Gohar AA. *Clove oil cream: a new effective treatment for chronic anal fissure.* Mansoura Faculty of Medicine, Surgery, Mansoura University Hospital, Mansoura, Dakahlia, Egypt. Colorectal Dis. 2007 Jul;9(6):549-52.

7 *Therapeutic Guide to Plant Pharmaceuticals and Honey Pharmaceuticals (Guia Terapeutica Dispensarial de Fitofarmacos y Apifarmacos* - Ministerio de Salud Publica, Ciudad de La Habana - Republica de Cuba 1992). Cuban Ministry of Public Health, Havana.

Inflammatory Diseases
Inflammation (in General)

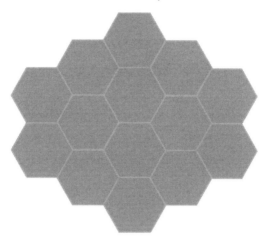

COMBINED NUMBER OF STUDIES: 14

COMBINED CHI VALUE   40

Inflamed tissue is a natural and necessary response of the healing process. Without inflammation, injuries would not heal. Inflammation occurs in response to the invasion of an organism, exposure to a toxin or to the presence of impaired or injured cells. The inflammatory response is a general intervention and not a specific intervention such as in the production of antibodies aimed to destroy a specific invader or threat. This general response involves swelling (accumulation of fluids), heat, redness (increased micro-blood supply), and the impairment of function and pain at the affected site, which serves as a constant reminder to guard the site until the healing process is complete.

Inflammation is classified as either acute or chronic. An acute inflammation is a temporary reaction to an organism's injury and ends when the affected tissue is healed. Chronic inflammation varies. It can result from the existence of a maintaining cause; when an invading organism or toxin cannot be expelled or continuously reappears; when an injury is not allowed to heal and instead is constantly agitated; due to the presence of a foreign object; or, lastly, from an over-reactive immune system that attacks itself such as in Crohn's Disease.

TAKE NOTICE

(E)-β-CARYOPHELLENE CONTAINING SPICES: BLACK "ASHANTI PEPPER" • WHITE "ASHANTI PEPPER" • INDIAN BAY-LEAF • ALLIGATOR PEPPER • BASIL • CINNAMON • ROSEMARY • BLACK CARAWAY • BLACK PEPPER • MEXICAN OREGANO • CLOVE.

CARYOPHYLLENE: (E)-β-Caryophyllene or (E)-BCP is a FDA-approved dietary plant-cannabinoid that activates CB2 receptor sites and initiates potent anti-inflammatory actions.[1,2]

For more information of these specific spices go to Chapter I "Cannabinoid Research."

OTHER SPICES WHICH MAY AID THE INFLAMMATORY CONDITION

CAYENNE • COCOA • COCONUT • GARLIC • MYRRH • NIGELLA • TURMERIC

CAYENNE: Cayenne stimulates peripheral circulation. In Cuba, a topical tincture and cream is used to treat chronic aches and pains of lumbago, arthritis and rheumatism.[3]

GARLIC: Garlic is used in Cuba for the treatment of thrombophlebitis and other inflammations.[4]

MYRRH: A study from the University of Cincinnati, Ohio, confirmed the physiological benefits of myrrh, used for thousands of years in the treatment of arthritis. Myrrh modulates inflammatory responses.[5]

NIGELLA: An experiment from Yüzüncü Yil University, Turkey, demonstrated that the volatile oil of nigella can suppress artificially induced arthritis in rats. Nigella has historically been used in the treatment of arthritis and other chronic inflammatory conditions.[6]

TURMERIC: In a meta-study, scientists gave an overview of decades of scientific studies on turmeric. They found that turmeric's anti-inflammatory properties effectively supported the healing of wounds, arthritis, inflammatory bowel disease (IBS), ulcerative colitis (colon inflammation with ulcers), atherosclerosis, pancreatitis, psoriasis, chronic anterior and uveitis (inflammation of the middle layer of the eye).[7]

1 Béla Horvátha, Partha Mukhopadhyaya, Malek Kechrida, Vivek Patela, Gali Tanchiana, David A. Winkb, Jürg Gertschc, Pál Pachera. *β-Caryophyllene ameliorates cisplatin-induced nephrotoxicity in a cannabinoid 2 receptor-dependent manner.* a Laboratory of Physiologic Studies, National Institute on Alcohol Abuse and Alcoholism, National Institutes of Health, Bethesda, MD 20892, USA. b Radiation Biology Branch, National Cancer Institute, National Institutes of Health, Bethesda, MD 20892, USA. c Institute of Biochemistry and Molecular Medicine, University of Bern, 3012 Bern, Switzerland. Free Radical Biology and Medicine. Volume 52, Issue 8, 15 April 2012, Pages 1325–133.

2 Gertsch J, Leonti M, Raduner S, Racz I, Chen JZ, Xie XQ, Altmann KH, Karsak M, Zimmer A. *Beta-caryophyllene is a dietary cannabinoid.* Institute of Pharmaceutical Sciences, Department of Chemistry and Applied Biosciences, Eidgenössische Technische Hochschule (ETH) Zurich, 8092 Zürich, Switzerland. Proc Natl Acad Sci U S A. 2008 Jul 1;105(26):9099-104.

3 *Therapeutic Guide to Plant Pharmaceuticals and Honey Pharmaceuticals (Guia Terapeutica Dispensarial de Fitofarmacos y Apifarmacos* - Ministerio de Salud Publica, Ciudad de La Habana - Republica de Cuba 1992). Cuban Ministry of Public Health, Havana.

4 Ibid.

5 Khanna D, Sethi G, Ahn KS, Pandey MK, Kunnumakkara AB, Sung B, Aggarwal A, Aggarwal BB. *Natural products as a gold mine for arthritis treatment.* Division of Immunology, Department of Medicine, University of Cincinnati, Cincinnati, OH, USA. Curr Opin Pharmacol. 2007 Jun;7(3):344-51.

6 Tekeoglu I, Dogan A, Ediz L, Budancamanak M, Demirel A. *Effects of thymoquinone (volatile oil of black cumin) on rheumatoid arthritis in rat models.* Yuzuncu Yil University, Medical School, Department of Rehabilitation and Rheumatology, Turkey. Phytother Res. 2007 Sep;21(9):895-7.

7 Goel A, Kunnumakkara AB, Aggarwal BB. *Curcumin as "Curecumin": From kitchen to clinic.* Gastrointestinal Cancer Research Laboratory, Department of Internal Medicine, Charles A. Sammons Cancer Center and Baylor Research Institute, Baylor University Medical Center, Dallas, TX, United States. Biochem Pharmacol. 2007 Aug 19.

Inflammatory Diseases
Arthritis

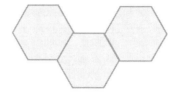

NUMBER OF STUDIES: 3

CHI VALUE: 6

Arthritis is inflammation of a joint connecting two bones such as the fingers, wrists, hips, back and knee joints. People suffering from arthritis often complain of pain in the affected joint, which is commonly accompanied by redness, a sensation of heat, and minor swelling. Arthritis typically develops gradually over many years. Initially, it presents as an occasional mild ache in the joints which progresses into chronic pains, stiffness and swelling. The arthritis sufferer begins to avoid certain painful movements so as to guard against the pain, resulting in further stiffness, limited in range of motion, and decreased mobility. Arthritis has become the leading cause of disability in the U.S. with more than 46 million people suffering various forms of physical difficulties.[1]

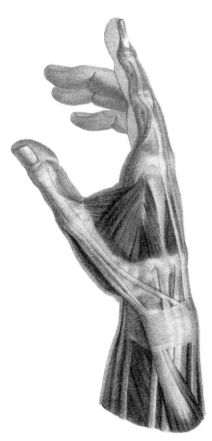

Western medicine claims little knowledge of the causes or cures of this ailment. However, over one-hundred different causes for arthritis are considered, including gout and scleroderma, and viral, bacterial, or fungal infections. Limited treatments focus on suppressing pain or diminishing inflammation flare-ups.

One of the major pharmaceutical drugs for arthritis, nonsteroidal anti-inflammatory drugs (NSAIDs), can result in serious consequences and should be taken with caution. "Each year 41,000 older adults are hospitalized, and 3,300 of them die from ulcers caused by NSAIDs. Thousands of younger adults are hospitalized."[2]

CANNABIS AND ARTHRITIS

In one animal study, researchers from the U.K., U.S. and Israel (2000) discovered that cannabidiol (CBD) treatment in rats effectively blocked progression of both acute and chronic arthritis.[3]

In a variety of animal assays (a procedure for testing effectiveness of a drug), cannabinoid-derived ajulemic acid showed efficacy in models for pain and inflammation. In a Worcester, Massachusetts study, on rat adjuvant arthritis, ajulemic acid displayed a remarkable action to prevent destruction of inflamed joints.[4]

Researchers from Calgary, Canada, (2011) injected the synthetic cannabinoid URB597 into the osteoarthritic knees of rodents and discovered that it significantly reduced pain. This mechanism was mediated via CB1 receptors. Scientists consider cannabinoids a possible novel approach to treating osteoarthritis pain.[5]

STUDY SUMMARY:

Drugs	Type of Study	Published Year, Place, and Key Results	CHI
URB597	Animal study (Rodents)	2011 – University of Calgary, Calgary, Canada. Injecting URB597 into the osteoarthritic knees of rodents significantly reduced pain.	2
Cannabinoid derived ajulemic acid	Animal study (Rats)	2005 – Worcester, University of Massachusetts Medical School. Cannabinoid derived ajulemic acid reduces pain, inflammation and protected joints from damage in arthritis.	2
Cannabidiol (CBD)	Animal study (Rats)	2000 – International Scientific Institutions. Protection of joints from damage. Cannabidiol (CBD) at 25 mg/kg per day orally was optimal in blocking progression of disease.	2

Total CHI Value   6

STRAIN SPECIFIC CONSIDERATIONS

Pre-clinical trials have explored URB597, cannabinoid-derived ajulemic acid (HU239) and the plant cannabinoid CBD to reduce arthritis in rodents.

URB597 is an inhibitor of an enzyme (fatty acid amide hydrolase or FAAH), which breaks down anandamide, thereby increasing anandamide presence and activity in the body. The endocannabinoid anandamide binds relatively equally to CB1 and CB2. Ajulemic acid (HU239) is a synthetic cannabinoid hypothesized to be a CB1 agonist while CBD has a greater affinity for CB2 than CB1.

Basic strain, the sativa and indica strains all each contain CB1 and CB2 activating cannabinoids. Indicas and indica heavy strains usually contain lower THC:CBD ratios, thereby favoring CB2 activation.

EXPLORING MIND–BODY CONSCIOUSNESS

For many years, psychosomatic theories have emerged to suggest the mind's impact on the genesis, progression and management of arthritis. One study considered psychological stress factors as a causative influence in the development of rheumatoid arthritis. In this model researchers attribute the loss of muscle tone to increased muscle tension associated with psychosomatic stress. Stress reportedly interferes with signals from a central nervous system-based (CNS) neurological feedback loop (fusimotor frequency) necessary in maintaining muscle tone.[6]

In another experiment, researchers examined 266 osteoarthritis (OA) patients for possible correlations between their mental health and OA affecting the knees and/or the hips. Researchers discovered that the intensity and type of pain experienced by patients related directly to the quality of their mental health. The authors of the study suggested that mental health measures could be employed to manage chronic and flare-up pain associated with the disease.[7]

SUGGESTED BLESSING

May the spirit of reconciliation and forgiveness grease your joints so you can reach and stretch for your dreams and for the stars.

QUESTIONS

What is tucked away inside the affected joint?
Why does it hurts to reach and stretch to become taller than I really am?
What limiting belief(s) is keeping me contracted?
What belief says it hurts to reach and stretch?
Where am I emotionally inflexible?
What feeling is keeping me from reaching for the stars?
Where am I inflexible in my thinking?
What thoughts are limiting my reach?

AGGRAVATING FACTORS

Psychological stressors / repressed emotions / suppressed emotions / hurt and anger in combination.

HEALING FACTORS

Discovering and releasing repressed or suppressed feelings and emotions / developing an appreciation of our emotional nature and the entire emotional spectrum of which humans are capable.

ANECDOTE

Jonathan was diagnosed with arthritis by age 53. It started with an occasional stiffness in his left knee but over time graduated into a pain he felt deep inside his joint. He would have occasional flare-ups and swelling especially after sitting for a longer period or when the temperature dropped. He had been given numerous pharmaceutical medications over the years, including steroid injections into the joint, but no intervention really touched the pain. On top of that he began feeling depressed.

One winter night the pain escalated, and a friend suggested he try some cannabis. At this point, willing to try anything, he did something he had never thought he would do. He inhaled. After a few minutes, Jonathan felt relaxed and, to his surprise, the pain diminished. He noticed more flexibility in his joint and was able to enjoy a deep and restful night's sleep. An experience with cannabis a few months later helped move him beyond mere pain management toward deeper healing.

This time, when Jonathan treated himself for the pain as usual, he felt his visual attention drawn into his left knee. He saw the lining of the joint covered in a sand-like dirty dust. He was curious and his imagination drew ever closer to the dusty residue. He felt himself entering a single grain of dust and instantly felt tense. Somehow, his sense of wonder kept him exploring rather than retreating from the unpleasant sensation. He felt hurt. But it was a hurt from long ago, a vivid memory of a friend telling his secret to another. He remembered it like it was yesterday. Jonathan felt that it was right to stay with the hurt for what must have been perhaps 10 or 20 minutes. Suddenly, the hurt released. He was left feeling lighter and with what he considered his "real hurt".

He subsequently turned this experience into a healing meditation where he would imagine himself (without the help of cannabis) enter his left knee, visualize the dirty dust, select an individual grain and enter it. Each time he would find another scene, another hurt, or sometimes a sensation of anger. Each time he would let himself feel it until it was no more. Little by little, Jonathan noticed a significant and sustained improvement, not just with the arthritic knee but also in how he felt about himself. His depression began to lighten, and he described himself as happier and more confident in dealing with whatever feeling or emotion came his way.

TAKE NOTICE

CAYENNE • MYRRH • NIGELLA • (E)-B-CARYOPHYLLENE

CAYENNE: Cayenne stimulates peripheral circulation. In Cuba, a topical tincture and cream is used to treat chronic aches and pains of lumbago, arthritis and rheumatism.[8]

MYRRH: A study from the University of Cincinnati, Ohio, discovered physiological benefits of myrrh, used for thousands of years in the treatment of arthritis. Myrrh modulates inflammatory responses.[9] Scientists from the King Saud University, Kharj, Saudi Arabi confirmed that myrrh treatment via drinking water increased white blood cell count.[10] These results may serve as an explantion for the time-proven efficacy of myrrh in the treatment of wounds and inflammation.

NIGELLA: An experiment from Yüzüncü Yil University, Turkey, demonstrated that the volatile oil of nigella can suppress artificially induced arthritis in rats. Nigella has historically been used in the treatment of arthritis and other chronic inflammatory conditions.[11]

(E)-β-CARYOPHELLENE or (E)-BCP: This FDA-approved dietary plant-cannabinoid activates CB2 receptor sites and initiates potent anti-inflammatory actions. Spice plants known to contain significant amounts of (E)-BCP include: BLACK "ASHANTI PEPPER" • WHITE "ASHANTI PEPPER" • INDIAN BAY-LEAF • ALLIGATOR PEPPER • BASIL • CINNAMON • ROSEMARY • BLACK CARAWAY • BLACK PEPPER • MEXICAN OREGANO • CLOVE.

For more information on these specific spices go to Chapter I "CANNABINOID RESEARCH."

3 A. M. Malfait,*† R. Gallily,†‡ P. F. Sumariwalla,* A. S. Malik,* E. Andreakos,* R. Mechoulam,‡ and M. Feldmann*§ *The nonpsychoactive cannabis constituent cannabidiol is an oral anti-arthritic therapeutic in murine collagen-induced arthritis.* *Kennedy Institute of Rheumatology, 1 Aspenlea Road, Hammersmith, London W6 8LH, United Kingdom; and ‡Hebrew University, Hadassah Medical School, P.O.B. 12272, Jerusalem 91120, Israel. †A.M.M. and R.G. contributed equally to this work. Edited by Anthony Cerami, The Kenneth S. Warren Laboratories, Tarrytown, NY. Proc Natl Acad Sci U S A. 2000 August 15; 97(17): 9561–9566.

4 Summer Burstein. *Ajulemic acid (IP-751): Synthesis, proof of principle, toxicity studies, and clinical trials.* Department of Biochemistry and Molecular Pharmacology, University of Massachusetts Medical School, 364 Plantation Street, 01605 Worcester, MA. AAPS J. 2005 March; 7(1): E143–E148.

5 Schuelert N, Johnson MP, Oskins JL, Jassal K, Chambers MG, McDougall JJ. *Local application of the endocannabinoid hydrolysis inhibitor URB597 reduces nociception in spontaneous and chemically induced models of osteoarthritis.* Department of Physiology & Pharmacology, University of Calgary, Calgary, AB, Canada T2N 4N1. Pain. 2011 May;152(5):975-81.

6 Schiel KA. *A proposed psychosomatic etiologic model for rheumatoid arthritis.* Med Hypotheses. 1999 Oct;53(4):305-14.

7 Wise BL, Niu J, Zhang Y, Wang N, Jordan JM, Choy E, Hunter DJ. *Psychological factors and their relation to osteoarthritis pain.* University School of Medicine, Boston, MA, USA. Osteoarthritis Cartilage. 2010 Jul;18(7):883-7.

8 *Therapeutic Guide to Plant Pharmaceuticals and Honey Pharmaceuticals (Guia Terapeutica Dispensarial de Fitofarmacos y Apifarmacos* - Ministerio de Salud Publica, Ciudad de La Habana - Republica de Cuba 1992). Cuban Ministry of Public Health, Havana.

9 Khanna D, Sethi G, Ahn KS, Pandey MK, Kunnumakkara AB, Sung B, Aggarwal A, Aggarwal BB. *Natural products as a gold mine for arthritis treatment.* Division of Immunology, Department of Medicine, University of Cincinnati, Cincinnati, OH, USA. Curr Opin Pharmacol. 2007 Jun;7(3):344-51.

10 Haffor AS. *Effect of myrrh (Commiphora molmol) on leukocyte levels before and during healing from gastric ulcer or skin injury.* Department of Radiological Science, King Saud University, Kharj, Saudi Arabia. J Immunotoxicol. 2010 Mar;7(1):68-75.

11 Tekeoglu I, Dogan A, Ediz L, Budancamanak M, Demirel A. *Effects of thymoquinone (volatile oil of black cumin) on rheumatoid arthritis in rat models.* Yuzuncu Yil University, Medical School, Department of Rehabilitation and Rheumatology, Turkey. Phytother Res. 2007 Sep;21(9):895-7.

Inflammatory Diseases
Atherosclerosis

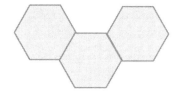

NUMBER OF STUDIES: 3

CHI VALUE: 6

In the past, atherosclerosis was largely defined in terms of the accumulation of plaque or bad cholesterol (LDL) within the arterial walls leading to obstructions.However, it is now understood as more than a simple build-up of plaque. This obstruction is actually a physical response to injuries in the walls' lining. Causes of arterial wall injuries include high blood pressure, infectious microbes or excessive presence of a certain amino acid called homocysteine. Studies have demonstrated that inflammatory molecules stimulate events leading to the development of atherosclerotic lesions. Some researchers consider atherosclerosis a natural type of band-aid approach to cover an injury or inflammation. When the band-aid becomes too thick or breaks loose, symptoms of a chronic or acute nature occur. In mild cases, this can lead to diminished oxygen supply to the tissue on the other side of the occlusion; in acute cases, it can cause severe stokes or heart attacks.

Atherosclerosis develops slowly over many years. If extant in the limbs (called peripheral artery disease), it may present as a pain in the legs or arms, especially when exercising. Atherosclerosis in arteries in the torso may produce signs and symptoms similar to heart disease or strokes: primarily chest pain, shortness of breath or loss of sensation and function (speech and movement of limbs).

In addition to a careful examination and patient history, doctors may request several tests to determine the risk of atherosclerosis. Doctors may scan blood samples for levels of cholesterol(s), the concentration of fibrinogen, a blood protein involved in clotting (too much fibrinogen may mean atherosclerosis); homocysteine (too much may contribute to atherosclerosis); and C-reactive protein (CRP) produced by the liver. These factors could indicate the presence of inflammation and might be associated with atherosclerosis. Other diagnostic examinations range from such safe tests as stress tests, ultrasound, the ankle-brachial index (a test that helps to determine if atherosclerosis is present in the legs), or electrocardiogram (EKG), to those tests with the potential for severe side-effects such as CT-scans, cardiac catheterization and angiograms involving arterial invasion, injection of dye and the use of x-rays (ionizing radiation).

Orthodox treatment includes surgery and numerous pharmacological interventions. Life-style recommendations may include stress reduction, appropriate exercise, and the control of contributing factors such as weight-loss, poor food avoidance or the cessation of smoking.

In 2006 researchers acknowledged some important benefits of cannabis use. "Habitual cannabis use has been shown to positively affect the human immune system, and recent advances in endocannabinoid research provide a basis for understanding these immunomodulatory effects. Cell-based experiments or in vivo animal testing suggest that regulation of the endocannabinoid circuitry can impact almost every major function associated with the immune system." The scientists tested numerous novel molecules that exert their biological effects through the endocannabinoid system. The result of this exploration suggested the therapeutic potential of cannabinoids on inflammatory diseases such as atherosclerosis.[1]

Researchers observed that the enzyme 15-LOX could oxygenate low-density lipoprotein (LDL), which leads to the production of oxidized LDL. They understood that this in turn might play a factor in developing atherosclerosis. So in 2009, researchers from Kanazawa, Japan, conducted an experiment examining the impact of cannabinoids on 15-LOX. Results indicated that the cannabinoids cannabidiol (CBD) and its derivatives CBD-2'-monomethyl ether and CBD-2',6'-dimethyl ether (CBDD) inhibit 15-LOX enzyme activity to varying degrees. Researchers thus suggested that (CBDD), which had the strongest enzyme inhibitory effects, could be a useful prototype for producing medicines for atherosclerosis.[2]

A group of scientists from Shaanxi, China, (2010) examined the impact of a synthetic cannabinoid (WIN55212-2) on the development of atherosclerosis in an animal study using mice. Results revealed a significant and direct reduction in the size of aortic atherosclerotic lesions.[3]

STUDY SUMMARY:

Drugs	Type of Study	Published Year, Place, and Key Results	CHI
Synthetic cannabinoid (WIN55212-2)	Animal study	2010 – Department of Cardiovascular Medicine, First Affiliated Hospital of Medical School, Xi'an Jiaotong University, Shaanxi, China. Significant and direct reduction in the size of aortic atherosclerotic lesions.	2
The cannabinoids cannabidiol (CBD) and its derivatives CBD-2'-monomethyl ether and CBD-2',6'-dimethyl ether (CBDD)	Laboratory	2009 – Department of Hygienic Chemistry, Faculty of Pharmaceutical Sciences, Hokuriku University, Kanazawa, Japan. (CBDD) may be a useful prototype for producing medicines for atherosclerosis.	1
Cannabinoids	Laboratory and animal	2006 – Center for Drug Discovery, Northeastern University, Boston, MA. Potential reduction of inflammation.	1+2

Total CHI Value 6

STRAIN AND FORM SPECIFIC CONSIDERATIONS

In two pre-clinical studies, researchers examined the synthetic cannabinoid

WIN 55212-2, the plant cannabinoid cannabidiol (CBD) and its derivatives CBD-2'-monomethyl ether and CBD-2',6'-dimethyl ether (CBDD) in the context of atherosclerosis.

WIN 55212-2 binds to both receptors but with higher affinity to CB2 than CB1. The same is true for CBD. Indica and indica heavy strains tend to possess a lower THC:CBD ratio, thus favoring CB2 expression. Raw cannabis, fresh leaf and leaf juice contain CBD-acid and thus favor CB2 activation.

EXPLORING MIND–BODY CONSCIOUSNESS

While the connection between psychological factors and cardiovascular disease has been well demonstrated in numerous meta-analyses,[4] fewer experiments exist to date to elucidate this connection in the context of atherosclerosis. In fact, those available show different results. One such study conducted on 1,592 men and women during a period of five years determined that social deprivation and hostility were significantly associated with the progression of atherosclerosis.[5] Data used from the Multi-Ethnic Study of Atherosclerosis (MESA), a study of 6,814 persons aged 45 to 84 years with no history of clinical cardiovascular disease, revealed that pessimism relates to higher levels of inflammation.[6] Opposing study results failed to find connections between psychological factors and the disease's development.[7]

One theory holds that if plaque build-up is a response to an inflammation of the artery lining, that caused the body to respond with deposits in a "band-aid" attempt to contain the damage, the original inflammation likely still lingers beneath it. Thus, an underlying emotional architecture of social deprivation/isolation or loneliness could be a wall we build around ourselves to keep away emotions such as pain and shame seem too difficult to confront. While initially the wall of isolation may be effective as a protective barrier, over time, it can become a problem larger than the one it was build to contain.

Alternatively, it can be argued that blood has to do with family and, since veins and arteries serve to carry blood, it may be helpful to look for intolerable emotions and experiences related to family.

SUGGESTED BLESSING

May your need to cover-up or hide perceived past transregressions or mistakes transcend into the experience of complete safety and trust.

SUGGESTED AFFIRMATION

I now choose to heal instead of judging.

I now choose to flush all hurt, pain and shame from the core of my being.

QUESTIONS

How does your family respond to the presence of something intolerable?
How do I respond to the presence of something intolerable?
Does your family brush intolerable experiences under the carpet?
Do I use the barrier of loneliness to shelter myself from pain?
Where is belonging associated with pain or shame?
What resource do I have today that allows me to deal with what before was intolerable?

AGGRAVATING FACTORS

Social deprivation and hostility / loneliness / isolation / pessimism.

Undoing the internal architecture of loneliness, social isolation and deprivation / optimism / safe and meaningful social interaction / contact and mutual support in problem solving / releasing suppressed and repressed emotions / and developing a tendencies for positive affect.

TAKE NOTICE

CARDAMOM • COCOA • COCONUT • GARLIC • ROSEMARY • TURMERIC

• (E)-B-CARYOPHYLLENE

CARDAMON: Scientists from the city of Mysore, India discovered that cardamon extract protects platelets (blood particles involved in clotting) from aggregation and lipid peroxidation associated cardio-vascular disease.[8]

COCOA: Scientists at the McGill University School of Dietetics and Human Nutrition in Quebec, Canada cautiously suggest that the consumption of dark chocolate may have a protective impact on heart and vascular illness and their connection to oxidized bad cholesterol (LDL).[9]

COCONUT: Researcher Hans Kaunitz correlated data from several laboratory animal studies with the findings from the United Nations. He reported that death from ischemic heart disease is lowest where coconut fat intake is highest.[10]

GARLIC: Garlic may be helpful when peripheral signs and symptoms of heart disease are present. These include water retention, spasms, thrombophlebitis, inflammations, viral infections and hypertension.[11]

German Commission E approved garlic as a treatment for vascular concerns: "Supportive to dietary measures at elevated levels of lipids in blood. Preventative measures for age-dependent vascular changes."[12]

For the first time, Japanese scientists have been able to scientifically prove what many traditional practitioners have suspected, namely that garlic, or specifically allicin, has potent antioxidant properties.[13]

Another study from Japan suggests that odorless garlic powder can play a beneficial role in preventing destructive thrombus (clot) formation such as in heart attacks. It apparently does so, according to the researchers, by suppressing the formation of clots and by destroying fibrin, a protein involved in the clotting of blood.[14]

ROSEMARY: In an experiment from Taichung Hsien, Taiwan, scientists concluded that: "…rosemary is an excellent multifunctional therapeutic herb; by looking at its potentially potent antiglycative bioactivity, it may become a good adjuvant medicine for the prevention and treatment of diabetic, cardiovascular, and other neuro-degenerative diseases."[15]

TURMERIC: In this meta-study, scientists presented an overview of decades of scientific studies on turmeric. A long list of turmeric's potential therapeutic properties included beneficial effects in cardio-vascular disease.[16]

(E)-β-CARYOPHELLENE or (E)-BCP: This FDA-approved dietary plant-cannabinoid that activates CB2 receptor sites and initiates potent anti-inflammatory actions. Spice plants known to contain significant amounts of (E)-BCP in include: BLACK "ASHANTI PEPPER" • WHITE "ASHANTI PEPPER" • INDIAN BAY-LEAF • ALLIGATOR PEPPER • BASIL • CINNAMON • ROSEMARY • BLACK CARAWAY • BLACK PEPPER • MEXICAN OREGANO • CLOVE.

For more information on these specific spices go to Chapter I "Cannabinoid Research."

1 Lu, Dai1; Kiran Vemuri, V.1; Duclos, Richard I.1; Jr.1; Makriyannis, Alexandros.1 *The Cannabinergic System as a Target for Anti-inflammatory Therapies.* 1 Center for Drug Discovery, Northeastern University, 360 Huntington Avenue, 116 Mugar Hall, Boston, MA, 02115, USA. Current Topics in Medicinal Chemistry, Volume 6, Number 13, July 2006 , pp. 1401-1426(26). Bentham Science Publishers.

2 Takeda S, Usami N, Yamamoto I, Watanabe K. *Cannabidiol-2',6'-Dimethyl Ether, a Cannabidiol Derivative, Is a Highly Potent and Selective 15 Lipoxygenase Inhibitor.* Department of Hygienic Chemistry, Faculty of Pharmaceutical Sciences, Hokuriku University, Ho-3 Kanagawa-machi, Kanazawa, Japan. Drug Metab Dispos. 2009 Aug;37(8):1733-7.

3 Zhao Y, Yuan Z, Liu Y, Xue J, Tian Y, Liu W, Zhang W, Shen Y, Xu W, Liang X, Chen T. *Activation of Cannabinoid CB2 Receptor Ameliorates Atherosclerosis Associated with Suppression of Adhesion Molecules.* Department of Cardiovascular Medicine, First Affiliated Hospital of Medical School, Xi'an Jiaotong University, Shaanxi, China. J Cardiovasc Pharmacol, 9. Januar 2010.

4 Miller TQ, Smith TW, Turner CW, Guijarro ML, Hallet AJ. *A meta-analytic review of research on hostility and physical health.* Psychol Bull 1996;119:322– 48.

5 MARTHA C. WHITEMAN, PHD, IAN J. DEARY, FRCPE, AND F. GERALD R. FOWKES, FRCPE. *Personality and Social Predictors of Atherosclerotic Progression: Edinburgh Artery Study.* Wolfson Unit for Prevention of Peripheral Vascular Diseases (M.C.W., F.G.R.F.), Public Health Sciences, and Department of Psychology (M.C.W., I.J.D.), University of Edinburgh, Edinburgh, Scotland. Psychosomatic Medicine 62:703–714 (2000)

6 Brita Roy, MD, MPH, MS, Ana V. Diez-Roux, MD, PhD, Teresa Seeman, PhD, Nalini Ranjit, PhD, Steven Shea, MD and Mary Cushman, MD. *Association of Optimism and Pessimism With Inflammation and Hemostasis in the Multi-Ethnic Study of Atherosclerosis (MESA).* Center for Social Epidemiology and Population Health (B.R., A.V.D.-R., N.R.), University of Michigan, Ann Arbor, Michigan; Division of Geriatrics (T.S.), School of Medicine, UCLA, Los Angeles, California; Division of General Medicine (S.S.), College of Physicians and Surgeons, and Division of Epidemiology, School of Public Health, Columbia University New York, New York; and the Department of Medicine (M.C.), University of Vermont, Burlington, Vermont. Psychosomatic Medicine February/March 2010 vol. 72 no. 2 134-140.

7 Alan Rozanski, MD, Heidi Gransar, MS, Laura D. Kubzansky, PhD, Nathan Wong, MD, Leslee Shaw, PhD, Romalisa Miranda-Peats, MPH, Louise E. Thomson, MBChB, Sean W. Hayes, MD, John D. Friedman, MD, MPH and Daniel S. Berman, MD. *Do Psychological Risk Factors Predict the Presence of Coronary Atherosclerosis?* Division of Cardiology and Department of Medicine (A.R.), St. Luke's Roosevelt Hospital and the Department of Medicine, Columbia University College of Physicians and Surgeons, New York, New York; Departments of Imaging and Medicine and the Burns and Allen Research Institute (H.G., R.M.P., L.E.T., S.W.H., J.D.F., D.S.B.), Cedars-Sinai Medical Center, Los Angeles, California, and the Department of Medicine, David Geffen School of Medicine, University of California, Los Angeles, Los Angeles, California; Department of Society, Human Development and Health (L.D.K.), Harvard School of Public Health, Boston, Massachusetts; the Heart Disease Prevention Program (N.W.), University of California, Irvine, Irvine, California; and the Division of Cardiology (L.S.), Department of Medicine, Emory University School of Medicine, Atlanta, Georgia. Psychosomatic Medi-

cine January 2011 vol. 73 no. 1 7-15.

8 Suneetha WJ, Krishnakantha TP. *Cardamom extract as inhibitor of human platelet aggregation.* Department of Biochemistry and Nutrition, Central Food Technological Research Institute, Mysore 570 020, India. Phytother Res. 2005 May;19(5):437-40.

9 Rudkowska I, Jones PJ. *Functional foods for the prevention and treatment of cardiovascular diseases: cholesterol and beyond.* School of Dietetics and Human Nutrition McGill University, St-Anne-de-Bellevue, Quebec, Canada. Expert Rev Cardiovasc Ther. 2007 May;5(3):477-90.

10 Kaunitz H. *Medium chain triglycerides (MCT) in aging and arteriosclerosis.* J Environ Pathol Toxicol Oncol. 1986 Mar-Apr;6(3-4):115-21.

11 *Therapeutic Guide to Plant Pharmaceuticals and Honey Pharmaceuticals (Guia Terapeutica Dispensarial de Fitofarmacos y Apifarmacos* - Ministerio de Salud Publica, Ciudad de La Habana - Republica de Cuba 1992). Cuban Ministry of Public Health, Havana.

12 *Monographien der E-Kommission* (Phyto-Therapie) (380 monographs). A therapeutic guide to herbal medicine evaluating the safety and efficacy of herbs for licensed medical prescribing in Germany. Published between 1984 and 1994 in the Bundesanzeiger (official publication by the Federal Republic of Germany). Copies of the monographs are available at the Heilpflanzen-Welt Bibliothek: http://buecher.heilpflanzen-welt.de/BGA-Commission-E-Monographs/

13 Okada Y, Tanaka K, Sato E, Okajima H. *Kinetic and mechanistic studies of allicin as an antioxidant.* Department of Analytical Chemistry, Faculty of Health Sciences, Kyorin University, 476 Miyasita-cho, Hachioji, Tokyo, 192-8508, Japan. Org Biomol Chem. 2006 Nov 21;4(22):4113-7.

14 Fukao H, Yoshida H, Tazawa Y, Hada T. *Antithrombotic effects of odorless garlic powder both in vitro and in vivo.* Department of Nutritional Sciences, Faculty of Food Culture, Kurashiki Sakuyo University, Japan. Biosci Biotechnol Biochem. 2007 Jan;71(1):84-90.

15 Hsieh CL, Peng CH, Chyau CC, Lin YC, Wang HE, Peng RY. *Low-density lipoprotein, collagen, and thrombin models reveal that Rosemarinus officinalis L. exhibits potent antiglycative effects.* Department of Food and Nutrition, Research Institute of Biotechnology, and Division of Basic Medical Sciences, Hung-Kuang University, No. 34 Chung-Chie Road, Shalu County, Taichung Hsien, Taiwan. J Agric Food Chem. 2007 Apr 18;55(8):2884-91.

16 Goel A, Kunnumakkara AB, Aggarwal BB. *Curcumin as "Curecumin": From kitchen to clinic.* Gastrointestinal Cancer Research Laboratory, Department of Internal Medicine, Charles A. Sammons Cancer Center and Baylor Research Institute, Baylor University Medical Center, Dallas, TX, United States. Biochem Pharmacol. 2007 Aug 19.

Inflammatory Diseases
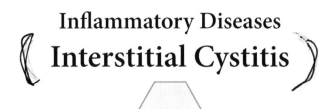
Interstitial Cystitis

NUMBER OF STUDIES: 1

CHI VALUE: 3

Interstitial cystitis (IC; painful bladder syndrome) predominantly affects women. The disease presents with chronic burning bladder pains due to inflammation and thinning of the urinary bladder lining. Other common symptoms include pain in the pelvic region particularly (vagina, perineum), the chronic sensation of having to urinate, or having voided incompletely, painful burning upon urination and polyuria (high frequency of urination). The chronic pain may also present as acute flare-ups, which are often triggered by stress, menses, bacteria or sex. Cystitis can be a debilitating condition that may severely reduce the quality of life in patients who are often depressed, have relationship and emotional difficulties or are unable to sleep or work but otherwise function normally.

Bacteria do not typically cause IC. Within orthodox medicine, the cause of the infection remains unknown; but it is hypothesized that IC is an autoimmune disease where the body's own defenses attack the lining of the bladder. Diagnostic tests may include a physical examination, a careful patient history, urine testing, cytoscope (a camera tube inserted into the urethra and extended into the bladder), and bladder tissue biopsies.

IC has no known cure within orthodox medicine. Management techniques include pharmaceuticals, external nerve stimulation (TENS units), physical bladder stretching (using water or a gas), and surgery. Urologists may also use a wood pulp by-product, dimethylsulfoxide (DMSO) injected into the bladder to alleviate symptoms.

CANNABIS AND CYSTITIS

Researchers (2003) reported on the case of a 31-year-old female patient suffering for 20 years from chronic cystitis.[1] Her persistent burning sensation grew so great that it interfered with sleeping. She tried pharmaceutical pain control (opioids and others) and a variety of alternative treatments, all without success. She was given nabilone (1 mg by mouth), which significantly reduced her burning pain by about a third but also caused confusion, psychotic sensations and bad dreams. Dose reduction did not resolve the adverse effects. Doctors switched to dronabinol (2.5mg by mouth), which further reduced her pain by another third without adverse effects, with the exception of "feeling strange." She was able to sleep and function without impediment. The dose, reduced to 2.5 mg by mouth every other day, continued to manage her pain without any side effects. After a period of 6 months, the therapeutic progress appeared well maintained.

STUDY SUMMARY:

Drugs	Type of Study	Published Year, Place, and Key Results	CHI
Nabilone and Dronabinol	One female patient with chronic cystitis	2003 - Nabilone reduced pain but cause adverse effects. Dronabinol reduced pain further without adverse effects.	3

Total CHI Value   3

STRAIN SPECIFIC CONSIDERATIONS

Dronabinol is a synthetic cannabinoid very similar to THC (isomer) while nabilone is a synthetic cannabinoid with some of the same properties as THC.

EXPLORING MIND–BODY CONSCIOUSNESS

One experiment conducted on patients with interstitial cystitis showed significantly greater startle responses during non-imminent threat conditions when compared to healthy human subjects.[2] The enhanced responsiveness in IC patients was associated with affective (feeling/emotion) circuits that included the amygdala, the portion of the limbic brain that is responsible for intense emotions and emotional memory. It is this discovery that suggests a possible psychosomatic connection related to an intense and likely early traumatic memory or experience.

Researchers at Tufts University School of Medicine conducted a meta-analysis of 713 mostly original papers published between 1990 to August 2008. One of the resulting discoveries suggested that stress played a significant role in IC and should be targeted to better understand and manage the disease.[3]

Both the location of the primary symptoms of IC, the bladder and its function of storing and voiding urine, chronic burning and ineffective void lend themselves to possible interpretations from a psychosomatic perspective.

QUESTIONS

How do I feel when I cannot completely void my urine?
What am I holding onto that hurts or burns?
What burning anger will not end?
Is there an emotion or memory that is constantly irritating me?
Which anger is causing me so much pain not to feel?
What feeling is starting to dribble out of me? Can I let it flow?

AGGRAVATING FACTORS

Stress / suppressed or repressed emotions.

HEALING FACTORS

Stress prevention / stress management / learning positive coping skills / emotional release work.

SUGGESTED BLESSING

May you relax enough to realize that anger, hurt, rage or shame only cause lasting damage when you pretend they do not exist.

SUGGESTED AFFIRMATION

It is okay to be pissed off.

I can release my anger with ease and harm to none. I can change any belief that says, "It's not okay to be angry."

I can change any belief that says, "It hurts to be angry."

TAKE NOTICE

For more information on alternative medical perspectives and natural treatment possibilities, consider looking at a book written by Amrit Willis RN, entitled *Solving the Interstitial Cystitis Puzzle: A Guide to Natural Healing.* Published by Holistic Life Enterprises, Beverly Hills, California, 2001 & 2003.

1 Krenn H Daha LK Oczenski W Fitzgerald R D. *A case of cannabinoid rotation in a young woman with chronic cystitis.* J Pain Symptom Manage. 2003;25(1):3-4.

2 Twiss, Christian; Kilpatrick, Lisa; Craske, Michelle; Buffington, C.A. Tony; Ornitz, Edward; Rodríguez, Larissa V.; Mayer, Emeran A.; Naliboff, Bruce D. "*Increased Acoustic Startle Responses in IBS Patients During Abdominal and Non-Abdominal Threat*". The Journal of Urology 2009, 181 (5): 2127–33.

3 Theoharides TC, Whitmore K, Stanford E, Moldwin R, O'Leary MP. *Interstitial cystitis: bladder pain and beyond.* Tufts University School of Medicine, Department of Pharmacology and Experimental Therapeutics, Experimental Therapeutics 136 Harrison Avenue, Boston, MA 02111, USA. Expert Opin Pharmacother. 2008 Dec;9(17):2979-94.

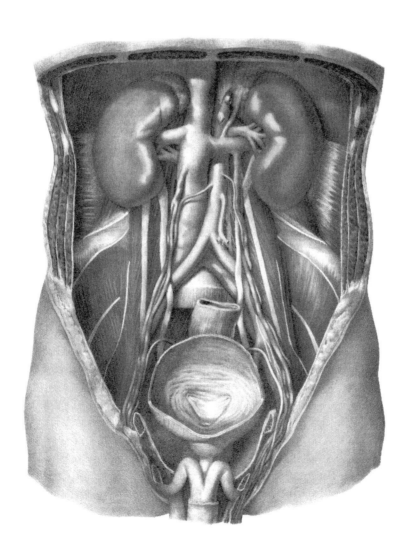

Inflammatory Diseases
Gastrointestinal Inflammatory Diseases
Inflammatory Bowel Disease (IBS)

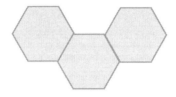

NUMBER OF STUDIES: 3

CHI VALUE: 8

Like the name suggests, this disease primarily affects the gastrointestinal tract but is also associated with inflammation. Orthodox medicine struggles to understand the causes for IBS and to date offers no cure. Possible reasons for developing IBS may include: stressful life events (mind–bowel axis), infections by yet to be identified pathogens or toxins, immune-dysfunction or unhealthy gut environments.

IBS is classified according to the primary symptoms displayed by each patient. Thus, diarrhea, constipation, alternating diarrhea with constipation and infection become the basis for diagnosing the disease as IBS-D, IBS-C, IBS-A, or post-infectious, IBS-PI respectively. Ulcerative colitis (UC) is a form of IBD that can affect other body parts as well. Crohn's disease, another form of IBD, is an autoimmune disorder affecting the gastrointestinal tract.

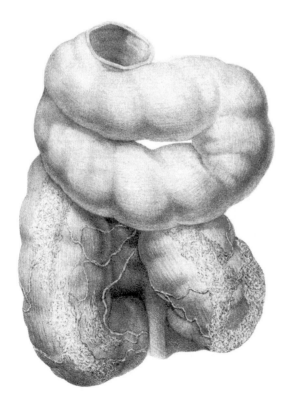

Other frequently observed symptoms may include abdominal discomfort (gas, bloating, cramps), the sensation of incomplete void of stool, gastroesophageal reflux disease (GERD), anxiety, depression, pain (abdominal, back, head, muscle), increased generalized weakness and lack of energy.

Orthodox diagnoses are performed by elimination. Doctors run a variety of tests to rule out diseases with similar symptoms. These may include: colonoscopies, screening for parasites (blood or stool tests), testing for lactose intolerance (hydrogen breath test) or the presence of infections (stool examinations), as well as tests for celiac disease (blood test screening for anti-bodies). If none of these diseases are responsible for the patient's symptoms, practitioners may follow one of several possible established diagnostic algorithms (a list of questions related to the patient's symptoms).

Physicians manage the disease with dietary modifications, pharmaceutical medications and referrals to psychotherapy. Canadian researchers conducted a meta-analysis of all randomized controlled trials published on Medline, Embase, and the Cochrane register up through April 2008.

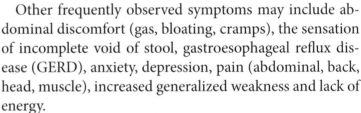

They reported that fiber, antispasmodics, and peppermint oil merited greater effectiveness than a placebo in the treatment of irritable bowel syndrome.[1]

CANNABIS AND INFLAMMATORY BOWEL DISEASE (IBD) OR SYNDROME (IBS)

Case reports from cannabis-using IBS patients suggest that cannabis may be effective in managing some symptoms, especially nausea, diarrhea, stress, cramps and lack of appetite. Human studies remain under way to determine a scientific basis for the use of marijuana in the treatment of IBS.

However, Italian researchers (2010) conducted a meta-analysis/review of the available pre-clinical studies related to cannabinoids and the gut. The authors wrote: "Anatomical, physiological and pharmacological studies have shown that the endocannabinoid system is widely distributed throughout the gut, with regional variation and organ-specific actions. It is involved in the regulation of food intake, nausea and emesis, gastric secretion and gastroprotection, GI motility, ion transport, visceral sensation, intestinal inflammation and cell proliferation in the gut."[2] Three pre-clinical studies give us more insights.

In 2006 Boston researchers tested numerous novel molecules that exert their biological effects through the endocannabinoid system. The results suggested a therapeutic potential of cannabinoids on inflammatory diseases such as IBD.[3]

Two years later, researchers from Alberta, Canada, similarly showed cannabinoids reduced colitis in test animals. The scientists concluded that: "...drugs targeting EC degradation offer therapeutic potential in the treatment of inflammatory bowel diseases."[4]

Another experiment conducted in 2008 in Naples, Italy, indicated that CBD could reduce hypermotility in mice. Based on these observations, scientists hypothesized that CBD normalizes motility in cases of inflammatory bowel disease.[5]

STUDY SUMMARY:

Drugs	Type of Study	Published Year, Place, and Key Results	CHI
CBD	Animal study (mice)	2008 – University of Naples, Italy. CBD could reduce hypermotility in mice.	2
Fatty acid amide hydrolase (FAAH) blocker URB597	Animal and Laboratory. (Mice and human DNA)	2008 – Division of Gastroenterology, Department of Medicine, University of Calgary, Alberta, Canada. EC membrane transport inhibitor VDM11 enhance the action of the ECS. Cannabinoids reduce colitis.	1+2
Cannabinoids	Laboratory and animal	2006 – Center for Drug Discovery, Northeastern University, Boston, MA. Potential reduction of inflammation.	2+1

Total CHI Value   8

STRAIN SPECIFIC CONSIDERATIONS

While research has discovered both CB1 and CB2 in parts of the gastro-intestinal tract, patients with Crohn's disease reported that indica strains worked especially well for them in reducing pain, nausea, vomiting, depression, low energy and lack of sleep. This observation may be supported, in part, by the

278

aforementioned pre-clinical trial from Naples, which showed that CBD could reduce hypermotility (abnormally high activity) in the guts of mice.

Inicas or indica heavy strains tend to have a lower THC:CBD ratio when compared to sativas resulting in a relative increase in CB2 activation.

EXPLORING MIND–BODY CONSCIOUSNESS

SUGGESTED BLESSING

May you discover the internal point of peace you need to feel the safety and security that you desire.

SUGGESTED AFFIRMATION

I compost all that is fear, worry and stress.

I now believe – the source and genesis for feeling safe and secure lie within me.

Two studies conducted by international teams of scientists using placebos demonstrated the significant therapeutic potential of belief in relieving IBS symptoms.[6,7] Similarly, a meta-analysis of studies on IBS located in Medline since 1996 revealed that, "Psychiatric disorders, especially major depression, anxiety, and somatoform disorders, occur in up to 94% of patients with IBS."[8]

In cases of IBS-C, consider the following observations: "Constipation occurs when an individual was grimly determined to carry on even though faced with a problem he could not solve." Typical statements were (17 patients with constipation): "I have to keep on with this, but I know I'm not going to like it. … It's a lousy job but it's the best I can do. … This marriage is never going to get any better but I won't quit … I'll have to keep on with this but I'm not going to like it. … I'll stick with it even though nothing good will come of it."[9] The authors concluded: "Constipation is a phenomenon of holding on without change." This corresponds to the patients' attitude of trying to continue with things as they are, without hope of immediate improvement or definite desire to do something different.

In cases of IBS-D, consider the following observations: "Diarrhea occurred when an individual wanted to be done with a situation or to have it over with, or to get rid of something or somebody." One man who developed severe diarrhea after he had purchased a defective automobile said: "If I could only get rid of it. … I want to dispose of it." Typical statements of others were: "If the war was only over with. … I wanted to get done with it. … I wanted to get finished with it."[10]

If nausea or vomiting is a persistent problem, consider the following observations: "Nausea and vomiting occurred when an individual was thinking of something which he wished had never happened. He was preoccupied with the mistake he had made, rather than with what he should have done instead. Usually he felt responsible for what happened." Typical statements: "I wish it hadn't happened. … I was sorry I did it. … I wish things were the way they were before. … I made a mistake. … I shouldn't have listened to him."[11] The authors concluded that: "Vomiting is a way of undoing something which has been done. It thus corresponds with the patients' wishes to restore things to their original situation, it is as if nothing ever happened."

AGGRAVATING FACTORS

Major depression / anxiety / somatoform disorders / tendency for negative affect / IBS-C: holding on without change / IBS-D: wanting to get rid of something or somebody / hyper focus on regret or remorse.

Anti-depressive measures / anti-anxiety measures / decipher message of the physical symptoms / tendency for positive affect / IBS-C: work on releasing with ease / IBS-D: work on reducing fear, worry and stress / focus instead on forgiveness, learning from the situatio, and initiating positive action.

TAKE NOTICE

ACACIA • TURMERIC • (E)-B-CARYOPHYLLENE

ACACIA: Research from Minneapolis, Minnesota, suggests acacia improves stool consistency and reduces the occurrence of fecal incontinence in adults.[12] Alternative practitioners in the U.S. have begun to use the highly soluble fiber to ease symptoms of irritable bowel syndrome (IBS). Further studies are under way to determine the mechanism whereby acacia appears to reduce sugar-induced weight gain.

TURMERIC: In this meta-study, scientists gave an overview of decades of scientific studies on turmeric. Turmeric's shared promise as a treatment for adenomatous polyposis (multiple polyps in the large intestines – precursor to colon cancer), inflammatory bowel disease (IBS), and ulcerative colitis (colon inflammation with ulcers).[13]

In a double-blind randomized placebo-controlled human study from Hamamatsu, Japan, scientists examined turmeric's ability to prevent relapse in patients with a history of dormant ulcerative colitis. They concluded that curcumin, an active ingredient in turmeric, seemed to be a safe medication for maintaining remission from ulcerative colitis.[14]

(E)-β-CARYOPHELLENE: is a FDA-approved dietary plant-cannabinoid that activates CB2 receptor sites and initiates potent anti-inflammatory actions. Spice plants known to contain significant amounts of (E)-BCP in include: BLACK "ASHANTI PEPPER" • WHITE "ASHANTI PEPPER" • INDIAN BAY-LEAF • ALLIGATOR PEPPER • BASIL • CINNAMON • ROSEMARY • BLACK CARAWAY • BLACK PEPPER • MEXICAN OREGANO • CLOVE.

For more information on these specific spices, go to Chapter I "Cannabinoid Research."

1 Ford AC, Talley NJ, Spiegel BM, Foxx-Orenstein AE, Schiller L, Quigley EM, Moayyedi P. *Effect of fibre, antispasmodics, and peppermint oil in the treatment of irritable bowel syndrome: systematic review and meta-analysis.* Gastroenterology Division, McMaster University, Health Sciences Centre, 1200 Main Street West, Hamilton, ON, L8N 3Z5, Canada. BMJ. 2008 Nov 13;337:a2313.

2 Izzo AA, Sharkey KA. *Cannabinoids and the gut: new developments and emerging concepts.* Department of Experimental Pharmacology, University of Naples Federico II and Endocannabinoid Research Group, Naples, Italy. Pharmacol Ther. 2010 Apr;126(1):21-38.

3 Lu, Dai1; Kiran Vemuri, V.1; Duclos, Richard I.1; Jr.1; Makriyannis, Alexandros.1 *The Cannabinergic System as a Target for Anti-inflammatory Therapies.* 1 Center for Drug Discovery, Northeastern University, 360 Huntington Avenue, 116 Mugar Hall, Boston, MA, 02115, USA. Current Topics in Medicinal Chemistry, Volume 6, Number 13, July 2006 , pp. 1401-1426(26). Bentham Science Publishers.

4 Storr MA, Keenan CM, Emmerdinger D, Zhang H, Yüce B, Sibaev A, Massa F, Buckley NE, Lutz B, Göke B, Brand S, Patel KD, Sharkey KA. *Targeting endocannabinoid degradation protects against experimental colitis in mice: involvement of CB(1) and CB (2) receptors.* Division of Gastroenterology, Department of Medicine, University of Calgary, 3280 Hospital Dr. N.W., Calgary, Alberta, T2N 4N1, Canada. J Mol Med. 2008 May 21.

5 R Capasso,1 F Borrelli,1 G Aviello,1 B Romano,1 C Scalisi,1,2 F Capasso,1 and A Izzo1* *Cannabidiol, extracted from Cannabis sativa, selectively inhibits inflammatory hypermotility in mice.* 1Department of Experimental Pharmacology, University of Naples Federico II and Endocannabinoid Research Group, Naples, Italy. *Author for correspondence: Email: aaizzo@unina.it 2Current address: Human Physiology Section, Department of Experimental Medicine, University of Palermo, corso Tukory 129, 90134 Palermo, Italy. Br J Pharmacol. 2008 July; 154(5): 1001–1008.

6 Ted J. Kaptchuk1,2*, Elizabeth Friedlander1, John M. Kelley3,4, M. Norma Sanchez1, Efi Kokkotou1, Joyce P. Singer2, Magda Kowalczykowski1, Franklin G. Miller5, Irving Kirsch6, Anthony J. Lembo1. *Placebos without Deception: A Randomized Controlled Trial in Irritable Bowel Syndrome.* 1 Beth Israel Deaconess Medical Center, Harvard Medical School, Boston, Massachusetts, United States of America, 2 Osher Research Center, Harvard Medical School, Boston, Massachusetts, United States of America, 3 Psychology Department, Endicott College, Beverly, Massachusetts, United States of America, 4 Massachusetts General Hospital, Harvard Medical School, Boston, Massachusetts, United States of America, 5 Department of Bioethics, National Institutes of Health, Bethesda, Maryland, United States of America, 6 Department of Psychology, University of Hull, Hull, United Kingdom. PLoS ONE 5(12): e15591. doi:10.1371/journal.pone.0015591

7 Ted J Kaptchuk, associate professor of medicine1, John M Kelley, assistant professor of psychology and statistics2, Lisa A Conboy, instructor of medicine1, Roger B Davis, associate professor of medicine and biostatistics3, Catherine E Kerr, instructor of medicine1, Eric E Jacobson, lecturer4, Irving Kirsch, professor of psychology5, Rosa N Schyner, research associate1, Bong Hyun Nam, research fellow1, Long T Nguyen, research fellow1, Min Park, research coordinator1, Andrea L Rivers, research coordinator1, Claire McManus, research coordinator1, Efi Kokkotou, assistant professor of medicine3, Douglas A Drossman, professor of medicine6, Peter Goldman, professor emeritus 7, Anthony J Lembo, assistant professor of medicine3 *Components of placebo effect: randomised controlled trial in patients with irritable bowel syndrome.* BMJ 336 : 999 doi: 10.1136/ bmj.39524.439618.25 (Published 3 April 2008).

8 Whitehead WE, Palsson O, Jones KR. *Systematic review of the comorbidity of irritable bowel syndrome with other disorders: what are the causes and implications?* Division of Digestive Diseases and Center for Functional Gastrointestinal and Motility Disorders, University of North Carolina, Chapel Hill, North Carolina 27599, USA. Gastroenterology. 2002 Apr;122(4):1140-56.

9 William J. Grace, M.D. and David T. Graham, M.D. *Relationship of Specific Attitudes and Emotions to Certain Bodily Diseases.* Dept. of Medicine, of the New York Hospital-Cornell Medical Center. Psychosomatic Medicine July 1, 1952 vol. 14 no. 4 243-251.

10 Ibid.

11 William J. Grace, M.D. and David T. Graham, M.D. *Relationship of Specific Attitudes and Emotions to Certain Bodily Diseases.* Dept. of Medicine, of the New York Hospital-Cornell Medical Center. Psychosomatic Medicine July 1, 1952 vol. 14 no. 4 243-251.

12 Bliss DZ, Jung HJ, Savik K, Lowry A, LeMoine M, Jensen L, Werner C, Schaffer K. *Supplementation with dietary fiber improves fecal incontinence.* School of Nursing, University of Minnesota, Minneapolis 55455, USA. Nurs Res. 2001 Jul-Aug;50(4):203-13.

13 Goel A, Kunnumakkara AB, Aggarwal BB. Curcumin as "Curecumin": From kitchen to clinic. Gastrointestinal Cancer Research Laboratory, Department of Internal Medicine, Charles A. Sammons Cancer Center and Baylor Research Institute, Baylor University Medical Center, Dallas, TX, United States. Biochem Pharmacol. 2007 Aug 19.

14 Hanai H, Iida T, Takeuchi K, Watanabe F, Maruyama Y, Andoh A, Tsujikawa T, Fujiyama Y, Mitsuyama K, Sata M, Yamada M, Iwaoka Y, Kanke K, Hiraishi H, Hirayama K, Arai H, Yoshii S, Uchijima M, Nagata T, Koide Y. *Curcumin maintenance therapy for ulcerative colitis: randomized, multicenter, double-blind, placebo-controlled trial.* Department of Endoscopic and Photodynamic Medicine, Hamamatsu University School of Medicine, and Center for Gastroenterology, Hamamatsu South Hospital, Hamamatsu, Japan. Clin Gastroenterol Hepatol. 2006 Dec;4(12):1502-6.

Inflammatory Diseases
Gastrointestinal Inflammatory Diseases
Gastro-esophageal Reflux Disease (GERD)

NUMBER OF STUDIES: 1

CHI VALUE: 7

Commonly known as heartburn and acid reflux disease, this illness is due to damage of the esophageal mucus membrane and the esophageal sphincter. Damage occurs when stomach acid reaches the lower part of the esophagus. Under normal conditions, the esophageal sphincter opens to allow food and drink to enter the stomach but closes right after to prevent stomach acid from affecting the tissue above. In GERD, however, the closing action is temporarily incomplete allowing acid to reach unprotected tissue causing damage. This mechanism is also referred to as transient lower esophageal sphincter relaxations (TLESRs). Symptoms include: heartburn, regurgitation (tasting ones stomach contents), pain when swallowing, nausea, vomiting (especially in children), and chest pains (often with burning sensation).

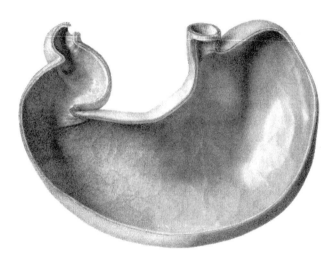

GERD-produced damage can lead to long-term problems and acute episodes. Allopathic treatments include pharmaceuticals and surgery, each with their own risks and side effects.

Effective management may include life style changes such as not eating for two hours before lying down, sleeping slightly elevated and a more alkaline diet.

CANNABIS AND GERD

As in other studies, the therapeutic effects of cannabinoids seems to have a dose specific therapeutic window warranting a cautious and gradual approach to using cannabinoids for treatment of GERD. Dutch researchers (2009) discovered that among the many controlling actions, cannabinoid receptors CB1 and CB2 aid in triggering TLESRs in humans. Additionally, researchers noted that while 10mg doses of THC significantly inhibited the increase in meal-induced TLESRs and reduced spontaneous swallowing in dogs and humans, dosage levels of 20mg caused some volunteers to experience nausea, vomiting, hypotension, rapid heart rates and other central effects. To protect the participants from the dose-dependent side effects, scientists discontinued dosage tests at 20mg before the study design reached its parameters.[1]

STUDY SUMMARY:

Drugs	Type of Study	Published Year, Place, and Key Results	CHI
THC (dogs) THC (humans) 10mg and 20mg	Trial on healthy human (placebo controlled) volunteers and dogs.	2009 – Academic Medical Centre, Department of Gastroenterology and Hepatology, Amsterdam, The Netherlands. THC significantly inhibited the increase in meal-induced TLESRs and reduced spontaneous swallowing in both dogs and humans. High doses produced side effects.	5+2

Total CHI Value 7

STRAIN SPECIFIC CONSIDERATIONS

Both CB1 and CB2 may be involved in triggering TLESRs in humans. THC binds with both CB1 and CB2 relatively equally.

Both sativas and indicas contain cannabinoids, which activate CB1 and CB2.

EXPLORING MIND–BODY CONSCIOUSNESS

One study conducted on 60 patients diagnosed with heartburn concluded that, "As with other chronic conditions such as irritable bowel syndrome (IBS), heartburn severity appears to be most responsive to major life events and not an accumulation of more minor stressors or fluctuations in mood. In addition, vital exhaustion, which may in part result from sustained stress, may represent the psychophysiological symptom complex most closely associated with heartburn exacerbation."[2]

Another experiment using 19 healthy volunteers demonstrated that the introduction of anxiety increases acid-induced esophageal hyperalgesia (increased sensitivity to pain).[3]

AGGRAVATING FACTORS

Major life events / vital exhaustion due to sustained stress or anxiety.

HEALING FACTORS

Healing the damage done by major life events / rest / anxiety intervention / reducing fear, worry and stress.

1 Beaumont H, Jensen J, Carlsson A, Ruth M, Lehmann A, Boeckxstaens GE. *Effect of Delta(9)-tetrahydrocannabinol, a cannabinoid receptor agonist, on the triggering of transient lower oesophageal sphincter relaxations in dogs and humans.* Academic Medical Centre, Department of Gastroenterology and Hepatology, Amsterdam, The Netherlands. Br J Pharmacol. 2009 Jan;156(1):153-62.

2 Bruce D. Naliboff, PhD, Minou Mayer, MA, MFT, Ronnie Fass, MD, Leah Z. Fitzgerald, RN, MS, Lin Chang, MD, Roger Bolus, PhD and Emeran A. Mayer, MD. *The Effect of Life Stress on Symptoms of Heartburn.* Center

for Neurovisceral Sciences & Women's Health, Departments of Medicine (M.M., L.C., L.Z.F., R.B., E.A.M.), Physiology (E.A.M.), Psychiatry & Biobehavioral Sciences (B.D.N., E.A.M.), UCLA, Los Angeles, CA; Greater Los Angeles Healthcare System, VA Medical Center (B.D.N.), Los Angeles, CA; and University of Arizona/VA Medical Center GI Division (R.F.), Tucson, AZ. Psychosomatic Medicine 66:426-434 (2004).

3 Abhishek Sharma, MD, PhD, Lukas Van Oudenhove, MD, PhD, Peter Paine, MD, PhD, Lloyd Gregory, PhD and Qasim Aziz, MD, PhD. *Anxiety Increases Acid-Induced Esophageal Hyperalgesia.* GI Science Group (A.S., P.P.), Salford Royal NHS Foundation Trust, Salford, United Kingdom; Department of Pathophysiology (L.V.O.), Gastroenterology Section, Department of Neurosciences, Psychiatry Division, University of Leuven, University Hospital Gasthuisberg, Leuven, Belgium; The University of Manchester (L.G.), Manchester Academic Health Science Centre, Salford Royal NHS Foundation Trust, R&D Directorate, Salford, United Kingdom; Centre for Digestive Diseases (Q.A.), Wingate Institute of Neurogastroenterology, Barts, and The London School of Medicine and Dentistry, Queen Mary, University of London, United Kingdom. Psychosomatic Medicine October 2010 vol. 72 no. 8 802-809.

Inflammatory Diseases
Pancreatitis

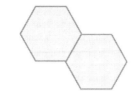

NUMBER OF STUDIES: 2

CHI VALUE: 3

The pancreas is both an endocrine gland secreting hormones such as insulin, glucagons, somatostatin and a digestive organ producing digestive juices containing enzymes vital to the break down of food particles and their molecular absorption in the small intestines. Pancreatitis, an inflammation of the pancreas, occurs when the digestive enzymes are activated while still in the pancreas, causing the breakdown of cells while still inside the organ. The resulting irritation and inflammation cause the symptoms associated with the disease.

The pancreas is a vital organ and the human body cannot exist without it. A damaged or impaired pancreas can lead to digestive difficulties and the development of diabetes. Orthodox medicine identifies numerous reasons for pancreatitis. The chief culprits leading the way are alcoholism and gallbladder stones. Other causes include toxic pharmaceutical medication such as those used to treat AIDS, abdominal surgeries or injuries and high concentrations of minerals, fats or parathyroid hormones.

Symptoms may vary between acute and chronic versions of the disease but usually include upper abdominal pains. Diagnostic tools may include: physical examinations, blood tests screening for concentrations of pancreatic enzymes, stool samples determining the presence of undigested fat, the use of imaging devices such as magnetic resonance imaging (MRI), CT-scans utilizing ionizing radiation (x-rays), ultrasound and endoscopic ultrasound. Treatment plans unfold depending on the underlying cause and may include intravenous fluids, pharmaceutical medications, surgeries or dietary restrictions (no alcohol, smoking or fat).

CANNABIS AND PANCREATITIS

While cannabinoids have been shown to ameliorate liver fibrosis, their effects in chronic pancreatitis and on pancreatic stellate cells mostly remain unknown. However, during recent investigations, an international group of scientists discovered that CB1 and CB2 receptors are found in the human pancreas and that the administration of synthetic cannabinoids constituted a novel option in treatment of inflammation and fibrosis in chronic pancreatitis.[1]

Study results inconsistent: it would appear that in some cases, cannabinoids such as anandamide have a therapeutic effect on acute pancreatitis; at other times, their treatment produced an aggravation of the acute inflammation. This international team of researchers (2008) explained the apparently paradoxical nature of earlier study results. They wrote: "… the effect of anandamide on the severity of acute pancreatitis depends on the phase of this disease. Administration of anandamide, before induction of pancreatitis, aggravates pancreatic damage; whereas anandamide administered after induction of pancreatitis, reduces the severity of acute pancreatitis."[2]

STUDY SUMMARY:

Drugs	Type of Study	Published Year, Place, and Key Results	CHI
Synthetic Cannabinoid	Laboratory	2008 – various International Scientific Institutions. Positive treatment option for inflammation and fibrosis in chronic pancreatitis.	1
Anandamide	Animal study (rats)	2008 – Department of Physiology, Jagiellonian University Medical College, Krakow, Poland. Effect of anandamide on the severity of acute pancreatitis depends on the phase of this disease.	2

Total CHI Value   3

STRAIN SPECIFIC CONSIDERATIONS

CB1 and CB2 receptors are present in the human pancreas. Research has shown that CB1 and CB2 activation may positively affect pancreatitis - at least in preclinical animal trials. Anandamide binds relatively equally to both CB1 and CB2 as does THC.

Sativa and sativa dominant strains contain higher THC:CBD ratios when compared to indicas or indica heavy hybrids.

EXPLORING MIND – BODY CONSCIOUSNESS

SUGGESTED BLESSING

May I discover a new depth of self-respect.

In a Japanese study conducted on 69 patients with chronic pancreatitis, researchers used a comparative analysis to examine potential psychosomatic influences.[3]

Suspicious type – (actual psychosomatic disease), primarily related to psychosomatic factors.	Definite type – (character psychosomatic disease), primarily manifested as chronic alcohol-drinking habits.
Significantly more psychological complaints, including neurotic reactions.	Significantly more compulsive tendencies and incidences of stern discipline, compulsive parents, dominant fathers and separation experiences.

SUGGESTED AFFIRMATION

I honor all of my emotions safely and appropriately.

If the heart is where we feel our emotions and the liver where we process them, then the pancreas represents the space where we gather, collect and store them. Difficulty with this organ may arise when we refuse to put our emotional life into perspective. Refusing to integrate our emotional experiences or being irritated/inflamed by the idea of having to give dimensions to our emotional reality may warrant a message. Emotions are central to the human experience. Emotions are normal and natural; and the degree to which we diminish their importance in life is the degree with which we diminish self-respect.

QUESTIONS

Do I feel like a victim to my feelings and emotions?
Do I place any value on feelings and emotions?
Do I want to numb myself to my emotions?

AGGRAVATING FACTORS

De-valuing emotions and ignoring the importance of our emotional experience.

HEALING FACTORS

Learning to feel and express all emotions appropriately, without hurting anyone.

TAKE NOTICE

TURMERIC

TURMERIC: In a large meta-study, scientists provided an overview of decades of scientific analysis on turmeric. Turmeric's potential therapeutic value in the treatment of pancreatitis was noted.[4]

1 Christoph W. Michalski,#1,2* Milena Maier,#2 Mert Erkan,#1 Danguole Sauliunaite,1 Frank Bergmann,3 Pal Pacher,4 Sandor Batkai,4 Nathalia A. Giese,2 Thomas Giese,5 Helmut Friess,1 and Jörg Kleeff.1 *Cannabinoids Reduce Markers of Inflammation and Fibrosis in Pancreatic Stellate Cells* 1Department of Surgery, Technische Universität München, Munich, Germany2Department of General Surgery, University of Heidelberg, Heidelberg, Germany 3Institute of Pathology, University of Heidelberg, Heidelberg, Germany 4Section of Oxidative Stress Tissue Injury, Laboratory of Physiologic Studies, National Institutes of Health, National Institute on Alcohol Abuse and Alcoholism (NIAAA), Bethesda, Maryland, United States of America 5Institute of Immunology, University of Heidelberg, Heidelberg, Germany. Christian Gluud, Academic Editor Copenhagen University Hospital, Denmark. #Contributed equally. PLoS ONE. 2008; 3(2): e1701.

2 Dembiński A, Warzecha Z, Ceranowicz P, Warzecha AM, Pawlik WW, Dembiński M, Rembiasz K, Sendur P, Kuśnierz-Cabala B, Tomaszewska R, Chowaniec E, Konturek PC. *Dual, time-dependent deleterious and protective effect of anandamide on the course of cerulein-induced acute pancreatitis. Role of sensory nerves.* Department of Physiology, Jagiellonian University Medical College, Krakow, Poland. mpdembin@cyf-kr.edu.pl Eur J Pharmacol. 2008 Sep 4;591(1-3):284-92.

3 Nakai Y, Araki T, Takahashi S, Shimada A, Nakagawa T. *Chronic pancreatitis as psychosomatic disorder.* Psychother Psychosom. 1983;39(4):201-12.

4 Goel A, Kunnumakkara AB, Aggarwal BB. *Curcumin as "Curecumin": From kitchen to clinic.* Gastrointestinal Cancer Research Laboratory, Department of Internal Medicine, Charles A. Sammons Cancer Center and Baylor Research Institute, Baylor University Medical Center, Dallas, TX, United States. Biochem Pharmacol. 2007 Aug 19.

Inflammatory Diseases
Peridontitis

NUMBER OF STUDIES: 1

CHI VALUE: 2

Periodontitis is an inflammation of the tissues that support the teeth. Thought to be caused by oral microbes and an overzealous immune response, it leads to the reduction of tissue support and alveolar bone-loss. The process of resorption initiates this deficiency where bone cells leak substances and become weak.

Symptoms may include painful swelling of the gums and tissue surrounding the teeth, tissue reduction, deep pockets around the teeth, bad breath (halitosis) and loose teeth. Periodontitis may also be implicated in the development of heart attacks, strokes and atherosclerosis.

Orthodox medical treatments include deep cleaning, surgical cleaning and interventions. Alternative treatments may involve solutions of hydrogen peroxide or other oral oxidants.

CANNABIS AND PERIODONTITIS

The first known study to examine the therapeutic effects of cannabidiol on resorption-produced periodontitis took place in Brazil in 2009. The analysis demonstrated that CBD-treated rats presented a reduction of alveolar bone loss. The authors wrote: "These results indicate that CBD may be useful to control bone resorption during progression of experimental periodontitis in rats."[1]

STUDY SUMMARY:

Drugs	Type of Study	Published Year, Place, and Key Results	CHI
Cannabidiol (CBD)	Animal study (rats)	2009 – Laboratory of Molecular Biology, University of Uberaba, Brazil. CBD may be useful to control bone resorption.	2

Total CHI Value   2

STRAIN SPECIFIC CONSIDERATIONS

CB1 and CB2 receptors are found in bone tissue. Anandamide is produced in bone and synovial tissue. The pre-clinical trial conducted on animals discovered that CBD aided in mitigating periodontitis, at least in animals. CBD has a greater affinity for CB2.

Indica and indica dominant stains tend to contain a lower THC:CBD ratio, resulting in a relatively higher activation of CB2.

EXPLORING MIND–BODY CONSCIOUSNESS

Studies have identified possible psychological, behavioral, physiological and demographic risk factors implicated in the progression of simple gingivitis to the development of periodontitis. Relationships have been observed between on-going stressors such as financial difficulties, grief, caring for a spouse with Alzheimer's disease (or other dementias), depressed mood, perceived and ongoing stress or hassles. Physiological responses included elevation in pro-inflammatory cytokines and a reduction of salivary flow. Both contributed to reducing the body's ability to properly respond to bacterial infection's role in increasing the risk for peridontitis.[2]

Taking a bite out of the apple of life has become an impossible or painful experience. Similarly being able to chew and enjoy solid foods has become an irritation or a thing of the past. Chronic stressors are eroding the substance of once solid bone tissue. Bones are a physiological foundation on which the layers of the body build and rely. When this foundation erodes, it may help to examine foundational issues related to family.

It is easy to imagine the chronic stress that comes with seeing your spouse slip away into the void. Scientists have determined that caregivers of spouses who suffer from dementia are more than twice as likely to develop oral bone loss as non-caregivers.[3] Studies of this nature may speak to the emotional impact of an eroding foundation of a family union.

SUGGESTED BLESSING:

May you reach for new depth, new horizons and expanded complexities of belonging.

SUGGESTED AFFIRMATION:

I release all that is not love from the core of my life.

QUESTIONS

Can I identify any on-going stressors eroding my sense of foundation/family?
Are the stressors man-made or unavoidable?
If they are avoidable, where can I ask for help through these trying times?
Could I infuse acceptance, forgiveness or gratitude into my process?
What new choice(s) may provide safe and new direction?

AGGRAVATING FACTORS

Chronic mental and emotional stressors / stress to family foundations (past or current).

HEALING FACTORS

Reducing fear, worry and stress / applying positive affect-producing-qualities such as forgiveness, acceptance, gratitude, etc., to the process involving significant life changes.

TAKE NOTICE

Floss your teeth regularly and consider this homemade, anti-inflammatory, anti-bacterial tooth powder for brushing your teeth after each meal:

Mix equal parts of the following: xylitol, a healthy and "tooth friendly" sugar, ideally made from birch bark, included for caries prevention and its anti-bacterial properties; And sodium bicarbonate ($NaHCO_3$/baking soda), used to increase oral pH, which acts as an antiseptic and neutralize the acidic environment of the mouth. Add cinnamon, cardamom, nutmeg or ginger for taste and for their combined anti-bacterial, anticaries[4] and anti-inflammatory properties. Moisten your toothbrush, dip it into the mixed powder and brush your teeth.

1 Napimoga MH, Benatti BB, Lima FO, Alves PM, Campos AC, Pena-Dos-Santos DR, Severino FP, Cunha FQ, Guimarães FS. *Cannabidiol decreases bone resorption by inhibiting RANK/RANKL expression and pro-inflammatory cytokines during experimental periodontitis in rats*. Laboratory of Molecular Biology, University of Uberaba, Brazil. Int Immunopharmacol. 2009 Feb;9(2):216-22.

2 Peter P. Vitaliano, PhD, Rutger Persson, DDS, PhD, Asuman Kiyak, PhD, Hardeep Saini, BS and Diana Echeverria, PhD. *Caregiving and Gingival Symptom Reports: Psychophysiologic Mediators*. Department of Psychiatry and Behavioral Sciences (P.P.V., H.S.), Department of Periodontics (R.P.), and Department of Oral and Maxillofacial Surgery (A.K.), University of Washington, Seattle, Washington; Battelle Centers for Public Health Research & Evaluation, Seattle, Washington (D.E.). Psychosomatic Medicine 67:930-938 (2005).

3 Ibid.

4 Gazzani G, Daglia M, Papetti A. *Food components with anticaries activity*. Department of Drug Sciences, Pavia University, Viale Taramelli 12, 27100 Pavia, Italy. Curr Opin Biotechnol. 2012 Apr;23(2):153-9.

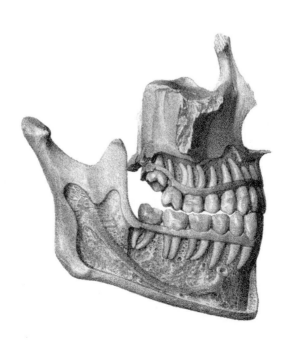

Inflammatory Diseases
Rheumatoid Arthritis

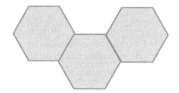

NUMBER OF STUDIES: 3

CHI VALUE: 10

Rheumatoid arthritis is the most crippling form of arthritis, deforming joints and bending bodies. It is considered an autoimmune disorder, which apparently occurs when something goes wrong with the body's immune system itself and it attacks healthy parts of the body such as joints. One can tell long-time rheumatoid arthritis sufferers from a distance. Their joints take on a gnarly appearance.

CANNABIS AND RHEUMATOID ARTHRITIS

In 2006, researchers from the UK enrolled 58 patients with RA in a double blind, placebo controlled study to determine the effect of cannabinoids on pain and other symptoms. The results indicated that patients who received the cannabinoids slept better and experienced a reduction in pain when compared to the placebo group. Researchers wrote: "In the first ever controlled trial of a CBM in RA, a significant analgesic effect was observed and disease activity was significantly suppressed following Sativex treatment."[1]

Boston scientists (2006) acknowledged that "Habitual cannabis use has been shown to [positively] affect the human immune system, and recent advances in endocannabinoid research provide a basis for understanding these immunomodulatory effects. Cell-based experiments, or in vivo animal testing, suggest that regulation of the endocannabinoid circuitry can impact almost every major function associated with the immune system." After testing numerous novel molecules that exert their biological effects through the endocannabinoid system, the researchers suggested the therapeutic potential of cannabinoids on inflammatory diseases such as rheumatoid arthritis.[2]

A 2009 Worcester, Massachusetts meta-analysis of studies on cannabinoids in the context of pain is instructive.[3] Results showed that all types of cannabinoids as well as noncannabinoid parts of the plant effectively reduce pain from inflammation found in post-surgery patients, rheumatism, rheumatoid arthritis, chronic neuropathic pain and fibromyalgia.

STUDY SUMMARY:

Drugs	Type of Study	Published Year, Place, and Key Results	CHI
All types of can-nabinoids (endog-enous, plant-based and synthetic)	Meta-analysis (2004-2009)	2009 – University of Massachusetts Medical School. Can-nabinoids effective in reducing pain from rheumatoid ar-thritis.	4
Cannabinoids	Laboratory	2006 – Center for Drug Discovery, Northeastern Univer-sity, Boston, MA. Potentially useful in reduction of inflam-mation.	1
Sativex (sublingual spray) daily in the evening		2006 – Multi-Institutional Study. Randomized, double-blind, parallel group study on patients with RA Improve-ment in sleep and reduction in pain.	5

Total CHI Value   10

STRAIN SPECIFIC CONSIDERATIONS

Sativex, produced by a large pharmaceutical corporation, is an oromucosal mouth spray consisting of roughly equal parts of THC(2.7mg) and CBD(2.5mg). Sativex is not synthetic, but rather made from cannabis. However, the formulation ratios are very similar when compared to actual cannabis sativa ratios.

Sativa and sativa prominent hybrids contain relatively higher THC:CBD ratios and thus activate CB1 and CB2.

EXPLORING MIND–BODY CONSCIOUSNESS

Researchers from Ann Arbor looking at psychological factors in the development of rheumatoid arthritis "…suggested that the rheumatoids communicate poorly with their relatives about their hurt feelings."[4]

Auto-immune diseases may mirror an intense and likely longstanding conflict of belief and the dueling emotions this elicits. H. Levitan, M.D. studied onset situa-tions in rheumatoid arthritis.[5] A case study of three female patients with the disease revealed two shared mental/emotional denominators. First, upon onset of the dis-ease, each woman was in a relationship that produced at once intense rage and love for her partner. These patients hated their relationships but were too dependent to leave them behind. Second, neither woman acted out her anger but had to endure the abuse that elicited the rage and also the impact of her own unexpressed feel-ings. Thus, the unexpressed intense emotions produced by conflicting beliefs such as 'without my husband I am on the street' or 'it is not OK to feel angry' might have contribtuted to an internal experience of dependency misinterpreted as love and silent rage respectively.

In another study of 33 patients (4 male, 29 female) with rheumatoid arthritis, researchers concluded, "In these cases the general psychodynamic background is a chronic inhibited hostile aggressive state as a reaction to the earliest masochistic dependence on the mother that is carried over to the father and all human relation-ships, including the sexual. The majority of these personalities learn to discharge hostility through masculine competition, physical activity, and serving, and also through domination of the family."[6]

What is eating away at me (in my affected joint(s)?
Also see ARTHRITIS.

AGGRAVATING FACTORS

Having to endure abuse perpetrated by a perceived authority (God, priest, leader, husband), leading to suppressed hurt and unexpressed rage with both, combining to form hostility / unexpressed feelings / conflicting beliefs / hostility comprised of anger and hurt directed at oneself.

HEALING FACTORS

Discover and release repressed and/or suppressed feelings and emotions / develop an appreciation of our emotional nature and the entire emotional spectrum of which humans are capable / Replace conflicting and unhealthy belief(s) with those that will engender love, caring and compassion / Find, embrace, feel, release and forgive all lingering hurt and angers.

TAKE NOTICE

CAYENNE • MYRRH • NIGELLA • ROSEMARY • TURMERIC

• (E)-β-CARYOPHYLLENE

CAYENNE: Cayenne stimulates peripheral circulation. In Cuba, a topical tincture and cream is used to treat chronic aches and pains of lumbago, arthritis and rheumatism.[7]

MYRRH: This study conducted by the University of Cincinnati, Ohio, confirmed physiological benefits of myrrh, used for thousands of years in the treatment of arthritis. Myrrh modulates inflammatory responses.[8]

NIGELLA: A study conducted at the Yüzüncü Yil University, Turkey, demonstrated that the volatile oil of nigella can suppress artificially induced arthritis in rats. Nigella has historically been used in the treatment of arthritis and other chronic inflammatory conditions.[9]

ROSEMARY: German Commission E has approved rosemary for "External: Supportive therapy for rheumatic diseases, circulatory problems."

TURMERIC: The World Health Organization (W.H.O.) Monographs on selected Medicinal Plants describes the uses of turmeric in pharmacopoeias and in traditional systems of medicine: "Treatment of … pain and inflammation due to rheumatoid arthritis…."

(E)-β-CARYOPHYLLENE This FDA-approved food-based plant-cannabinoid activates CB2 receptor sites and initiates potent anti-inflammatory actions.

Spice plants known to contain significant amounts of (E)-BCP in include: BLACK "ASHANTI PEPPER" • WHITE "ASHANTI PEPPER" • INDIAN BAY-LEAF • ALLIGATOR PEPPER • BASIL • CINNAMON • ROSEMARY • BLACK CARAWAY • BLACK PEPPER • MEXICAN OREGANO • CLOVE.

For more information on these specific spices, go to Chapter I "Cannabinoid Research."

1 D. R. Blake, P. Robson1, M. Ho2, R. W. Jubb3 and C. S. McCabe. *Preliminary assessment of the efficacy, tolerability and safety of a cannabis-based medicine (Sativex) in the treatment of pain caused by rheumatoid arthritis.* Royal National Hospital for Rheumatic Diseases, Bath, 1 Cannabinoid Research Institute, Oxford Science Park, Oxford, 2 Department of Rheumatology, Northampton General Hospital, Northampton and 3 Department of Rheumatology, Selly Oak Hospital, Birmingham, UK. Rheumatology 2006 45(1):50-52.

2 Lu, Dai1; Kiran Vemuri, V.1; Duclos, Richard I.1; Jr.1; Makriyannis, Alexandros.1 *The Cannabinergic System as a Target for Anti-inflammatory Therapies.* 1 Center for Drug Discovery, Northeastern University, 360 Huntington Avenue, 116 Mugar Hall, Boston, MA, 02115, USA. Current Topics in Medicinal Chemistry, Volume 6, Number 13, July 2006 , pp. 1401-1426(26). Bentham Science Publishers.

3 Sumner H. Burstein1,2 and Robert B. Zurier2. *Cannabinoids, Endocannabinoids, and Related Analogs in Inflammation.* 1Department of Biochemistry & Molecular Pharmacology, University of Massachusetts Medical School, 364 Plantation St., Worcester, Massachusetts 01605 USA. 2Department of Medicine, University of Massachusetts Medical School, 364 Plantation St., Worcester, Massachusetts 01605 USA. AAPS J. 2009 March; 11(1): 109–119.

4 Sidney Cobb M.D., Stanislav V. Kasl Ph.D., Edith Chen M.A. and Roger Christenfeld M.A. *Some psychological and social characteristics of patients hospitalized for rheumatoid arthritis, hypertension, and duodenal ulcer.* Institute for Social Research, The University of Michigan, Ann Arbor, Michigan, USA. Journal of Chronic Diseases. Volume 18, Issue 12, December 1965, Pages 1259-1278.

5 Stanley Cheren, M.D., Harold Levitan M.D. Psychosomatic Medicine: Theory, Physiology and Practice. Vol. 1. Chapter 4. *Onset Situation in Three Psychosomatic Illnesses.* 1989. International University Press, Inc. Madison, Connecticut.

6 DELAIDE JOHNSON, M.D., LOUIS B; SHAPIRO, M.D., and FRANZ ALEXANDER, M.D. *Preliminary Report on a Psychosomatic Study of Rheumatoid Arthritis.* Institute of Psycho-analysis, Chicago. September 1947.

7 *Therapeutic Guide to Plant Pharmaceuticals and Honey Pharmaceuticals (Guia Terapeutica Dispensarial de Fitofarmacos y Apifarmacos* - Ministerio de Salud Publica, Ciudad de La Habana - Republica de Cuba 1992). Cuban Ministry of Public Health, Havana.

8 Khanna D, Sethi G, Ahn KS, Pandey MK, Kunnumakkara AB, Sung B, Aggarwal A, Aggarwal BB. *Natural products as a gold mine for arthritis treatment.* Division of Immunology, Department of Medicine, University of Cincinnati, Cincinnati, OH, USA. Curr Opin Pharmacol. 2007 Jun;7(3):344-51.

9 Tekeoglu I, Dogan A, Ediz L, Budancamanak M, Demirel A. *Effects of thymoquinone (volatile oil of black cumin) on rheumatoid arthritis in rat models.* Yuzuncu Yil University, Medical School, Department of Rehabilitation and Rheumatology, Turkey. Phytother Res. 2007 Sep;21(9):895-7.

Insomnia

NUMBER OF STUDIES: 1

CHI VALUE: 5

Insomnia is the difficulty or inability to fall or stay asleep. While many possible causes exist for insomnia, it is interesting to note that its preceding symptoms mirror the condition's effects. Depending on the severity, insomnia affects mental and physical performance as well as emotional expressions (sufferers become moody or irritable). Insomnia may produce symptoms of anxiety, depression, low energy and affect, fatigue, hallucinations, lowered immunity, and hormone disruption - each with its own set of possible complications (i.e., hypertension or heart disease).

If insomnia follows acute pain, jet leg or a new work schedule, it is usually self-correcting with time. Insomnia due to other causes is more complex. Insomnia caused by anxiety or use of addictive substances (such as methamphetamines), require more time and active intervention to resolve.

Orthodox medicine's approach to dealing with insomnia includes diagnostics to determine underlying causes. Common pharmacological treatments for insomnia may include: psycho-active benzodiazepines such as valium (can be addictive), sedative-hypnotic drugs like ambien (can be addictive), opiates for the co-treatment of pain (can be addictive), and antidepressants (possible serious side effects). While these agents help manage the symptoms, none of these medications cure chronic insomnia, which usually returns once the medication is stopped.

CANNABIS AND INSOMNIA

Like cannabis, the majority of common pharmacological treatments for insomnia affect both the body as well as the mind. Most studies on the effects of cannabis and sleep took place in the 70s and 80s.[1] These early studies revealed that cannabis had a varied impact on sleep. The plant seems to act like a sedative in some ways but also reduced deep sleep. None of the early studies explained this paradoxical influence. However, the Farnborough study[2] revealed an apparent self-balancing mechanism between CBD and THC. Dose dependent THC appears to have sedative effects while dose dependent CBD appears to have some alerting properties.

STUDY SUMMARY:

Drugs	Type of Study	Published Year, Place, and Key Results	CHI
4 treatments were an oromucosal spray of either placebo or 15mg THC or 5 mg THC with 5 mg CBD or 15 mg THC with 15 mg CBD.	8 healthy human volunteers (4 males, 4 females; 21 to 34 years old)	2004 - QinetiQ Ltd, Centre for Human Sciences, Farnborough, Hampshire, UK. THC appears to have some sedative effects. CBD appears to have some alerting properties.	5

Total CHI Value 5

STRAIN SPECIFIC CONSIDERATIONS

Practical reports from patients using cannabis to improve their sleep have shown that the use of indica and indica dominant strains and their particular mix of cannabinoid ratios, namely a relatively lower THC:CBD combination, encourage sedation, relaxation and grounding effects.

EXPLORING MIND–BODY CONSCIOUSNESS

Researchers discovered that insomniac patient populations appear to have two characteristic traits, which may make them vulnerable to developing the disorder but also provide a potential basis for therapeutic interventions. Commonly noted traits of insomniacs include a poor mechanism for managing stress, and states of cognitive-emotional hyper arousal (exaggerated mental-emotional responses and/or tensions).[3]

Since both insomnia and hyper arousal are commonly noted symptoms in post-traumatic stress disorders, some clinicians suggest a potential similar connection with past traumatic events in cases of insomniacs.

Whatever the physical reasons for insomnia may be, a commonly observed thread is the inability to let go and relax. The mind is constantly engaged in thinking to a point where it could be considered excessive, suggesting a belief(s) that forces the mind to control and dominate the thinking process itself. Relaxation and surrender to sleep can happen only when everything is worked out perfectly, which of course will never happen. The mind can always come up with another thing that could go wrong. Within the insomniac's mind, undefined feelings produce on-going anxieties; omnipresent fears create the constant need for control; guilt induces the constant threat of imagined punishment and the need to protect one-self f; and self-depreciating self-talk seems endless.

Regular, deep and restful sleep usually returns once the person learns to trust the process of life.

QUESTIONS

What is going to happen if I let go and fall asleep?
I cannot trust myself because…?
I cannot trust life because…?
Can I let go of these definitions or beliefs?
What must I believe to have a peaceful slumber and restful sleep?

AGGRAVATING FACTORS

Chronic stress/ poor mechanisms for managing stress / unresolved past traumatic events (consider insomnia in the context of PTSD) / fear-based belief(s) / inappropriate trust.

SUGGESTED BLESSING:

May our flower help you to retrieve your imagination from the cesspool of fear.

May you remember that you are the director of your internal experiences.

Consider taking your imagination and boldly going where fear does not dare to tread.

SUGGESTED AFFIRMATION:

The day is over, this day is gone.

I release the day and all the good and bad that may have come with it.

I surrender to the night and trust that I will find a way to handle whatever comes my way.

HEALING FACTORS

Reduce fear, worry and stress / develop appropriate stress management skills / change fear-based beliefs / develop appropriate trust with self and people who are trustworthy.

1 Fujimori, M. and H. E. Himwich. Delta sup(9) Tetrahydrocannabinol and the sleep wakefulness cycle. 1973. Physiology and Behavior 11(3): 291-295

Freemon, F. R. The effect of Delta sup(9) tetrahydrocannabinol on sleep. Psychopharmacologia 1974. 35(1): 39-44

Adams, P. M. and E. S. Barratt. Effect of chronic marijuana administration on stages of primate sleep wakefulness. 1975. Biological Psychiatry 10(3): 315-322.

Feinberg, I., R. Jones, et al. Effects of high dosage delta-9-tetrahydrocannabinol on sleep patterns in man. 1975. Clinical Pharmacology and Therapeutics 17(4): 458-66

Feinberg, I., R. Jones, et al. Effects of marijuana extract and tetrahydrocannabinol on electroencephalographic sleep patterns. 1976. Clinical Pharmacology and Therapeutics 19(6): 782-94.

Freemon, F. R. The effect of chronically administered delta-9-tetrahydrocannabinol upon the polygraphically monitored sleep of normal volunteers. 1982. Drug and Alcohol Dependence 10(4): 345-353.

2 Nicholson AN, Turner C, Stone BM, Robson PJ. *Effect of Delta-9-tetrahydrocannabinol and cannabidiol on nocturnal sleep and early-morning behavior in young adults.* QinetiQ Ltd, Centre for Human Sciences, Cody Technology Park, Ively Road, Farnborough, Hampshire GU14 0LX, UK. annicholson@QinetiQ.com J Clin Psychopharmacol. 2004 Jun;24(3):305-13.

3 Julio Fernández-Mendoza, MSc, Antonio Vela-Bueno, MD, Alexandros N. Vgontzas, MD, María José Ramos-Platón, PhD, Sara Olavarrieta-Bernardino, MSc, Edward O. Bixler, PhD and Juan José De la Cruz-Troca, MSc. *Cognitive-Emotional Hyperarousal as a Premorbid Characteristic of Individuals Vulnerable to Insomnia.* Departments of Psychiatry (J.F.-M., A.V.-B., S.O.-B.) and Preventive Medicine (J.J.D.C.-T.), School of Medicine, Universidad Autónoma de Madrid, Spain; Department of Psychobiology (J.F.-M., M.J.R.-P.), School of Psychology, Universidad Complutense de Madrid, Spain; Sleep Research and Treatment Center (E.O.B.), Department of Psychiatry, College of Medicine, Penn State University, Hershey, Pennsylvania. Psychosomatic Medicine May 2010 vol. 72 no. 4 397-403.

Libido

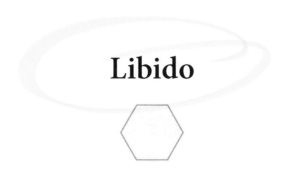

NUMBER OF STUDIES: 1

CHI VALUE: 2

Sigmund Freud and Carl Jung introduced the term libido into common usage via psychological theory. Today it is used to describe sexual virility and desire, biological drive or psychic-emotional force.

While some people with low libido may simply be asexual (not really interested in sex at all), others describe it as reduced frequency or complete absence of normal desire. It's no wonder researchers spend much time and energy seeking to discover the potential underpinnings of people complaining of low libido. Psychiatry even has a name for it: low libido hypoactive sexual desire disorders (HSDD). Non-physical or psychosomatic causes of the pathological type of low libido may include: subjective emotional reasons, anxieties, guilt, shame, stress, worry, chronic fears, sexual abuse, and post-traumatic stress syndrome (PTSD).

Orthodox medicine further defines underlying physical reasons of a low libido as pathological sexual desire disorders, erectile dysfunction, impotence (in males), frigidity (in women), female sexual arousal disorder, orgasm disorder, or simply sexual dysfunction. Physical causes of a low libido may include: pain, adverse effects of hundreds of common pharmacological medications (especially antidepressants), drug abuse, smoking, hormone imbalances, numerous chronic medical conditions (especially nervous system disorders and blood-flow/circulation disorders), surgeries (particularly in the region of the genitals), radiation therapy and chemotherapy.

Depending on underlying causes, modern medicine uses psychotherapy, pharmacological interventions, lifestyle changes, physical therapy and surgery to improve libido. Viagra, with world-wide annual sales exceeding billions of dollars, is by far the best-selling pharmaceutical drug brought to the market. This has held true since its introduction; despite reports of Viagra's adverse effects, including death. However, men hoping to regain youthful desires and long-lost intensities of romance, love and courtship soon realized this journey's limits. There is only so much that enhanced blood flow to the penis can do to resolve emotional deficits. While profits remain high, this realization may be responsible for the first reported decline of sales on all erectile dysfunction pharmaceuticals in 2010.

CANNABIS AND LIBIDO ENHANCEMENT

Some of the neurochemistry associated with sexual arousal and cannabis bear similarities. Both dilate pupils, elevate heart rates, alter endocrine releases, affect brain signaling, induce euphoria, relax muscles, produce changes in blood perfusion and shift respiratory patterns.

Hindu Tantric scriptures and practices dating back more than a thousand years reveal age-old uses of cannabis to enhance sexual pleasure and bring about enlightenment. In fact, several ancient cultures that deified sensuality and sexual practices in order to produce extraordinary states of consciousness and facilitate enlightenment used cannabis to achieve their goals.

Experiences from the latter two centuries present a picture of cannabis producing both libido stimulation and depression. Scientific studies today focus on this paradox of whether cannabis is a sexual stimulant or depressant. Researchers have gained insights by comparing accounts from modern users, historical records,[1] the world's therapeutic prescriptions manuals[2] and scientific studies on cannabinoids.[3]

The comparisons show that a properly dosed use of the plant may stimulate heightened sensations, increase stamina, deepen intensity of orgasms, and produce a more profound sense of intimacy. Furthermore, some people who feel anxious before lovemaking have discovered that the plant's anti-anxiety properties can ease the tension and stress often associated with performance problems. Males have reported harder erections while females described increases in lubrication and clitoral swelling during sex.

It is important to note that each of these properties depends on a very subjective therapeutic window. For instance, too high a dose can deepen anxieties and reduce sensations. While these effects fade as the body metabolizes the plant, user experience teaches to err on the side of caution and suggests beginning with low to medium doses gently and over time.

STUDY SUMMARY:

Drugs	Type of Study	Published Year, Place, and Key Results	CHI
Anandamide	Animal (rats)	2007 – University of Michigan. Enhances pleasure experience.	2

Total CHI Value 2

STRAIN SPECIFIC CONSIDERATIONS

The body's own anandamide activates CB1 and CB2 receptors relatively equally.

Sativas and sativa heavy hybrids present with a higher THC:CBD/CBN ratio, which, similar to anandamide, tend to activate both receptors relatively equally.

EXPLORING MIND–BODY CONSCIOUSNESS

An ebb and flow of libido is normal and natural. Asexuality is not an illness but rather a naturally occuring condition. However, if a person experiences loss of libido and desires a return or increase in virility and sexual arousal capacity, it is helpful to explore underlying causes.

Observations have shown that men who suppress anger or hostility toward their partner or all women in general, and men who recycle and harbor their anger or hostility have lower testosterone profiles and a lower libido. The resulting sexual dysfunction may bring these emotional tendencies to the surface.

QUESTIONS

Is there a part of me that wants to make my partner feel sexually unattractive? If so, why?

Where do I experience lack or loss of libido?

How do I feel about it?

How deep is that feeling?

How can I feel and release the feeling(s) appropriately and with harm to none?

What is at the bottom of the feeling(s)?

What belief do I find at the core of this feeling(s)?

Do I need to practice healing work regarding that belief?

Am I willing to replace this core belief(s)?

AGGRAVATING FACTORS

Suppressed or harbored anger, especially at the gender one feels attracted to; performance anxieties.

HEALING FACTORS

Appropriate release of anger and hostility toward the gender one feels attracted to; changing belief(s) that create feelings of anger at the gender one feels attracted to; reducing or ending performance-based anxieties.

ANECDOTES

Bill had performance problems in bed and as much as he said he wanted intimacy, he was terrified of it. He described his past relationships as difficult, always leaving him feeling ambivalent towards his ex-girlfriends and women in general. Typical statements were, "Women, you can't live with them, and you can't live without them." "First they love you, then they hurt you."

Eventually he realized that the only common denominator in all his relationships was himself. He pondered the thought as he inhaled. It wasn't long before a typical memory emerged; Gina had told him about an affair. And, while they had a relationship that made such events OK, he felt jealous and even envious but pretended not to be. After all, he had agreed to an open relationship. But now, examining his emotional reaction, he realized the fullness of his envy. He felt he could never have as much fun as women (Gina) had. However, instead of his usual knee-jerk reaction denying his envy, he relaxed. Bill looked deeper and longer until he unveiled his inability to create for himself what he thought Gina had. With that embrace of an otherwise intolerable emotion, he felt oddly empowered.

That night, he had a dream. He was watching a beautiful woman (not Gina) dancing sensuously. The dancer seemed to move to music only she could hear and feel; a music that moved her to orgasmic ecstasy that never seemed to end. After awhile, she approached him and simply said, "Would you like me to teach you how to do this?" Bill responded with a single word, "Yes."

Since that fateful night, Bill explained, sexual intimacy had new and intriguing dimensions he never before imagined and his troubles in bed vanished.

TAKE NOTICE

ANISE • CINNAMON • CLOVE • COCOA • GINGER • GRAINS OF PARADISE •
NUTMEG • MACA

ANISE: Greek herbalists have used anise to promote menstruation, increase breast milk production, facilitate birth and enhance libido. University of Athens' scientists have taken a closer look at anise in the context of finding a safe alternative to estrogen replacement therapies in the prevention of osteoporosis. Anise exhibits estrogen receptor modulator-like properties that produced bone-cell formation without causing breast and cervical cancer cells proliferation.[4]

CINNAMON: Neurologist Dr. Alan Hirsch, Director of Chicago's Smell and Taste Treatment and Research Foundation, established that male sexual stimulation increases with exposure to the scent of cinnamon. Furthermore, researchers from Washington concluded that cinnamon might also play a beneficial role in lowering high blood pressure, which can play a role in male sexual dysfunction.[5]

Barefoot Doctors in rural China use cinnamon sticks to prepare a decoction, which is used in the treatment of male sexual dysfunction.

CLOVE: Clove has long held a standing reputation in the Unani traditions as an aphrodisiac for males. Now, an Aligarh Muslim University study may provide further clues as to why it works in the treatment of male sexual dysfunction. Researchers noted that normal male rats given a 50% alcoholic extract of clove (between 100mg/kg to 500mg/kg) registered significantly enhanced sexual appetites without any noticeable side effects.[6]

COCOA: Similar to cinnamon, Dr. Hirsch, Director of Chicago's Smell and Taste Treatment and Research Foundation, also discovered that people's sexual stimulation increases when exposed to the scent of chocolate.

GINGER: Unani traditional medicine has long used ginger to enhance sexual function and fertility in males. Scientists from Riyadh, Saudi Arabia, used a rodent experiment to test the influence of ginger as part of their diet. The results showed that ginger significantly increased sperm motility (movement) and content without any toxic side effects.[7]

GRAINS OF PARADISE: Researchers from Yaoundé, Cameroon, using a rodent model, discovered that 115mg/kg of a water-based extract of grains of paradise significantly increased male arousal and sexual function.[8]

MACA: Sexual dysfunction and loss of sexual interest are all too common side-effects of selective-serotonin reuptake inhibitor (SSRI) pharmaceuticals, which are used in the treatment of depression. A study from Massachusetts General Hospital (2008) tested whether maca, a Peruvian high altitude vegetable, could mitigate (SSRI)-induced sexual dysfunction. The majority of study participants were women. Results showed a dose dependent (3gm daily) significant improvement with an increase in libido. Numerous other studies have confirmed the plant's libido enhancing properties in males as well.[9]

NUTMEG: Unani traditions boast nutmeg's long-standing reputation as a male aphrodisiac. An Aligarh Muslim University study found that when rats were given a 50% alcoholic extract of nutmeg as well as clove (500mg/kg), male rats experienced an increased sexual appetite without any noticeable side effects.[10]

1 Parker RC, Lux. *"Psychoactive Plants in Tantric Buddhism; Cannabis and Datura Use in Indo-Tibetan Esoteric Buddhism"*. Erowid Extracts. Jun 2008;14:6-11.

2 Sam'l O. L. Potter, M.A., M.D., M.R.C.P. (Lond,) *A Compend of Materia Medica and Therapeutics and Prescription Writing; with especial references to the physiological actions of drugs.* Based on the last revision of the U.S. Pharmacopeia. Fifth Edition. P.Blakiston, Son & Co., Philadelphia, 1012 Walnut St. 1892. Page #40.

3 Mahler SV, Smith KS, Berridge KC. *Endocannabinoid hedonic hotspot for sensory pleasure: anandamide in nucleus accumbens shell enhances 'liking' of a sweet reward.* Department of Psychology, The University of Michigan, Ann Arbor, MI 48109, USA. svmahler@umich.edu Neuropsychopharmacology. 2007 Nov;32(11):2267-78.

4 Kassi E, Papoutsi Z, Fokialakis N, Messari I, Mitakou S, Moutsatsou P. *Greek plant extracts exhibit selective estrogen receptor modulator (SERM)-like properties.* Department of Biological Chemistry, Medical School, University of Athens, 115 27 Athens, Greece. J Agric Food Chem. 2004 Nov 17;52(23):6956-61.

5 Preuss HG, Echard B, Polansky MM, Anderson R. *Whole cinnamon and aqueous extracts ameliorate sucrose-induced blood pressure elevations in spontaneously hypertensive rats.* Department of Physiology, Georgetown University Medical Center, Washington, DC 20057, USA. J Am Coll Nutr. 2006 Apr;25(2):144-50.

6 Tajuddin, Shamshad Ahmad, Abdul Latif and Iqbal A Qasmi. *Myristica fragrans Houtt. (nutmeg) and Syzygium aromaticum (L) Merr. & Perry. (clove) in male mice: a comparative study.* Department of Ilmul Advia (Unani Pharmacology), Faculty of Unani Medicine, Aligarh Muslim University, Aligarh-202002, India. BMC Complementary and Alternative Medicine 2003, 3:6.

7 Qureshi S, Shah AH, Tariq M, Ageel AM. *Studies on herbal aphrodisiacs used in Arab system of medicine.* Research Centre, College of Pharmacy, King Saud University, Riyadh, Saudi Arabia. Am J Chin Med. 1989;17(1-2):57-63.

8 Kamtchouing P, Mbongue GY, Dimo T, Watcho P, Jatsa HB, Sokeng SD. *Effects of Aframomum melegueta and Piper guineense on sexual behaviour of male rats.* Laboratoire de Physiologie Animale, Faculté des Sciences, Université de Yaoundé I, Yaoundé, Cameroun. mbongue@yahoo.com Behav Pharmacol. 2002 May;13(3):243-7.

9 Dording CM, Fisher L, Papakostas G, Farabaugh A, Sonawalla S, Fava M, Mischoulon D. *A double-blind, randomized, pilot dose-finding study of maca root (L. meyenii) for the management of SSRI-induced sexual dysfunction.* Depression Clinical and Research Program, Department of Psychiatry, Massachusetts General Hospital, Boston, MA 02114, USA. CNS Neurosci Ther. 2008 Fall;14(3):182-91.

10 Tajuddin , Ahmad S, Latif A, Qasmi IA. *Aphrodisiac activity of 50% ethanolic extracts of Myristica fragrans Houtt. (nutmeg) and Syzygium aromaticum (L) Merr. & Perry. (clove) in male mice: a comparative study.* Department of Ilmul Advia (Unani Pharmacology), Faculty of Unani Medicine, Aligarh Muslim University, Aligarh-202002, India. BMC Complement Altern Med. 2003 Oct 20;3:6.

Lung Diseases
Asthma

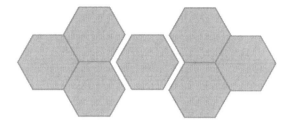

NUMBER OF STUDIES: 7

CHI VALUE: 24

Asthma is typically a chronic medical problem, which ranges from mild breathing problems similar to those from a head cold, to severe and life-threatening emergencies that require rapid 911 interventions and transport to the nearest open emergency room (ER).

Asthma does not discriminate. People from all walks of life suffer from asthma; however, children and senior citizens are the most vulnerable. Some children outgrow their asthma while others do not. The causes for asthma are poorly understood, and no pharmacological cure exists. Orthodox medicine focuses on diminishing occurrences and trying to control acute symptoms.

Physicians typically use oxygen and bronchodilators (such as Albuterol, Azmacourt, Ventolin, or Theo-Dur) to open constricted tubes leading to the lungs. However, there is evidence that regular use of inhalers contributes to making asthma worse over time. Other commonly used pharmaceuticals include steroids and drugs that stimulate beta-2 adrenergic receptor sites (receptors that enlist responses including the relaxation of the smooth muscles in the upper airways).

Some of the main triggers of an asthma attack include: emotional distress, dust, dust mites, molds, smoking, strong smells, pollution (indoor and outdoor), industrial chemicals, food additives, colds, coughs and strenuous exercise.

Common signs and symptoms include: difficulty breathing, wheezing, pale skin, diaphoresis (sweating), fear and anxiety, tightness in the chest, coughing (clear sputum), or spasms of the upper airways.

If you have an asthma attack, follow your doctor's advice or call 911.

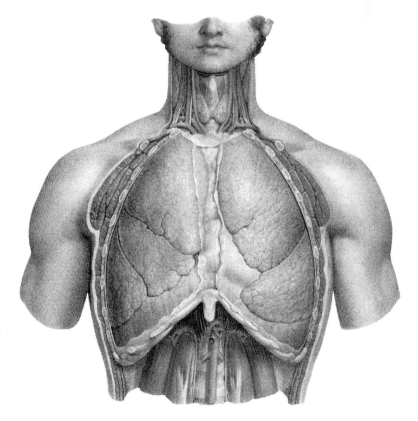

It has long been known that the inhalation of burned materials contributes to diseases of the lung. This is especially true when smoking commercial cigarettes. It is almost counterintuitive to believe that inhaling cannabis can reduce symptoms or be otherwise therapeutically beneficial to people with a lung disease such as asthma. However, if smoking can be tolerated without the spasm of coughing, the therapeutic effects of relaxation and upper airway expansion, both important goals in treating asthma, may arrive relatively quickly.

Since 1974, studies have been conducted to document the effects of cannabinoids on human patients with asthma. In the first of such trials (1974) researchers developed a double-blind placebo-controlled crossover study. Scientists enrolled ten patients with stable asthma to test and compare the efficacy of smoked cannabis, ingested THC, placebo, and a pharmaceutical (isoproterenol) commonly used in the 70s to treat asthma. Results showed that while the initial effect of isoproterenol was more pronounced, the effects of smoked cannabis and oral THC lasted longer. "These findings indicated that in the asthmatic subjects, both smoked marijuana and oral THC caused significant bronchodilation of at least 2 hours duration."[1]

By 1975, eight stable asthmatics were enrolled in another study to determine the effects of cannabis on asthma, both chemically and exercise induced. Results showed that in both cases, smoked cannabis (THC 2%) produced a prompt correction of the bronchospasms and associated hyperinflation, similar to isoproterenol.[2]

In 1976, another double-blind placebo-controlled study enlisted ten patients with asthma to learn more about the potential therapeutic properties of cannabinoids in controlling the disease. Results showed that: "Salbutamol and THC significantly improved ventilatory function. Maximal bronchodilation was achieved more rapidly with salbutamol, but at 1 hour both drugs were equally effective." The conducting scientist did not detect any variation in mood or heart rate during the application of THC and concluded that: "The mode of action of THC differs from that of sympathomimetic drugs (drugs which stimulate the sympathetic nervous system and increase heart rate and blood pressure), and it or a derivative may make a suitable adjuvant in the treatment of selected asthmatics."[3]

In the following year (1977), a study evaluated oral and smoked forms of THC compared to a placebo and isoproterenol in a random, double-blind trial conducted on eleven healthy people and five patients with asthma. Researchers measured airway dynamics and heart rates during the experiment. Results showed that aerolized THC was less pronounced than isoproterenol in producing bronchodilation in the short term (5 min.) but significantly better in the longer time ranges (1-3 hours). The authors wrote: "Aerosolized delta9-tetrahydrocannabinol caused significant bronchodilation in 3 of 5 asthmatic subjects, but caused moderate to severe bronchoconstriction associated with cough and chest discomfort in the other two. …These findings indicate that aerosolized delat9-tetrahydrocannabinol, although capable of causing significant bronchodilatation with minimal systemic side effects, has a local irritating effect on the airways, which may make it unsuitable for therapeutic use."[4]

These and the following study results have added more information about THC's ability to increase bronchodilation in asthma patients and highlight some of the differences in the available dosages, forms and routes of administration of cannabinoids.

In 1978, researchers administered an aerosol containing THC to asthmatic patients in a steady state of dosage ranging from 50-200 mcg. Results showed that the treatment increased the peak expiratory flow rate and forced expiratory volume in one second and that the onset, magnitude, and duration of the bronchodilator effect was dose related.[5]

Comparing the synthetic cannabinoid nabilone to the standard anti-asthmatic pharmaceutical terbutaline, researchers (1983) discovered that while nabilone had some bronchodilation effects in healthy patients it did not produce a therapeutic effect better than the placebo. The authors concluded that: "…oral nabilone (2 mg) does not result in significant acute bronchodilation in patients with asthma."[6]

Despite promising potential, for the next twenty years no studies on asthma and the therapeutics of cannabinoids appeared on the horizon of the usual publishing outlets.

However, by 2006 researchers from Boston had tested numerous novel molecules that exert their biological effects through the endocannabinoid system. The result of this exploration suggests the therapeutic potential of cannabinoids on inflammatory diseases such as asthma and allergic asthma.[7]

STUDY SUMMARY:

Drugs	Type of Study	Published Year, Place, and Key Results	CHI
Cannabinoids	Laboratory and animal	2006 –Boston, MA, United States. Potential reduction of inflammation in asthma and allergic asthma.	1+2
Nabilone (2mg) v. terbutaline sulfate v. placebo	6 healthy people and 6 asthmatic patients	1983 – Moderate bronchodilator action in healthy people but no difference compared to placebo in asthmatic patients.	0
Aerosolized THC 50--200 mcg	Asthmatic patients in 'steady state'	1978 – THC produces bronchodilatation in asthmatic patients.	3
Aerosolized THC, aerosolized placebo and isoproterenol and 20 mg of oral and smoked THC	11 healthy people and 5 patients with asthma	1977 – Bronchodilation lasts longer than isoproterenol in healthy subject. Among asthmatics 3 patients got better; 2 got worse.	5
THC 200 mcg in ethanol (inhaler) v. salbutamol 100 mcg (Ventolin inhaler) vs placebo ethanol	10 asthmatic patients	1976 – THC significantly improved ventilatory function.	5
Smoked cannabis 500mg with 2.0% THC v. 500 mg of smoked placebo marijuana	8 asthmatic patients	1975 – 2% cannbis and isoproterenol caused an immediate reversal of exercise-induced asthma and hyperinflation.	3
2% natural marijuana (7 mg per/kg) v. 15 mg of oral THC vs placebo v. isoproterenol	10 patients with stable bronchial asthma	1974 – Smoked cannabis and oral THC caused significant bronchodilation for at least 2 hours.	5

Total CHI Value 24

STRAIN SPECIFIC CONSIDERATIONS

The primary cannabinoid used in these asthma studies was THC, which binds to both CB1 and CB2 receptors.

Sativas or sativa dominant strains tend to contain a cannabinoid profile with a slightly higher THC:CBD/CBN ratio than indica or indica dominant strains.

EXPLORING MIND–BODY CONSCIOUSNESS

Grace and Graham examined the psychosomatic underpinning of 19 patients and discovered that in the case of the participating subjects, asthma occurred when a patient was faced with a life situation they wished would just go away. They wished someone else would take responsibility for the situation and make it disappear, or wished to avoid it altogether. Typical statements were: "I wanted them to go away." "I didn't want anything to do with it." "I wanted to blot it all out, I wanted to build a wall between me and him." "I wanted to hole up for the winter." "I wanted to go to bed and pull the sheets over my head."

The authors concluded that: "The reaction of the respiratory mucous membrane to a noxious agent is to exclude it by swelling of the membrane with consequent narrowing of the passageway, and to dilute it and wash it out by hypersecretion. When these changes are limited to the nose, the reaction is called vasomotor rhinitis (stuffy or runny nose from reasons other than allergies or infection); when they are sufficiently intense to include the bronchi, so that wheezing occurs, the name asthma is applied."[8]

Wheezing, a characteristic symptom of asthma, is an unmistakable sound. The tighter the airways, the higher the pitch. It appears akin to an internal smothering or a suppression of something that should not be released, which lies beneath the struggle to breathe in but especially to exhale.

Non-physical asthma triggers as well as non-physical asthma alleviators are well recognized and commonly noted in any emergency room (ER) setting. Most ER personnel know of cases in which a patient's respiratory distress was diminished or completely put to rest by 'talking the patient down.' Conversely, mental/emotional triggers of asthma have been studied.

One such study examined the emotional states during night dreams that ended in the patient waking up with wheezing and in respiratory distress. The common theme in all the dreams that produced an asthma attack focussed on intense overwhelming emotions: acts of violence (as victim or perpetrator), intense sexual dreams outside the bounds of what the patient considers normal, or dreams that bring up intense past traumas of abandonment, betrayal or humiliation.

QUESTIONS

Which feelings produce stress responses make me breathless?
Where do those feelings start?
What in life feels like it's smothering me?
Who smothers me but calls it love?
Are there tears I have not cried because I believe they must be kept inside at all cost?

AGGRAVATING FACTORS

Being faced with a life situation you wish would just go away, or wish that someone else would take responsibility for and make disappear / belief that avoidance would be the best course of (in)action.

HEALING FACTORS

Deep relaxation / trust in the trustworthy / develop trust in self / work with the paradox of relaxing in the presence of contricting emotions and experiences.

TAKE NOTICE

ANISE • BUSH TEA • COCOA • GARLIC • NIGELLA • TURMERIC

ANISE: Iranian scientists discovered a possible mechanism that explains why many traditional healers have been using anise extracts and oils in the treatment of certain respiratory ailments. Anise extracts and essential oils possess bronchodilatory qualities (they opens the upper airways).[10]

BUSHTEA: A recent study from Karachi, Pakistan, determined why Bush tea might be effective in cases of respiratory difficulties. Bush tea is a bronchodilator, antispasmodic and contains blood pressure-lowering properties. It apparently achieves this by Portassium (ATP) channel activation with a selective bronchodilatory effect.[11]

COCOA: A study from London, England, looked at a component of cocoa, theobromine, in the context of treating a persistent cough and determined it to be effective as an antitussive (reduces coughing).[12]

GARLIC: Garlic, an exceedingly versatile herb, is used for the treatment of asthma and to bring up phlegm during colds and flu.[13]

NIGELLA: Doctors from Mashhad University, Iran, evaluated the extracts from boiled nigella seeds on asthmatic adults and determined that patients using the extract reported a reduction in all asthma symptoms, including improved pulmonary function tests. Furthermore, patients experienced a reduced need for inhalers.[14]

TURMERIC: Based on the evidence of numerous laboratory and animal trials, scientists from Vandoeuvre-Lès-Nancy, France, contend "...that curcumin plays a protective role in chronic obstructive pulmonary disease, acute lung injury, acute respiratory distress syndrome, and allergic asthma; its therapeutic action being on the prevention or modulation of inflammation and oxidative stress." Furthermore, and based on the substance of these studies, "these scientists suggest the beginning of clinical trials using turmeric to treat human patients with a variety of chronic and acute lung disorders."[15]

For general immune support see TAKE NOTICE section in BACTERIAL and VIRAL INFECTIONS.

For anti-inflammatory support see TAKE NOTICE section in INFLAMMATORY DISEASE IN GENERAL.
For pain see TAKE NOTICE section in PAIN IN GENERAL.
For cough see BACTERIAL and IRAL INFECTIONS – COUGH.
For anti-spasm support see NEURO-PROTECTIVE IN GENERAL.

1 Tashkin DP, Shapiro BJ, Frank IM. *Acute effects of smoked marijuana and oral delta9-tetrahydrocannabinol on specific airway conductance in asthmatic subjects.* Am Rev Respir Dis. 1974 Apr;109(4):420-8.

2 Tashkin DP, Shapiro BJ, Lee YE, Harper CE. *Effects of smoked marijuana in experimentally induced asthma.* Am Rev Respir Dis. 1975 Sep;112(3):377-86.

3 Williams SJ, Hartley JP, Graham JD. *Bronchodilator effect of delta1-tetrahydrocannabinol administered by aerosol of asthmatic patients.* Thorax 1976;31(6):720-723.

4 Tashkin DP, Reiss S, Shapiro BJ, Calvarese B, Olsen JL, Lodge JW. *Bronchial effects of aerosolized delta 9-tetrahydrocannabinol in healthy and asthmatic subjects.* Am Rev Respir Dis. 1977 Jan;115(1):57-65.

5 Hartley JP, Nogrady SG, Seaton A. *Bronchodilator effect of delta1-tetrahydrocannabinol.* Br J Clin Pharmacol. 1978 Jun;5(6):523-5.

6 Gong H Jr, Tashkin DP, Calvarese B. *Comparison of bronchial effects of nabilone and terbutaline in healthy and asthmatic subjects.* Journal of Clinical Pharmacology 1983;23(4):127-133.

7 Lu, Dai1; Kiran Vemuri, V.1; Duclos, Richard I.1; Jr.1; Makriyannis, Alexandros.1 *The Cannabinergic System as a Target for Anti-inflammatory Therapies.* 1 Center for Drug Discovery, Northeastern University, 360 Huntington Avenue, 116 Mugar Hall, Boston, MA, 02115, USA. Current Topics in Medicinal Chemistry, Volume 6, Number 13, July 2006 , pp. 1401-1426(26). Bentham Science Publishers.

8 William J. Grace, M.D. and David T. Graham, M.D. *Relationship of Specific Attitudes and Emotions to Certain Bodily Diseases.* Dept. of Medicine, of the New York Hospital-Cornell Medical Center. Psychosomatic Medicine July 1, 1952 vol. 14 no. 4 243-251.

9 William Ernest Henley (1849-1903). *Invictus*

10 Boskabady MH, Ramazani-Assari M. *Relaxant effect of Pimpinella anisum on isolated guinea pig tracheal chains and its possible mechanism(s).* Department of Physiology, Ghaem Medical Centre, Mashhad University of Medical Sciences, 91735, Mashhad, Iran. J Ethnopharmacol. 2001 Jan;74(1):83-8.

11 Khan AU, Gilani AH. *Selective bronchodilatory effect of Rooibos tea (Aspalathus linearis) and its flavonoid, chrysoeriol.* Dept. of Biological and Biomedical Sciences, The Aga Khan University Medical College, Karachi, 74800, Pakistan. Eur J Nutr. 2006 Dec; 45(8):463-9.

12 Usmani OS, Belvisi MG, Patel HJ, Crispino N, Birrell MA, Korbonits M, Korbonits D, Barnes PJ. *Theobromine inhibits sensory nerve activation and cough.* Department of Thoracic Medicine, National Heart and Lung Institute, Imperial College London, London, UK. FASEB J. 2005 Feb;19(2):231-3.

13 *Therapeutic Guide to Plant Pharmaceuticals and Honey Pharmaceuticals (Guia Terapeutica Dispensarial de Fitofarmacos y Apifarmacos* - Ministerio de Salud Publica, Ciudad de La Habana - Republica de Cuba 1992). Cuban Ministry of Public Health, Havana.

14 Boskabady MH, Javan H, Sajady M, Rakhshandeh H. The possible prophylactic effect of Nigella sativa seed extract in asthmatic patients. Department of Physiology, Ghaem Medical Centre, Mashhad University of Medical Sciences, Mashhad 91735, Iran. Fundam Clin Pharmacol. 2007 Oct;21(5):559-66.

15 Venkatesan N, Punithavathi D, Babu M. *Protection from acute and chronic lung diseases by curcumin.* Faculte de Medecine, UMR-7561, CNRS UHP, Vandoeuvre lès Nancy, France. vnar12@yahoo.com Adv Exp Med Biol. 2007;595:379-405.

Lung Diseases
Chronic Obstructive Pulmonary Disease

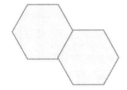

NUMBER OF STUDIES: 2

CHI VALUE: 3

This type of lung disease is characterized by the narrowing of the airways, which decreases the possible passage of gas exchange in and out of the lungs. In the paradigm of orthodox medicine, the major culprit of chronic obstructive pulmonay disease (COPD) is cigarette smoking. The constant presence of toxic gases produces an initial low-grade inflammation of the lung tissue. As the inflammation slowly progresses, the lungs develop chronic bronchitis, and symptoms such as chronic coughing occur. Burned carbon deposits deep inside the lung ultimately cause the slow destruction of alveoli (the lung structure that exchanges gases with the blood) leading to further deterioration and resulting in emphysema. At this stage of the disease, even the slightest exertion causes shortness of breath.

CANNABIS AND COPD

In 2005, researchers enrolled 18 patients with COPD, secondary weight loss and limited exertion potential. To measure the potential therapeutic impacts of cannabinoids on these physical limitations, patients were given twice daily orally administered oil containing between 3.3-4.2 mg THC. After 16 days, results indicated an average weight gain of 1.5 kg and a 36% average increase in walking distance.[1] This is a significant achievement especially when compared to orthodox treatment protocols.

Canadian scientists (2009) examined the effects of tobacco, tobacco with cannabis and cannabis alone on COPD. Researchers interpret the resulting data: "Smoking both tobacco and marijuana synergistically increased the risk of respiratory symptoms and COPD. Smoking only marijuana was not associated with an increased risk of respiratory symptoms or COPD."[2]

STUDY SUMMARY:

Drugs	Type of Study	Published Year, Place, and Key Results	CHI
Smoking cannabis alone and smoking cannabis with tobacco.	Population based study	2009 – Centre for Cardiovascular and Pulmonary Research, St. Paul's Hospital and the University of British Columbia, Vancouver, Canada. Tobacco with cannabis increases risk of COPD. Smoking cannabis alone does not increase risk of COPD.	0

Drugs	Type of Study	Published Year, Place, and Key Results	CHI
Cannabis oil	Human case study	2005 – Presentation at the 2005 Conference of the German Society for Pneumology, Berlin, Karl-Christian Bergmann, Allergie- und Asthmaklinik, Bad Lippspringe, Germany. Increase in walking distance and significant weight gains.	3

Total CHI Value   3

STRAIN AND FORM SPECIFIC CONSIDERATIONS

The human case study from Bad Lippspringe, Germay, used THC dissolved in oil. THC binds to CB1 and CB2 relatively equally.

Sativa and Sativa prominent strains contain higher THC:CBD ratios. Organic sativa oil extracts are made easily or may be purchased at your local dispensary.

EXPLORING MIND–BODY CONSCIOUSNESS

The barrel chest, a common symptom in patients with emphysema, merits interpretation. An impressive hyper inflated, dominant body part mimics that of a person inflating his chest to look bigger and perhaps feel strong and in control. Vulnerability is generally interpreted as feared feelings (especially sadness, grief, hurt, love or fear), which are often not expressed but rather held in. Un-exhaled feelings linger in the chest pressing against the ribs and causing constant pressure that ultimately contributes to a barrel chest. A difficulty exhaling is another common symptom for emphysema patients. Ironically, this strategy, to appear strong and in control all the time, ultimately produces very weak and actually physically vulnerable people who cannot leave the house without an oxygen tank or take a few steps without having to stop and try to catch their breath.

> **SUGGESTED BLESSING:**
>
> *May you relax and release your fears.*
>
> *May you find true strength and allow yourself to walk with ease.*

QUESTIONS

Are there tears that have never been shed?
What grief have I refused to release?
Which love has never been allowed to blossom?
What hurt still lingers after oh so many years?

AGGRAVATING FACTORS

Repressed emotions / belief system that demands a denial of certain feelings and emotions.

HEALING FACTORS

Emotional release work / challenge and change any belief that demands repression of emotions.

> **SUGGESTED AFFIRMATION:**
>
> *It is safe to feel everything with strength and intensity.*
>
> *My emotions are a gift and part of what it means to be human.*
>
> *I can relax and release my breath fully and with ease.*
>
> *I am safe and I am free.*

TAKE NOTICE

See TAKE NOTICE section in chapter on ASTHMA.

For general immune support see TAKE NOTICE section in BACTERIAL and VIRAL INFECTIONS.

For anti-inflammatory support see TAKE NOTICE section in INFLAMMATORY DISEASE IN GENERAL.

For pain see TAKE NOTICE section in PAIN IN GENERAL.

For cough see BACTERIAL and IRAL INFECTIONS – COUGH.

For anti-spasm support see NEURO-PROTECTIVE IN GENERAL.

1 Karl-Christian Bergmann. *Dronabinol - eine mögliche neue Therapieoption bei COPD-Patienten mit pulmonaler Kachexie.* Presentation at the 2005 Conference of the German Society for Pneumology, Berlin, 17 March 2005. Karl-Christian Bergmann, Allergie- und Asthmaklinik, Bad Lippspringe, Germany.

2 Tan WC, Lo C, Jong A, Xing L, Fitzgerald MJ, Vollmer WM, Buist SA, Sin DD; *Vancouver Burden of Obstructive Lung Disease (BOLD)* Research Group. Marijuana and chronic obstructive lung disease: a population-based study. iCapture Centre for Cardiovascular and Pulmonary Research, St. Paul's Hospital and the University of British Columbia, Vancouver, Canada. wtan@mrl.ubc.ca CMAJ. 2009 Apr 14;180(8):814-20.

Mental Disorders

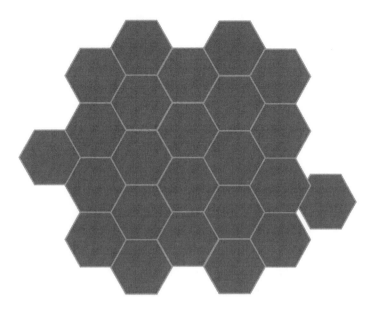

COMBINED NUMBER OF STUDIES: 24

COMBINED CHI VALUE: 68

The Diagnostic and Statistical Manual of Mental Disorders (DSM) published by the American Psychiatric Association stands as the primary system for mental illness diagnoses in the U.S. It contains about 400 different types of mental diseases and provides guidelines of specific signs and symptoms to determine diagnoses, possible causes, and treatment options.

Indeed, many techniques exist for exploring the differences amongst mentally ill patients, especially those with acute episodes or those who are chronically debilitated. However, for those in search of a mystical experience, still another set of methods remain for determining similarities. Those patients who have achieved a lasting cure often describe an evolution from the psychotic state of mind into one of mystical revelations. Many a mystic, monk or ascetic has similarly described experiences of a psychotic nature on their path to enlightenment.

Mental Disorders
Anxieties

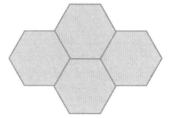

NUMBER OF STUDIES: 4

CHI VALUE: 14

Generally speaking, anxiety is a normal reaction to the subjective experience of stress such as in 'performance anxiety.' It also occurs when anticipation of future events is associated in one's mind with thoughts and feelings not rooted in the present moment. While anxieties can be considered a normal part of life, chronic or constant anxiety can be debilitating to one's quality of life. In fact, such interference can produce very real physiological changes in the short and long term. It is estimated that almost two out of ten people in the U.S. suffers from some kind of anxiety disorders.[1]

Western medicine considers anxiety disorders mood disorders and defines five basic types: generalized anxiety disorder (GAD), obsessive-compulsive disorder (OCD), panic disorder, post-traumatic stress disorder (PTSD) and social anxiety disorder (social phobias).

Generalized Anxiety Disorder (GAD): GAD patients present with chronic worry about anticipated events constructed by their mind. Symptoms often include 'feeling the other shoe is about to drop,' unreasonable worry, tense and aching muscles (e.g. neck, shoulders), headaches, trembling and diaphoresis (sweating).

Obsessive-Compulsive Disorder (OCD): OCD patients are characterized by compulsive, often odd, behavior that can be described as personal rituals such as filling in all the letter O's when writing, not stepping on any cracks on the sidewalk or constantly needing to wash their hands. Continuously occupying the mind with such trivial activities provides a sense for control who otherwise would focus on anticipated but unwanted thoughts or feelings.

Panic Disorder: Patients with panic disorder anxiety are prone to panic attacks. Acute short term symptoms may begin as rapid heart rates, rapid breathing (hyperventilation) and a dry mouth, but can progress to an anxiety attack with restlessness, chest tightness, palpitations, chest pain, shortness of breath, tingling, numbness (in the hands, feet or lips), diaphoresis (sweating), feelings of impending doom or death and inconsolability.

Post-Traumatic Stress Disorder (PTSD): PTSD develops after undergoing or witnessing a significant traumatic event. Patients frequently re-experience the trauma in their mind, either when dreaming or triggered by an external stimulus. S/he will often try to avoid all feelings and attempt to numb oneself against a constant dread of the return of the event. Some symptoms include 'feeling on edge,' flashbacks, constant fearful thoughts, sudden outbursts of anger and an aversion to being close to anyone.

Social Anxiety Disorder: Social phobia patients are often defined by their anticipation of severely humiliating events. This type of anxiety disorder is often isolated to a very narrow context such as being extremely self-conscious about turning red in public and than feeling judged by everybody in the room. Physical symptoms include blushing, trembling, sweating, nausea and difficulty forming words or sentences.

Doctors often prescribe pharmaceuticals (e.g. anti-anxiety drugs, anti-depressants) or psychological intervention to treat anxiety absent underlying physical causes. Adverse effects of pharmaceutical anti-anxiety medication range from mild to fatal. A thorough risk versus benefit analysis is advisable before committing to such a regimen.

CANNABIS AND ANXIETY (IN GENERAL)

Various medical traditions use cannabis extracts because of their time-proven calming and sedative effects. Today, numerous studies confirm that cannabinoids modulate mood states and can reduce anxiety. However, evidence has also shown that anxiety-reducing effects of cannabis are subjectively dose specific. Too little can be sub-optimal while too much can actually increase anxious feelings.

In 2005, teams from China, Canada and the U.S. conducted a review of the available scientific literature on the topic of cannabinoids and anxiety and found that "Cannabis and its major psychoactive component (-)-trans-Delta-tetrahydrocannabinol, have profound effects on mood and can modulate anxiety and mood states."[2] In the same year, another international team of scientists examined the impact of a potent synthetic cannabinoid (HU210) in an experiment on rats. Most illegal substances have been reported to decrease the growth of new nerve cells in the hippocampus. However, chronic HU210 treatment promoted neurogenesis in the hippocampal regions of the rodents, which was likely to produce both an anxiolytic and antidepressant-like effect.[3]

In 2009, researchers from Boston collected data from 775 patients living with HIV/AIDS and suffering from six common symptoms associated with them: anxiety, depression, fatigue, diarrhea, nausea and peripheral neuropathy. Study participants came from Kenya, South Africa, Puerto Rico and ten different U.S. locations. Results showed that while the differences were relatively small, cannabis was considered somewhat more effective than standard prescription and over-the-counter medications in treating anxiety, depression, diarrhea, fatigue, and neuropathy. However it proved less effective in cases of nausea.[4]

In 2010, researchers from Sao Paulo, Brazil reviewed available studies on two cannabinoids, CBD and THC, and their impact on the psychiatric patient. Researchers considered CBD's therapeutic potential as an antipsychotic, anxiolytic, and antidepressant while THC was considered a potential adjuvant in the treatment of schizophrenia. The authors concluded that: "Cannabinoids may be of great therapeutic interest to psychiatry; however, further controlled trials are necessary to confirm the existing findings and to establish the safety of such compounds."

STUDY SUMMARY:

Drugs	Type of Study	Published Year, Place, and Key Results	CHI
Canna-bidiol and THC	Meta-analysis	2010 – Universidade de São Paulo, Brasil. Cannabidiol therapeutic potential: antipsychotic, anxiolytic, and antidepressant. THC: adjuvant in the treatment of schizophrenia.	4
Cannabis	775 Humans living with HIV/AIDS	2009 – MGH Institute of Health Professions, School of Nursing, Boston. Cannabis considered effective in treating anxiety and depression and other symptoms in AIDS patients.	3
HU210	Animal and laboratory study (rats)	2005 – Multi-institutional and international study. Hypocampal cell are immunoreactive for CB1 receptors. Cannabinoids may induce hippocampal neurogenesis, which may explain their anxiolytic and antidepressant-like effects.	2+1
Cannabis, cannabinoids	Literature review (meta-analysis)	2005 – Psychiatric Drug Discovery, Lilly Research Laboratories, Eli Lilly and Company, Indianapolis, Indiana. Cannabis can modulate anxiety and mood states.	4

Total CHI Value   14

STRAIN SPECIFIC CONSIDERATIONS

Cannabis, CBD, THC and HU210 underwent testing in these trials in the context of anxiety. Cannabis contains the full spectrum of cannabinoids' and non-cannabinoids' biologically active ingredients activating CB1 and CB2. CBD has greater affinity for CB2. THC binds relatively equally with both CB1 and CB2 receptors. HU210 possesses a higher affinity for CB1.

It appears that both signaling pathways (CB1 and CB2) individually as well as in combination - modulate anxiety. Indicas and indica dominant hybrids, which tend to present with a lower THC:CBD/CBN ratio are preferred. In fact, many cannabis-using patients suffering from anxiety prefer such treatment due to its sedating, relaxing and grounding effects.

EXPLORING MIND–BODY CONSCIOUSNESS

SUGGESTED BLESSING:

May you discover the natural confidence that comes from trusting yourself to be calm and quiet until action is required.

May you always find your natural balance between tension and relaxation.

In the depths of anxiety reside the keys to our imagination and access to the power of our creativity. Thus, anxious people can imagine anything and everything that can go wrong. And most patients suffering from anxiety disorders know very well the power of their creativity, which when driven by anxiety can often produce the very thing so feared.

Mild forms of anxiety occurs when the mind anticipates challenging feelings. Anxieties progress to their debilitating forms when this anticipation interferes with normal daily functions and quality of life. Although most commonly associated with constricting feelings or emotions such as fear, anxiety can be triggered by anticipation of expansive emotions such as an unprecedented love or joy.

QUESTIONS

What was the 'accident' or event that caused you to become a nervous wreck?
What trigger event(s) sets off your anxiety?
Who or what is getting on your nerves?
What can you learn about your anxiety?

Can you befriend your anxiety?

Can you have compassion for yourself when feeling anxious?

What belief(s) is locking your imagination on the object(s) of your anxiety?

What is the worst that could happen?

Can you come up with a plan B if the worst occurs?

When was the last time you felt relaxed, quiet, calm, secure or confident?

AGGRAVATING FACTORS

Fear-based beliefs.

HEALING FACTORS

Replacing fear-based beliefs.

ANECDOTE

Maria was a self-described worrywart. She worried excessively and needlessly until her constant anticipation of the worst possible scenario began to erode her health. She felt anxious, uncertain, uneasy and irritable, which eventually produced a constant fatigue, insomnia, indigestion and episodes of rapid heartbeats, hypertension, hyperventilation and panic attacks. She sought a cannabis prescription for help with her disorder.

Maria describes her experience taking cannabis: "After a few minutes, I felt relaxed for what felt like the first time ever. I saw my worry like a dark cloud or mist right in front of me; but my reaction to it was noticeably different. I remained relaxed and curious where I normally would feel overwhelmed and panicky. Wherever I turned my mind's eye, my worry snapped into place in front me. I started to realize that I was the one pulling it with me at every turn of my imagination. I realized that I used my worry as a shield to protect myself from enemies sprung from my own imagination. I could see that my worry rose from the belief I held so dear that 'the world was a scary place' and that almost 'everybody was out to get me' in some way or another. I was a victim, thinking I had no power to do anything about it. Then I saw that I used my worry to separate myself from a memory I did not want to experience, an experience I pretended did not really exist.

But what was it that I was so worried about? As I asked the question, I remembered an accident when I was little. I had run into traffic and was sideswiped by a car. I was ok but for a few abrasions. However, my parents were freaking out. 'I told you it is too dangerous to be out here by yourself.' 'People don't care and they will hurt you if you don't watch it.' I was kept inside for a long while and later strictly limited and supervised when outside. I saw how my parents used worry to excessively control my life. However, I also understood that that was then and this was now. I became aware that just because my parents did this does not mean I need to continue the behavior. I heard myself saying: I don't have to hide behind my worry any

SUGGESTED AFFIRMATION:

I take back my imagination from the clutches of my anxieties and fears.

I imagine trusting myself.

I can relax, be calm and feel safe.

I can imagine the good, the truth and the beauty in this world.

I imagine what can go right.

longer. I don't have to keep the world apart from me any longer."

This case demonstrated a relatively quick resolution engaging the underlying body-mind aspects of Maria's symptoms. Once Maria had understood and answered the message of her chronic worry, the physical symptoms went away. Now-a-days Maria hardly has any worries at all and during those times when they do appear, she knows with a sense of confidence that she'll get through it just fine. In those moments, Maria does not succumb to them; she merely acknowledges the anxiety as part of the human experience that can be handled with a bit of mindfulness and attention. Maria considers herself cured.

1 Ronald C. Kessler, PhD; Wai Tat Chiu, AM; Olga Demler, MA, MS; Ellen E. Walters, MS. *Prevalence, Severity, and Comorbidity of 12-Month DSM-IV Disorders in the National Comorbidity Survey* Replication. Arch Gen Psychiatry. 2005;62:617-627.

2 Witkin JM, Tzavara ET, Nomikos GG. *A role for cannabinoid CB1 receptors in mood and anxiety disorders.* Psychiatric Drug Discovery, Lilly Research Laboratories, Eli Lilly and Company, Indianapolis, Indiana 46285-0510, USA. Behav Pharmacol. 2005 Sep;16(5-6):315-31.

3 Wen Jiang1,2, Yun Zhang1, Lan Xiao1, Jamie Van Cleemput1, Shao-Ping Ji1, Guang Bai3 and Xia Zhang1. *Cannabinoids promote embryonic and adult hippocampus neurogenesis and produce anxiolytic- and antidepressant-like effects.* 1Neuropsychiatry Research Unit, Department of Psychiatry, University of Saskatchewan, Saskatoon, Saskatchewan, Canada. 2Department of Neurology, Xijing Hospital, Fourth Military Medical University, Xi'an, People's Republic of China. 3Department of Biomedical Sciences, Dental School, Program in Neuroscience, University of Maryland, Baltimore, Maryland, USA. J Clin Invest. 2005;115(11):3104–3116.

4 Corless IB, Lindgren T, Holzemer W, Robinson L, Moezzi S, Kirksey K, Coleman C, Tsai YF, Sanzero Eller L, Hamilton MJ, Sefcik EF, Canaval GE, Rivero Mendez M, Kemppainen JK, Bunch EH, Nicholas PK, Nokes KM, Dole P, Reynolds N. *Marijuana Effectiveness as an HIV Self-Care Strategy.* MGH Institute of Health Professions, School of nursing, Boston, Massachusetts 02129, USA. icorless@mghihp.edu Clin Nurs Res. 2009 May;18(2):172-93

Mental Disorders
Autism

NO MODERN CANNABIS STUDIES AVAILABLE

Thirty years ago few people had ever heard the word autism. By 1975, only one in 5,000 children had been diagnosed with this condition.[1] Nowadays it is a household word, and almost everybody knows of someone suffering from the disease. The allopathic community considers autism a neuro-developmental disorder that begins in very early childhood.

Among many psychological approaches applied to autism, applied behavioral analysis (ABA), developed by O.I. Lovaas Ph.D.,[2] appears to stand out in reported efficacies. Using ABA, improvements were seen in IQ, social skills, adaptive behavior and academic progress.[3,4,5] However, while proven effective, ABA's one-on-one teaching conditions remain a 'full-time job' at about 40 hours a week, making it cost prohibitive for many parents.

Pharmaceutical medications (such as Ritalin, an amphetamine-like drug), are given to millions of children every year to control symptoms. This leaves many parents little choice but to accept the risks of possible adverse effects, with reported deaths in the hundreds. No cure exists, resulting in an ever-growing number of autistic patients. Government statistics suggest the prevalence rate of autism is increasing 10-17% annually, doubling roughly every five years since 1980.[6] The facts are starkly clear: the pervasiveness of autism is growing exponentially. If current trends continue and no cure is found, we could be looking at a future reality where, by 2047, one in two people will be diagnosed as autistic.

Outwardly, autistic patients may look perfectly normal, but a closer look at their behavior demonstrates obvious differences from those unaffected. Autism is considered a spectrum disorder in which signs and symptoms range from mild to severe. Symptoms of autism include impaired social interaction and language skills, difficulty in relating to others including peers, reduced or altered emotional or behavioral responses, difficulty making eye contact, no interest in sharing experiences and repetitive focus and actions (ritualistic behavior such as lining up items are commonly noted). Depending on the severity, autistic patients are frequently socially isolated and often considered social outcasts by the rest of society, which does not know how to relate to them.

The reasons for autism's development and its exponential growth remain a mystery within the modern medical system, which generally hypothesizes that genetic and environmental conditions are at play. More specific origination theories include: bio-chemical causes, psychiatric causes, possible food components (e.g. gluten, casein, Vitamin D deficiency), the overuse of pharmaceutical drugs (e.g. the use of antibiotics or oxytocin during birth), parent's compromised immune-systems, vaccinations, neuro-inflammatory conditions, auto-immune conditions, imbalances of neuro-transmitters, toxins (e.g. lead, mercury, pesticides), microbes (e.g. mold, viral load) or electromagnetic pollution.

"Autism is a very expensive disorder costing our society upwards of $35 billion in direct (both medical and non-medical) and indirect costs to care for all individuals diagnosed each year over their lifetimes."[7] As it stands, many autistic children will likely need life-long care. Parents and caretakers need to make specific and practical long-term care plans that continue beyond their own lifetimes.

CANNABIS AND AUTISM

Scientists have learned much from communicative autistic people. For one, autistic individuals process sensory information differently, thus producing an altered perception, and by extension, meaning to reality.

Some cannabis users have reported similar experiences when using more than the therapeutically appropriate dose. For example, experiences of sensory disconnect between the eye and the ear, not unlike the disjointed soundtrack of a poorly dubbed foreign movie, have been noted to cause people to temporarily withdraw and display symptoms similar to those observed in autistic persons.

Based on these observations, it is hypothesized that dose-specific cannabinoids may somehow be involved in calibrating the connectivity between sensory input, perception, meaning and the ability to respond and function.

Many parents have found themselves up against a wall. Feeling hopeless in the face of modern medicine's iinability to understand the disease and its origin, perhaps lacking lack of safe and effective assistance, many have turned to cannabis.[8] Based on anecdotal reports by some physicians, pediatricians, caretakers and patients themselves that using cannabis had significant positive effects on patients suffering from autism, efforts are under way to learn more about if and how these reported therapeutic effects take place.

Positive results have been reported from ingestion of appropriate doses of cannabis or their pharmaceutical version of isolated cannabinoids, even in some extremely difficult cases where pharmaceutical treatment had proven ineffective or destructive. Reported results included reductions in tantrums, rage, self-injury and property destruction, and improved happiness, an increased ability to learn, and flexibility in altering norms.

While it is known that the body's own endocannabinoid system is involved in mood regulation, no clinical study results exist to confirm or deny the anecdotally positive experiences of autistics.

Cannabis and isolated cannabinoids can both have adverse effects, especially outside their appropriate therapeutic dosage; this must be cautiously considered, especially when dealing with children. However, parents faced with repeated ineffectiveness from prescribed pharmaceuticals may benefit in working with a qualified health care professional experienced in evaluating possible benefits of metered cannabis or prescription cannabinoids.

EXPLORING MIND–BODY CONSCIOUSNESS

Most differences between autistic and 'normal' people are defined by the ability to function according to socially 'normal' criteria. For most autistic people, their own symptoms are natural, and autism is nothing to be ashamed about. This is remarkable, and in contrast to many fully functioning 'normal' people who often feel ashamed for something as simple as their face, height or name. In this sense, it would seem that a majority of autistic people may have a more centered sense of their worth than a 'normal' person.

Along the spectrum of ability to function, some autistics display extraordinary abilities in relatively narrow fields. Professor Treffert,[9] researcher at the University of Wisconsin Medical School, discovered in his research on savant syndrome that over half of all savants are autistics. Abilities include: total musical recall,[10] total visual recall,[11] synesthesia,[12] and animal empathy.[13] A study by Patricia Howlin of King's College, London, suggests that as many as one-third of autistic people have some sort of savant-like capability[14] in areas such as calculation or music. Savant syndrome then is a case where the politically correct euphemism "differently abled" has real meaning. Autistic savants displaying super-natural ability alongside their sub-normal limitations demonstrate new possibilities for the human mind.

Since the senses of each autistic person seem in tune with realities different from those of non-autistic people, learning how these senses function may provide insights to better understand, communicate and relate to a person with an autistic mind.

QUESTIONS

How do the senses of this autistic person function?
What purpose does this extraordinary autistic state of mind serve?
What does this autistic person perceive that we do not?
Might there be a message inherent in autism?

While the impact on parents, caretakers and society at large is omnipresent and understood, we are left with questions about autism's alarming numbers, unknown possible environmental causes and psychosomatic influences. this mystery still in need of much exploring.

Since autistics are usually oblivious to the music, motion and symbology of neuro-typical or 'normal' human-to-human communication using gesture, voice, body language and facial muscles, answering the following questions may be useful.

How can I add voice and body to mere words?
How can I learn to understand facial expressions?
How can I make my facial expressions understood?
How can I add theatre to my message?

1 http://www.autismspeaks.org/docs/Prevalence_Graph_12_18_2009.pdf

2 Lovaas OI. *Behavioral treatment and normal educational and intellectual functioning in young autistic children.* Consult Clin Psychol. 1987 Feb;55(1):3-9.

3 Cohen, Howard, Amerine-Dickens, Mila, Smith, Tristram. *Early Intensive Behavioral Treatment: Replication of the UCLA Model in a Community Setting. 2006.* Journal of Developmental & Behavioral Pediatrics, 27 (2), 145-155.

4 Sallows, Glen O. & Graupner, Tamlynn D. *Intensive Behavioral Treatment for Children with Autism: Four-Year Outcome and Predictors.* 2005. American Journal on Mental Retardation, 110 (6), 417-438.

SUGGESTED BLESSING:

May you find supportive teachers who can direct the autistic gaze and focus in fruitful directions.

May you be like a Hollywood Star and learn easy and practical ways to add meaningful theatre to your expressions.

May you discover a way to add gesture, voice, body language and facial expressions to linguistics, so as to be more fluent with others.

5 Myers SM, Johnson CP. *Management of children with autism spectrum disorders.* American Academy of Pediatrics Council on Children With Disabilities. Pediatrics. 2007 Nov;120(5):1162-82.

6 Ibid.

7 Ganz M.L., MS, Phd. *The Lifetime Distribution of the Incremental Societal Costs of Autism.* Arch Pediatr Adolesc Med. 2007;161(4):343-349.

8 Autism Research Institute. 4182 Adams Ave., San Diego, CA 92116. *Medical Marijuana: A Valuable Treatment for Autism?* Autism Research Review International, 2003, Vol. 17, No. 1, page 3.

9 Darold A. Treffert. *Extraordinary People: Understanding Savant Syndrome,* iUniverse.com, 2000.

10 Derek Paravicini (Born July, 1979) can play any piece of music after hearing it but once.

11 Richard Wawro (Born April, 1952) Wawro's phenomenal and extremely detailed and vivid land and seascape drawings are rendered from memory after seeing them but once.

12 Daniel Tammet. (Born January, 1979) Tammet is well-known for his vivid and complex ability to see positive integer up to 10,000 with its own unique shape, color, texture and feeling.

13 Temple Grandin. (Born August, 1947) is an American doctor of animal science and Professor at Colorado State University.

14 Howlin P, Goode S, Hutton J, Rutter M. *Savant skills in autism: psychometric approaches and parental reports.* Department of Psychology, Institute of Psychiatry, King's College London, London SE5 8AF, UK. Philos Trans R Soc Lond B Biol Sci. 2009 May 27;364(1522):1359-67.

Mental Disorders
Depression

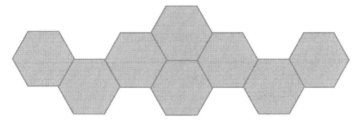

NUMBER OF STUDIES: 8

CHI VALUE: 23

While brief episodes of 'feeling depressed' are part of the human experience, severe or clinical depression can make it very difficult or even impossible to get out of bed in the morning and function normally. An estimated 120-million-plus people suffer from depression worldwide.[1] Symptoms vary but may include: low energy or lack of interest in life, work or pleasure.

Western medicine does not claim to know the causes for depression, but hypothesizes that genetic predisposition, certain underlying medical conditions (e.g. hypothyroidism), toxins or nutritional deficiencies which alter normal neurochemistry, stressful life events (deep and sudden changes) or a combination of these and other factors are causal agents.

Treatment varies. Psychiatrists prescribe antidepressant medications, while psychologists employ psychotherapy. Some patients with milder forms of the disease find help in using the herb St. John's Wort. Depression during longer nights in winter may also respond well to an exposure of full spectrum light at home.

It is estimated that about 15% of clinically depressed patients will succeed in committing suicide. This morbidity combined with the other debilitating symptoms make treatment of the disease and support of patients paramount.

Ironically, antidepressant drugs, marketed to treat depression and prevent suicides and sold sold by the billions in the U.S. alone reportedly contribute to a significant rise in suicide rates. In fact, the FDA has commissioned major antidepressants like paxil, prozac or zoloft to post black box warning labels regarding rise of suicidality.

CANNABIS AND DEPRESSION

Cannabinoids have proven effective in laboratory studies and rodent tests for antidepressant activity. These effects appear to share a similar mechanism of action as current antidepressant drugs such as the selective-serotonin reuptake inhibitors (SSRI's). Human trials have confirmed the antidepressant effects and mood elevating properties of cannabis.

More specifically, in both a Tulsa study[2] (1995) and an experiment from Miami[3] (2002), researchers discovered that cannabinoids might play a therapeutic role in improving mood and reducing signs of depression. In 2005, an international team of scientists examined the impact of a potent synthetic cannabinoid (HU210) in an experiment on rats. Most illegal substances have been reported to decrease the growth of new nerve cells in the hippocampus. However, chronic HU210 treatment promoted neurogenesis in the hippocampal regions of the study rodents and appeared likely to produce both an anxiolytic and antidepressant-like effect.[4]

A Vancouver study (2007) confirmed the potential antidepressant effect of cannabinoids; specifically, enhanced CB1 activity in the hippocampus region of the brain produced an antidepressant-like effect in rats.[5] Scientists from Montreal, Canada (2007) lent further support for the hypothesis that cannabis modulates moods and possesses antidepressant-like properties via CB1 receptors.[6]

A Boston trial (2009) involved data collected from 775 patients living with HIV/AIDS and the manifestation of depression. Results revealed that cannabis was more effective in treating depression when compared with standard prescription and over-the-counter medications given for the same condition.[7]

Scientists from Sao Paulo, Brazil (2010) conducted a review of available studies on two cannabinoids (CBD and THC) and their impact on the psychiatric patient. Cannabidiol showed a therapeutic tendency as an antipsychotic, anxiolytic, and antidepressant while THC emerged as a potential adjuvant in the treatment of schizophrenia.[8] In addition, an Oxford, Mississippi, experiment demonstrated that THC exerted antidepressant-like actions, and thus might contribute to the overall mood-elevating properties of cannabis."[9]

STUDY SUMMARY:

Drugs	Type of Study	Published Year, Place, and Key Results	CHI
Δ9-THC, Δ8-THC, CBG, CBN, CBC, CBD	Animal study (mice)	2010 – University of Mississippi. THC and other cannabinoids exert antidepressant-like actions and mood elavation.	2
CBD and THC	Meta-analysis	2010 – Universidade de São Paulo, Brasil. Cannabidiol therapeutic potential: antipsychotic, anxiolytic, and antidepressant. THC: adjuvant in the treatment of schizophrenia.	4
Cannabis	775 Humans living with HIV/AIDS	2009 – MGH Institute of Health Professions, School of Nursing, Boston. Cannabis considered effective in treating anxiety and depression and other symptoms in AIDS patients.	3
WIN55,212-2 (synthetic CB1 agonist)	Animal study (rats)	2007 – Montreal, Canada. Central CB1 modulates mood and has antidepressant-like effects.	2
HU-210 (CB1 receptor agonist), URB597 (the fatty acid amide hydrolase inhibitor), AM251 (CB1 receptor antagonist)	Animal study (rats)	2007 – Department of Psychology, University of British Columbia, Vancouver, Canada. Enhanced CB1 activity in the hippocampus region of the brain produces an antidepressant-like effect.	2
HU210 (CB1 receptor agonist)	Animal and laboratory study (rats)	2005 – Multi-institutional and international study. Hippocampal cells are immunoreactive for CB1 receptors. Cannabinoids may induce hippocampal neurogenesis, which may explain the anxiolytic and antidepressant-like effects.	2
Oral doses of Delta-9-THC 2.5mg to 5mg	Human Clinical Study (3 patients)	2002 – Department of Medicine, University of Miami, Florida. Decrease in itching, improvement in sleep and resolution of depression in patients with pruritus due to cholestatic liver disease.	3
2.5 mg of dronabinol twice daily or placebo	139 patients living with AIDS	1995 – St. John's Hospital, Tulsa, Oklahoma, USA. Improvement in mood (10% vs -2% for placebo).	5

Total CHI Value 23

STRAIN SPECIFIC CONSIDERATIONS

In these various studies, cannabinoids demonstrated the ability to modulate mood in depression via different pathways or mechanisms, chiefly among them THC and whole spectrum cannabis. THC binds with both CB1 and CB2 relatively equally. It is hypothesized that cannabis, containing 70 cannabinoids and hundreds of non-cannabinoid ingredients, may work in concert to induce mood improvement via CB1 and CB2 activation as well as through the balancing influences of whole plant constituents.

Δ9-THC, Δ8-THC, CBG, CBN, CBC, CBD, Cannabis, WIN55,212-2, HU-210 and dronabinol have been tested for treatment of depression. THC binds with both CB1 and CB2 relatively equally. Cannabigerol (CBG) binds with both CB1 and CB2. Cannabinol (CBN) has higher affinity for CB2. Cannabichromene's (CBC) underlying mechanism of action may not involve CB1 or CB2 receptors. Cannabidiol (CBD) has a greater affinity for CB2. WIN55,212-2 has a grater affinity for CB2. HU-210 has a higher affinity for CB1 receptors. Dronabinol is an isomer (same molecular formula but different structural formula) of Δ9-tetrahydrocannabinol.

Sativas and sativa dominant strains tend to have a higher THC:CBD/CBN ratio and are generally sought after by cannabis-using patients suffering from depression for their stimulating, energizing and uplifting potential.

EXPLORING MIND–BODY CONSCIOUSNESS

The emotional realities of a depressed person often include feeling weighed down by layers upon layers of unexpressed emotions such as hurt or anger. This accumulative emotional burden often results in low energy and lack of interest in life, work or pleasure. The prospect of expending energy to do some emotional house cleaning when depressed can be depressing in and of itself. Healing depression requires patients to deal with and feel the layers of emotions that so depress the body, mind and spirit. This is especially true when considering anger and hurt.

Anger is generally judged because of its direct association with violent expressions. Therefore, many consider it as something not OK to feel, or at least not for very long or with any real intensity. However, when discerning the complexities of anger, it is important to realize that as with any real feeling it can be liberating or imprisoning. For example, expressions of anger can be authentic or dramatic performances. Authentic anger is felt and released while performing anger is harbored and stored. Anger can either be used to communicate or to manipulate others. Anger can be focused on the impact of an action which is easily correctable or it can be used to shame a person into thinking there is something wrong with them. Few role models exist that demonstrate how to express and release anger with intensity, focused appropriately for positive impact.

QUESTIONS

Is it OK for you to feel angry?
How do you deal with your anger?
How intense do you allow your anger to get?

SUGGESTED BLESSING:

May you find a reason to get intricately involved with something that produces vibrant thoughts and juicy feelings.

May the process of thinking and feeling release the heaviness that so consumes your energy.

May you discover an omnipresent help to make this process easy or at least as easy as possible.

Does your anger leave a wave of destruction in its wake?

Similarly, for many people, it is not okay to feel hurt. Hurt is seen as a liability or vulnerability and considered a sign of weakness. Hurt diminishes trust and has the ability to destroy a healthy love of self, reduce the experience of one's worth, and otherwise negatively affect self-esteem and self-confidence.

Can you identify when your self-love suffers?
Do you notice when your self-esteem has taken a hit?
Do you see what reduces your self-confidence?
Is it OK for you to feel hurt?
How do you deal with your hurt?
Can you show hurt to others?
Can you show it to yourself?
Does hurt heal you?

TAKE NOTICE

COCOA • NUTMEG

COCOA: Scientists from Tucson, Arizona, reported that chocolate is likely to be involved in increasing low levels of serotonin and dopamine (neurotransmitters involved in 'mood regulation).[10]

NUTMEG: An extract of nutmeg seeds (10mg/kg) has been found - in a mouse model - to have antidepressant properties similar to those of pharmacological antidepressants such as imipramine (15 mg/kg) and fluoxetine (20 mg/kg). The researchers from Guru Jambheshwar University in Hisar, India, stated: "The antidepressant-like effect of the extract seems to be mediated by interaction with the adrenergic, dopaminergic, and serotonergic systems."

1 World Health Organization (WHO). Mental Health. *Depression. 2011.* http://www.who.int/mental_health/management/depression/definition/en/

2 Beal JE, Olson R, Laubenstein L, Morales JO, Bellman P, Yangco B, Lefkowitz L, Plasse TF, Shepard KV. *Dronabinol as a treatment for anorexia associated with weight loss in patients with AIDS.* St. John's Hospital, Tulsa, Oklahoma, USA. Journal of Pain and Symptom Management 1995;10(2):89-97

3 Neff GW, O'Brien CB, Reddy KR, Bergasa NV, Regev A, Molina E, Amaro R, Rodriguez MJ, Chase V, Jeffers L, Schiff E. *Preliminary observation with dronabinol in patients with intractable pruritus secondary to cholestatic liver disease.* Department of Medicine, University of Miami, Florida, USA. Am J Gastroenterol. 2002 Aug; 97(8):2117-9.

4 Wen Jiang1,2, Yun Zhang1, Lan Xiao1, Jamie Van Cleemput1, Shao-Ping Ji1, Guang Bai3 and Xia Zhang1. *Cannabinoids promote embryonic and adult hippocampus neurogenesis and produce anxiolytic- and antidepressant-like effects.* 1Neuropsychiatry Research Unit, Department of Psychiatry, University of Saskatchewan, Saskatoon, Saskatchewan, Canada. 2Department of Neurology, Xijing Hospital, Fourth Military Medical University, Xi'an, People's Republic of China. 3Department of Biomedical Sciences, Dental School, Program in Neuroscience, University of Maryland, Baltimore, Maryland, USA. J Clin Invest. 2005;115(11):3104–3116.

5 McLaughlin RJ, Hill MN, Morrish AC, Gorzalka BB. Local enhancement of cannabinoid CB1 receptor signalling in the dorsal hippocampus elicits an antidepressant-like effect. Department of Psychology, University of British Columbia, Vancouver, Canada. Behav Pharmacol. 2007 Sep;18(5-6):431-8.

6 Bambico FR, Katz N, Debonnel G, Gobbi G. Cannabinoids elicit antidepressant-like behavior and activate serotonergic neurons through the medial prefrontal cortex. Neurobiological Psychiatry Unit, Department of Psychiatry, McGill University, Montréal, Quebec, Canada H3A 1A1. Published 25 October 2007 in J Neurosci, 27(43): 11700-11.

7 Corless IB, Lindgren T, Holzemer W, Robinson L, Moezzi S, Kirksey K, Coleman C, Tsai YF, Sanzero Eller L, Hamilton MJ, Sefcik EF, Canaval GE, Rivero Mendez M, Kemppainen JK, Bunch EH, Nicholas PK, Nokes KM, Dole P, Reynolds N. Marijuana Effectiveness as an HIV Self-Care Strategy. MGH Institute of Health Professions, School of nursing, Boston, Massachusetts 02129, USA. icorless@mghihp.edu Clin Nurs Res. 2009 May;18(2):172-93

8 Crippa JA, Zuardi AW, Hallak JE. Therapeutical use of the cannabinoids in psychiatry. Departamento de Neurociências e Ciências do Comportamento, Faculdade de Medicina de Ribeirão Preto, Universidade de São Paulo, Ribeirão Preto, SP, Brasil. Rev Bras Psiquiatr. 2010 May;32 Suppl 1:S56-66.

9 Abir T. El-Alfya, , , Kelly Iveya, Keisha Robinsona, Safwat Ahmedb, 1, Mohamed Radwanb, Desmond Sladeb, Ikhlas Khanb, c, Mahmoud ElSohlyb, d and Samir Rossb, c *Antidepressant-like effect of Δ9-tetrahydrocannabinol and other cannabinoids isolated from Cannabis sativa L*. a Pharmacology Department, School of Pharmacy, University of Mississippi, University, MS 38677, USA. b National Center for Natural Products Research, University of Mississippi, University, MS 38677, USA. c Pharmacognosy Department, School of Pharmacy, University of Mississippi, University, MS 38677, USA. d Pharmaceutics Department, School of Pharmacy, University of Mississippi, University, MS 38677, USA. Pharmacology Biochemistry and Behavior. Volume 95, Issue 4, June 2010, Pages 434-442.

10 Bruinsma K, Taren DL. *Chocolate: food or drug?* Arizona Prevention Center, University of Arizona, College of Medicine, Tucson 85719, USA. J Am Diet Assoc. 1999 Oct;99(10):1249-56.

11 Dhingra D, Sharma A. *Antidepressant-like activity of n-hexane extract of nutmeg (Myristica fragrans) seeds in mice*. Pharmacology Division, Department of Pharmaceutical Sciences, Guru Jambheshwar University, Hisar, Haryana, India. J Med Food. 2006 Spring;9(1):84-9.

Mental Disorders
Manic-Depressive Disorder or Bipolar Affective Disorder (BAD)

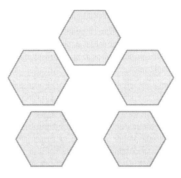

NUMBER OF STUDIES: 5

CHI VALUE: 8

Psychiatry considers manic-depressive disorder to be a chronic mental illness characterized by dramatic and sudden mood swings ranging from manic to depressed and back. Onset of the illness is usually observed in late adolescents or early adulthood but has also been noted in younger people. While normal ups and downs in mood are part of being human, pathological mood swings severely reduce quality of life and the ability to function and maintain social relations. Subgroups of the illness are identified on a spectrum by severity of the disease and frequencies of mood swings.

The scientific community believes bipolar disorders has a variety of causes. These include genetic, environmental (childhood trauma or abuse)[1] and physiological (e.g. brain, endocrine irregularities) origins. Diagnosis is based on observation and clinical evaluation. Tests may be performed to rule out possible underlying causes or contributing diseases.

Western treatment consists of pharmacological interventions and talk therapy. The most commonly used pharmaceutical is an alkali metal – lithium - which functions as a potent mood stabilizer and has been proven to significantly prevent suicides in bi-polar patients.[2]

CANNABIS AND MANIC-DEPRESSIVE DISORDER

Scientists have conducted numerous studies to examine the effects of cannabis and cannabinoids on individuals with manic-depressive disorder. Results revealed that the body's own endocannabinoid system is involved in mood regulation. While some case studies reported possible beneficial effects vis a vis manic episodes, available evidence was too small and narrow to warrant using cannabis/cannabinoids for treatment. However, the plant and its products have been found to therapeutically influence the depressive aspect of the disease.

STUDY SUMMARY:

Drugs	Type of Study	Published Year, Place, and Key Results	CHI
Δ9-THC, Δ8-THC, CBG, CBN, CBC, and CBD	Animal study (mice)	2010 – University of Mississippi. THC and other cannabinoids exert antidepressant-like actions and mood elevation.[3]	2
Cannabidiol (CBD)	Placebo controlled human case study (2 patients with BAD)	2010 – Department of Neuropsychiatry and Medical Psychology, Faculty of Medicine, University of São Paulo, Ribeirão Preto, São Paulo, Brazil. Ineffective for the manic episode of BAD.[4]	- 5
Cannabis	Human case study, one patient diagnosed with BAD.	2007 – University of Louisville School of Medicine, Louisville, Kentucky. Cannabis reduced the number of depressed days and increased the number of hypomanic days.[5]	3
Cannabis and various other cannabinoids	Literature review	2005 – Department of Psychiatry, University of Newcastle upon Tyne, Royal Victoria Infirmary, Newcastle upon Tyne, UK. Some patients claim that cannabis relieves symptoms of mania and/or depression.[6]	4
Cannabis	Human case studies	1998 – Department of Psychiatry, Harvard Medical School, Boston, Massachusetts. Positive therapeutic impact based on individual case studies only.[7]	4

Total CHI Value   8

STRAIN SPECIFIC CONSIDERATIONS

Only whole plant cannabis and CBD (rather than other forms) have been tested for treatment of bipolar disorder. CBD was not proven effective while whole herb constituents could be supportive. CBD has a greater affinity for CB2. Whole cannabis contains cannabinoids activating CB1 and CB2.

Sativas and sativa-dominant strains tend to contain a higher THC:CBD ratio, which may slightly reduce CBD influence.

Some patients have reported on alternate strains of cannabis used during either the manic or depressive phase. During depressive phases, cannabis-using patients may benefit from sativas; while during manic phases, they might benefit more from an indica strain.

EXPLORING MIND–BODY CONSCIOUSNESS

In a manic-depressive patient, the mind can swing relatively quickly between excessive excitement (mania) and feeling low in energy or spirit (depression). Both depression and mania can be a consequence of early childhood trauma or abuse. In that sense, the disease might work as a coping mechanism to separate the present state of mind from the encroachment of thoughts and feelings associated with a trigger event. A trigger can be anything the patient associates with the underlying trauma - weather, a certain song, a specific memory, a holiday or a distinct smell.

It is well known that manic-depressive patients are more sensitive to stress than the normal person. External stress seems to draw the trigger event closer to the forefront of the mind and in so doing, can become a source of stress itself. Together, external and internal stress can create a loop-like experience that can severely threaten the well-being of the patient and can give rise to manic-depressive episodes. The patient might believe that an episode of the disease is preferable to dealing with the

SUGGESTED BLESSING:

May you have compassion for your manic-depressive responses.

May you be able to recognize your triggers.

May you embrace and befriend your triggers.

May you find a way to learn from your situation.

May you find a way to turn a liability into a present power or strength.

trigger event that resides deep in the recesses of the unconscious.

Others have suggested that the rhythmic appearances of bi-polar episodes may be an effort of the unconscious to bring the underlying trauma to conscious awareness in thin layers so that the conscious mind can process it. Thus, each episode may be one layer of an onion, only truly processed and transcended when the last layer is peeled away.

1 Gabriele S. Leverich, Robert M. Post. *Course of bipolar illness after history of childhood trauma.* Biological Psychiatry Branch, NIMH, NIH, DHHS, Bethesda, MD 20892, USA. The Lancet, Volume 367, Issue 9516, Pages 1040 - 1042, 1 April 2006.

2 Baldessarini RJ, Tondo L, Davis P, Pompili M, Goodwin FK, Hennen J. *Decreased risk of suicides and attempts during long-term lithium treatment: a meta-analytic review.* International Consortium for Research on Bipolar Disorders, Department of Psychiatry and Neuroscience Program, Harvard Medical School, Boston, MA, USA. Bipolar Disord. 2006 Oct;8(5 Pt 2):625-39.

3 Abir T. El-Alfya, , , Kelly Iveya, Keisha Robinsona, Safwat Ahmedb, 1, Mohamed Radwanb, Desmond Sladeb, Ikhlas Khanb, c, Mahmoud ElSohlyb, d and Samir Rossb, c *Antidepressant-like effect of Δ9-tetrahydrocannabinol and other cannabinoids isolated from Cannabis sativa L.* a Pharmacology Department, School of Pharmacy, University of Mississippi, University, MS 38677, USA. b National Center for Natural Products Research, University of Mississippi, University, MS 38677, USA. c Pharmacognosy Department, School of Pharmacy, University of Mississippi, University, MS 38677, USA. d Pharmaceutics Department, School of Pharmacy, University of Mississippi, University, MS 38677, USA. Pharmacology Biochemistry and Behavior. Volume 95, Issue 4, June 2010, Pages 434-442.

4 Zuardi A, Crippa J, Dursun S, Morais S, Vilela J, Sanches R, Hallak J. *Cannabidiol was ineffective for manic episode of bipolar affective disorder.* Department of Neuropsychiatry and Medical Psychology, Faculty of Medicine, University of São Paulo, Ribeirão Preto, São Paulo, Brazil. awzuardi@fmrp.usp.br J Psychopharmacol. 2010 Jan;24(1):135-7.

5 El-Mallakh RS, Brown C. *The effect of extreme marijuana use on the long-term course of bipolar I illness: a single case study.* Mood Disorders Research Program, Department of Psychiatry and Behavioral Sciences, University of Louisville School of Medicine, Louisville, Kentucky 40202, USA. J Psychoactive Drugs 2007;39(2):201-2.

6 Ashton CH, Moore PB, Gallagher P, Young AH. *Cannabinoids in bipolar affective disorder: a review and discussion of their therapeutic potential.* Department of Psychiatry, University of Newcastle upon Tyne, Royal Victoria Infirmary, Newcastle upon Tyne, UK. J Psychopharmacol. 2005 May;19(3):293-300.

7 Grinspoon L, Bakalar JB. *The use of cannabis as a mood stabilizer in bipolar disorder: anecdotal evidence and the need for clinical research.* Department of Psychiatry, Harvard Medical School, Boston, Massachusetts 02115, USA. J Psychoactive Drugs. 1998 Apr-Jun;30(2):171-7.

Mental Disorders
Post Traumatic Stress Disorder

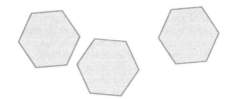

NUMBER OF STUDIES: 3

CHI VALUE: 7

Post Traumatic Stress Disorder (PTSD) is a debilitating condition affecting the body, mind and spirit. The condition results from direct or witnessed exposure to an extreme traumatic event such as war, police action, famine, earthquake, tsunami, assault, abuse, rape, kidnapping, torture, plane crash, explosions, life-threatening illness, or any situation involving the threat of death, extreme fears, dread and helplessness. PTSD most often results from sudden trauma that happens without warning, was repeated and over long periods of time, amd included intentional violence to body and psyche, involved grotesque injury and death, rape, or the loss of a close friend or relative.

While history brims with cases describing patients suffering from the symptoms of PTSD, the allopathic health care system, including hospitals charged with caring for veterans, has been very slow to acknowledge the disease. During WWI and WWII, it was called "battle fatigue" or "shell shock," respectively. The British military placed more than 300 soldiers in front of a firing squad and shot them to death ostensibly for cowardice before the enemy or desertion, when most of them were likely suffering from PTSD. The current term, PTSD, was formulated during the Vietnam War when thousands of soldiers came home suffering from a collection of common symptoms including guilt, depression, flashbacks, insomnia, or the inability to be close to loved ones. It was not until 1980 that PTSD was codified and included in the DSM.

With the advent of new imaging techniques, researchers discovered new insights pertinent to PTSD. A meta-analysis of available neuroimaging research suggests measurable physiological changes in the limbic system in patients with PTSD; namely the amygdala, responsible for the processing of fear, the medial prefrontal cortex involved in decision making, and the hippocampus, needed for the formation of long-term memories. The analysis suggests that during episodes of activated PTSD, the hippocampus is diminished in size, neuronal integrity, and functional integrity. Furthermore, the medial prefrontal cortex appears to be volumetrically smaller and is hyporesponsive during symptomatic PTSD. Lastly, neuroimaging research reveals heightened amygdala responsivity in PTSD during symptomatic states.[1]

Not surprisingly, people exposed to the same traumatic events tend to respond differently. Some may only experience mild and passing symptoms while others may feel numb, depressed and suicidal or progress to developing full-blown PTSD. Symptoms often begin within three months after the traumatic event and may include: profound lack of care for anything, emptiness, hopelessness, helplessness, worthlessness, shame, emotional numbness, distrust, paranoid behavior with hypervigilance, inexplicable fear, anxiety, lost memories, passivity, withdrawing, fits of anger with little or no provocation, irritability, impatience, lack of focus, insomnia, fitful sleep with sweating, nightmares, generalized weakness or fatigue, flashbacks and avoidance of anything associated with the traumatic event.

Avoidance strategies themselves can become an additional problem for patients with PTSD. The compounding effects of detachments and unhealthy tension-reducing behaviors such as substance/food abuse, cutting or promiscuous sex can make recovery more challenging.

The primary treatments within orthodox medicine are talk-therapy and pharmaceutical medications, primarily antidepressants and anxiolytics. However, misuse of prescription drugs and possible severe adverse effects with these classes of medication frame the clear and present limitations of pharmaceutical intervention. In addition, despite success from behavioral-cognitive therapies in the treatment of PTSD, patients often show vulnerability to reversal of progress by exposure to stress and stress triggers.

CANNABIS AND POST TRAUMATIC STRESS DISORDER

Recent discoveries (2009) from Haifa, Israel, show that the fear-processing center of the brain (amygdala) contains a significant number of endogenous cannabinoid receptors (CB1). Observation demonstrated that when the synthetic cannabinoid WIN55,212-2 was injected into the amygdala of rats, the cannabinoid modulated anxiety responses, especially extinction learning via regulation of the hypothalamic-pituitary-adrenal axis.[2] The Israeli study results further suggested that the cannabinoid supported inhibitory avoidance conditioning and extinction (the goal in PTSD therapies) by reducing the negative effects of stress.[3] Moreover, the same study from Haifa demonstrated that: "microinjecting WIN55,212-2 into the basolateral amygdala (BLA) before exposing the rats to a stressor reversed the enhancing effects of the stressor on inhibitory avoidance (IA) conditioning and its impairing effects on IA extinction." This observation might explain why cannabinoids can modulate panic responses not just after extremely painful and traumatic events but also before.

An Ottawa study (2009) reported that cannabis could remove fear responses to stressors such as nightmares, poor sleep, night sweats and flashbacks. Forty-seven PTSD patients suffering from nightmares that failed to adequately respond to standard pharmaceutical antidepressants and hypnotics received the synthetic cannabinoid nabilone. Researchers wrote: "The majority of patients (72%) receiving nabilone experienced either cessation of nightmares or a significant reduction in nightmare intensity. Subjective improvement in sleep time, the quality of sleep, and the reduction of daytime flashbacks and night sweats were also noted by some patients."[4]

Researchers (2008) from Richmond, Virginia, worked to determine the effect of the endocannabinoid system on learning and forgetting pleasant and unpleasant experiences. After analyzing the tests, the authors wrote: "…these results provide compelling support for the hypothesis that the endogenous cannabinoid system plays a necessary role in the extinction of aversively motivated behaviors but is expendable for appetitively motivated behaviors."[5]

STUDY SUMMARY:

Drugs	Type of Study	Published Year, Place, and Key Results	CHI
WIN55,212-2	Animal study (rats)	2009 – Israel, Haifa. WIN55,212-2 microinjected into the BLA reduced stress-induced elevations in corticosterone levels.	2
Nabilone	Human case study 47 Patients diagnoses with PTSD	2009 – Canada – Ottawa. Reduction in nightmares, night sweats, daytime flashbacks and improved sleep.	3
Rimonabant (CB 1 antagonist)	Animal study	2008 – United States – Richmond. Endogenous cannabinoid system is involved in forgetting painful events.	2

Total CHI Value   7

STRAIN SPECIFIC CONSIDERATIONS

WIN55,212-2, nabilone and rimonabant have been tested for the treatment of PTSD. WIN 55212-2 binds with higher affinity to CB2. Nabilone is a synthetic cannabinoid similar to THC, which binds with both CB1 and CB2 relatively equally. Rimonabant is a CB1 antagonist known to disrupt extinction learning (fear extinction).

While the human case study cited above relied on nabilone, a synthetic cannabinoid similar to THC, many cannabis using-patients prefer indicas or indica dominant hybrids with a relatively lower THC:CBD/CBN ratio, favoring the more relaxing and grounding properties of these strains.

EXPLORING MIND–BODY CONSCIOUSNESS

Psychosomatic researchers reported that WWII combat veterans who suffered from PTSD for decades possessed a chronically different thyroid hormone profile than normal men.[6] This was especially true for T3 concentrations, which were found in higher than normal concentrations. T3 is a potent, fast-acting hormone that readily enters the brain and is involved in fight or flight. Scientists hypothesized that this constantly elevated hormone profile associated with stress and fear is involved in the mechanism of PTSD.

Scientists describe PTSD as a temporary breakdown of a natural and balanced response reaction between body and mind, between imagination and will, or between one's feeling and action.

Many of the symptoms or behaviors commonly seen in PTSD are coping mechanisms in the presence of an otherwise intolerable traumatic situation or memory of trauma. Irrational fears or anxieties, overly aggressive behaviors, substance abuse, pacing, rocking, isolating or unsafe behaviors are set in motion to cope with the intolerable. However, while these coping mechanisms may be initially practical and useful in avoiding the key event, over time they become a liability.

In a way, PTSD symptoms physically manifest into a message that cannot be denied. Suppressed emotions can harm you. Emotional release can contribute to your healing.

SUGGESTED BLESSING:

May you embrace yourself just as you are right now.

May you consider the possibility that all forgiveness benefits your health and aids in your healing.

SUGGESTED AFFIRMATION:

I am okay just as I am right now.

I can feel and release even the most powerful emotions.

I am safe now, I feel safe now, and I know I am safe now.

It takes time to heal, but it will not take forever.

Hypervigilant behavior is but one way I can make myself feel safe.

Anger is a sign that my values have been violated.

I can use that anger constructively and without hurting anyone.

AGGRAVATING FACTORS

Unresolved emotional trauma(s) / beliefs that suggest feeling and emotion are a weakness or liability / maintaining negative coping strategies.

HEALING FACTORS

Practice of forgiveness and acceptance / change in beliefs that devalue emotional experiences / use of positive coping skills.

ANECDOTE

Jack talked his girlfriend Daniela into a bike ride through downtown San Francisco. While Jack was used to the traffic and pace of the city, Daniela was new to it. As they rode south on Market on their way to see the gold plated roof of City Hall, a tractor-trailer slowly passed both of them. Jack saw Daniela wavering. Jack recalled, "She was getting really scared at the large wheels passing us. Daniela wobbled and flipped the bike. The large wheel rolled over the very top of her head and with a loud pop spilled its contents onto the street." Jack was still screaming uncontrollably when the Paramedics arrived. He kept repeating: "I'll never forget that sound, I'll never forget that sound."

Jack initially received treatment with pharmaceutical medication, but after a few days, he discontinued them because he felt in a constant fog, with dizziness and blurred vision. He could not sleep, and when he did manage to get some sleep, he would wake up drenched in sweat. The nightmares came almost every night. Jack told his therapist that his heart would start racing, he'd break into a sweat and shake every time he saw a tractor-trailer passing by. Worse were the nightmares and terrifying sounds of himself screaming silently as if falling helplessly into an abyss. In contrast, during therapy sessions, Jack was unwilling to remember details of the event. He had difficulty expressing his feelings, and the symptoms persisted. One time at work when somebody opened a champagne bottle, the sudden sound triggered a fit. He was hard to console and a co-worker took him home. Jack believed that safety and security were but an illusion.

After months of slow progress, a friend suggested that he obtain a cannabis prescription. He did, and for the first time in weeks, he relaxed into a deep and restful sleep, void of nightmares or night sweats. He felt more able to articulate and express the variety of his feelings about the event, especially his guilt. Over time he noticed that his guilt gave way to anger, which gave way to sorrow about Daniela's death, and slowly a sense of empathy and compassion became his new companions. Instead of, " I never forget that sound," he now kept repeating, "as long as I hear the sound of my breath, I am safe."

1 Shin LM, Rauch SL, Pitman RK. *Amygdala, medial prefrontal cortex, and hippocampal function in PTSD*. Department of Psychology, Tufts University, 490 Boston Avenue, Medford, MA 02155, USA. Ann N Y Acad Sci. 2006 Jul;1071:67-79.

2 Ganon-Elazar E, Akirav I.. *Cannabinoid receptor activation in the basolateral amygdala blocks the effects of stress on the conditioning and extinction of inhibitory avoidance*. Department of Psychology, University of Haifa, Haifa 31905, Israel. J Neurosci. 2009 Sep 9;29(36):11078-88.

3 Ibid.

4 Fraser, G.A. *The use of a synthetic cannabinoid in the management of treatment-resistant nightmares in post-traumatic stress disorder (PTSD)*. Operational Trauma and Stress Support Centre, Canadian Forces Health Services Centre, 1745 Alta Vista Drive, Ottawa, Ontario, Canada. fraser.ga2@forces.gc.ca CNS Neurosci Ther. 2009 Winter;15(1):84-8.

5 Harloe JP, Thorpe AJ, Lichtman AH. *Differential endocannabinoid regulation of extinction in appetitive and aversive Barnes maze tasks*. Department of Pharmacology and Toxicology, Medical College of Virginia Campus, Virginia Commonwealth University, Richmond, Virginia 23284, USA. Learn Mem. 2008 Oct 28;15(11):806-9.

6 Wang S, Mason J. *Elevations of serum T3 levels and their association with symptoms in World War II veterans with combat-related posttraumatic stress disorder: replication of findings in Vietnam combat veterans*. Psychosom Med 1999; 61: 131–138.

Mental Disorders
Schizophrenia

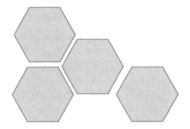

NUMBER OF STUDIES: 4

CHI VALUE: 16

Schizophrenia remains one of the most common and serious yet least understood mental illnesses in the world today. Swiss psychiatrist Eugene Bleuler first used the word schizophrenia, which he derived from the Greek words 'schizo' (to split) and 'phren' (brain or mind). However, unlike common usage suggests, it does not necessarily refer to a split personality (-ies) but rather a split or disconnect between thinking and feeling. Symptoms often include hallucinations involving the senses making it difficult for patients to communicate or connect to others and the world. These symptoms typically emerge in adolescence or early adulthood. Bleuler divided schizophrenic symptoms into positive and negative symptoms.

Positive symptoms (abnormal functions) may include: hallucinations (involving one or several of the senses but most commonly hearing voices), misunderstanding or misinterpreting internal or sense-based experiences, difficulty expressing oneself verbally, lack of insight, social awkwardness (disorganization, inappropriate behavior), grandiosity, hostility and feeling persecuted or suspicious.

Negative symptoms (reduction or absence of normal functions) may include: amotivation, lack of affect, lack of eye-contact, inappropriate emotional expressions, social isolation, poor hygiene, poor planning abilities, poor follow-through.

The allopathic tradition considers this type of mental illness a chronic condition that requires lifelong treatment. In this paradigm, no cure exists and treatment consists of managing symptoms, employing antipsychotic pharmaceutical drugs and psychological or social support. While antipsychotic drugs can help with some symptoms, they also significantly increase the risks of developing a wide variety of adverse effects. This causes a majority of patients to discontinue use. Adverse effects, especially from long-term use, may include: impotence, weight gain, and especially extrapyramidal[1] symptoms such as spasms of the neck, jaw, mouth, tongue, face, restlessness, inability to hold still or maintain a posture, and rigidity. Serious adverse effects may include brain damage, low blood pressure, cardiac toxicity, diabetes, seizures or death. However, considering the grave and often debilitating nature of this disease and in spite of considerable adverse effects, treatment enables many patients to live a relatively normal life.

Causes are not known but are considered to include a combination of environmental and genetic reasons. Scientists have conducted tens of thousands of studies to better understand the reasons for this elusive disease. Modern science learned that pre-natal stress could trigger subtle developmental changes, which might later develop into the disease. Prenatal stress,[2] family history,[3] social isolation,[4] inner city life,[5] sudden life altering events such as migration[6] or psychotic episodes are each commonly found in schizophrenia patients. Toxins, nutritional deficiencies, and other biological influences may also contribute and thus provide an opportunity for therapeutics such as detoxification and nutritional support.

Schizophrenic patients have excessive dopamine (neurotransmitter) in their brain's mesolimbic system. Drugs such as methamphetamines or cocaine produce similar patient presentations in chemistry and behavior. Intense life-changing events can trigger the onset of the illness especially in those who came from a schizophrenic family. Early child abuse has been identified with the development of certain mental disorders and some mental health practitioners suggest a strong link to schizophrenia as well.[7]

Diagnosis involves an observation and thorough history guided by the Diagnostic and Statistical Manual of Mental Disorders (DSM) to rule out underlying causes.

A variety of psychological traditions have taken their own views on schizophrenia. C. G. Jung, who believed schizophrenia related to unresolved early traumas, worked effectively with schizophrenic patients using non-authoritarian psychiatric work, free of drugs. Stanislav Grof's work on extraordinary states of consciousness and prenatal experiences describes schizophrenia as a type of spiritual crisis or emergency. Therapists associated with many disciplines around the world use numerous non-drug approaches to treat schizophrenia with varying degrees of success or cure rates. However, former schizophrenic patients who have healed their schizophrenic episode or spiritual emergency can be an invaluable help to people still stuck in the process.

CANNABIS AND SCHIZOPHRENIA

While other studies on cannabis and schizophrenia exist, I have selected two meta-analyses containing all or most of them and two other relevant experiments for the purpose of providing a relevant and general overview.

In the year 2004, University of California, Irvine, scientists discovered that the body's own cannabinoid anandamide levels in the cerebral spinal fluids (CSF) of untreated first-episode paranoid schizophrenics were eight times higher than healthy control subjects. Such an alteration remained absent in schizophrenics treated with 'typical' antipsychotics. These results suggest that anandamide increases in acute paranoid schizophrenia patients and may be a compensatory adaptation to the disease state.[8] This might indicate a potential role of the endocannabinoid system in schizophrenia pathology and treatment.

Many schizophrenic patients have never been exposed to cannabis and the vast majority of cannabis users do not develop psychotic events or subsequent schizophrenia. However, some observational studies present data demonstrating that cannabis use by still developing adolescents presents a statistical risk factor for developing schizophrenia. While cannabis is not a necessary or sufficient cause, in some cases, it may be a co-factor.

To better understand why certain users may be vulnerable when the majority are not, it may be helpful to examine some studies. London researchers (2005) looked at specific genetic expressions between similar patients and discovered that those who carried a specific allele[9] (one of two or more versions of a gene) were most likely to exhibit psychotic symptoms.[10]

It is hypothesized that an experience with cannabis may combine with an existing genetic vulnerability to induce psychosis. "There are two ways to measure genetic liability to psychosis—directly and indirectly—and studies with both measures provide growing evidence that an underlying mechanism of gene–environment interaction explains the association between cannabis and psychosis."[11]

Based on the current evidence, it would be prudent for adolescents and young adults with a known family history of psychosis or schizophrenia to stay away from cannabis, or any other mind altering substance, especially alcohol and speed-based drugs such as cocaine and methamphetamines.

Selected studies illuminate aspects of the interplay of genetic and environmental influences on developing schizophrenia. In 2009, German and U.S. researchers conducted a double-blind crossover clinical trial with 42 patients. Fulfilling DSM-IV criteria of acute paranoid schizophrenia, they compared the effectiveness of CBD with that of the antipsychotic amisulpride for the treatment of acute schizophrenia. Results revealed that the CBD reduced symptoms similar to that of amisulpride but with significantly lower incidence of side effects. The authors of the study concluded: "Cannabidiol revealed substantial antipsychotic properties in acute schizophrenia. This is in line with our suggestion of an adaptive role of the endocannabinoid system in paranoid schizophrenia, and raises further evidence that this adaptive mechanism may represent a valuable target for antipsychotic treatment strategies."[12]

Brazilian and Italian researchers conducted a meta-analysis of relevant literature in 2010 and suggested that THC was a potential adjuvant in the treatment of schizophrenia.[13] Additionally, CBD emerged with the most constant antipsychotic properties in dopamine- and glutamate-based models of schizophrenia[14] respectively.

STUDY SUMMARY:

Drugs	Type of Study	Published Year, Place, and Key Results	CHI
Cannabidiol (CBD) and SR141716A (CB1 antagonist)	Meta-analysis	2010 – University of Insubria, Italy. Potential novel approach for treating schizophrenia. CBD and THC Meta-analysis. THC: adjuvant in the treatment of schizophrenia.[15]	4
CBD	Meta-analysis	2010 – Universidade de São Paulo, Brasil. CBD therapeutic potential: antipsychotic, anxiolytic, and antidepressant.[16]	4
CBD vs amisulpride	42 patients fulfilling DSM-IV criteria of acute paranoid schizophrenia.	2009 – Multi-national research team, Cologne, Germany, Irvine, California. Decrease in symptoms not different between both substances. CBD induced significantly less side effects.[17]	5
Ananda-minde	Antipsychotic-naive first-episode paranoid schizophrenics.	2004 – Department of Pharmacology, University of California, Irvine. Anandamide elevation in acute paranoid schizophrenia may be a compensatory mechanism.[18]	3

Total CHI Value 16

STRAIN SPECIFIC CONSIDERATIONS

CBD, THC and endogenous anandamide were examined in the context of schizophrenia. CBD has a greater affinity for CB2. THC and anandamide bind with CB1 and CB2 relatively equally.

Cannabis-using patients suffering from schizophrenia often choose a strain relative to their needs. If a generally more stimulating or uplifting effect is needed, patients tend to consider sativa or sativa dominant strains. Those in need of a generally more relaxing or grounding effect tend to prefer indicas or indica-dominant strains with a relatively lower THC:CBD ratio, which likely favors CB2 activation.

EXPLORING MIND–BODY CONSCIOUSNESS

Schizophrenia is described by some patients as a loss of connection between thinking and feeling and with a sense of loss of soul.

QUESTIONS

What was the trigger event?
What happened?
Has the negative loop ever been interrupted?
By what?
Is it possible to bring in other resources?

AGGRAVATING FACTORS

Prenatal stress / family history / social isolation / inner city life / sudden life altering events such as migration / toxins / nutritional deficiencies / other biological influences.

HEALING FACTORS

Nutritional support / detoxification / support group(s) or therapy.

SUGGESTED BLESSING:

May you recover from the sense of loss of soul.

SUGGESTED AFFIRMATION:

I can discover peace and solitude, good friends and practical help. I accept myself. I have compassion for myself.

---

1 The extrapyramidal system is the part of the brain involved in reflexes, movements, and positional control. It is located outside the normal pyramidal pathways responsible for motion leading from the brain into the spinal cord.

2 Marco M Picchioni and Robin M Murray. *Schizophrenia*. King's College London, Institute of Psychiatry, Division of Psychological Medicine, London. BMJ. 2007 July 14; 335(7610): 91–95.

3 Ibid.

4 Ibid

5 Ibid.

6 Ibid.

7 Read J, van Os J, Morrison AP, Ross CA. *Childhood trauma, psychosis and schizophrenia: a literature review with theoretical and clinical implications.* Department of Psychology, The University of Auckland, Auckland, New Zealand. Acta Psychiatr Scand. 2005 Nov;112(5):330-50.

8 Giuffrida A, Leweke FM, Gerth CW, Schreiber D, Koethe D, Faulhaber J, Klosterkotter J, Piomelli D. *Cerebro-spinal anandamide levels are elevated in acute schizophrenia and are inversely correlated with psychotic symptoms.* Department of Pharmacology, University of California, Irvine, CA, USA. Neuropsychopharmacology. 2004 Nov;29(11):2108-14.

9 Catechol-O-methyltransferase (COMT) valine (an amino acid) 158 allele

10 Caspi A, Moffitt TE, Cannon M, McClay J, Murray R, Harrington H, Taylor A, Arseneault L, Williams B, Braithwaite A, Poulton R, Craig IW. *Moderation of the effect of adolescent-onset cannabis use on adult psychosis by a functional polymorphism in the catechol-O-methyltransferase gene: longitudinal evidence of a gene X environment interaction.* Social, Genetic, and Developmental Psychiatry Centre, Institute of Psychiatry, King's College London, London, United Kingdom. Biol Psychiatry. 2005 May 15;57(10):1117-27.

11 Cécile Henquet, Robin Murray, Don Linszen, Jim van Os. *The Environment and Schizophrenia: The Role of Cannabis Use.* Department of Psychiatry and Neuropsychology, South Limburg Mental Health Research and Teaching Network, European Graduate School of Neuroscience, Maastricht University, Maastricht, the Nether-lands. Division of Psychological Medicine, Institute of Psychiatry, De Crespigny Park, London. Department of Psychiatry, University Medical Hospital, Amsterdam. Department of Psychiatry and Neuropsychology, South Limburg Mental Health Research and Teaching Network, European Graduate School of Neuroscience, Maas-tricht University, Maastricht, the Netherlands Division of Psychological Medicine, Institute of Psychiatry, De Crespigny Park, London. Schizophr Bull (July 2005) 31 (3): 608-612.

12 F.M. Leweke1, D. Koethe1, F. Pahlisch1, 2, D. Schreiber1, 2, C.W. Gerth1, B.M. Nolden1, J. Klosterkötter1, M. Hellmich3 and D. Piomelli2 S39-02 *Antipsychotic effects of cannabidiol.* 1Dept. of Psychiatry and Psychotherapy, University of Cologne, Cologne, Germany. 2Depts. of Pharmacology and Biological Chemistry, University of California, Irvine, USA. 3Institute for Medical Statistics, Informatics, and Epidemiology, University of Cologne, Cologne, Germany. European Psychiatry. Volume 24, Supplement 1, 2009, Page S207.

13 Crippa JA, Zuardi AW, Hallak JE. *Therapeutical use of the cannabinoids in psychiatry.* Departamento de Neurociências e Ciências do Comportamento, Faculdade de Medicina de Ribeirão Preto, Universidade de São Paulo, Ribeirão Preto, SP, Brasil. Rev Bras Psiquiatr. 2010 May;32 Suppl 1:S56-66.

14 Parolaro D, Realini N, Vigano D, Guidali C, Rubino T. *The endocannabinoid system and psychiatric disorders.* DBSF and Neuroscience Center, University of Insubria, Via A. da Giussano 10, 21052 Busto Arsizio (Varese), Italy. Exp Neurol. 2010 Jul;224(1):3-14.

15 Parolaro D, Realini N, Vigano D, Guidali C, Rubino T. *The endocannabinoid system and psychiatric disorders.* DBSF and Neuroscience Center, University of Insubria, Via A. da Giussano 10, 21052 Busto Arsizio (Varese), Italy. Exp Neurol. 2010 Jul;224(1):3-14

16 Crippa JA, Zuardi AW, Hallak JE. *Therapeutical use of the cannabinoids in psychiatry.* Departamento de Neurociências e Ciências do Comportamento, Faculdade de Medicina de Ribeirão Preto, Universidade de São Paulo, Ribeirão Preto, SP, Brasil. Rev Bras Psiquiatr. 2010 May;32 Suppl 1:S56-66.

17 F.M. Leweke1, D. Koethe1, F. Pahlisch1, 2, D. Schreiber1, 2, C.W. Gerth1, B.M. Nolden1, J. Klosterkötter1, M. Hellmich3 and D. Piomelli2 S39-02 *Antipsychotic effects of cannabidiol.* 1Dept. of Psychiatry and Psychotherapy, University of Cologne, Cologne, Germany. 2Depts. of Pharmacology and Biological Chemistry, University of California, Irvine, USA. 3Institute for Medical Statistics, Informatics, and Epidemiology, University of Cologne, Cologne, Germany. European Psychiatry. Volume 24, Supplement 1, 2009, Page S207.

18 Giuffrida A, Leweke FM, Gerth CW, Schreiber D, Koethe D, Faulhaber J, Klosterkotter J, Piomelli D. *Cere-brospinal anandamide levels are elevated in acute schizophrenia and are inversely correlated with psychotic symp-toms.* Department of Pharmacology, University of California, Irvine, CA, USA. Neuropsychopharmacology. 2004 Nov;29(11):2108-14.

Neurological Diseases

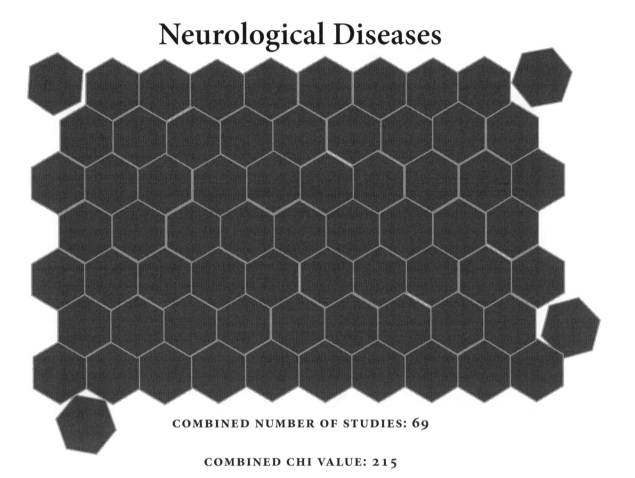

COMBINED NUMBER OF STUDIES: 69

COMBINED CHI VALUE: 215

To date, hundreds of different neurological disease classifications exist within orthodox medicine. While specific and unique in their presentation of signs, symptoms and damages caused, they each share a common inability to properly transmit nerve impulses. This inability may be due to damages to the conduction network itself (nerve fibers) or from difficulties in transmitting nerve impulses/signals at the energetic/ electrical, molecular or chemical levels. Specific disease manifestation largely depends on how and which aspect or part of the nervous system is affected.

Modern medicine basically divides the nervous system into the central nervous system (CNS), comprised of the brain, spinal cord and the optic nerve, and the peripheral nervous system (PNS), consisting of nerve pathways from the spine extending outward toward the periphery of the body. The PNS is further divided into the autonomic nervous system (ANS) and the enteric nervous system (ENS), responsible for gastrointestinal or gut reactions. The ANS also sub-divides into the sympathetic and parasympathetic nervous systems, which up or down regulate automatic (involuntary) responses such as heartbeat, blood pressure, and hormonal release.

Orthodox medicine has identified a variety of possible culprits in the promotion of neurological diseases. They include: toxins, lack of nutrition, infectious pathogens, radiation, accidents, as well as genetic and autoimmune causes. In many cases, though, both an exact causation and cure have so far escaped modern medicine. An arsenal of tests may provide insights into some of the specifics of disease development, and by extension, manage progression. However, treatment is often limited to pharmaceutical medication or surgery. In addition, most of the neurological disorders are chronic and the patient deteriorates over time.

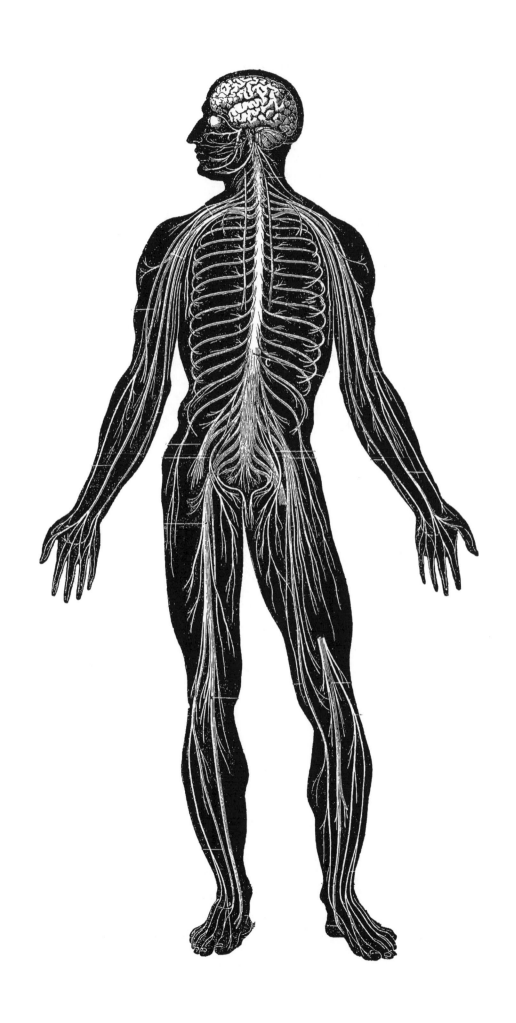

Neurological Diseases
Cannabis and Neuroprotection in General

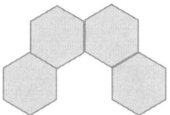

NUMBER OF STUDIES: 4

CHI VALUE: 11

Cannabinoids assist in regulating functions associated with endocannabinoid receptor sites found in the human body. Endocannabinoid receptor sites (CB1 & CB2) are firmly embedded in all parts of the nervous system. More specifically, CB1 receptor sites are especially prominent in those parts of the brain (CNS) related to motor control, cognition, emotional responses, motivation and homeostasis. While CB2 receptor sites often sit outside the brain in the periphery, they relate to the autonomic nervous system (ANS), immune system, cellular circulation, hormonal regulation and gastrointestinal function. Scientists suspect that other undiscovered receptor sites exist in endothelial cells (cells that line the inside of blood vessels), which are referred to as non-CB1 or non-CB2.

By 2003, the U.S. Federal Government had issued itself a patent on a newly found property of cannabis making it: "…useful in the treatment and prophylaxis of a wide variety of oxidation associated diseases such as ischemic, age-related, inflammatory and autoimmune diseases. The cannabinoids are found to have particular application as neuroprotectants; for example, in limiting neurological damage following ischemic insults such as stroke and trauma, or in the treatment of neurodegenerative diseases such as Alzheimer's disease, Parkinson's disease and HIV dementia."[1]

A multi-disciplinary Bethesda, Maryland, research team further examined the neuroprotective properties of cannabinoids by designing an experiment inducing rats to binge drink alcohol. This activity causes substantial neurodegeneration in the brain, especially the hippocampus and the entorhinal cortex. Concurrently, the rats received CBD, a non-psychoactive cannabinoid. Results indicated that CBD could protect nerve cells from alcohol-induced toxicity in a dose dependent manner.[2] Laboratory studies in Italy[3] and Spain echoed these results on the neuroprotective properties of cannabinoids. Researchers discovered that while the drug ecstasy (MDMA) produces hyperthermia, oxidative stress and neuronal damage, especially at higher room temperatures, THC causes the opposite (namely hypothermic, anti-inflammatory and antioxidant effects). Thus, researchers concluded that THC protects against MDMA neurotoxicity, at least in mice.[4]

STUDY SUMMARY:

Drugs	Type of Study	Published Year, Place, and Key Results	CHI
MDMA, THC	Animal study (Mice)	2010 – Departament de Ciències Experimentals i de la Salut, Grup de Recerca en Neurobiologia del Comportament, Universitat Pompeu Fabra, Barcelona, Spain. THC may have a neuroprotective effect against MDMA-induced neurotoxicity.	2
JWH-015	Laboratory	2009 – Santa Lucia Foundation Istituto di Ricovero e Cura a Carattere Scientifico, Rome, Italy. Endocannabinoids are neuroprotective.	1
CBD	Animal study (rats)	2005 – Multi-institutional, Bethesda, U.S. CBD was neuroprotective in a dose dependent manner.	2
Cannabinoids	In vitro and in vivo laboratory, animal and human studies.	2003 – The United States of America as represented by the Department of Health and Human Services. Cannabinoids are neuroprotectants.	1+2+3

Total CHI Value   11

STRAIN AND FORM SPECIFIC CONSIDERATIONS

Large cannabis leaves eaten in a salad or made into a juice may contain preventative properties in the context of neurological disorders. William L. Courtney, MD, a physician working with fresh cannabis, considers raw cannabis a dietary essential that provides potent preventative influences on several degenerative processes often involved with neurological diseases. These preventative features include: neuroprotection, anti-inflammatory and anti-oxidant properties. These properties are echoed in the overall results of studies reviewed here and throughout this chapter.

EXPLORING MIND–BODY CONSCIOUSNESS

The breakdown of communication between command central (the brain) and the rest of the body may indicate a breakdown between the mind and body, between spirit and nature, between heaven and earth, between dreams and reality, between the future and past, between destiny and free will, between victimhood and responsibility, between the two brain hemispheres, between logic and intuition, between doing and feeling or between will and imagination.

QUESTIONS

What is getting on my nerves?
Who is getting on my nerves?
What hurts to communicate?
What is too dangerous to be communicated?
What must not be communicated?
Does it feel safer to withold information?
Do I feel I cannot handle certain topics in my life?
What would happen if I talked about a taboo or charged topic?
Like a deer in the headlights, what has frozen my face?
Is my body shaking to express denied fear or terror?
Why do I shake when I am still?

Why do I shake less when I move?
Can I find a balance between stillness and movement?
How do I feel when I find it?
How do I feel if I cannot find it?
When did I freeze the expression of my thought and feelings?
Why did they need to be halted at all cost?
What would happen without my poker face?
What is my body showing me about my frozen affect?
What is my body telling me about my lack of motion?
Where am I inflexible and frozen deep inside myself?
When did I lose my face?
Have I resigned myself to die?

TAKE NOTICE

GARLIC • ROSEMARY • TURMERIC

GARLIC: Aged garlic extract may prevent the progression of Alzheimer's disease, according to the results of a rodent experiment that examined garlic to treat Alzheimer's.[5]

ROSEMARY: In a Hung-Kuang University, Taiwan, scientists concluded that: "… rosemary is an excellent multifunctional therapeutic herb; by looking at its potentially potent antiglycative bioactivity, it may become a good adjuvant medicine for the prevention and treatment of diabetic, cardiovascular, and other neurodegenerative diseases."[6]

TURMERIC: In a meta-study, scientists provided an overview of decades of scientific studies on turmeric. Turmeric was noted as a therapeutic agent in Alzheimer's and Parkinson's diseases.[7]

Curcumin is a naturally occurring compound found in the rhizome of turmeric. Now researchers from Nashville, Tennessee have examined the compound's ability to affect mice with multiple sclerosis (MS). Results of the study suggest that the amount of curcumin used to protect the mice from artificially induced MS corresponds to the amount found in the typical Indian diet. One author of the study reported that MS in India is very rare; and, while no human studies to date confirm the results, it certainly can't hurt to add some turmeric to your food.[8]

For general immune support, see BACTERIAL and VIRAL INFECTION.
For anti-inflammatory support, see INFLAMMATORY DISEASES.
For pain, see PAIN IN GENERAL.

1 The United States of America as represented by the Department of Health and Human Services. (Aidan J. Hampson, Julius Axelrod and Maurizio Grimaldi) Patent No. 09/674028 filed on 02/02/2001. *Patent 6630507 issued on October 7, 2003.* Estimated expiration date: 2021. Cannabinoids as antioxidants and neuroprotectants. http://www.patentstorm.us/patents/6630507.html

2 Carol Hamelink1, Aidan Hampson1, David A. Wink, Lee E. Eiden and Robert L. Eskay. *Comparison of Cannabidiol, Antioxidants, and Diuretics in Reversing Binge Ethanol-Induced Neurotoxicity.* Section on Molecular Neuroscience, Laboratory of Cellular and Molecular Regulation, National Institute of Mental Health (C.H., A.H., L.E.E.); Section of Neurochemistry and Neuroendocrinology, Laboratory of Clinical Studies, National Institute on Alcohol Abuse and Alcoholism (R.L.E.); and Radiology and Biology Branch, National Cancer Institute (D.A.W.), National Institutes of Health, Bethesda, Maryland. JPET August 2005 vol. 314 no. 2 780-788.

3 Viscomi MT, Oddi S, Latini L, Pasquariello N, Florenzano F, Bernardi G, Molinari M, Maccarrone M. *Selective CB2 Receptor Agonism Protects Central Neurons from Remote Axotomy-Induced Apoptosis through the PI3K/Akt Pathway.* Santa Lucia Foundation Istituto di Ricovero e Cura a Carattere Scientifico, Rome, Italy. J Neurosci. 2009 Apr 8;29(14):4564-70.

4 Touriño C, Zimmer A, Valverde O. *THC Prevents MDMA Neurotoxicity in Mice.* Departament de Ciències Experimentals i de la Salut, Grup de Recerca en Neurobiologia del Comportament (GRNC), Universitat Pompeu Fabra, Barcelona, Spain. PLoS One. 2010 Feb 10;5(2):e9143.

5 Chauhan NB, Sandoval J. *Amelioration of early cognitive deficits by aged garlic extract in Alzheimer's transgenic mice.* Research and Development (151), Jesse Brown VA Medical Center Chicago, Department of Anesthesiology, University of Illinois at Chicago, IL 60612, USA. Phytother Res. 2007 Jul;21(7):629-40.

6 Hsieh CL, Peng CH, Chyau CC, Lin YC, Wang HE, Peng RY. *Low-density lipoprotein, collagen, and thrombin models reveal that Rosemarinus officinalis L. exhibits potent antiglycative effects.* Department of Food and Nutrition, Research Institute of Biotechnology, and Division of Basic Medical Sciences, Hung-Kuang University, No. 34 Chung-Chie Road, Shalu County, Taichung Hsien, Taiwan. J Agric Food Chem. 2007 Apr 18;55(8):2884-91.

7 Goel A, Kunnumakkara AB, Aggarwal BB. *Curcumin as "Curecumin": From kitchen to clinic.* Gastrointestinal Cancer Research Laboratory, Department of Internal Medicine, Charles A. Sammons Cancer Center and Baylor Research Institute, Baylor University Medical Center, Dallas, TX, United States. Biochem Pharmacol. 2007 Aug 19.

8 Natarajan C, Bright JJ. *Curcumin inhibits experimental allergic encephalomyelitis by blocking IL-12 signaling through Janus kinase-STAT pathway in T lymphocytes.* Division of Neuroimmunology, Department of Neurology, Vanderbilt University Medical Center, Nashville, TN 37212, USA. J Immunol. 2002 Jun 15;168(12):6506-13.

Neurological Diseases
Alcohol Dependence/Abuse

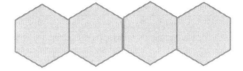

NUMBER OF STUDIES: 4

CHI VALUE: 9

Alcohol abuse is one of the most common contributing factors to a great deal of pain and suffering. A neurological and mental illness, alcohol abuse causes or exacerbates a variety of serious social problems: domestic violence, child abuse, spousal abuse, homicide, suicide, purposeful injuries, falls, accidents, fatal overdose, loss of work and increased poverty.

Alcohol abuse affects the entire body. Doctors name cardio-vascular disease as the primary cause of death associated with alcohol abuse. Other health problems connected to alcohol abuse include: poor absorption of food, cancer, cirrhosis of the liver, pancreatitis, gastritis, alcohol poisoning or overdose, aspiration of vomit, burns, drowning, damage to the nervous system, depression, dementia and symptoms such as seizures, psychosis and withdrawal delirium tremens (DT's).

A worldwide health problem, alcohol dependence impacts more males than females. However, women's bodies endure more rapid damage from the disease than do males. In this author's experience as a paramedic, alcohol abuse-related health problems generate a majority of 911 emergencies followed by nicotine-related health problems. Additionally, no antidote exists for the acute alcohol overdose common in binge drinking. In fact, orthodox medicine suggests no cure for chronic alcoholism. In this paradigm, patients remain alcoholics for life and must learn to manage the urge and stay abstinent.

Long-term alcohol abuse induces neurochemical changes in brain physiology and structure, which serve to reinforce the psychological and physical need for alcohol and may lead to dependence. Therapy is basically two-fold. First, patients begin a process of detoxification and treatment through the initial withdrawal phases, followed by nutritional support consisting mainly of thiamine (vitamin B1). Second, doctors prescribe therapy, conducted usually in a peer group setting.

CANNABIS AND ALCOHOLISM

In 1970, Tod H. Mikuriya, MD, published a case involving an alcohol dependent patient who significantly benefited from cannabis' ability to reduce his alcohol consumption.[1] Thirty-four years later, Dr. Mikuriya followed up with a larger study incorporating 92 alcoholic patients. Forty-five patients found the treatment "very effective"; 38 found it "effective"; and nine patients reported that they had been able to give up alcohol altogether.[2]

Since then, studies conducted on mice suggest that blocking the CB1 receptor appears to effectively reduce the preference for alcohol and actual alcohol intake. Researchers speculate that medications targeting the CB1 receptors may be beneficial for the treatment of alcoholism.[3,4]

While this research involved the body's own endocannabinoid receptor system (CB1), another experiment examined the neuroprotective properties of a specific cannabinoid (CBD) in the context of binge drinking. A multi-disciplinary research team from Bethesda, Maryland, designed an experiment inducing rats to binge drink alcohol - an activity causing substantial neurodegeneration in the brain, especially the hippocampus and the entorhinal cortex. Concurrently, rats received CBD, a non-psychoactive cannabinoid, and results indicated that CBD could protect nerve cells from alcohol-induced toxicity in a dose dependent manner.[5]

STUDY SUMMARY:

Drugs	Type of Study	Published Year, Place, and Key Results	CHI
CB1 antagonist	Animal study (mice)	2008 – Division of Analytical Psychopharmacology, Orangeburg, New York. CB(1) antagonists receptor may reduce ethanol dependence.	2
CBD	Animal study (rats)	2005 – Multi-institutional, Bethesda, US. CBD was able to protect nerve cells from alcohol-induced toxicity.	2
CB1 antagonist	Animal study (rats)	2005 – Behavioral Pharmacology Lab, Department of Medicine, Upton, New York. Blocking CB1 receptors may be beneficial for the treatment of alcoholism.	2
Cannabis	Case study on 92 alcoholics.	2004 – California Cannabis Research Medical Group, Berkeley. 45 patients found the treatment "very effective"; 38 found it "effective"; and 9 patients reported that they had been able to give up alcohol altogether.	3

Total CHI Value   9

STRAIN SPECIFIC CONSIDERATIONS

The drugs reviewed in these studies included: cannabis (whole plant material), the isolated cannabinoid CBD and CB1 antagonists. Cannabis contains cannabinoids that bind with both CB1 and CB2. CB1 antagonists block CB1 expression.

Indica strains and indica dominant hybrids tend to have lower THC:CBD ratios favoring CB2 expression.

EXPLORING MIND–BODY CONSCIOUSNESS

While not all stress-exposed children go on to develop alcoholism, severe childhood stressors have been associated with increased vulnerability to addiction. Researchers also suggest a genetic-environmental connection, which may contribute to one's vulnerability to later develop alcohol dependence.[6]

QUESTIONS

How or where have I lost the spirit I am trying to find in this bottle of spirit?
What is so intolerable in my life that I have to numb myself?
What is the crisis that always seems to loom at the edge of my reality?
What is too much for me to own?

SUGGESTED BLESSING:

May you receive the vision needed to move through hopelessness and despair.

May you find the will and determination to manifest the vision.

Where am I convinced I cannot change?
What happened to my trust and my hope?
Who do I blame for my life?
Can I see what matters to me on the other side of blame?
Can I see my ability to forgive on the other side of blame?
Can I see my passion on the other side of blame?

AGGRAVATING FACTORS

Self-pity / hopelessness / shame / guilt / judgments / hard-heartedness / blame.

HEALING FACTORS

Self-acceptance / forgiveness / gratitude / love / intimacy / a connection with something larger than myself / finding what matters / passion / hope / trust.

1 Tod H. Mikuriya M.D. *Cannabis substitution. An adjunctive therapeutic tool in the treatment of alcoholism.* Medical Times 1970;98(4):187-91.

2 Tod H. Mikuriya M.D. *Cannabis as a Substitute for Alcohol: A Harm-Reduction Approach.* Journal of Cannabis Therapeutics, Vol. 4(1) 2004.

3 Thanos PK, Dimitrakakis ES, Rice O, Gifford A, Volkow ND. *Ethanol self-administration and ethanol conditioned place preference are reduced in mice lacking cannabinoid CB1 receptors.* Behavioral Pharmacology Lab, Department of Medicine, Brookhaven National Laboratory, Building 490, 30 Bell Avenue, Upton, NY 11973-5000, USA. Behav Brain Res. 2005 Nov 7;164(2):206-13.

4 Vinod KY, Yalamanchili R, Thanos PK, Vadasz C, Cooper TB, Volkow ND, Hungund BL. *Genetic and pharmacological manipulations of the CB(1) receptor alter ethanol preference and dependence in ethanol preferring and nonpreferring mice.* Division of Analytical Psychopharmacology, Nathan Kline Institute for Psychiatric Research, Orangeburg, New York, USA. Synapse. 2008 Aug;62(8):574-81.

5 Carol Hamelink1, Aidan Hampson1, David A. Wink, Lee E. Eiden and Robert L. Eskay. *Comparison of Cannabidiol, Antioxidants, and Diuretics in Reversing Binge Ethanol-Induced Neurotoxicity.* Section on Molecular Neuroscience, Laboratory of Cellular and Molecular Regulation, National Institute of Mental Health (C.H., A.H., L.E.E.); Section of Neurochemistry and Neuroendocrinology, Laboratory of Clinical Studies, National Institute on Alcohol Abuse and Alcoholism (R.L.E.); and Radiology and Biology Branch, National Cancer Institute (D.A.W.), National Institutes of Health, Bethesda, Maryland. JPET August 2005 vol. 314 no. 2 780-788.

6 Enoch MA. *Genetic and environmental influences on the development of alcoholism: resilience vs. risk.* Laboratory of Neurogenetics, National Institute on Alcohol Abuse and Alcoholism, NIH, Bethesda, Maryland, USA. Ann N Y Acad Sci. 2006 Dec;1094:193-201.

Neurological Diseases
Alzheimer's Disease

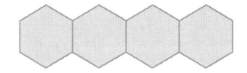

NUMBER OF STUDIES: 4

CHI VALUE: 10

Alzheimer's disease (AD), a chronic degenerative illness that affects the mind and brain, is partially characterized by selective neuronal loss (AD kills brain cells) and cognitive deficits. Early symptoms include forgetfulness or a decrease in cognitive function, which eventually progresses to a gradual loss of communication abilities and significant behavioral changes. Eventually, the patient becomes completely dependent and bedridden. Death usually occurs from secondary sources such as trauma or chronic infections. The disease affects more women than men and usually begins between ages 50 and 60. AD is the main culprit for dementia. In 2007, it was the sixth leading cause of death in the U.S.[1]

Within the modern medical system, the causes of the disease remain unknown. In addition, the disease lacks a cure or effective treatment. Management of AD involves a multi-disciplinary approach of supportive care, pharmaceutical medications, exercise, nutrition and an assurance of the patient's safety through supervision. Depending on the progression of the disease, feeding tubes may be used to assure adequate nutritional intake.

Generally speaking, scientists believe AD originates in part from genetic, environmental and lifestyle causes. Established risk factors include lack of exercise, obesity, hypertension, diabetes, depression and smoking. More specifically, one hypothesis proposes beta-amyloid plaque as a factor, partially due to doctors observing higher concentrations in the brain cells of Alzheimer patients. Another discovery in AD involves a protein called tau, which in AD, tangles and twists, preventing the delivery of nutrients to brain cells. Scientists believe these plaques and tangles induce neurochemical and inflammatory changes responsible for the development of the disease.

No test exists, with the exception of an autopsy, to diagnose AD. However, the presence of dementia can be determined via a combination of cognitive and neurological examinations as well as various brain imaging techniques.

While unable to explain the reason, observational studies reveal that higher levels of education, life-long interests in learning, challenging activities and social interactions can reduce the risk of the disease.[2]

CANNABIS AND ALZHEIMER'S

Recent experiments suggest that the endocannabinoid system may play a significant role in the development of AD. One study (2005) from Madrid, Spain, discovered that "… cannabinoid receptors are important in the pathology of AD and that cannabinoids succeed in preventing the neurodegenerative process occurring in the disease."[3] Another experiment from Madrid (2009) demonstrated that the CB2 agonist JWH-015 could induce the removal of native beta-amyloid from frozen human tissue.[4] Using available data from prior studies and experiments, scientists from Naples, Italy, conducted a meta-analysis (2008). Their results suggested that endocannabinoids likely produce a response that might counteract both the neurochemical and inflammatory consequences of beta-amyloid-induced tau protein hyperactivity. This might possibly be the most important underlying cause of AD.[5] While clinical trials are still lacking, researchers from British Columbia, Canada (2008) tested a patient with Alzheimer's related behavioral symptoms, such as agitation and aggression, who failed to respond to such pharmaceuticals as neurontin, trazodone, quetiapine and olanzapine. Scientists then gave the patient 0.5mg of nabilone, which significantly reduced his agitation levels. After doubling the dose, his symptoms were further reduced without any side effects.[6]

STUDY SUMMARY:

Drugs	Type of Study	Published Year, Place, and Key Results	CHI
CB2 agonist JWH-015	Laboratory	2009 – Laboratorio de Apoyo a la Investigación, Hospital Universitario Fundación Alcorcón and Centro de Investigación Biomédica en Red sobre Enfermedades Neurodegenerativas, Madrid, Spain. Removal of native beta-amyloid.	1
Cannabinoids in the context of AD, especially CBD.	Meta-analysis and literature review.	2008 – Endocannabinoid Research Group, Institute of Biomolecular Chemistry, Consiglio Nazionale delle Ricerche, Naples, Italy. Results suggest a possible novel approach to AD. Might counteract neurochemical and inflammatory consequences of beta-amyloid-induced tau protein hyperactivity.	4
Nabilon 0.5mg X 1 pm and 0.5mg X 2 daily.	Human (1 patient).	2008 – Division of Geriatric Psychiatry, Department of Psychiatry, University of British Columbia, Canada. Dramatic reduction in the severity of agitation and other behavioral symptoms.	3
WIN55,212-2, HU-210 and JWH-133	Rodent study	2005 – Neurodegeneration Group, Cajal Institute, Consejo Superior de Investigaciones Científicas, Madrid, Spain. Neuroprotective in AD. Intracerebroventricular administration of the synthetic cannabinoid WIN55,212-2 to rats prevented beta-amyloid peptide-induced microglial activation, cognitive impairment, and loss of neuronal markers.	2

Total CHI Value 10

STRAIN AND FORM SPECIFIC CONSIDERATIONS

The cannabinoids used in this study review include CBD, nabilone, JWH-015, WIN55,212-2, HU-210 and JWH-133.

CBD has a greater affinity for CB2. JWH-015 is a CB2 agonist. WIN55,212-2 has a greater affinity for CB2. JWH-133 is a potent CB2 agonist. Out of this group of cannabinoids, only HU 210 has a higher affinity for CB1, and nabilone is a synthetic cannabinoid similar to THC, which likely binds relatively equally to CB1 and CB2.

Indica and indica dominant hybrids tend to present with a lower THC:CBD ratio, thus potentially favoring CB2 activation. Furthermore, raw use of fresh leaf or juice contains biologically active cannabinoids in the form of relatively non-psychoactive THC-acid and CBD-acid, which according to William L. Courtney MD, a physician working with fresh cannabis as a dietary essential, can deliver a much higher concentration of CBD before any mind altering effect may occur.

EXPLORING MIND–BODY CONSCIOUSNESS

The AD patient typically experiences a gradual loss of physical and mental abilities until s/he becomes completely dependent on others to care for basic bodily functions. Based on the image presented by the body, it would appear that AD is an attempt to return to the source of all life by way of the infant. Other options to return to the source of all life, such as the return through wisdom, appear nonexistent.

Physiologically, two parts of the brain are especially vulnerable to aggregation - the hippocampus (memory) and the amygdala (emotional reactions). This possibly suggests that clogged up memories and related emotional reactions interfere with life. A part of the patient has given up on conscious growing and learning and seems to seek a return, little by little, to a womb-like existence where all one's needs are met without conscious involvement or responsibility.

QUESTIONS

Where do I refuse to be responsible even at the cost of freedom?
What do wise men have that children do not?
Where am I averse to learning new perspectives?
Where am I averse to learning new ways of being and doing things?

AGGRAVATING FACTORS

Social isolation / poor nutritional support / new skill or learning avoidance / a belief that says 'as the body ages the mind must fade away'.

HEALING FACTORS

Continuing education and learning opportunities / new activities or experiences / mental excercise and acquisition of new skills / new friendships and close relationships / belief in your ability to continue to grow even as your body grows older.

TAKE NOTICE

GARLIC • TURMERIC • INFRA-RED LIGHT (670NM)

GARLIC: A rodent experiment to examine the impact of ingesting garlic on Alzheimer's disease concluded that aged garlic extract has a potential for preventing the progression of Alzheimer's disease.[7]

TURMERIC: In a meta-study, scientists provide an overview of decades of scientific studies on turmeric. They summarized a long list of turmeric's potential therapeutic properties including positive benefits for Alzheimer's patients.[9]

INFRA-RED LIGHT (670NM): A multi-institutional laboratory research project (2012) brought together scientists from nanotechnology, molecular medicine and numerous other medical specialties. Using a laser emitting infrared light at a frequency of 670 nm, scientists significantly reduced intra cellular beta-amyloid aggregation with no ill effects on cell proliferation. Researchers noted that infrared light at 670nm can penetrate skull bone and underlying tissue beneath to a depth of several centimeters, making infrared light a potentially novel and non-invasive treatment for AD.[10]

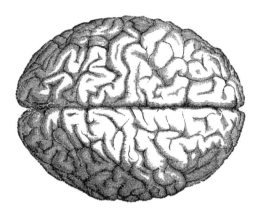

1 Jiaquan Xu, M.D.; Kenneth D. Kochanek, M.A.; Sherry L. Murphy, B.S.; and Betzaida Tejada-Vera, B.S.; *National Vital Statistics Reports. Deaths: Final Data for 2007*. Volume 58, Number 19. May 20, 2010. U.S. DEPARTMENT OF HEALTH AND HUMAN SERVICES. Centers for Disease Control and Prevention. National Center for Health Statistics. National Vital Statistics System.

2 Stern Y. *Cognitive reserve and Alzheimer disease*. Cognitive Neuroscience Division of the Taub Institute, 630 W. 168th Street, New York, NY 10032, USA. Alzheimer Dis Assoc Disord. 2006 Jul-Sep;20(3 Suppl 2):S69-74.

3 Ramírez BG, Blázquez C, Gómez del Pulgar T, Guzmán M, de Ceballos ML. *Prevention of Alzheimer's disease pathology by cannabinoids: neuroprotection mediated by blockade of microglial activation*. Neurodegeneration Group, Cajal Institute, Consejo Superior de Investigaciones Científicas, 28002 Madrid, Spain. J Neurosci. 2005 Feb 23;25(8):1904-13.

4 Tolón RM, Núñez E, Pazos MR, Benito C, Castillo AI, Martínez-Orgado JA, Romero J. *The activation of cannabinoid CB2 receptors stimulates in situ and in vitro beta-amyloid removal by human macrophages*. Laboratorio de Apoyo a la Investigación, Hospital Universitario Fundación Alcorcón and Centro de Investigación Biomédica en Red sobre Enfermedades Neurodegenerativas, 28922 Alcorcón, Madrid, Spain. Brain Res, 5. Juni 2009.

5 Bisogno T, Di Marzo V. *The role of the endocannabinoid system in Alzheimer's disease: facts and hypotheses*. Endocannabinoid Research Group, Institute of Biomolecular Chemistry, Consiglio Nazionale delle Ricerche, Via Campi Flegrei 34, Pozzuoli (Naples), Italy. Curr Pharm Des. 2008;14(23):2299-3305.

6 Passmore MJ. *The cannabinoid receptor agonist nabilone for the treatment of dementia-related agitation*. Division of Geriatric Psychiatry, Department of Psychiatry, University of British Columbia, Canada. Int J Geriatr Psychiatry 2008;23(1):116-7.

7 Chauhan NB, Sandoval J. *Amelioration of early cognitive deficits by aged garlic extract in Alzheimer's transgenic mice*. Research and Development (151), Jesse Brown VA Medical Center Chicago, Department of Anesthesiology, University of Illinois at Chicago, IL 60612, USA. Phytother Res. 2007 Jul;21(7):629-40.

8 Goel A, Kunnumakkara AB, Aggarwal BB. *Curcumin as "Curecumin": From kitchen to clinic*. Gastrointestinal Cancer Research Laboratory, Department of Internal Medicine, Charles A. Sammons Cancer Center and Baylor Research Institute, Baylor University Medical Center, Dallas, TX, United States. Biochem Pharmacol. 2007 Aug 19.

9 Aggarwal BB, Kumar A, Bharti AC. *Anticancer potential of curcumin: preclinical and clinical studies.* Cytokine Research Section, Department of Bioimmunotherapy, University of Texas M. D. Anderson Cancer Center, 1515 Holcombe Boulevard, Box 143, Houston, TX, USA. Anticancer Research. 2003 Jan-Feb;23(1A):363-98.

10 Andrei P. Sommer, Jan Bieschke, Ralf P. Friedrich, Dan Zhu, Erich E. Wanker, Hans J. Fecht, Derliz Mereles, and Werner Hunstein. *670 nm Laser Light and EGCG Complementarily Reduce Amyloid-β Aggregates in Human Neuroblastoma Cells: Basis for Treatment of Alzheimer's Disease?* Photomedicine and Laser Surgery. January 2012, 30(1): 54-60.

Neurological Diseases
Amyotrophic Lateral Sclerosis (ALS) or Lou Gehrig's Disease

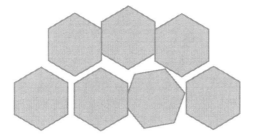

NUMBER OF STUDIES: 7

CHI VALUE: 19

Lou Gehrig's Disease is considered a chronic degenerative neurological illness associated with the selective loss of only those nerve cells needed for muscular motion located in the brain and spinal cord. A-myo-trophic, derived from ancient Greek, translates into no-muscle-nourishment respectively. Lateral refers to muscles on either side of the affected nerve and sclerosis means hardening. Without nourishment, a muscle wastes away and with it so does the ability to initiate movements.

The disease often begins spontaneously, and otherwise healthy adults suddenly show symptoms ranging from isolated muscle weakness, twitching, difficulty voicing speech, muscle cramps and spasms, periods of uncontrollable laughter or crying, and progressing to advanced stage symptoms, namely difficulty swallowing. Breathing, while a mostly non-voluntary function, is also somewhat subject to will and, thus, ultimately affected by ALS. Most ALS patients eventually die of respiratory failure. While late stage ALS patients descend into total paralysis, their minds for the most part remain unaffected. One study estimated that, in the U.S. alone, about two people in 100,000 die of the disease.[1] While some patients survive for up to ten years, the majority of ALS patients die within three to five years after the onset of symptoms. However, one of the more famous ALS patients, Stephen Hawking, considered by many one of the most brilliant scientific minds to date, has shattered all life-expectancy statistics. He has not just survived ALS but has, in spite of his illness, produced a body of work earning him unprecedented international acclaim in both academia and the public domain.

Orthodox medicine does not know the exact causes of ALS and offers no cure. Although mostly observed in the elderly, ALS can affect anyone. While the vast majority of ALS patients have no family history of the disease, reports show two population groups with higher incidence of ALS. During the 1950s, ALS occurred at high rates in the U.S. territory of Guam.[2] More recently, military veterans, especially those who served in the Gulf War,[3] proved twice as likely to develop ALS than other population groups.[4] The last two observations have lead to the hypothesis that ALS development may involve environmental components such as exposure to nerve toxins, both present in Guam in the 50s and during the Gulf War.

Doctors diagnose the disease by neurological examination, review of a patient's symptom progression and results of nerve and muscle function tests. In the rare case of a possible hereditary link, genetic testing might be performed. Observing that ALS patients possess higher levels of glutamate in their spinal fluid, doctors have taken to one treatment currently available. The pharmaceutical drug riluzole is used to reduce glutamate levels, which may extend one's life span by up to two months. However, the drug does not reverse nerve damage, can be liver toxic and initiates a host of other adverse affects.

CANNABIS AND ALS

The number of studies examining the endocannabinoid system in the context of ALS continues to grow steadily. Researchers suggest that marijuana, with its pain killing, muscle relaxant, bronchodilating, saliva reducing, appetite stimulating, sleep inducing, anti-oxidative and neuroprotective properties, may be a practical therapeutic agent in the management of ALS. A 2010 Seattle trial conducted on mice lead scientists to suggest that an optimal treatment regimen for ALS would include, "glutamate antagonists, antioxidants, a centrally acting anti-inflammatory agent, microglial cell modulators (including tumor necrosis factor alpha [TNF-alpha] inhibitors), an antiapoptotic agent, 1 or more neurotrophic growth factors, and a mitochondrial function-enhancing agent would be required to comprehensively address the known pathophysiology of ALS. Remarkably, cannabis appears to have activity in all of those areas."[5]

STUDY SUMMARY:

Drugs	Type of Study	Published Year, Place, and Key Results	CHI
Patients were randomly assigned to receive 5 mg THC twice daily followed by placebo or vice versa.	27 ALS patients suffering from daily cramps	2010 – Neuromuscular Diseases Unit, Kantonsspital St Gallen, Switzerland. No change in cramps.[7]	0
Cannabinoids	Mice	2010 – Muscular Dystrophy Association/Amyotrophic Lateral Sclerosis Center, University of Washington Medical Center, Seattle, WA. Cannabinoids exhibited prolonged neuronal cell survival, delayed onset of ALS symptoms and slower progression of the disease.[8]	2
Cannabinoids	Review	2010 – Clinica Neurologica, Dipartimento di Neuroscienze, Università Tor Vergata, Rome, Italy. Cannabinoids regulate immune responses and protect nerve cell function and integrity.[9]	4
Cannabinoids	Review	2007 – Department of Neurosciences, University of Rome Tor Vergata, Rome. The endocannabinoid system is involved in modulating neurodegeneration and neuroinflammation.[10]	4
CBN was delivered via subcutaneously implanted osmotic mini-pumps (5 mg/kg/day) over a period of up to 12 weeks.	Mice	2005 – Department of Neurology, University of Washington. Treatment significantly delays disease onset by more than two weeks while survival was not affected.[11]	2

Drugs	Type of Study	Published Year, Place, and Key Results	CHI
Cannabis	131 ALS patient survey	2004 – Department of Rehabilitation Medicine, University of Washington School of Medicine, Seattle, Washington. Cannabis may be moderately effective at reducing symptoms of appetite loss, depression, pain, spasticity, and drooling but not helpful with speech, swallowing or sexual dysfunction.[12]	3
Cannabis	A review of preclinical and anecdotal data.	2001 – Muscular Dystrophy Association Neuromuscular Disease Clinic, University of Washington School of Medicine, Seattle, Washington. ALS patients may benefit from analgesia, muscle relaxation, bronchodilation, saliva reduction, appetite stimulation and sleep induction effects of cannabis. In addition, marijuana's strong antioxidative and neuroprotective effects may prolong neuronal cell survival.[13]	4

Total CHI Value   19

STRAIN SPECIFIC CONSIDERATIONS

The reviews, pre-clinical trials and human case surveys analyzed in this section seem to generally suggest an employment of full spectrum cannabinoids, which bind with both endocannabinoid receptors. More specifically, CBN has proven effective in delaying the onset of symptoms in mice. To date, no human trial has been conducted to discover if these findings translate to the human experience.

Some cannabis-using patients suffering from ALS prefer to employ indicas or indica dominant strains that tend to present with a higher CBD/CBN:THC profile than sativas or sativa dominant hybrids.

Other cannabis-using ALS patients have reportedly benefited from prioritizing their symptoms and choosing a strain that addresses the top items.

EXPLORING MIND–BODY CONSCIOUSNESS

Many physicians and caregivers alike often assume that those with ALS must feel depressed and that this state of mind only increases as the disease takes its course. However, a recent study involving 56 ALS patients and many of their caregivers concluded that, "clinical depression or significant depressive symptomatology is not an inevitable or common outcome of life-threatening illness, even in the presence of major disability."[6] In his 1939 farewell speech to fans, Lou Gehrig expressed nothing but gratitude for his life. He succumbed to ALS two years later. In a recent interview, Hawkins responded to a question about fear of death: "I have lived with the prospect of an early death for the last 49 years. I'm not afraid of death, but I'm in no hurry to die. I have so much I want to do first…"

In ALS, the widening rift between the diminishing body and a fully functioning mind may offer some insight into its feedback or message. Worldly things fade away leaving the inner world of mind fully functioning. Some neurologists refer to this unique condition as "locked-in syndrome." Research conducted on developing brainwave – computer interface technology hopes to enable "locked in" minds to somewhat open the door to the world and interact.

SUGGESTED BLESSING:

May you learn to enjoy the nature and beauty of body and mind.

SUGGESTED AFFIRMATION:

I can complete my inner work and enjoy the gifts my body has to offer.

QUESTIONS

Do I believe my body is keeping me from my mind's work or focus?
What does a separation between body and mind serve?
Do I consider my body a limitation or obstacle?
Why must I be locked in?
What would happen if the door stayed open?
What would happen if I came and went as I please?

AGGRAVATING FACTORS

Second Gulf war / environmental toxins.

HEALING FACTORS

Grattitude / long-term projects / passion for life.

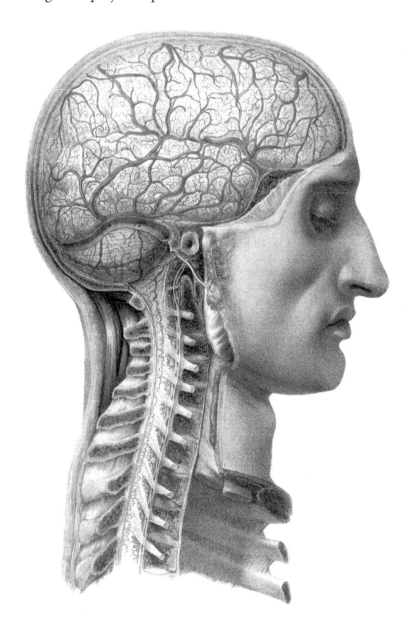

1 Sejvar JJ, Holman RC, Bresee JS, Kochanek KD, Schonberger LB. *Amyotrophic lateral sclerosis mortality in the United States, 1979-2001*. Division of Viral and Rickettsial Diseases, National Center for Infectious Diseases, Centers for Disease Control and Prevention, Atlanta, GA 30333, USA. Neuroepidemiology. 2005;25(3):144-52.

2 Pablo J, Banack SA, Cox PA, Johnson TE, Papapetropoulos S, Bradley WG, Buck A, Mash DC. *Cyanobacterial neurotoxin BMAA in ALS and Alzheimer's disease*. Department of Neurology, Miller School of Medicine, University of Miami, Miami, FL 33136, USA. Acta Neurol Scand. 2009 Oct;120(4):216-25.

3 Horner RD, Kamins KG, Feussner JR, Grambow SC, Hoff-Lindquist J, Harati Y, Mitsumoto H, Pascuzzi R, Spencer PS, Tim R, Howard D, Smith TC, Ryan MA, Coffman CJ, Kasarskis EJ. *Occurrence of amyotrophic lateral sclerosis among Gulf War veterans*. National Institute of Neurological Disorders and Stroke, Bethesda, MD 20852, USA. Neurology. 2003 Sep 23;61(6):742-9.

4 Haley RW. *Excess incidence of ALS in young Gulf War veterans*. Epidemiology Division, Department of Internal Medicine, University of Texas Southwestern Medical Center, Dallas, TX 75390-8874, USA. Neurology. 2003 Sep 23;61(6):750-6.

5 Carter GT, Abood ME, Aggarwal SK, Weiss MD. *Cannabis and amyotrophic lateral sclerosis: hypothetical and practical applications, and a call for clinical trials*. Muscular Dystrophy Association/Amyotrophic Lateral Sclerosis Center, University of Washington Medical Center, Seattle, WA, USA. Am J Hosp Palliat Care. 2010 Aug;27(5):347-56.

6 Judith G. Rabkin, PhD, Glenn J. Wagner, PhD and Maura Del Bene, RN, BSN. *Resilience and Distress Among Amyotrophic Lateral Sclerosis Patients and Caregivers*. Department of Psychiatry (J.G.R.), College of Physicians and Surgeons, Columbia University; New York State Psychiatric Institute (J.G.R., G.J.W.); and The Eleanor and Lou Gehrig MDA/ALS Center (M.D.), New York Presbyterian Hospital, New York, NY. Psychosomatic Medicine 62:271-279 (2000).

7 M Weber1,2, B Goldman1, S Truniger2 *Tetrahydrocannabinol (THC) for cramps in amyotrophic lateral sclerosis: a randomised, double-blind crossover trial*. 1Neuromuscular Diseases Unit/ALS Clinic, Kantonsspital St Gallen, St Gallen, Switzerland. 2Department of Neurology, University Hospital Basel, Basel, Switzerland J.Neurol. Neurosurg.Psychiatry. 81:1135-1140.

8 Carter GT, Abood ME, Aggarwal SK, Weiss MD. *Cannabis and amyotrophic lateral sclerosis: hypothetical and practical applications, and a call for clinical trials*. Muscular Dystrophy Association/Amyotrophic Lateral Sclerosis Center, University of Washington Medical Center, Seattle, WA, USA. Am J Hosp Palliat Care. 2010 Aug;27(5):347-56.

9 Rossi S, Bernardi G, Centonze D. *The endocannabinoid system in the inflammatory and neurodegenerative processes of multiple sclerosis and of amyotrophic lateral sclerosis*. Clinica Neurologica, Dipartimento di Neuroscienze, Università Tor Vergata, Rome, Italy. Exp Neurol. 2010 Jul;224(1):92-102.

10 Centonze D, Finazzi-Agrò A, Bernardi G, Maccarrone M. *The endocannabinoid system in targeting inflammatory neurodegenerative diseases*. Neurological Clinics, Department of Neurosciences, University of Rome Tor Vergata, Rome 00133, Italy. Trends Pharmacol Sci. 2007 Apr;28(4):180-7.

11 Weydt P, Hong S, Witting A, Möller T, Stella N, Kliot M. *Cannabinol delays symptom onset in SOD1 (G93A) transgenic mice without affecting survival*. Department of Neurology, University of Washington, Seattle, WA 98195, USA. Amyotroph Lateral Scler Other Motor Neuron Disord. 2005 Sep;6(3):182-4.

12 Amtmann D, Weydt P, Johnson KL, Jensen MP, Carter GT. *Survey of cannabis use in patients with amyotrophic lateral sclerosis*. Department of Rehabilitation Medicine, University of Washington School of Medicine, Seattle, Washington, USA. Am J Hosp Palliat Care. 2004 Mar-Apr;21(2):95-104.

13 Carter GT, Rosen BS. *Marijuana in the management of amyotrophic lateral sclerosis*. Muscular Dystrophy Association (MDA), Neuromuscular Disease Clinic, Department of Rehabilitation Medicine, University of Washington School of Medicine, Seattle, Washington, USA. Am J Hosp Palliat Care. 2001 Jul-Aug;18(4):264-70.

Neurological Diseases
Epileptic Seizure (Status Epilepticus)

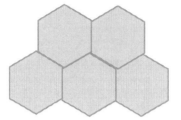

NUMBER OF STUDIES: 5

CHI VALUE: 13

An emergency room definition for status epilepticus (SE) is: a continuous seizure activity lasting longer than five minutes or multiple seizures without regaining consciousness in between the seizures. This is a true emergency. SE, a potentially life threatening condition, involves the brain and by extension the entire nervous system in a state of excessive nerve cell activity. Some people liken it to a short in the electrical system.

Several patients have reported an aura just prior to the onset of a seizure. This aura can be a smell, a visual shift in color or a sense of psychic perceptions such as déjà vu or the sensation of shifting into 'slow motion'. It is a practical and useful sensation that helps the patient prepare for a coming event and allows her to reduce the risk of trauma and complications.

Other symptoms range from thrashing movements to loss of consciousness. They may include: involuntary spasms of the body or parts of it, rapid heart rates, oral trauma from involuntarily biting cheek or tongue, incontinence and confusion. Caution should be heeded due to possible secondary trauma acquired from a fall.

Causes may include: nerve toxins, hypoglycemia (low sugar), very high fevers (most common cause of SE in children), septic condition, trauma (especially to the head or spinal cord), tumors (especially brain and spinal cord), metabolic imbalances, acquired tolerance to anti-seizure medications, alcohol withdrawal, pharmaceutical drugs, street drugs, stroke (CVA), hereditary or brain diseases.

Allopathic treatment consists of diagnosing and correcting, if possible, underlying causes. Diagnosed epileptic patients are given anti-seizure pharmaceuticals to reduce seizures and their intensity. Orthodox medicine currently has no cure for epilepsy.

CANNABIS AND STATUS EPILEPTICUS

Researchers (2009) from the University of Reading, England, wrote that, "Early studies suggested that cannabidiol (CBD) has anticonvulsant properties in animal models and reduced seizure frequency in limited human trials." Based on these early results, researchers conceived a study in which mice received a chemical substance (pentylentetrazol) known to produce generalized spasms similar to epileptic seizures. Cannabidiol (CBD), administered at a dose of 100 mg/kg, produced a significant reduction in the frequency of spasms and overall mortality,[1] thus confirming earlier findings.

The endocannabioid system in the human body helps maintain an up/down (excitatory/inhibitory) balance within the central nervous system (CNS). With this understanding, neuroscientists (2009) from Rome, Italy, explored the relationship between epileptic activity and the amount of endocannabioids present in cerebrospinal fluid (CSF). Doctors withdrew cerebrospinal fluid from patients suffering from diagnosed temporal lobe epilepsy (TLE) and from healthy individuals. They measured the presence of two cannabinoids, anandamide and 2-arachidonoylglycerol (2-AG). Results revealed a significantly lower amount of anandamide in TLE patients when compared with the healthy controls, thus suggesting that the presence of anandamide, or lack thereof, may play a part in epilepsy.[2]

Based on prior research establishing the endocannabinoid system's involvement in hyperexcitability, particularly in the causation and control of seizures and status epilepticus (SE), scientists from the Commonwealth University in Virginia (2009) conducted an experiment to learn more about the endocannabinoid system during SE. Scientists discovered that chemically induced SE caused a redistribution of cannabinoid receptor site (CB1) in the hippocampus suggesting a role for dysregulation of the endocannabinoid system during epileptogenesis.[3]

Pediatricians in Germany (2003) conducted the first human trial using pediatric patients suffering from a variety of neurological disorders including seizures. Doctors treated patients with Delta-9-THC with dosages ranging from 0.04 mg/kg body weight to 0.14 mg/kg body weight. The authors concluded: "In severely disabled children and adolescents, Delta-9-THC medication can have positive psychotropic effects, influences the degree of spasticity and dystonia and-occasionally-seems to have an anticonvulsant action."[4]

In 2005, a group of international researchers from Leiden, Holland, and Rome, Italy, conducted a second and similar human trial on pediatric patients suffering from epileptic seizures who failed to respond to traditional pharmaceutical anti-seizure medications. Pediatric patients received an oil-based solution of cannabidiol (CBD). Each of the patients responded positively. The authors of the study concluded: "So far, obtained results in our open study appear encouraging for various reasons: 1) no side effects of such a severity were observed as to require CBD discontinuation; 2) in most of the treated children, an improvement of the crises was obtained equal to, or higher than, 25% in spite of the low CBD doses administered; 3) in all CBD- treated children, a clear improvement of consciousness and spasticity (whenever present) was observed."[5]

STUDY SUMMARY:

Drugs/Focus	Type of Study	Published Year, Place, and Key Results	CHI
Cannabidiol (CBD) 100 mg/kg	Animal study (mice)	2009 – School of Pharmacy, University of Reading, Whiteknights, Reading, UK. Antispasmodic.	2
Anandamide and 2-arachidonoylglycerol (2-AG)	Human patients with epilepsy.	2009 – Dipartimento di Neuroscienze, Università degli Studi di Roma Tor Vergata, Roma, Italy. Anandamide may prevent epilepsy.	3
Cannabinoid receptor CB1 studied.	Animal study (epileptic rats)	2009 – Department of Neurology, Virginia Commonwealth University, Richmond, VA, USA. Authors suspect redistribution of cannabinoid receptors CB1 in hippocampus may play a role in epilepsy.	2

Drugs/Focus	Type of Study	Published Year, Place, and Key Results	CHI
Cannabidiol (CBD)	18 children suffering from epileptic seizures who had no success with traditional pharmaceutical anti-seizure medications.	2005 – Multi-institutional research team from Holland and Italy. Safe and clear improvement of consciousness and spasticity.	3
Delta-9-THC at dosages ranging from 0.04 mg/kg body weight to 0.14 mg/kg body weight	8 pediatric patients suffering from a variety of neurological disorders including seizures.	2003 – Pediatrician, Brunnenstrasse 54, Bad Wildungen, Germany. Positive psychotropic effects, influences the degree of spasticity and dystonia and occasionally seems to have an anticonvulsant action.	3

Total CHI Value   13

STRAIN SPECIFIC CONSIDERATIONS

The relevant cannabinoids used in these trials against epilepsy include CBD, anandamide and THC. Anandamide and THC bind relatively equally to CB1 and CB2. CBD has a greater affinity for CB2. The largest study to date (2005) from Leiden, Holland, and Rome, Italy, used a CBD infused oil on their pediatric seizure patients.

Indicas or indica dominant strains tend to have a higher CBD:THC ratio than sativa or sativa heavy hybrids, thus favoring relative CB2 activation.

EXPLORING MIND–BODY CONSCIOUSNESS

SUGGESTED
BLESSING:

May you find a place in you where peace reigns supreme.

Julius Cesar suffered from epilepsy. In those days, people believed that epileptics were communing with the gods during a seizure event. Today some researchers echo this belief and past experience. The occurrences of temporal lobe seizure activity have been associated with religious vision and hyperreligiosity.[6]

The tonic-clonic jarring movements during an epileptic seizure simulate a short circuit without the circuit breaker present. The sparks simply continue to fly. Electrical energy keeps firing, overwhelming the nervous system, and the body responds in fits. The mental-emotional equivalent is overwhelming intense thoughts and feelings which the person refuses to consciously experience.

SUGGESTED
AFFIRMATION:

I release all fear.

Studies exploring the significance of psychological tension in connection with seizure activity suggest that this tension, not immediately soluble in reality, can contribute to the occurrence of seizures. However, the resolution of such tension in a therapeutic setting could ameliorate seizure activities.[7]

Another researcher noted that seizure responses from relatively minor petit mal seizures to full-blown status epilepticus may appear as specific responses within the central nervous system, "…which abolishes consciousness when awareness of the discrepancy in the immediate situation between consciously acceptable responses and the true unconscious reactions threatens to disrupt the patient's existing pattern of integration."[8] This last finding suggests a conflict between the conscious and unconscious mind, a short due to crossed wires of conflicting beliefs, intentions or experiences.

Another study examined the relationship between emotionally disturbed children and seizure activity. Researchers learned that sometimes the children would use the seizure activities as an unconscious defense mechanism; for instance, when witnessing the parents destroy each other psychologically. In such moments, the child would often succeed, temporarily ending the marital conflict. However, at other times, the child would display seizure activities to seek sympathy or attention and employ an avoidance mechanism such as procrastination when not wanting to do a certain task. This suggests that in some cases the frequency of seizure activity and the underlying psychodynamics were intertwined. "For example, greater passivity increased the frequency, and greater aggression decreased the frequency of petit mal attacks in two children; whereas increased anxiety probably caused more frequent psychomotor seizures in another child."[9]

A physician compiled the following examples. A patient never had seizures in college classes that he actively engaged in and liked when compared to classes he disliked. A trapeze artist had regular seizures except when he was working at the trapeze. A baseball player had seizures on the sidelines but never when playing ball. Another patient had regular seizures except when swimming. Based on these examples, this researcher suggested that mental activity, which engages and appeals to the person, might be employed in the treatment and prevention of seizure events.[10]

Given the rather elusive origin of seizures, those dealing with epilepsy might consider exploring the metaphysical underpinnings in order to better understand, cope and hopefully diminish seizures. Many patients with epilepsy perceive an aura just prior to an epileptic event. The aura can be a particular scent, a sound, a halo or color or a specific sensation that signals the imminent seizure.

Another helpful mechanism includes increasing one's awareness of the trigger mechanisms involved in seizure development. Some epileptics have found success in this task by approaching it as a mindfullness exercise. Learning which signals from the environment such as sounds, music[11] or lights can trigger a seizure is another way to be more aware of the complexities of this disease picture.

QUESTIONS

What thoughts or feelings overwhelm me?
What is too much for me to handle?
What is so intense that I want to throw in the towel?

AGGRAVATING FACTORS

Psychological tension from repressed memories and emotions / increased anxiety and passivity / negative affect / lack of connection with the spiritual.

HEALING FACTORS

Integrating and healing childhood traumas / accepting and appropriately releasing repressed content / increasing assertiveness (appropriately expressed and without hurting anyone) / engaging in profound spiritual connections or intensely enjoyed activities / finding positive persective.

1 Jones NA, Hill AJ, Smith I, Bevan SA, Williams CM, Whalley BJ, Stephens GJ. *Cannabidiol displays anti-epileptiform and anti-seizure properties in vitro and in vivo*. School of Pharmacy, University of Reading, Whiteknights, Reading RG6 6AJ, UK. J Pharmacol Exp Ther, 11. November 2009.

2 Romigi A, Bari M, Placidi F, Marciani MG, Malaponti M, Torelli F, Izzi F, Prosperetti C, Zannino S, Corte F, Chiaramonte C, Maccarrone M. *Cerebrospinal fluid levels of the endocannabinoid anandamide are reduced in patients with untreated newly diagnosed temporal lobe epilepsy*. Dipartimento di Neuroscienze, Università degli Studi di Roma Tor Vergata, Roma, Italy. a_romigi@inwind.it Epilepsia, 8. Oktober 2009.

3 Falenski KW, Carter DS, Harrison AJ, Martin BR, Blair RE, DeLorenzo RJ. *Temporal characterization of changes in hippocampal cannabinoid CB(1) receptor expression following pilocarpine-induced status epilepticus*. Department of Neurology, Virginia Commonwealth University, PO Box 980599, Richmond, VA 23298, USA. Brain Res. 2009;1262:64-72.

4 Lorenz R. *Experiences with THC-treatment in children and adolescents*. Abstract, IACM 2nd Conference on Cannabinoids in Medicine, September 12-13, 2003, Cologne. Paediatrician, Brunnenstrasse 54, 34537 Bad Wildungen, Germany.

5 Pelliccia A, Grassi G, Romano A, Crocchialo P. *Treatment with CBD in oily solution of drug-resistant paediatric epilepsies*. 9-10 September, 2005 Congress on Cannabis and the Cannabinoids, Leiden, The Netherlands: International Association for Cannabis as Medicine, p. 14. in cooperation with Institute of Biology, Pharmacognosy/Metabolomics, Leiden University. Office of Medicinal Cannabis, Ministry of Health, Welfare and Sports. II Facoltà di Medicina, Università "La Sapienza", 00100 Rome, Italy, Istituto Sperimentale Colture Industriali, Sezione di Rovigo, Italy, American University of Rome, 00100, Italy.

6 Blumer D. E*vidence supporting the temporal lobe epilepsy personality syndrome*. Department of Psychiatry, University of Tennessee Medical School, Memphis 38105, USA. Neurology. 1999;53(5 Suppl 2):S9-12.

7 ARTHUR W. EPSTEIN M.D. and FRANK ERVIN M.D. *Psychodynamic Significance of Seizure Content in Psychomotor Epilepsy*. Department of Psychiatry and Neurology, Tulane University School of Medicine, New Orleans, La. Psychosomatic Medicine 18:43-55 (1956).

8 WAYNE BARKER M.D. *Studies on Epilepsy: The Petit Mal Attack as a Response Within the Central Nervous System to Distress in Organism-Environment Integration*. New York Hospital and the Department of Medicine, Cornell University Medical College New York, N.Y. Psychosomatic Medicine 10:73-94 (1948).

9 J. P. KEMPH M.D., L. S. ZEGANS M.D., K. A. KOOI M.D., and R. W. WAGGONER M.D. *The Emotionally Disturbed Child with a Convulsive Disorder*. Department of Psychiatry, University of Michigan, Ann Arbor, Mich. Psychosomatic Medicine 25:441-449 (1963).

10 HANS STRAUSS M.D. *The Effect of Mental Activity on the Incidence of Seizures and the Electroencephalographic Pattern in some Epileptic*. Neurological Service of Dr. I. S. Wechsler, The Mount Sinai Hospital, New York City. Psychosomatic Medicine 6:141-145 (1944).

11 DAVID D. DALY M.D. and MAURICE J. BARRY JR. M.D. Musicogenic Epilepsy: Report of Three Cases. Sections of Neurology and Psychiatry, Mayo Clinic and Mayo Foundation, Rochester, Minn. Psychosomatic Medicine 19:399-408 (1957).

Neurological Diseases
Huntington's Disease

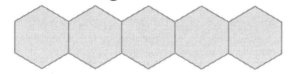

NUMBER OF STUDIES: 5

CHI VALUE: 10

Huntington's disease (HD) or Huntington's chorea (abnormal twisting and writhing movements) is a degenerative genetic disease that affects the brain and nervous system leading to loss of muscle control and dementia. A mutated form of the Huntington gene (HTT), found significantly more in Western Europeans, is thought to be responsible for disease development. The gene can be passed on to offspring. One parent with the mutation on one of the two DNA strand pairs is associated with a 50% chance any offspring will develop the disease. If both parents have a single pair mutation, the risk for the offspring increases to 75%, and if both parents have dual pair mutation, development of Huntington's is a virtual certanty. Parents who may carry this gene may want to consider genetic testing.

Researchers currently ponder a variety of questions about Huntington's disease: how does the disease start? What causes or maintains the mutation? What activates the gene? Why does HD develop at a certain time after years of apparent dormancy? Why does HD begin earlier in some people and later in others?

Some scientists believe that the mutated gene codes for a protein that rather than forming and folding into functional protein molecules causes protein aggregation. These aggregated proteins clump together, collect, and eventually corrupt certain portions of the brain causing the characteristic signs and symptoms of HD.

Once HD begins, the illness takes a predictable course for most patients. Symptoms usually begin with lack of coordination and ataxia (unsteady gait). They soon progress to chorea, dystonia (muscle contraction, twisting and abnormal posturing), dementia, behavioral difficulties and eventually death. No treatment exists within orthodox medicine for HD. However, to manage some of the disease complications, doctors may certain treatments using a multidisciplinary approach comprised of physical and speech therapies, neuroleptics (tranquilizing psychiatric pharmaceuticals) and other medication. If eating or drinking becomes too difficult, gastric tubes may be used. Huntington mortality statistics suggest the leading causes of death are the development of pneumonia and heart disease followed by nutritional deficiencies, mental and cerebrovascular disorders, accidents, poisoning and violence.[1]

CANNABIS AND HUNTINGTON'S DISEASE

As early as 1986, researchers enrolled three patients suffering from HD whose disease progression continued to deteriorate and who did not respond to pharmaceuticals. Each received an oral form of the non-psychoactive cannabinoid CBD. After the first week of treatment, results revealed a mild improvement of 5 to 15% in objective and subjective tests. After week two, the improvement of 20 to 40% was observed using the same tests. The results remained stable for the following two weeks. The only adverse effect noted was a mild and transient hypotension.[2]

Five years later, researchers from the University of Arizona conducted a double-blind, randomized cross-over trial testing the effects of oral CBD and placebo on 15 neuroleptic-free patients with HD. In this case, CBD proved only as effective as the placebo.[3]

In 2007, Spanish scientists examined the neuroprotective potential of CBD in the context of Huntington's disease. Results indicated that: "...CBD provides neuroprotection against 3NP-induced striatal damage, which may be relevant for Huntington's disease, a disorder characterized by the preferential loss of striatal projection neurons. ... This capability seems to be based exclusively on the anti-oxidant properties of CBD."[4]

Two more experiments published in 2011 examined the effects of cannabinoids on HD. Researchers from Madrid, Spain examined whether Sativex (THC/CBD) was able to protect animals from HD progression and development. The authors observed, "In conclusion, this study provides preclinical evidence in support of a beneficial effect of the cannabis-based medicine Sativex as a neuroprotective agent capable of delaying disease progression in HD, a disorder that is currently poorly managed in the clinic, prompting an urgent need for clinical trials with agents showing positive results in preclinical studies."[5]

In another study, scientists also in Madrid, Spain, acknowledged cannabinoids as promising medicines for slowing the chronic degenerative progression of both Parkinson's disease and HD. Researchers examined in more detail the affects of CB1 and CB2 receptor activation on disease progression. Results demonstrated that "...activation of CB(2) receptors leads to a slower progression of neurodegeneration in both disorders." Furthermore, "... cannabinoids like $\Delta(9)$ -tetrahydrocannabinol or cannabidiol protect nigral or striatal neurons in experimental models of both disorders in which oxidative injury is a prominent cytotoxic mechanism." Researchers concluded that, "...the evidence reported so far supports that those cannabinoids having antioxidant properties and/or capability to activate CB(2) receptors may represent promising therapeutic agents in HD and PD, thus deserving a prompt clinical evaluation."[6]

STUDY SUMMARY:

Drugs/Focus	Type of Study	Published Year, Place, and Key Results	CHI
THC and CBD containing Sativex.	Animal model (rats)	2011 – Departamento de Bioquímica y Biología Molecular, Instituto Universitario de Investigación en Neuroquímica, Facultad de Medicina, Universidad Complutense, Madrid, Spain. Sativex is a neuroprotective agent capable of delaying disease progression in HD.	1
Endocannabinoid system and cannabinoids especially THC and CBD.	Meta-analysis and review.	2011 – Departamento de Bioquímica y Biología Molecular III, Instituto Universitario de Investigación en Neuroquímica, Facultad de Medicina, Universidad Complutense, Madrid, Spain. The endocannabinoid system behaves as an endogenous neuroprotective system in both PD and HD.	4

Drugs/Focus	Type of Study	Published Year, Place, and Key Results	CHI
Arachidonyl-2-chloro-ethylamide (ACEA) a CB1 agonist; HU-308 a CB2 agonist; and can-nabidiol (CBD)	Animal study (rats)	2007 – Departamento de Bioquímica y Biología Molecular III, Universidad Complutense. CBD provides neuroprotection, which may be relevant to Hunting-ton's disease.	2
Oral CBD (10 mg/kg/day for 6 weeks) and placebo (sesame oil for 6 weeks).	15 patients with Hunting-ton's Disease	1991 – Department of Pharmacology/Toxicology, University of Arizona, Tucson. CBD was neither symptom-atically effective nor toxic, relative to placebo.	0
Orally administered CBD was initiated at 300 mg/d and increased 1 week later to 600 mg/d for the next 3 weeks.	Three patients, ages 30 to 56, had HD for 7 to 12 years' duration.	1986 – Decreased choreic movements and severity.	3

Total CHI Value   10

STRAIN SPECIFIC CONSIDERATIONS

The relevant cannabinoids examined in this set of pre-clinical and human case studies include primarily CBD, THC and Sativex. CBD has a greater affinity for CB2. THC binds relatively equally to CB1 and CB2. Sativex is a standardized plant cannabis extract containing THC and CBD in ratios similar to those in cannabis flowers.

Indica and indica dominant strains or hybrids usually contain lower THC:CBD ratios, thus favoring CB2 activation when compared to sativas or sativa leaning strains.

EXPLORING MIND–BODY CONSCIOUSNESS

The threat of progression of HD and the relative certainty that the beginning of the end is near forces one focus on living in the moment. The value of life is associated with youth and the rest with pain and inevitable death. The archetype of youth rebelling against the predetermined destiny comes to mind. In a way, HD engages and sometimes challenges supernatural authorities such as destiny or the unconscious. It engages us in the intense choices ahead. Will I be choosing to look at life with gratitude for what I have now, or choosing to blame others and feel hopeless? Another strong component of HD is that of family burden and shared destiny in a movement towards less conscious control while uncontrollable unconscious dance-like movement increases. As consciousness retreats, it is apparently replaced by an unconscious release of energy.

To some people with HD, another choice may present itself: What if I were to embrace the inevitable unconscious dance of twisting, writhing energy exploding into my reality? What if I surrender consciously to the unconscious?

SUGGESTED BLESSING:

May all my blame turn to forgiveness.

May all my future fear become a present and creative love.

May all my hopelessness transcend into a creative vision carried by a determined will into the arms of loving possibilities.

QUESTIONS

What comes up for me when looking at the past, present and the future?
What is my relationship to the conscious and the unconscious mind?

What is my relationship to the bridge between the conscious and the unconscious mind?

How do I feel about the unconscious?

What do I think of destiny?

Could I surrender to whatever emerges?

Could I embrace the emerging?

How do I feel about outside controlling forces?

How would I feel if I learned that those forces were set in motion by me for a good reason that I have purposefully forgotten?

Can I make peace with the coming unconscious dance?

1 Lanska DJ, Lavine L, Lanska MJ, Schoenberg BS. *Huntington's disease mortality in the United States.* Department of Neurology, University Hospitals of Cleveland, OH 44106. Neurology. 1988 May;38(5):769-72.

2 Reuven Sandyk, Paul Consroe, Lawrence Z. Stern, and Stuart R. Snider, Tucson, AZ. *EFFECTS OF CANNABIDIOL IN HUNTINGTON'S DISEASE.* Neurology 36 (Suppl 1) April 1986 p. 342.

3 Consroe P, Laguna J, Allender J, Snider S, Stern L, Sandyk R, Kennedy K, Schram K. *Controlled clinical trial of cannabidiol in Huntington's disease.* Department of Pharmacology and Toxicology, University of Arizona, Tucson 85721. Pharmacol Biochem Behav. 1991. Nov;40(3):701-8.

4 Sagredo O, Ramos JA, Decio A, Mechoulam R, Fernández-Ruiz J. *Cannabidiol reduced the striatal atrophy caused 3-nitropropionic acid in vivo by mechanisms independent of the activation of cannabinoid, vanilloid TRPV1 and adenosine A2A receptors.* Departamento de Bioquímica y Biología Molecular III, Universidad Complutense, 28040-Madrid, Spain. Eur J Neurosci. 2007 Aug;26(4):843-51.

5 Sagredo O, Pazos MR, Satta V, Ramos JA, Pertwee RG, Fernández-Ruiz J. *Neuroprotective effects of phytocannabinoid-based medicines in experimental models of Huntington's disease.* Departamento de Bioquímica y Biología Molecular, Instituto Universitario de Investigación en Neuroquímica, Universidad Complutense, Madrid, Spain. J Neurosci Res. 2011 Sep;89(9):1509-18.

6 Fernández-Ruiz J, Moreno-Martet M, Rodríguez-Cueto C, Palomo-Garo C, Gómez-Cañas M, Valdeolivas S, Guaza C, Romero J, Guzmán M, Mechoulam R, Ramos JA. *Prospects for cannabinoid therapies in basal ganglia disorders.* Departamento de Bioquímica y Biología Molecular III, Instituto Universitario de Investigación en Neuroquímica, Facultad de Medicina, Universidad Complutense, Madrid, Spain. Br J Pharmacol. 2011 Aug;163(7):1365-78.

Neurological Diseases
Multiple Sclerosis (MS)

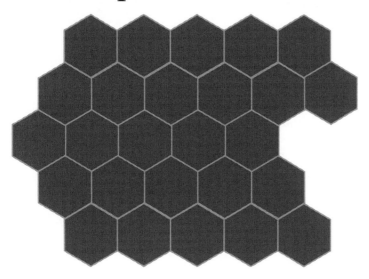

NUMBER OF STUDIES: 26

CHI VALUE: 91

Orthodox medicine considers multiple sclerosis (MS) a chronic, inflammatory, and degenerative neurological illness with no cure and no exact cause. In fact, MS is one of the most common neurological diseases.

The meaning of the word multiple sclerosis provides a clue about the general picture of this illness. It derives from the Latin words 'multi' and 'plus,' which together translate into 'manifold,' and the Greek word 'sclerosis' which translates as 'hardness'. Place the words together and we get 'many folded hardness.' Apply 'manifold hardness' to the brain and spinal cord and we have a description of MS.

Multiple sclerosis is a chronic inflammatory disease characterized by the breakdown of some of the thin sheets which cover the brain and spinal cord. These fat-based myelin sheets normally provide insulation and protection, but when lesions occur, nerve impulses misfire across the broken insulation causing a variety of debilitating symptoms.

Scientists speculate that MS might be an autoimmune disease that inadvertently prompts adhesion molecules, which summon immune cells to fight an inflammation, and thus contribute to the destruction of myelin sheets.[1] Other likely culprits include a combination of genetic factors, infections and environmental influences such as decreased sun exposure and subsequent insufficient vitamin D.

Some pharmaceutical medications exist to manage symptoms as they develop or worsen, but they come with a steep price of significant side effects. MS may initially appear as only acute attacks or it may progress to its chronic degenerative form in which symptoms accumulate and gradually worsen. Some of the most common symptoms include: muscular spasms affecting the eyes, bladder and bowels, numbness, increased weakness, ataxia, slurred speech or acute and chronic pain.

Due to limited success within the allopathic model, many MS patients have turned to other healing methodologies in the hope of finding help and relief.

CANNABIS AND MS

The earliest study listed in the National Library of Health took place in 1981 when researchers found motivation in anecdotal accounts of MS patients who reported that inhaling cannabis gave relief from spasticity. This, combined with the scientific discovery that THC was able to inhibit spasms in animal studies, opened the door to a multitude of scientific inquiries.

While initial studies merely focused on observing the effect of cannabis on the most common symptoms of MS, later studies worked to discover the mechanisms underlying the observed therapeutic effects.

The scientific community began to build on the data accumulated. The therapeutic frame of cannabis in the context of MS became more clear and defined. A reduction in spasticity was recognized as only the first of many benefits. Cannabis use also reduced pain, depression, anxiety, paresthesia, neuropathic pains, sleep disturbances, urge incontinence and nocturnal polyuria.

Even the U.S. Federal Government issued itself a patent on the neuroprotective properties of cannabinoids employed in the treatment of several diseases involving inflammation and the nervous system such as MS.

One of the latest animal studies on the cannabinoid receptor systems alludes to the involvement of cannabinoids in the inhibition of brain adhesion molecules, which in turn may be responsible for some therapeutic effects on MS. If clinical trials can confirm these results, scientists may be able to partly understand how to slow or even reverse the progression of MS.

While the focus of 26 studies differs in approach, scope and methodology, the results share a common denominator. For patients suffering from MS, cannabis may be a potent and powerful ally in alleviating the disease's symptoms. Furthermore, cannabinoids may slow the progression of the illness itself, and thus provide an improvement to long-term survival and quality of life.

WARNING: Most clinical studies reported adverse effects of cannabis use in addition to benefits dependant on dose and form. Those included reduced balance and posture, nausea and dizziness; and at high dosages, negative psychological symptoms such as anxiety. These studies indicated that when used within the proper subjective therapeutic dose, cannabinoids' potential adverse effects are usually well tolerated and negligible especially when compared to the beneficial effects.

To determine the best possible therapeutic window for you, seek advise from peers with MS who have used cannabis themselves, and consult a licensed health care professional familiar with cannabinoids.

STUDY SUMMARY:

Drugs/Focus	Type of Study	Published Year, Place, and Key Results	CHI
WIN55,212-2	Animal study (mice)	2009 – Neuroimmunology Group, Functional and Systems Neurobiology Department, Cajal Institute (CSIC), Madrid, Spain. Inhibition of brain adhesion molecules may produce therapeutic effects in MS.[7]	2
Free-dose cannabis plant extract (Sativex)	17 patients with MS. Double-Blind, Placebo Controlled, Cross-over Study.	2009 – "Sapienza" University, Rome, Italy. Within therapeutic doses, no impairment or negative psychological symptoms noted. However, at high dosages, negative psychological symptoms noted.[8]	5
THC:CBD as an oral spray	18 Patients with MS. Randomized, double-blind, placebo-controlled, cross-over study	2009 – Department of Neurological Sciences, University of Rome "Sapienza", Rome, Italy. RIII reflex threshold increased and RIII reflex area decreased plus pain reduction.[9]	5
Anandamide AEA, PEA, 2-AG and OEA levels.	50 patients with MS and 20 control subjects	2008 – Centre for Study of Demyelinating Diseases, Department of Medical and Surgical Specialities and Public Health, Ospedale S Maria della Misericordia, University of Perugia, Perugia, Italy. Significantly reduced levels of all the tested eCBs were found in the CSF of patients with MS compared to control subjects…"[10]	3
Dronabinol	Case study of a 52-year-old woman with MS, paroxysmal dystonia, complex vocal tics, and marijuana dependence.	2008 – Mental Health Service Line, Department of Veterans Affairs Medical Center, Washington, DC, USA. Improvement in sleep, decreased anxiety, decreased frequency of paroxysmal dystonia and "a dramatic reduction of craving and illicit use".[11]	3
Sativex (THC:CBD)	66 patients with MS	2007 – Walton Centre for Neurology and Neurosurgery, Liverpool, United Kingdom. THC/CBD was effective to reduce pains with no evidence of tolerance for the 2 years tested.[12]	5
THC:CBD daily	189 patients with MS	2007 – Royal Berkshire and Battle NHS Trust, Reading. Reduction in spasms.[13]	5
Endocannabinoids (AEA) & (2-AG) levels, metabolism, binding, and physiological activities.	26 patients with MS, 25 healthy controls and an animal study (mice).	2007 – Multi-Departmental study from Italy. Clinica Neurologica, Dipartimento di Neuroscienze, Università Tor Vergata, Rome, Italy. Targeting the endocannabinoid system might be useful for the treatment of MS.[14]	5
Endocannabinoid agonists	Animal study (mice)	2007 – Department of Neuro-inflammation, Institute of Neurology, University College London, London, UK. CB(1) receptor is the main cannabinoid target for an anti-spastic effect.[15]	2
Cannabinoids studied.	Laboratory	2006 – Center for Drug Discovery, Northeastern University, Boston, MA, USA. Results suggest a therapeutic potential of cannabinoids on inflammatory diseases such as MS.[16]	1
Cannabis extract, THC or placebo.	630 MS patients	2006 – Urogynaecology Unit, Derriford Hospital, Plymouth, Devon, UK. Both Cannabis extract and THC showed significant reductions in urge incontinence.[17]	5

Drugs/Focus	Type of Study	Published Year, Place, and Key Results	CHI
Sativex as an oromucosal spray. Each spray delivers 2.7 mg THC and 2.5 mg CBD. Average use in this study I 22-32 mg/day THC and 20-30 mg/day for CBD.	Patients with MS	2006 – Hunters Moor Regional Neurological Rehabilitation Centre, Newcastle upon Tyne, UK. Reduction in spasticity, neuropathic pain, and neuropathic pain of other etiologies.[18]	3
Cannabinoid HU210	Animal study (rats)	2006 – Department of Physical Medicine and Rehabilitation, University of Saskatchewan, Saskatoon, Canada . "HU210 dramatically reduced peroxynitrite-induced axonal injury…"[19]	2
Cannabinoids	A meta-analysis of human, animal and laboratory studies	2005 – Neurologische Klinik mit Klinischer Neurophysiologie, Medizinische Hochschule Hannover, Germany."…there is reasonable evidence for the therapeutic employment of cannabinoids in the treatment of MS related symptoms."[20]	4
Whole-plant cannabis-based medicine, containing (THC:CBD) & delivered via an oromucosal spray.	66 patients with MS.	2005 – Walton Centre for Neurology and Neurosurgery, University of Liverpool, Liverpool, United Kingdom. Reduction of pain and sleep disturbance in MS.[21]	5
Oromucosal spray sativex containing (THC:CBD)	Meta-analysis on 368 human patients with various neurological disorders including MS	2005 – In some trials, THC:CBD spray significantly reduced neuropathic pain, spasticity, muscle spasms and sleep disturbances.[22]	4
Whole-plant cannabis-based medicine, containing (THC:CBD) and delivered via an oromucosal spray, as adjunctive analgesic treatment. Each spray delivered 2.7 mg of THC and 2.5 of CBD, and patients could gradually self-titrate to a maximum of 48 sprays in 24 hours.	66 patients with MS	2005 – Walton Centre for Neurology and Neurosurgery, University of Liverpool, Liverpool, United Kingdom. "Cannabis-based medicine is effective in reducing pain and sleep disturbance in patients with multiple sclerosis related central neuropathic pain and is mostly well tolerated."[23]	3
Oromucosal spray (Sativex) containing a Cannabis based extract (THC:CBD) at 2.5-120 mg of each daily in divided doses.	160 outpatients with MS	2004 – Oxford Centre for Enablement, Windmill Road, Oxford, UK. Significant reduction of spasms.[24]	5
THC and CBD; 2.5mg of each per spray for eight weeks followed by THC-only (2.5 mg THC per spray).	15 MS patients with lower urinary tract symptoms (LUTS)	2004 – Dept of Uro-Neurology, Institute of Neurology and National Hospital for Neurology and Neurosurgery, London, UK. Urinary urgency, the number and volume of incontinence episodes, frequency and nocturia all decreased significantly. Pain, spasticity and quality of sleep improved significantly.[25]	3
Cannabis, inhaled.	420 patients with MS	2003 – Office of Medical Bioethics, University of Calgary, Canada. Reduced anxiety, depression, spasticity and chronic pain.[26]	3
Cannabis, inhaled.	112 patients with MS	1997 – University of Arizona Health Sciences Center, Tucson, USA. Reduced spasticity, pain, tremor, depression, anxiety and paresthesia.[27]	3
Nabilone 1mg every 2nd day	1 patient with MS	1995 – Reduced muscle spasms and nocturia.[28]	3

Drugs/Focus	Type of Study	Published Year, Place, and Key Results	CHI
One marijuana cigarette containing 1.54% THC	10 MS patients and 10 normal volunteers.	1994 – Department of Neurology, University of Michigan, Ann Arbor. Inhaled cannabis reduced balance in MS patients.[29]	3
One marijuana cigarette	1 MS patient	1989 – Department of Clinical Neurophysiology, University of Göttingen, Germany. Chronic motor handicaps improved while smoking a marijuana cigarette. [30]	3
THC oral 2.5-15 mg once or twice daily	13 MS patients	1987 – Department of Psychiatry, U.C.L.A. School of Medicine, Califonrnia. At doses greater than 7.5mg, significant improvement in patient ratings of spasticity compared to placebo.[31]	3
Either 10 or 5 mg THC or placebo once daily	9 patients suffering from spasticity from various etiologies incl. MS	1981 – 10 mg THC significantly reduced spasticity.[32]	3

Total CHI Value   88

STRAIN SPECIFIC CONSIDERATIONS

The majority of the studies reviewed in this section used whole plant matter or the pharmaceutical plant derivative sativex, a cannabinoid combination containing THC and CBD in similar proportions as in the strain cannabis sativa. Whole flower cannabis and sativex activate both CB1 and CB2 receptors.

Similarly, sativa or sativa dominant hybrids usually contain a higher THC:CBD ratio activating both CB1 and CB2 receptors, while indicas or indica dominant strains usually contain a lower THC:CBD ratios, favoring CB2 signaling.

EXPLORING MIND–BODY CONSCIOUSNESS

A cross-cultural study of patients with MS from the US and Israel showed that both patient groups experienced similar concurrent psychological challenges at the time of the emergence of MS symptoms. These challenges were 'characterized as a psychologically stressful situation involving difficulty in coping and feelings of helplessness'.[2] Later studies revealed emotional stress as a potential trigger for the onset, exacerbations, and relapses of disease activity.[3,4]

QUESTIONS

How do I turn my energies on myself?
What do I try to control in my reality even though I know I can't?
How do I have impact in life when I don't want to participate?
Why am I so hardhearted with myself, others and the whole world?
Why am I so rigid with what I perceive as right and wrong?
What other perspectives can help me melt my stubbornness away?
Where are my tears wanting and where are they wasted?
What keeps me from facing changes and unforeseen events?
What paralyzes my courage and substance?
How do I love myself so as to allow a world where I am free and where I am safe?

SUGGESTED BLESSING:

May our buds and leaves assist you in the calming of your fears.

May they elevate your mood and help dispel numbness, anxiety and depression.

May we help relax the tension, the spasms and diminish the exhaustion.

Relax; release the grip of your mental fists, release control and surrender to a calming night of blissful sleep.

Why does it hurt to move or to show backbone?
How do I numb my senses or myself?
Why is life so exhausting?

AGGRAVATING FACTORS

Difficulty in coping / feelings of helplessness / emotional stress.

HEALING FACTORS

Learning / adapting positive coping mechanisms to reduce trigger events.

TAKE NOTICE

TURMERIC • VITAMIN D

TURMERIC: Ayurvedic practitioners, herbalists and naturopaths have long known about the multitudes of potent therapeutic properties of curcuma longa or turmeric. Curcumin is a naturally occurring compound found in the rhizome of the plant. Now researchers from Nashville, Tennessee, have examined the compound's ability to affect mice with MS. Results of the study revealed a similarity between the amount of curcumin used to protect the mice from artificially induced MS and that found in the typical Indian diet. One author of the study reported that MS in India is very rare, and while no human studies to date confirm the results, it certainly can't hurt to add some turmeric to your food.[5]

VITAMIN D: Researchers in Stockholm, Sweden, suggest that vitamin D is important for MS patients. "One of the environmental factors that has been implicated in MS and autoimmune diseases, such as type 1 diabetes, is vitamin D deficiency."[6]

If applicable, see also INFLAMMATORY DISEASES or the chapter on PAIN.

1 Irina Elovaara, MD, PhD; Maritta Ukkonen, MD; Minna Leppakynnas, MD; Terho Lehtimaki, MD, PhD; Mari Luomala, MSc; Jukka Peltola, MD; Prasun Dastidar, MD. *Adhesion Molecules in Multiple Sclerosis - Relation to Subtypes of Disease and Methylprednisolone Therapy.* Neuroimmunology Unit, Department of Neurology (Drs Elovaara, Ukkonen, Leppakynnas, and Peltola and Ms Luomala), and the Department of Diagnostic Radiology (Dr Dastidar), Tampere University Hospital, and the Laboratory of Atherosclerosis Genetics, Department of Clinical Chemistry, Center for Laboratory Medicine, Medical 3 School of Tampere University (Dr Lehtimaki and Ms Luomala), Tampere, 4 Finland. Arch Neurol. 2000;57:546-551.

2 VARDA MEI-TAL MD1, SANFORD MEYEROWITZ MD1, and GEORGE L. ENGEL MD2 *The Role of Psychological Process in a Somatic Disorder: Multiple Sclerosis1. The Emotional Setting of Illness Onset and Exacerbation.* 1 Departments of Psychiatry and Medicine, University of Rochester, School of Medicine, Rochester, NY 14620. 2 Departments of Psychiatry and Medicine, University of Rochester, School of Medicine, Rochester, NY 14620; Research Career Awardee, NIMH US Public Health Service. Psychosomatic Medicine 32:67-86 (1970).

3 Kurt D. Ackerman, MD, PhD, Rock Heyman, MD, Bruce S. Rabin, MD, PhD, Barbara P. Anderson, PhD, Patricia R. Houck, MSH, Ellen Frank, PhD and Andrew Baum, PhD. Stressful *Life Events Precede Exacerbations of Multiple Sclerosis.* Departments of Psychiatry (K.D.A., B.P.A., P.R.H., E.F., A.B.), Neurology (R.H.), Pathology (B.S.R.), and Psychology

(A.B.), University of Pittsburgh, Pittsburgh, Pennsylvania. Psychosomatic Medicine 64:916-920 (2002).

4 G. S. PHILIPPOPOULOS M.D., E. D. WITTKOWER M.D., and A. COUSINEAU M.A. *The Etiologic Significance of Emotional Factors in Onset and Exacerbations of Multiple Sclerosis.* A Preliminary Report. Allan Memorial Institute of Psychiatry, McGill University, the Montreal Neurological Institute, the Montreal General Hospital, and the Queen Mary Veterans' Hospital Montreal, Que., Canada. Psychosomatic Medicine 20:458-474 (1958).

5 Natarajan C, Bright JJ. *Curcumin inhibits experimental allergic encephalomyelitis by blocking IL-12 signaling through Janus kinase-STAT pathway in T lymphocytes.* Division of Neuroimmunology, Department of Neurology, Vanderbilt University Medical Center, Nashville, TN 37212, USA. J Immunol. 2002 Jun 15;168(12):6506-13

6 Sundqvist E, Bäärnhielm M, Alfredsson L, Hillert J, Olsson T, Kockum I. *Confirmation of association between multiple sclerosis and CYP27B1.* Neuroimmunology Unit, Department of Clinical Neuroscience, Center for Molecular Medicine, Karolinska Institutet, Stockholm, Sweden. Eur J Hum Genet. 2010 Jul 21.

7 Mestre L, Docagne F, Correa F, Loría F, Hernangómez M, Borrell J, Guaza C. *A cannabinoid agonist interferes with the progression of a chronic model of multiple sclerosis by downregulating adhesion molecules.* Neuroimmunology Group, Functional and Systems Neurobiology Department, Cajal Institute (CSIC), Av. Doctor Arce 37, 28002 Madrid, Spain. Mol Cell Neurosci. 2009 Feb;40(2):258-66.

8 Aragona M, Onesti E, Tomassini V, Conte A, Gupta S, Gilio F, Pantano P, Pozzilli C, Inghilleri M. *Psychopathological and Cognitive Effects of Therapeutic Cannabinoids in Multiple Sclerosis: A Double-Blind, Placebo Controlled, Crossover Study.* "Sapienza" University, Rome, Italy. Clin Neuropharmacol. 2009 Jan-Feb;32(1):41-7.

9 Conte A, Bettolo CM, Onesti E, Frasca V, Iacovelli E, Gilio F, Giacomelli E, Gabriele M, Aragona M, Tomassini V, Pantano P, Pozzilli C, Inghilleri M. *Cannabinoid-induced effects on the nociceptive system: A neurophysiological study in patients with secondary progressive multiple sclerosis.* Department of Neurological Sciences, University of Rome "Sapienza", Viale dell'Università 30, 00185 Rome, Italy. Eur J Pain. 2009 May;13(5):472-7.

10 Di Filippo M, Pini LA, Pelliccioli GP, Calabresi P, Sarchielli P. *Abnormalities in the cerebrospinal fluid levels of endocannabinoids in multiple sclerosis.* Centre for Study of Demyelinating Diseases, Department of Medical and Surgical Specialities and Public Health, Ospedale S Maria della Misericordia, University of Perugia, Perugia, Italy. J Neurol Neurosurg Psychiatry. 2008 Nov;79(11):1224-9.

11 Deutsch SI, Rosse RB, Connor JM, Burket JA, Murphy ME, Fox FJ. *Current status of cannabis treatment of multiple sclerosis with an illustrative case presentation of a patient with MS, complex vocal tics, paroxysmal dystonia, and marijuana dependence treated with dronabinol.* Mental Health Service Line, Department of Veterans Affairs Medical Center, Washington, DC, USA. stephen.deutsch@med.v CNS Spectr. 2008 May;13(5):393-403.

12 Rog DJ, Nurmikko TJ, Young CA. *Oromucosal delta9-tetrahydrocannabinol/cannabidiol for neuropathic pain associated with multiple sclerosis: an uncontrolled, open-label, 2-year extension trial.* Walton Centre for Neurology and Neurosurgery, Liverpool, United Kingdom. djrdjr@doctors.org.uk Clin Ther. 2007 Sep;29(9):2068-79.

13 Collin C, Davies P, Mutiboko IK, Ratcliffe S; Sativex Spasticity in MS Study Group. *Randomized controlled trial of cannabis-based medicine in spasticity caused by multiple sclerosis.* Department of Neurorehabilitation, Royal Berkshire and Battle NHS Trust, Reading, UK. christine.collin@rbbh-tr.nhs.uk Eur J Neurol. 2007 Mar;14(3):290-6.

14 Centonze D, Bari M, Rossi S, Prosperetti C, Furlan R, Fezza F, De Chiara V, Battistini L, Bernardi G, Bernardini S, Martino G, Maccarrone M. *The endocannabinoid system is dysregulated in multiple sclerosis and in experimental autoimmune encephalomyelitis.* Clinica Neurologica, Dipartimento di Neuroscienze, Università Tor Vergata, Rome, Italy. centonze@uniroma2.it Brain. 2007 Oct;130(Pt 10):2543-53.

15 G. Pryce & D. Baker. *Control of Spasticity in a Multiple Sclerosis Model is mediated by CB1, not CB2, Cannabinoid Receptors.* Department of Neuroinflammation, Institute of Neurology, University College London, London, UK. British Journal of Pharmacology (2007) 150, 519–525.

16 Lu, Dai1; Kiran Vemuri, V.1; Duclos, Richard I.1; Jr.1; Makriyannis, Alexandros.1 *The Cannabinergic System as a Target for Anti-inflammatory Therapies.* 1 Center for Drug Discovery, Northeastern University, 360 Huntington Avenue, 116 Mugar Hall, Boston, MA, 02115, USA. Current Topics in Medicinal Chemistry, Volume 6, Number 13, July 2006 ,

pp. 1401-1426(26). Bentham Science Publishers.

17 Freeman RM, Adekanmi O, Waterfield MR, Waterfield AE, Wright D, Zajicek J. *The effect of cannabis on urge incontinence in patients with multiple sclerosis: a multicentre, randomised placebo-controlled trial (CAMS-LUTS)*. Urogynaecology Unit, Derriford Hospital, Plymouth, Devon, UK. robert.freeman@phnt.swest.nhs.uk Int Urogynecol J Pelvic Floor Dysfunct. 2006 Nov;17(6):636-41.

18 Barnes MP. *Sativex: clinical efficacy and tolerability in the treatment of symptoms of multiple sclerosis and neuropathic pain.* Hunters Moor Regional Neurological Rehabilitation Centre, Newcastle upon Tyne, NE2 4NR, UK. m.p.barnes@btinternet.com Expert Opin Pharmacother. 2006 Apr;7(5):607-15.

19 Yang C, Hader W, Zhang X. *Therapeutic action of cannabinoid on axonal injury induced by peroxynitrite.* Department of Physical Medicine and Rehabilitation, University of Saskatchewan, 701 Queen Street, Saskatoon, SK, Canada S7K 0M7. Brain Res. 2006 Mar 3;1076(1):238-42.

20 Trebst C, Stangel M. *Cannabinoids in multiple sclerosis -- therapeutically reasonable?* Neurologische Klinik mit Klinischer Neurophysiologie, Medizinische Hochschule Hannover. Fortschr Neurol Psychiatr. 2005 Aug;73(8):463-9.

21 Rog DJ, Nurmikko TJ, Friede T, Young CA. *Randomized, controlled trial of cannabis-based medicine in central pain in multiple sclerosis.* Walton Centre for Neurology and Neurosurgery, University of Liverpool, Liverpool, United Kingdom. djrdjr@doctors.org.uk Neurology. 2005 Sep 27;65(6):812-9.

22 Perras C. *Sativex for the management of multiple sclerosis symptoms.* Issues Emerg Health Technol. 2005 Sep;(72):1-4.

23 Rog DJ, Nurmikko TJ, Friede T, Young CA. *Randomized, controlled trial of cannabis-based medicine in central pain in multiple sclerosis.* Walton Centre for Neurology and Neurosurgery, University of Liverpool, Liverpool, United Kingdom. djrdjr@doctors.org.uk Neurology. 2005 Sep 27;65(6):812-9.

24 Wade DT, Makela P, Robson P, House H, Bateman C. *Do cannabis-based medicinal extracts have general or specific effects on symptoms in multiple sclerosis? A double-blind, randomized, placebo-controlled study on 160 patients.* Oxford Centre for Enablement, Windmill Road, Oxford OX3 7LD, UK. derick.wade@dsl.pipex.com Mult Scler. 2004 Aug;10(4):434-41.

25 Brady CM, DasGupta R, Dalton C, Wiseman OJ, Berkley KJ, Fowler CJ. *An open-label pilot study of cannabis-based extracts for bladder dysfunction in advanced multiple sclerosis.* Dept of Uro-Neurology, Institute of Neurology and National Hospital for Neurology and Neurosurgery, Queen Square, London WC1N 3BG, UK. Multiple Sclerosis 2004;10(4):425-33.

26 Page SA, Verhoef MJ, Stebbins RA, Metz LM, Levy JC. *Cannabis use as described by people with multiple sclerosis.* Office of Medical Bioethics, University of Calgary, Calgary, AB, Canada. Can J Neurol Sci 2003;30(3):201-5.

27 Consroe P, Musty R, Rein J, Tillery W, Pertwee R. *The perceived effects of smoked cannabis on patients with multiple sclerosis.* Department of Pharmacology/Toxicology, University of Arizona Health Sciences Center, Tucson, USA. European Neurology 1997;38(1):44-48.

28 Martyn CN, Illis LS, Thom J. N*abilone in the treatment of multiple sclerosis.* Lancet 1995;345(8949):579.

29 Greenberg HS, Werness SAS, Pugh JE, Andrus RO, Anderson DJ, Domino EF. *Short-term effects of smoking marijuana on balance in patients with multiple sclerosis and normal volunteers.* Clinical Pharmacology and Therapeutics 1994;55:324-328. Department of Neurology, University of Michigan, Ann Arbor.

30 Meinck HM, Schönle PW, Conrad B. *Effect of cannabinoids on spasticity and ataxia in multiple sclerosis.* Department of Clinical Neurophysiology, University of Göttingen, Germany. Journal of Neurology 1989;236(2):120-122.

31 Ungerleider JT, Andrysiak T, Fairbanks L, Ellison GW, Myers LW. *Delta-9-THC in the treatment of spasticity associated with multiple sclerosis.* Department of Psychiatry, U.C.L.A. School of Medicine 90024. Advances in Alcohol and Substance Abuse 1987;7(1):39-50

32 Petro DJ, Ellenberger C Jr. *Treatment of human spasticity with delta 9-tetrahydrocannabinol.* Journal of Clinical Pharmacology 1981;21(8-9 Suppl):413S-416S.

Neurological Diseases
Parkinson's Disease

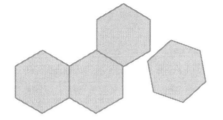

NUMBER OF STUDIES: 4

CHI VALUE: 14

Western medicine considers Parkinson's disease a chronic degenerative brain/nervous system disorder. An estimated 50,000 new cases of Parkinson's arise in the U.S. every year. Scientists believe that this degenerative disease results from the loss of specific nerve cells which produce the chemical dopamine (a natural occurring neuro-transmitter), causing symptoms like shaking extremities, stiffness, loss of balance, shuffling steps, difficulty swallowing, insomnia, blank expressions and emotional problems.

CANNABIS AND PARKINSON'S DISEASE

U.S. Department of Health and Human Services (2003) researchers received a patent on cannabinoids as antioxidants and neuroprotectants. Based on a multitude of earlier studies, these scientists noted in their U.S. patent abstract that: "...cannabinoids are found to have particular application as neuroprotectants, for example in limiting neurological damage following ischemic insults, such as stroke and trauma, or in the treatment of neurodegenerative diseases, such as Alzheimer's disease, Parkinson's disease and HIV dementia."[1]

A study (2004) from Hradec Kralove, Czech Republic, reports that almost half of all patients who used cannabis to treat symptoms associated with their Parkinon's reported a reduction in resting state tremors, reduced bradykinesia (slowed ability to start and/or continue movements), less muscle rigidity and decreased side-effects from levodopa (common Parkinson's medication) induced dyskinesias (repetitive spasmic motions). It took an average reported time of 1.7 months for these effects to take hold.[2]

East Lansing, Michigan, researchers (2009) reported on the case of a 24-year-old woman suffering from hyperkinetic movement disorder presenting with tremors, generalized dystonia, unstable standing position, dysarthria (speech disorder) and mild anorexia. The patient reportedly tried the usual pharmacological medications such as benztropin, clonazepam und tetrabenazin, but these failed to achieve the desired therapeutic impact. Doctors at the Department for Neurology, University of Michigan then treated the woman with a cannabinoid during her pregnancy, after which her symptoms improved significantly.[3]

European scientists (2009) from Naples, Italy, know very well that neurodegenerative diseases remain one of the main causes of death in the industrialized world. They are also keenly aware that very few allopathic therapies currently exist for most neurodegenerative diseases. Thus in searching for novel approaches, they studied cannabinoids. Their research concluded that: "…among Cannabis compounds, cannabidiol (CBD), which lacks any unwanted psychotropic effect, may represent a very promising agent with the highest prospect for therapeutic use."[4]

STUDY SUMMARY:

Drugs/Focus	Type of Study	Published Year, Place, and Key Results	CHI
Cannabidiol (CBD).	Meta-analysis	2009 – Department of Experimental Pharmacology, Faculty of Pharmacy, University of Naples Federico II, Naples, Italy. Cannabidiol (CBD) may represent a very promising agent with the highest prospect for therapeutic use in the treatment of neuro-degenerative illness.[5]	4
Dronabinol 5mg 3x daily.	Human case study	2009 – Department for Neurology, University of Michigan. Reduction of hyperkinetic movement disorder.[6]	3
Cannabis, taken orally or inhaled.	Patients with Parkinson's	2004 – Department of Pharmacology and Toxicology, Faculty of Pharmacy, Charles University, Hradec Kralove, Czech Republic. Reduction in resting state tremors, bradykinesia muscle rigidity and side-effect of levodopa induced dyskinesias.[7]	3
Cannabinoids, esp. cannabidiol (CBD).	Meta-analysis	2003 – United States Federal Government. Useful in the treatment of neuro-degenerative diseases such as Parkinson's disease.[8]	4

Total CHI Value   14

STRAIN SPECIFIC CONSIDERATIONS

The cannabinoids reviewed in these studies focus especially on CBD but also include dronabinol and whole cannabis (taken by mouth or inhaled). CBD has a higher affinity for CB2. Dronabinol, a synthetic cannabinoid prescription medication, is an isomer (same molecular formula but different structural formula) of Δ9-tetrahydrocannabinol. No information was given as to the strain used in the whole cannabis case study. Both the prior meta-analysis conducted by U.S. Government researchers from the Department of Health and Human Services (2003) and that of a team of Italian scientists (2009) highlight CBD as "…a very promising agent with the highest prospect for therapeutic use."

Indica and indica dominant hybrids tend to contain lower THC:CBD ratios thus favoring CB2 signaling.

EXPLORING MIND–BODY CONSCIOUSNESS

SUGGESTED BLESSING:

May all fears fade away like dew in the morning sun.

May love replace all that is fear.

Emotions commonly associated with the body language expressed by Parkinson's disease may offer some insights into the underlying body-mind influences. For instance: shaking extremities (extreme fear); stiffness (fear of pain or movement); aphasia (frozen speech – too shocked to talk); loss of balance (paradoxical emotions pulling in different directions); shuffling steps (chronic exhaustion); difficulty swallowing (shock/fear-frozen expression); insomnia (inability to let go of the thought process); blank expressions (hiding behind a facade); and emotional problems (unresolved experiences).

QUESTIONS

Shaking extremities (extreme fear): What is the chronic and age-old fear my body is demonstrating to me? What fear or dread is shaking me to the core?

Stiffness (fear of pain or movement): What do I believe will happen to me when I move forward in life?

Aphasia (frozen speech; too shocked to talk): What has taken away my voice?

Loss of balance/ataxia (paradoxical emotions pulling in different directions): What emotions are pulling me in opposite directions? What keeps me off balance?

Shuffling steps (chronic exhaustion): What causes my internal exhaustion? What keeps me from walking though life with virility?

Difficulty swallowing (shock/fear; frozen expression): What emotion sticks in my throat? What keeps me from easily swallowing nurturing food?

Insomnia (inability to let go of the thought process): Why can't I surrender my mind to the darkness of the night?

Blank expressions (hiding behind a facade): What shock has paralyzed my facial expression? What is a numb face protecting me from?

Long-standing emotional problems (unresolved experiences): What emotional luggage demands release?

SUGGESTED AFFIRMATION:

I trust myself. I trust those that are trustworthy.

I release all forms of control and doubt.

I can make room for any contradicting feelings until something completely new emerges.

TAKE NOTICE

TURMERIC

TURMERIC: In a large meta-study, scientists reviewed decades of scientific studies on turmeric. They summarize a list of turmeric's potential therapeutic properties including in cases of Parkinson's disease.[9]

1 The United States of America as represented by the Department of Health and Human Services. (Aidan J. Hampson, Julius Axelrod and Maurizio Grimaldi) Patent No. 09/674028 filed on 02/02/2001. *Patent 6630507 issued on October 7, 2003.* Estimated expiration date: 2021. Cannabinoids as antioxidants and neuroprotectants. http://www.patentstorm.us/patents/6630507.html

2 Venderova K, Ruzicka E, Vorisek V, Visnovsky P. *Survey on cannabis use in Parkinson's disease: subjective improvement of motor symptoms.* Department of Pharmacology and Toxicology, Faculty of Pharmacy, Charles University, Hradec Kralove, Czech Republic. Movement Disorders 2004;19(9):1102-6.

3 Farooq MU, Ducommun E, Goudreau J. *Treatment of a hyperkinetic movement disorder during pregnancy with dronabinol.* Parkinsonism Relat Disord. 2009 Mar;15(3):249-51.

4 Iuvone T, Esposito G, De Filippis D, Scuderi C, Steardo L. *Cannabidiol: a promising drug for neurodegenerative disorders?* Department of Experimental Pharmacology, Faculty of Pharmacy, University of Naples Federico II, Via D. Montesano 49, Naples, Italy. CNS Neurosci Ther. 2009 Winter;15(1):65-75.

5 Iuvone T, Esposito G, De Filippis D, Scuderi C, Steardo L. *Cannabidiol: a promising drug for neurodegenerative disorders?* Department of Experimental Pharmacology, Faculty of Pharmacy, University of Naples Federico II, Via D. Montesano 49, Naples, Italy. CNS Neurosci Ther. 2009 Winter;15(1):65-75.

6 Farooq MU, Ducommun E, Goudreau J. *Treatment of a hyperkinetic movement disorder during pregnancy with dronabinol.* Parkinsonism Relat Disord. 2009 Mar;15(3):249-51.

7 Venderova K, Ruzicka E, Vorisek V, Visnovsky P. *Survey on cannabis use in Parkinson's disease: subjective improvement of motor symptoms.* Department of Pharmacology and Toxicology, Faculty of Pharmacy, Charles University, Hradec Kralove, Czech Republic. Movement Disorders 2004;19(9):1102-6.

8 The United States of America as represented by the Department of Health and Human Services. (Aidan J. Hampson, Julius Axelrod and Maurizio Grimaldi) Patent No. 09/674028 filed on 02/02/2001. *Patent 6630507 issued on October 7, 2003.* Estimated expiration date: 2021. Cannabinoids as antioxidants and neuroprotectants. http://www.patentstorm.us/patents/6630507.html

9 Aggarwal BB, Kumar A, Bharti AC. *Anticancer potential of curcumin: preclinical and clinical studies.* Cytokine Research Section, Department of Bioimmunotherapy, University of Texas M. D. Anderson Cancer Center, 1515 Holcombe Boulevard, Box 143, Houston, TX, USA. Anticancer Research. 2003 Jan-Feb;23(1A):363-98.

Neurological Diseases
Tourette Syndrome

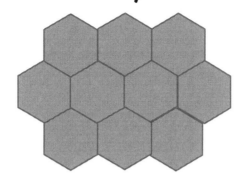

NUMBER OF STUDIES: 10

CHI VALUE: 38

Gilles de la Tourette Syndrome (GTS), more commonly referred to as Tourette syndrome (TS), is considered a developmental (most likely inherited), neurological and psychiatric disorder characterized by the presence of chronic motor and phonic tics. Tics (uncontrollable, repetitive and non-rhythmic movements of select muscle groups including those needed to speak), provoke involuntary sounds, phrases, taboo words or oddly appearing jerking motions such as slapping or grimacing. Tics range from a minor inconvenience to completely debilitating. Most people with tics perceive their onset as similar to sensing when one needs to sneeze or yawn. Some tics can be controlled while others cannot. Interestingly, even controllable tics appear irresistible like an itch that demands scratching.

TS usually develops during childhood, though some kids do outgrow the syndrome later in life. Although orthodox medicine has not pinpointed a root cause for the syndrome, scientists suggest that genetic, environmental, metabolic factors and/or the neurotransmitters dopamine and serotonin may play a leading role. In mild cases, reassurance and education can be enough to provide the practical resources for coping with and managing the condition. TS does not affect intelligence or life span and, unlike many other neurological disorders, TS is not degenerative. TS affects males significantly more often than females, but is relatively equally distributed across all ethnic groups. TS may disappear for periods of time and then reappear.

Physicians diagnose TS by conducting a thorough history, neurological examination and using a process of elimination of other diseases with similar symptoms. If doctors suspect abnormalities of the central nervous system, they might perform an MRI to examine the patient's brain physiology. Pharmaceutical medications used in TS prove mostly ineffective with intolerable side effects.

CANNABIS AND TOURETTE SYNDROME

Researchers from the University of Texas suggested as early as 1989 that cannabinoids could prove helpful in enhancing the effects of pharmaceuticals (neuroleptics) in relieving tics.[1] In addition: "High densities of cannabinoid receptors were found in the basal ganglia and hippocampus, possibly indicating a functional role of cannabinoids in movement and behavior."[2] Four randomized, double-blind, placebo-controlled studies have significantly calmed tics compared to placebos.[3,4,5,6] No serious adverse reactions occurred.

STUDY SUMMARY:

Drugs/Focus	Type of Study	Published Year, Place, and Key Results	CHI
THC	Case study (15 year old boy with TS)	2010 – Department of Psychiatry and Psychotherapy, Georg-August-University Göttingen, Göttingen, Germany. Administration of Delta 9-THC improved tics considerably without adverse effects.[7]	3
THC	A review of two double-blind trials on cannabinoids and TS	2009 – Birmingham and Solihull Mental Health Trust, Birmingham, UK. Although both trials reported a positive effect from Delta(9)THC, the improvements in tic frequency and severity were small.[8]	0
Up to 10 mg/day of THC	Randomized, double-blind, placebo-controlled study of 24 patients with TS.	2003 – Department of Clinical Psychiatry and Psychotherapy, Medical School of Hanover, Hanover, Germany. Results provide more evidence that THC is effective and safe in the treatment of tics.[9]	5
Up to 10 mg THC.	Randomized double-blind placebo-controlled study on 24 patients suffering from TS.	2003 – Department of Clinical Psychiatry and Psychotherapy, Medical School Hanover, Hanover, Germany. Trends toward significant improvement during and after treatment.[10]	5
THC 5.0, 7.5 or 10.0 mg	Randomized double-blind placebo-controlled crossover single-dose trial of Delta(9)-THC (5.0, 7.5 or 10.0 mg) used on 12 adult TS patients	2001 – Department of Clinical Psychiatry and Psychotherapy, Medical School Hanover, Germany. Significant improvement of tics when compared to placebo. No serious adverse reactions occurred.[11]	5
THC 5 to 10mg	12 patients with TS in a randomized double-blind placebo-controlled crossover trial.	2001 – Department of Clinical Psychiatry and Psychotherapy, Medical School Hanover, Germany. A single-dose treatment with delta9-THC in patients suffering from TS does not cause cognitive impairment.[12]	5
Endogeneous endocannabinoids system.	Review	2000 – Cannabis-Forschungs-Gruppe in der Medizinischen Hochschule, Abt. Klinische Psychiatrie und Psychotherapie. Dysregulation in the endogenous cannabinoid/anandamide system could possibly play an import role in the etiology of TS.[13]	4
Cannabinoids	Review	1999 – Department of Clinical Psychiatry and Psychotherapy, Medical School Hanover, Germany. Evidence that cannabinoids are of therapeutic value in the treatment of tics in Tourette syndrome.[14]	4
Cannabis	64 patients with TS	1998 – Department of Clinical Psychiatry and Psychotherapy, Medical School Hanover, Germany. Reduction or complete remission of motor and vocal tics and an amelioration of premonitory urges and obsessive-compulsive symptoms.[15]	3
Cannabinoids	Review	1989 – Laboratory of Psychobio-chemistry, University of Texas, El Paso. May significantly enhance the therapeutic value of neuroleptics in motor disorders.[16]	4

Total CHI Value 38

STRAIN SPECIFIC CONSIDERATIONS

The majority of the studies reviewed in this section on TS primarily used THC. However, whole plant cannabis THC also binds relatively equally to both CB1 and CB2 receptor sites.

Sativa and sativa dominant hybrids usually contain a higher THC:CBD ratio.

EXPLORING MIND–BODY CONSCIOUSNESS

TS begins during childhood. Like a self-fulfilling prophecy, the fear of public awkwardness often materializes. Fear of being seen with tics often precedes the awkward tics in movement or sudden outbursts of verbal shouts. Patients frequently describe the anticipation as similar to the sensation of a sneeze building-up followed by a release of the pre-sneeze tension.

SUGGESTED BLESSING:

May you learn to shift dread to anticipation.

QUESTIONS

Are there other ways to realize that which I focus on or manifest?
Are there other ways to deal with my fears of humiliation besides manifesting them?

AGGRAVATING FACTORS

Stress from chronic fears / anxiety / negative expectations.

SUGGESTED AFFIRMATION:

I have a powerful imagination and I get to choose the focus of my creativity moment by moment.

HEALING FACTORS

Positive stress coping mechanisms / learning to replace negative expectations with positive ones.

1 Moss DE, Manderscheid PZ, Montgomery SP, Norman AB, Sanberg PR. *Nicotine and cannabinoids as adjuncts to neuroleptics in the treatment of Tourette syndrome and other motor disorders.* Laboratory of Psychobiochemistry, University of Texas El Paso 79968. Life Sci. 1989;44(21):1521-5.

2 Müller-Vahl KR, Kolbe H, Schneider U, Emrich HM. *Cannabinoids: possible role in patho-physiology and therapy of Gilles de la Tourette syndrome.* Department of Clinical Psychiatry and Psychotherapy, Medical School Hanover, Germany. Acta Psychiatr Scand. 1998 Dec;98(6):502-6.

3 Müller-Vahl KR, Schneider U, Koblenz A, Jöbges M, Kolbe H, Daldrup T, Emrich HM. *Treatment of Tourette's syndrome with Delta 9-tetrahydrocannabinol (THC): a randomized crossover trial.* Department of Clinical Psychiatry and Psychotherapy, Hanover Medical School, Germany. Pharmacopsychiatry. 2002 Mar;35(2):57-61.

4 Müller-Vahl KR, Koblenz A, Jöbges M, Kolbe H, Emrich HM, Schneider U. *Influence of treatment of Tourette syndrome with delta9-tetrahydrocannabinol (delta9-THC) on neuropsychological performance.* Department of Clinical Psychiatry and Psychotherapy, Medical School Hanover, Germany. Pharmacopsychiatry. 2001 Jan;34(1):19-24.

5 Müller-Vahl KR, Prevedel H, Theloe K, Kolbe H, Emrich HM, Schneider U. *Treatment of Tourette syndrome*

with delta-9-tetrahydrocannabinol (delta 9-THC): no influence on neuropsychological performance. Department of Clinical Psychiatry and Psychotherapy, Medical School Hanover, Hanover, Germany. Neuropsychopharmacology. 2003 Feb;28(2):384-8.

6   Curtis A, Clarke CE, Rickards HE. *Cannabinoids for Tourette's Syndrome.* Cochrane Database Syst Rev. 2009 Oct 7;(4):CD006565. Neuropsychiatry, Birmingham and Solihull Mental Health Trust, Birmingham, UK.

7   Hasan A, Rothenberger A, Münchau A, Wobrock T, Falkai P, Roessner V. *Oral delta 9-tetrahydrocannabinol improved refractory Gilles de la Tourette syndrome in an adolescent by increasing intracortical inhibition: a case report.* Department of Psychiatry and Psychotherapy, Georg-August-University Göttingen, Göttingen, Germany. J Clin Psychopharmacol. 2010 Apr;30(2):190-2.

8   Curtis A, Clarke CE, Rickards HE. *Cannabinoids for Tourette's Syndrome.* Cochrane Database Syst Rev. 2009 Oct 7;(4):CD006565. Neuropsychiatry, Birmingham and Solihull Mental Health Trust, Birmingham, UK.

9   Müller-Vahl KR, Schneider U, Prevedel H, Theloe K, Kolbe H, Daldrup T, Emrich HM. *Delta 9-tetrahydrocannabinol (THC) is effective in the treatment of tics in Tourette syndrome: a 6-week randomized trial.* Department of Clinical Psychiatry and Psychotherapy, Medical School of Hanover, Hanover, Germany. J Clin Psychiatry. 2003 Apr;64(4):459-65.

10   Müller-Vahl KR, Prevedel H, Theloe K, Kolbe H, Emrich HM, Schneider U. *Treatment of Tourette syndrome with delta-9-tetrahydrocannabinol (delta 9-THC): no influence on neuropsychological performance.* Department of Clinical Psychiatry and Psychotherapy, Medical School Hanover, Hanover, Germany. Neuropsychopharmacology. 2003 Feb;28(2):384-8.

11   Müller-Vahl KR, Schneider U, Koblenz A, Jöbges M, Kolbe H, Daldrup T, Emrich HM. *Treatment of Tourette's syndrome with Delta 9-tetrahydrocannabinol (THC): a randomized crossover trial.* Department of Clinical Psychiatry and Psychotherapy, Hanover Medical School, Germany. Pharmacopsychiatry. 2002 Mar;35(2):57-61.

12   Müller-Vahl KR, Koblenz A, Jöbges M, Kolbe H, Emrich HM, Schneider U. *Influence of treatment of Tourette syndrome with delta9-tetrahydrocannabinol (delta9-THC) on neuropsychological performance.* Department of Clinical Psychiatry and Psychotherapy, Medical School Hanover, Germany. Pharmacopsychiatry. 2001 Jan;34(1):19-24.

13   Schneider U, Muller-Vahl KR, Stuhrmann M, Gadzicki D, Heller D, Seifert J, Emrich HM. *The importance of the endogenous cannabinoid system in various neuropsychiatric disorders.* Cannabis-Forschungs-Gruppe in der Medizinischen Hochschule, Abt. Klinische Psychiatrie und Psychotherapie. Fortschr Neurol Psychiatr. 2000 Oct;68(10):433-8.

14   Müller-Vahl KR, Kolbe H, Schneider U, Emrich HM. *Cannabis in movement disorders.* Department of Clinical Psychiatry and Psychotherapy, Medical School Hanover, Germany. Forsch Komplementarmed. 1999 Oct;6 Suppl 3:23-7.

15   Müller-Vahl KR, Kolbe H, Schneider U, Emrich HM. *Cannabinoids: possible role in patho-physiology and therapy of Gilles de la Tourette syndrome.* Department of Clinical Psychiatry and Psychotherapy, Medical School Hanover, Germany. Acta Psychiatr Scand. 1998 Dec;98(6):502-6.

16   Moss DE, Manderscheid PZ, Montgomery SP, Norman AB, Sanberg PR. *Nicotine and cannabinoids as adjuncts to neuroleptics in the treatment of Tourette syndrome and other motor disorders.* Laboratory of Psychobiochemistry, University of Texas El Paso 79968. Life Sci. 1989;44(21):1521-5.

Obstetrical and Gynecological Difficulties and Concerns (OBGYN)

Obstetricians specialize in the care of women during pregnancy while gynecologists specialize in women's health. In practice, many physicians specialize in both obstetrics (OB) and gynecology (GYN) and OBGYN clinics are generally set up to examine, diagnose and treat women in the areas of family planning (contraception), menstruation, chronic pelvic pain, fertility, pregnancy and prenatal care, sexually transmitted diseases, preventative care (pap smear, cancer screening) and menopausal concerns.

OBGYN AND CANNABIS

Plants used to assist women in managing their reproductive freedom and health have been around since Eve and the apple. Religious control mainly and sadly has prevented and destroyed much of this time-proven wisdom of the ages. However, many ideas still exist in the collective memory of the wise women and men who found means to carry on the natural ways of old.

Cannabis was once a plant consistently employed across a wide range of cultures to manage and treat gynecological issues by healers, midwives, herbalists and doctors versed in the art of natural healing. Used by Sumerian physicians and later by their Egyptian counterparts, the plant has made its way into many other cultures to ease difficult childbirth, menstrual difficulties, threatened abortion, morning sickness, postpartum bleeding, eclampsia, urinary difficulties, gonorrhea, menopausal symptoms, decreased libido, and as a possible abortifacient.[1]

A physician's Nineteenth Century Materia Medica describes one of the plant's efficacious properties as a stimulant to uterine muscle fibers. As such, it was used in the treatment of subinvolution (the uterus' inability to return to its normal size after delivery), menorrhagia (heavy menstrual bleeding), dysmenorrhia (painful menses) and to diminish uterine pain in general.[2]

---

1 Ethan Russo, MD. Clinical Assistant Professor of Medicine, University of Washington, Adjunct Associate Professor of Pharmacy, University of Montana, and Clinical Child and Adult Neurologist, Montana Neurobehavioral Specialists, 900 North Orange Street, Missoula, MT 58902 USA. *Cannabis Treatments in Obstetrics and Gynecology: A Historical Review. Journal of Cannabis Therapeutics* (The Haworth Integrative Healing Press, an imprint of The Haworth Press, Inc.) Vol. 2, No. 3/4, 2002, pp. 5-35; and: Women and Cannabis: Medicine, Science, and Sociology (ed: Ethan Russo, Melanie Dreher, and Mary Lynn Mathre) The Haworth Integrative Healing Press, an imprint of The Haworth Press, Inc., 2002, pp. 5-35.

2 Sam'l O. L. Potter, M.A., M.D., M.R.C.P. (Lond,) *A Compend of Materia Medica and Therapeutics and Prescription Writing; with especial references to the physiological actions of drugs.* Based on the last revision of the U.S. Pharmacopeia. Fifth Edition. P.Blakiston, Son & Co., Philadelphia, 1012 Walnut St. 1892. Page #123.

OBGYN

CANNABIS, ABORTION, MISCARRIAGE AND FERTILITY

Certain plant cannabinoids bind to the same set of receptors as the body's own cannabinoid anandamide. They similarly exert influence on the earliest processes of conception and egg implantation in the uterine wall and thus play a significant role in fertility. While studies have shown that low levels of anandamide enhance egg implantation and higher levels diminish egg implantation,[1,2] few physicians are able to translate these discoveries into practical and therapeutic applications.

These dose-dependent and opposing properties of cannabis are not new to researchers and are commonly found in other therapeutic contexts such as pain or mental states modulation. These opposing properties may also explain the historical medical references to cannabis in the prevention of miscarriage and at the same time its use as an early abortifacient.

Although reports exist about the adverse effects of cannabinoids on pregnancies, the discovery of endocannabinoids and their receptors in the female reproductive organs in rodents suggest the system's role in modulating pregnancy. Recently, in a trial conducted on mice, scientists from the Vanderbilt University Medical Center (2002) examined the role the endocannabinoid system plays during normal pregnancy. Results revealed that levels of anandamide in the uterus and CB1 receptors on the fertilized egg work together towards a successful implantation in the uterine wall.[3] If these discoveries are confirmed in other mammals and in humans, the endocannabinoid system may well turn out to play a significant role in the success or failure of pregnancies.

Either way, historical observation and a review of medical records suggest caution with opportunity for those wishing to get pregnant or those wishing to avoid pregnancy altogether.

Once the fetus is implanted, it is most vulnerable to the impact of environmental substances during the first trimester.

1 Daniele Piomelli. *THC: moderation during implantation.* Daniele Piomelli is in the Department of Pharmacology, University of California, Irvine, 360 MSR II, Irvine, California 92697-4625, USA. Nature Medicine 10, 19 - 20 (2004).

2 Paria, B.C., H. Song, X. Wang, P.C. Schmid, R.J. Krebsbach, H.H. Schmid, T.I. Bonner, A. Zimmer, and S.K. Dey. *Dysregulated cannabinoid signaling disrupts uterine receptivity for embryo implantation.* Department of Pediatrics, Ralph L. Smith Research Center, University of Kansas Medical Center, Kansas City, Kansas 66160-7338, USA. J Biol Chem. 2001 Jun 8;276(23):20523-8.

3 Paria BC, Wang H, Dey SK. *Endocannabinoid signaling in synchronizing embryo development and uterine receptivity for implantation.* Department of Pediatrics, Vanderbilt University Medical Center, Nashville, TN 37232-2678, USA. Chem Phys Lipids. 2002 Dec 31;121(1-2):201-10.

OBGYN

CANNABIS AND CHILDBIRTH PAINS

Nineteenth Century medical records describe the plant's effects on childbirth as being able to reduce pain, increase uterine contractions, modulate lactation and reduce inflammation associated with vaginal pains or mastitis.

Anecdotal evidence[1] from observations and surveys on cannabis clinics, patients and physicians supports historical records that describe the efficacy of cannabis in easing childbirth and childbirth pains.

Based on time proven safety records and the discoveries of the body's own natural endocannabinoid system and its role in the modulation of spasms, pain and inflammation, it is easy to see why obstetric and gynecological (OBGYN) treatments employed cannabis for cramps, pains and inflammation. However, while historical records are available, no modern data exists to better understand how the plant constituents specifically affect childbirth pains or other OBGYN related problems.

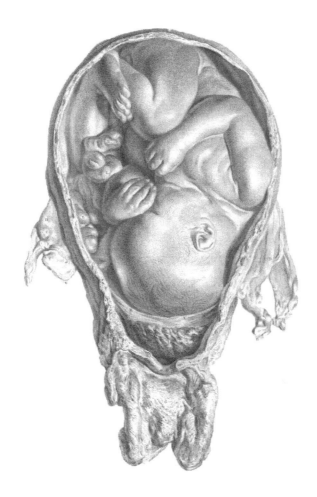

1 L. Grinspoon, M.D., James Bakalar, *Marijuana, The Forbidden Medicine*. 1997. Revised and expanded edition. Yale University Press, New Haven and London.

OBGYN
Endometriosis

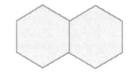

NUMBER OF STUDIES: 2

CHI VALUE: 5

The endometrium, the interior lining of the uterus, is governed by hormonal changes. Endometriosis is a proliferation of interior cells outside of the uterus. Displaced cells continue to respond to hormonal changes and behave as they would inside the uterus; however, without an easy exit, they remain causing growth and adhesions. This can be extremely painful. Growths and adhesions may spread throughout the pelvic cavity and form attachments on the ovaries, bowels or any other surrounding tissue.

Primary symptoms often include generalized pelvic pains, difficult periods, painful sexual intercourse and bleeding. Tests to determine endometriosis include a pelvic examination and ultra-sound; however, the only way to be certain of endometrial tissue growth outside the uterus is via a laparoscopy. Under full anesthesia, a physician inserts an instrument (laparoscope) into the woman's abdomen to visually check.

The exact causes of endometriosis remain unclear. Doctors hypothesize that a cause of endometriosis lies in unexpelled menstrual blood containing endometrial cells that returns via the fallopian tubes to the pelvic cavity. This process is called retrograde menstruation. Orthodox treatments include pain management, hormonal supplementation and surgery.

CANNABIS AND ENDOMETRIOSIS

Researchers discovered that the endocannabinoid system (ECS) plays a part in uterine function and dysfunction. This understanding combined with the historical application of phyto-cannabinoids to alleviate endometrial pain suggests that the endocannabinoid system may also be involved in alleviating pain and disease development.

Researchers from Florida State University (2010) discovered that CB1 receptors are present in nerve cells that innervate endometrial growths and that CB1 activation reduces pain sensation.[1] The authors wrote, "Together these findings suggest that the endocannabinoid system contributes to mechanisms underlying both the peripheral innervation of the abnormal growths and the pain associated with endometriosis, thereby providing a novel approach for the development of badly-needed new treatments."

Another laboratory experiment (2010) in Paris, France, conducted on human endomitriotic cell line confirmed in vivo (on rodents), reported several discoveries. Scientists noted that the synthetic cannabinoid WIN 55212-2 abrogated the growth of endometriotic tissue and exerted an anti-proliferative effect in mice implanted with endometrial tissue. This finding suggests a possible link between the ECS and possible novel treatments.[2]

STUDY SUMMARY:

Drugs/Focus	Type of Study	Published Year, Place, and Key Results	CHI
CB1 agonists and antagonists	Animal Study (Rats)	2010 – Florida State University. CB1 decreases endometriosis-associated hyperalgesia.	2
WIN 55212-2	Animal Study (Mice)	2010 – Université Paris Descartes, Paris, France. Abrogated the growth of endometriotic tissue and exerted an anti-proliferative effects.	1+2

Total CHI Value   5

STRAIN SPECIFIC CONSIDERATIONS

WIN 55212-2 binds with higher affinity to CB2 than CB1 receptor.

Indicas and indica-dominant strains generally present with a lower THC:CBD ratio thus favoring CB2 expression.

EXPLORING MIND–BODY CONSCIOUSNESS

Endometriosis is one of many underlying physical conditions that can cause chronic pelvic pain. Researchers have examined the psychological profiles of women with chronic pelvic pain. Results suggest a connection between changes in hormone profiles and exposure to chronic stress or posttraumatic stress disorders, especially in those patients who were victims of physical or sexual abuse.[3]

The disease picture of endometriosis may suggest a misplaced creativity. Cells leave the natural seat of biological creation and instead grow where they are not meant to grow, causing pain and damage. This may reflect the difference between creating life versus controlling life. Whenever we create life by making changes within, we create life from a natural and sustainable position. However, when we want to create life by trying to control others, we leave our natural domain and create, more often than not, very difficult circumstances that can harm us and the other people around us.

QUESTIONS

Do you feel you have nothing to say about what happens in the bedroom?
If so, do you blame your partner for that situation?
Do you feel like you have to control others to get what you want?
Is there an aspect of your sexuality that you don't like, hate, resent or feel guilty about?
Are you financially dependent on another, and how do you feel about it?
Do you feel the need to lie in the bedroom?

AGGRAVATING FACTORS

Chronic stress / exposure to severe traumatic events such as sexual or physical abuse (PTSD) / guilt.

SUGGESTED BLESSING:

May you realize that women who create change within are healers.

SUGGESTED AFFIRMATION:

I decide what to think or feel! I create change without controlling anybody.

HEALING FACTORS

Learning positive coping mechanisms / releasing guilt and its destructiveness.
  See also PTSD.

1 Dmitrieva N, Nagabukuro H, Resuehr D, Zhang G, McAllister SL, McGinty KA, Mackie K, Berkley KJ. *Endocannabinoid involvement in endometriosis.* Program in Neuroscience, Florida State University, Tallahassee, FL32306-4301, USA. Pain. 2010 Dec;151(3):703-10.

2 Leconte M, Nicco C, Ngô C, Arkwright S, Chéreau C, Guibourdenche J, Weill B, Chapron C, Dousset B, Batteux F. *Antiproliferative effects of cannabinoid agonists on deep infiltrating endometriosis.* Laboratoire d'immunologie, Université Paris Descartes, Paris, France. Am J Pathol. 2010 Dec;177(6):2963-70.

3 C. Heim, U. Ehlert, J.P. Hanker, H.H. Hellhammer. *Abuse-related posttraumatic stress disorder and alteration of the hypothalamic-pituitary-adrenal axis in women with chronic pelvic pain.* Center for Psychobiological and Psychosomatic Research, University of Trier, Germany. Psychosomatic Medicine May 1, 1998 vol. 60 no. 302-318.

OBGYN
Menstrual Pain

NUMBER OF STUDIES: 1

CHI VALUE: 3

The Latin word for month, mensis, is the basis for the term menses or menstruation. The average duration of one complete cycle is about 28 days coinciding with the approximate amount of time it takes for the moon to wax and wane. At the end of a cycle, a women's body regenerates a new lining inside the uterus. It discharges the old lining.

Many women have noticed that when the color of their menstrual blood is fairly dark, thick, and clotted, more cramps occur than when it is more liquid and bright red. Brighter blood is more oxygenated and generates an easy flow while thick, clotted and poorly oxygenated blood is more difficult to expel.

Typical allopathic treatments for menstrual cramps include nonsteroidal anti-inflammatory drugs (NSAIDs) such as ibuprofen or Aleve®.

CANNABIS AND MENSTRUAL PAIN

While the specifics of cannabis-based pain control are well established, little information exists to date to elucidate the impact of cannabinoids on menstrual pain. However, the proven antispasmodic effects of the plant alongside with its analgesic and anti-inflammatory properties may form the historical basis for its use in the treatment of menstrual cramps. The single human case study published by researchers from Hürth, Germany, suggests that menstrual pain is among the many painful conditions for which cannabis is used as analgesia.[1]

STUDY SUMMARY:

Drugs/Focus	Type of Study	Published Year, Place, and Key Results	CHI
Cannabis	Case study	2003 - Nova-Institute, Germany. Cannabis is used to treat menstrual pain.	3

Total CHI Value 3

EXPLORING MIND–BODY CONSCIOUSNESS

Women who give life are mothers. The primordial cyclical rhythms of nature such as birth, death and regeneration are part of the feminine power. Guided by subtle hormonal changes, the monthly flow of blood washes away the old mucosal lining of the uterus to prepare for its renewal.

Difficulties in embracing the power of the feminine may get expressed in

SUGGESTED BLESSING:

I embrace the feminine power of creation in my body and my mind.

difficult menstruations (dysmenorrhea). Women's blogs, dealing with dysmenorrhea, report similar stories of 'not being heard by my doctor,' and 'feeling disrespected' or 'belittled' by their health care providers when searching for relief from menstrual pain. These stories reveal an underlying theme of power and powerlessness.

This theme is further confirmed by women who empowered themselves through their own research or by joining other women with the same problems in their search for solutions to menstrual pain. These women discovered the importance of listening to subtle and not so subtle changes in their bodies. Some now view this monthly activity as a beautiful way of getting rid of toxins.

QUESTIONS

Do I buy into the notion that my period is punishment for being female?
How do I feel about my menses and why?
Where do I reject my feminine energy?
Where do I judge my feminine?
Where are my male and female energy out of balance?

AGGRAVATING FACTORS

Dehydration / unhealthy food choices / denial or judgments of femine energy.

HEALING FACTORS

Drinking more water about seven days before the start of menstruation / limiting unhealthy foods / embracing and cherishing the feminine in yourself.

TAKE NOTICE

ANISE • FENNEL

ANISE: Greek herbalists have used anise and fennel to promote menstruation, increase breast milk production, facilitate birth and enhance libido. University of Athens' scientists have taken a closer look at anise in order to find a safe alternative to estrogen replacement therapies to prevent osteoporosis. In their study anise exhibited estrogen receptor modulator-like properties that produce bone-cell formation without causing breast and cervical cancer cells to proliferate.[2]

FENNEL: Fennel extract was found to be a more potent pain relief agent than mefenamic acid (such as Ponstel) in primary dysmenorrhea of high-school girls whose age averaged thirteen. In fact, it proved so effective that 80% of the fennel group no longer needed to rest in order to cope with the aches and pain.[3] Fennel is a safe plant to use, while mefenamic acid can produce serious side effects.

1 Grotenhermen F, Schnelle M. *Survey on the medical use of cannabis and THC in Germany.* Nova-Institut, Goldenbergstraße 2, D-50354 Hürth, Germany. J Cannabis Ther 2003;3(2):17-40.

2 Kassi E, Papoutsi Z, Fokialakis N, Messari I, Mitakou S, Moutsatsou P. *Greek plant extracts exhibit selective estrogen receptor modulator (SERM)-like properties.* Department of Biological Chemistry, Medical School, University of Athens, 115 27 Athens, Greece. J Agric Food Chem. 2004 Nov 17;52(23):6956-61.

3 Modaress Nejad V, Asadipour M. *Comparison of the effectiveness of fennel and mefenamic acid on pain intensity in dysmenorrhoea.* Department of Obstetrics and Gynaecology, Kerman University of Medial Sciences and Health Services, Kerman, Islamic Republic of Iran. East Mediterr Health J. 2006 May-Jul;12(3-4):423-7.

OBGYN
Morning Sickness

NUMBER OF STUDIES: 1

CHI VALUE: 3

An estimated 50% of all pregnant women develop some kind of morning sickness, usually starting in the middle of the first trimester (at about 6 weeks). Normally, these episodes of nausea and vomiting are self-limiting and disappear toward the end of the first trimester (3 months). While women can experience nausea and vomiting at any time of the day, these symptoms more commonly occur in the morning hours.

One hypothesis for morning sickness and the associated heightened senses of smell and taste is a fetal protection mechanism. Foods normally harmless to the mother may contain substances that could easily harm a developing fetus. When substances are detected by smell or taste that could harm the fetus, nausea develops to prevent the mother from ingestion or to produce vomiting after ingestion. Midwives often advise their clients to go with their desires for certain food items and avoid those that produce revulsion.

CANNABIS AND MORNING SICKNESS

After an egg is fertilized, it stays in the fallopian tube for three days, than moves into the uterus for implantation. Morning sickness generally begins weeks after successful implantation. As mentioned earlier in the section on abortion, miscarriage and fertility, levels of endogenous anadamide via CB1 and CB2 play a deciding role in the process of implanting the fertilized egg to the uterine wall. The cannabinoid THC binds to the same receptors and therefore may also play a significant role in egg implantation.

University researchers (2006) from Victoria, Canada, collected self-assessment data from 51 pregnant women who inhaled cannabis to alleviate their symptoms of morning sickness. Their analysis indicated that the 40 women who chose to treat morning sickness with inhaled cannabis found it to be either 'extremely effective' or 'effective.'[1]

STUDY SUMMARY:

Drugs/Focus	Type of Study	Published Year, Place, and Key Results	CHI
Cannabis inhaled	51 pregnant women with morning sickness	2006 – Michael Smith Foundation for Health Research Post-doctoral Fellow, Department of Sociology, University of Victoria, Victoria, BC, Canada. 'Effective' or 'extremely effective.'	3

Total CHI Value   3

EXPLORING MIND–BODY CONSCIOUSNESS

Changes during pregnancy can be intense experiences caused by vastly different hormone profiles, physiological and psychological changes. Women may feel disconcerted by the simple fact that generally liked foods now produce aversions, yet they develop cravings for items normally despised. Pondering these changes in lifestyles and identities combined with the necessary preparations for the newcomer may increase the impact of disruption to normal routines. A sense of overwhelm and being out of control may set in.

The body produces the involuntary and rapid development of nausea and vomiting as a protective mechanism in the presence of a threat such as poison. The emotional underpinnings for nausea and vomiting, even when no physical threat is present, are very similar. When a perceived threat to the normal sense of self is detected or when the anticipation of mental-emotional upheaval is part of the experience, people often respond with fear and anxiety followed by symptoms of nausea. If intense enough, vomiting occurs.

See also chapters on NAUSEA and VOMITING.

1 Westfall RE, Janssen PA, Lucas P, Capler R. *Survey of medicinal cannabis use among childbearing women: patterns of its use in pregnancy and retroactive self-assessment of its efficacy against 'morning sickness'*. Complement Ther Clin Pract 2006;12(1):27-33. Michael Smith Foundation for Health Research Postdoctoral Fellow, Department of Sociology, University of Victoria, Victoria, BC, Canada V8W 3P5. rachelw@uvic.ca

SUGGESTED BLESSING:

May you find delightful wonder as you ponder the unknown.

May you relax with ease and throw away the clinging blanket of fear.

May you walk through the web of anxiety as easy as one, two, three.

SUGGESTED AFFIRMATION:

I am the author of my thoughts.

I am the architect of my perspectives.

I only choose beliefs that produce a feeling of safety.

OBGYN
Cannabis and Pregnancy

Much controversy surrounds the use of cannabis during pregnancy. Discoveries indicate that the presence of the brain's own cannabinoid, anandamide, triggers the endocannabinoid systems (CB1 and CB2). CB1 and CB2 receptors are present in reproductive glands and organs and, thus, may play a role in the modulation of conception, pregnancy, pain relief and the birth experience itself.[1]

A study from 1983 enrolled 313 women who decided to home deliver their children.[2] Of these, 41 women reported using marijuana. Researchers compared these two groups, and results showed that while both groups were generally similar, those women using marijuana made less money on average and were more likely to consume alcohol and cigarettes during pregnancy than non-users. Statistical evaluations revealed that the 41 women experienced slightly increased rates of difficulty at time of labor.

1 El-Talatini MR, Taylor AH, Konje JC. *The relationship between plasma levels of the endocannabinoid, anandamide, sex steroids, and gonadotrophins during the menstrual cycle.* Department of Cancer Studies and Molecular Medicine, University of Leicester, Leicester, United Kingdom. Fertil Steril. 2010 Apr;93(6):1989-96.

2 Greenland S, Richwald GA, Honda GD. *The effects of marijuana use during pregnancy. II. A study in a low-risk home-delivery population.* Drug Alcohol Depend. 1983 Jun;11(3-4):359-66.

Osteoporosis

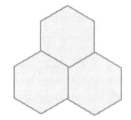

NUMBER OF STUDIES: 3

CHI VALUE: 5

Osteoporosis directly translates from Greek as the disease of 'porous bones' where the density of the bones diminishes over time. Cells that destroy aged bone cells are normally offset by cells that form new bones of proper strength and density. In osteoporosis, the balance shifts and more cells are destroyed than are born.

Once porous, the bones are vulnerable to stress fractures. The disease is most common in women, especially after hormone balances shift during menopause, and in patients who received steroids for chronic conditions.

Although there are limited known symptoms, orthodox medicine identifies numerous preventable risk factors (e.g. smoking) and underlying diseases that may contribute to osteoporosis. Within this model of medicine, treatment consists of mainly pharmaceuticals, some nutritional modification (minerals, Vitamin D) and exercise. Doctors diagnosis the disease via dual energy x-ray absorptiometry (DXA), which measures bone mineral density. Other imaging options include quantitative CT-scans and quantitative ultra sound. Unlike with the other imaging machines, ultra sound provides the added benefits of no harmful ionizing radiation. Other tests may be included to rule out underlying contributing diseases.

CANNABIS AND OSTEOPOROSIS

A German study (2005) discovered that cannabinoids binding with CB1 and CB2 receptors regulate osteoclast (cells that remove bone tissue) activity and bone mineral density alike; thus, partaking in the balance of removing old bone cells and sustaining bone density. The same experiment also revealed that the activation of CB2 receptors plays a role in the development of osteoporosis. The data from two Israeli studies (2006, 2009) confirmed that cannabinoids help maintain bone density and prevent age-related bone-loss.

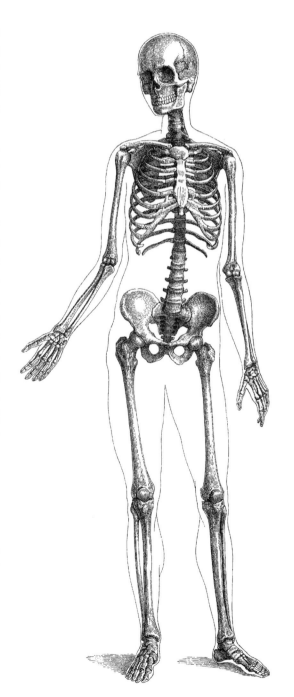

All three studies provide the potential basis for new methods in prevention and treatment of age-related bone-loss in both genders as well as postmenopausal osteoporosis.

STUDY SUMMARY:

Drugs/Focus	Type of Study	Published Year, Place, and Key Results	CHI
THC	Preclinical study	2009 – Bone Laboratory, the Hebrew University of Jerusalem, Jerusalem, Israel. Maintains bone remodeling and protects against age-related bone-loss.[1]	1
Endogenous cannabinoids system	Animal study (mice).	2006 – Bone Laboratory, the Hebrew University of Jerusalem, Jerusalem, Israel. Diminished endocannabinoid receptors increase bone loss.[2]	2
Endogenous cannabinoids receptors (CB1) and (CB2).	Animal study (mice)	2005 – Department of Psychiatry, Life and Brain Center, University of Bonn, Germany. (CB1) and (CB2) can regulate osteoclast activity and bone mineral density and CB2 receptors play a role in the development of osteoporosis.[3]	2

Total CHI Value   5

STRAIN SPECIFIC CONSIDERATIONS

The pre-clinical trials in this section suggest potential involvement of both receptor sites in modulating osteoporosis. Scientists focused their research on cannabinoid THC, which binds with both CB1 and CB2.

Sativa or sativa dominant strains generally contain a higher THC:CBD ratio.

EXPLORING MIND–BODY CONSCIOUSNESS

The skeleton functions to protect vital organs and produce a rigid support system. This enables the attached flexible counter system of muscles to exert force and allows the body to contract and expand, thus producing movement and enabling physical tasks.

The hollowness of bones provides strength despite their relatively light weight. An exterior of collagen and minerals protects the interior contents of soft and spongy yellow and red bone marrow. The red marrow produces blood cells while the yellow marrow stores fat cells as energy reserves.

In the disease picture of osteoporosis, the structure of life has become porous or brittle. At any time, a simple misstep can result in serious bone fractures. Hip and backbone fractures are most common, followed by broken ribs or wrists. In the internal architecture of patients with the disease, life may appear to offer no support; or if some support is still present, it appears transient and temporary. The patient is left dreading the inevitable end and resignation and hopelessness may ensue. Giving up on life may suck the marrow of the bone until the remaining hollow house of cards collapses.

Osteoporosis often becomes a concern during menopause when we have the opportunity to shift more of our attention from the body to the inner workings of our spiritual nature and design.

SUGGESTED BLESSING:

May you find strength and support in the wisdom of your mind, spirit and soul.

May you find the juice of life in places you never thought to look.

SUGGESTED AFFIRMATION:

I can choose to think of life as supporting me as gracefully as the air supports the flight of the eagle.

TAKE NOTICE

ANISE

ANISE: Greek herbalists use anise and fennel to promote menstruation, increase breast milk production, facilitate birth and enhance libido. University of Athens' scientists took a closer look at anise hoping to find a safe alternative to estrogen replacement therapy to prevent osteoporosis. Anise exhibited estrogen receptor modulator-like properties that produced bone-cell formation without causing breast and cervical cancer cells to proliferate.[4]

1 Bab I, Zimmer A, Melamed E. *Cannabinoids and the skeleton: from marijuana to reversal of bone loss.* Bone Laboratory, the Hebrew University of Jerusalem, Jerusalem, Israel. babi@cc.huji.ac.il Ann Med. 2009;41(8):560-7.

2 Orr Ofek, Meliha Karsak, Nathalie Leclerc, Meirav Fogel, Baruch Frenkel, Karen Wright, Joseph Tam, Malka Attar-Namdar, Vardit Kram, Esther Shohami, Raphael Mechoulam, Andreas Zimmer, and Itai Bab. *Peripheral cannabinoid receptor, CB2, regulates bone mass. Bone* Laboratory, Hebrew University of Jerusalem, P.O.B. 12272, Jerusalem 91120, Israel. E-mail: babi@cc.huji.ac.il PNAS January 17, 2006 vol. 103 no. 3 696-701

3 Karsak M, Cohen-Solal M, Freudenberg J, Ostertag A, Morieux C, Kornak U, Essig J, Erxlebe E, Bab I, Kubisch C, de Vernejoul MC, Zimmer A. *Cannabinoid receptor type 2 gene is associated with human osteoporosis.* Department of Psychiatry, Life and Brain Center, University of Bonn, Germany. Hum Mol Genet. 2005 Nov 15;14(22):3389-96.

4 Kassi E, Papoutsi Z, Fokialakis N, Messari I, Mitakou S, Moutsatsou P. *Greek plant extracts exhibit selective estrogen receptor modulator (SERM)-like properties.* Department of Biological Chemistry, Medical School, University of Athens, 115 27 Athens, Greece. J Agric Food Chem. 2004 Nov 17;52(23):6956-61.

Pain (in General)

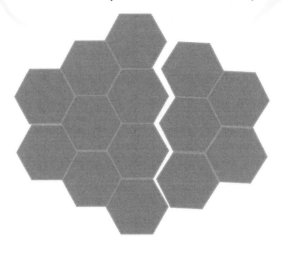

COMBINED NUMER OF STUDIES: 14

COMBINED CHI VALUE: 50

(FOR MORE INFORMATION ON SPECIFIC CANNABINOID AND PAIN STUDIES GO TO THE SUBSEQUENT PAIN CHAPTERS)

Pain affects the body, mind, one's quality of life and overall well-being. It is a highly subjective experience, and people have significantly different thresholds for pain, an aspect influenced by many cultural factors. Pain produces unpleasant sensory and emotional experiences due to injury or even threat of injury. Tiny sensory organs called nociceptors present throughout the skin, blood vessels, muscle tissue, organs and other strategic parts of the body stand ready to immediately signal the threat or presence of pain. Once the nociceptors are stimulated by the threat or presence of tissue damage from heat, pressure or chemicals, rapid signals produce complex changes to the affected tissue and central nervous system (CNS). In turn, this increases respiration, heartbeat and blood pressure. The whole organism, body and mind, quickly respond to stop or minimize pain and ensure survival.

Pain is the main reason people seek medical attention. While many describe pain with terms like sharp, dull, burning, or radiating, physicians specializing in pain distinguish between two basic types: neuropathic pain (usually chronic) and nociceptive pains (usually time limited). Further, differentiation includes referred pain, visceral pain and parietal pain. Referred pain is present at a distance from the point of origin. Sometimes a person with a heart attack experiences pains radiating down the left arm or up into the neck. Visceral pains are associated with specific organs such as the liver or bowels but are usually not specifically localized. Parietal pains normally present at a precise location and claim association with inflammation at the lining of organs.

Traditional allopathic treatment begins with a search for underlying causes. Depending on the results of diagnostic tests, care consists of pharmaceutical medications addressing the underlying cause and then targeting the pain itself (analgesics). Major analgesic groups include acetaminophen, non-steroidal anti-inflammatory drugs (NSAID) and opioids.

Doctors believe acetaminophen acts on the brain to reduce pain. Sold in the form of many brand names such as Tylenol®, the drug breaks down in the liver, which is also the reason for its more serious adverse effects - liver toxicity. "Acetaminophen overdose is the leading cause for calls to Poison Control Centers (>100,000/year) and accounts for more than 56,000 emergency room visits, 2,600 hospitalizations, and an estimated 458 deaths due to acute liver failure each year."[1]

Besides NSAIDs pain killing properties, they also reduce fever and inflammation. Over a hundred million NSAID's with brand names like aspirin or ibuprofen are sold every year in the U.S. alone.[2] Scientists hypothesize that NSAIDs inhibit enzymes (COX) involved in the neuro-chemical reaction needed for pain to occur. Major adverse affects include internal bleeding from gastrointestinal ulcers, heart attacks, strokes and renal failure. "Each year 41,000 older adults are hospitalized, and 3,300 of them die from ulcers caused by NSAID's. Thousands of younger adults are hospitalized."[3]

Opioids are effective painkillers because they bind to the body's opioid receptors in the nervous system and thus reduce or eliminate pain. Derived from the poppy plant, opioids are one of the oldest analgesics known to mankind. Patients report simultaneous experiences of mood altering sedation, constipation, constricted pupils and a reduction in respiratory rates. While short-term use of opioids can be an effective means to obtaining pain control, long-term use can lead to addiction. Two of the deadliest prescription drugs for pain in the U.S. include the opioids oxycodone and fentanyl, responsible for nearly ten thousand fatalities within seven years.[4]

CANNABIS AND PAIN

For the last 5,000 years, cannabis has been used as an analgesic in nearly all ancient cultures from Sumeria and China, to Babylon, the Indus Valley, Judean, Greek, Roman and Islamic civilizations.[5] The plant's prominent role and presence in medicine continued in early western medicine. In addition to pain relief, cannabis serves as an anti-inflammatory and relaxing agent to body and mind to the present day. Recent discoveries confirm that cannabis as safe and effective when used properly to treat both neuropathic pain and in some cases nociceptive pain.[6]

While hundreds of studies and modern scientific data confirm the ancient time-proven analgesic properties of the plant, they also elucidate some of the complex neurochemical workings of cannabinoids on pain within the human nervous system.

Foremost, scientists point to a relatively recent discovery that the human body contains its own naturally occurring endocannabinoid system. Naturally occurring cannabinoids or external cannabinoids, like those found in marijuana, signal cannabinoid receptors to regulate a wide variety of physiological processes including that of the sensation of pain. Two types of receptors Cannabinoid Receptor I and II (CB1 and CB2) employ specific regulatory functions.

Broadly speaking, CB1 receptors are located in the Central Nervous System (brain and spinal cord), which controls information received by the senses and enables response reactions and behaviors. These receptors are located in parts of the brain that regulate motor control, attention, emotion, thinking (cerebellum), habits (basal ganglia and limbic system), memory functions (hippocampus) and in both the male and female reproductive systems.

Here it is perhaps important to note that CB1 receptors are absent in the part of the brain (medulla oblongata) that regulates heart and respiratory function. This makes using cannabinoids as pain management safer than opiates, which can cause damage and death from respiratory deficiencies or arrests. Cannabinoids cannot replace opiates' strong analgesic properties, especially in cases of new trauma or injuries. However, in conjunction with a reduced amount of opiates, cannabinoids can produce a synergy of effective pain control while reducing the risk of adverse effects and the habit forming potential of opiates. "Preclinical studies indicate that Delta(9)-THC and morphine can be useful in low dose combination as an analgesic."[7]

CB2 receptors cluster in the periphery, especially in tissue involved in proper immune responses. The spleen houses a high concentration of CB2 receptors for example. CB2 receptor engagement thus becomes important for treatment of chronic pain associated with autoimmune diseases in which the body's own immune system turns on itself.

Numerous plant-based cannabinoids, other plant-based (noncannabinoid) constituents, synthetic cannabinoids and those produced naturally by the human body engage significantly in reducing inflammation, which often goes hand-in-hand with autoimmune disease. An overview of existing studies (2004-2009) determined that cannabinoids effectively relieve pain involving inflammation such as in post-surgery patients, rheumatism, rheumatoid arthritis, chronic neuropathic pain and fibromyalgia.[8]

Acetaminophen, non-steroidal anti-inflammatory drugs (NSAID) and opioids possess many therapeutic applications. However, patients in need of pain control, particularly those concerned about habit forming substances and adverse effects, may benefit from a broader risk benefit analysis, especially in cases of pain for which cannabinoids have proven efficacy.

Cannabis can induce unwanted results. It is important to remember that using cannabis in excess of the subjective therapeutic dosage window can induce adverse effects including an increase in pain,[9,10] anxiety, paranoia or irritability. However, when compared to other options, "cannabis has a unique distinction of safety over four millennia of analgesic usage: no deaths due to direct toxicity of cannabis have ever been documented in the medical literature."[11]

Beyond the anti-inflammatory properties, analgesia, and potential to reduce the use of opiates, cannabis reduces painful spasms, diminishes anxieties associated with the anticipation of pain, induces rest and sleep and can gently elevate mood - all essential elements to healing.

We list only three of many studies on the effects of cannabis and pain sensations to illustrate some interesting results and their implication for treatment.

A Worcester, MA study cast a wide net for relevant studies on cannabinoids used for pain management: "…published in the last 5 years on the activities of all classes of cannabinoids, including the endogenous cannabinoids such as anandamide, related compounds such as the elmiric acids (EMAs), and noncannabinoid components (200-250 constituents) of Cannabis that show anti-inflammatory action."[12] Results indicated that all types of cannabinoids as well as noncannabinoid parts of the plant effectively reduce pain from inflammation such as in post-surgery patients, rheumatism, rheumatoid arthritis, chronic neuropathic pain and fibromyalgia.

Multiple studies reveal that cannabinoids reduce neuropathic pains. A randomized, double blind, placebo-controlled, crossover study from Rome, Italy, on humans with Multiple Sclerosis (MS) was first to examine their impact on nociceptive pains using noxious stimulation via reflex tests. The authors observed "...that cannabinoids modulate the nociceptive system in patients with MS."[13]

San Diego-based scientists demonstrated the importance of dose in relation to therapeutic efficacy. In a randomized, double blind, placebo-controlled, crossover human trial, 15 healthy volunteers received capsaicin (the ingredient in cayenne pepper that makes it hot) injections in opposite forearms. The injections were spaced at 5- and 45-minute intervals after smoking cannabis of three different concentrations (2%, 4% and 8% THC by weight). Scientists measured their pains levels and pain thresholds. The results supported the importance of dose dependency in pain reduction. "Five minutes after cannabis exposure, there was no effect on capsaicin-induced pain at any dose. By 45 min after cannabis exposure, however, there was a significant decrease in capsaicin-induced pain with the medium dose and a significant increase in capsaicin-induced pain with the high dose."[14]

WARNING/DISCUSSION

While the analgesic effects of cannabis are time proven and empirically established, the study from San Diego adds a unique perspective to this common knowledge base. As a result, for those wishing to use cannabis to reduce pain, it is advisable to start out at a low dose and work up slowly to determine the most effective and appropriate therapeutic window.

EXPLORING MIND-BODY CONSCIOUSNESS

Pain gets our attention. It can save our lives and prevent or minimize damage. Beyond the positive attributes of pain as feedback and protective device, man-made belief(s) in punishment demands pain, as does guilt with its constant insistence on using pain as a means of making amends.

Pain can motivate new choices and inspires us to avoid choices that lead to pain in the first place. Pain lets you know where attention is immediately needed. The worse the pain, the more acute the demand for attention. This is true for acute or sudden pain as well as chronic pain. Pain demands change.

Normally, once pain receives attention, new choices are quickly implemented. The hand that nears fire is removed and the pain stops. The individual creates a strong memory to be more careful with fire in the future. The dentist drills into a nerve motivating healthier choices about sugar and flossing habits. A relationship ends and may break the proverbial heart leading to reflections on learning more about loving and intimacy.

While each person's experience with pain is unique, a common thread is simultaneous separation from, and longing for someone or something. We experience pain in the physical, emotional, mental and spiritual realm. A child falls and scrapes her knees. Separated from her sense of well-being while crying innocent tears, she yearns to return to it. A young man loses his first love and longs to hold her again. An author inadvertently pushes the wrong button on her computer losing her entire

SUGGESTED BLESSING:

May you forgive yourself or another for the pain.

SUGGESTED AFFIRMATION:

I have healed pain before and I can do it again.

manuscript; she feels a part of her has died with it. A Rabbi finds himself in a pit of despair, wondering about his normally unshakable faith.

Everybody has pain at one point or another in his or her life's journey. It is a part of the human experience. Pain can be a terribly destructive emotion, a terrifying state of being that produces isolation and exhaustion. It is for these and other reasons that many people want to numb themselves to pain by ignoring it, denying it or masking it. However, these perhaps understandable reactions to pain do not produce healing but sadly assure its continuation, re-emergence and eventual amplification. Pain will continue to exist somewhere in the complexity of being until it is healed.

Pain begins as an emotional reality. If dealt with and healed in the non-physical theatre, its existence will dissolve. If, however, pain is ignored, denied, masked or otherwise avoided, the emotion will seek healing through more forceful and solidified means. For instance, avoided pain born of betrayal and humiliation may develop into an auto-immune disease where the body's own defense mechanism turns on itself. Thus the drame of pain that previously played on an emotional stage is moved to the more dense physical form in a renewed effort to draw more conscious understanding of where internal change, forgiveness and healing is needed.

QUESTIONS

What is my pain keeping me from doing?
How do I feel about it?
What am I separated from and what am I longing for?
Is this pain pointing to some unfinished loss or grief?
Am I masking pain with punishing guilt?
Am I avoiding pain with numbing judgments or prejudices?
Am I denying pain by numbing it with self-pity?
Am I constantly avoiding pain with numbing medications?
Am I avoiding pain with imprisoning depression?
Am I running from pain by becoming addicted or obsessed?
Am I avoiding pain through focusing on blame and betrayal?

AGGRAVATING FACTORS

Guilt / belief(s) in punishment.

HEALING FACTORS

Releasing guilt / grief / pain / hurt in the emotional realm / employing forgiveness.

TAKE NOTICE

CAYENNE • CLOVE • COCOA • FENNEL • GARLIC • GRAINS OF PARADISE •
MYRRH • NIGELLA • ROSEMARY • TURMERIC

CAYENNE: In a meta-analysis of studies, University of Toronto doctors determined that cayenne cream used as a topical ointment treated the symptoms of chronic back pain better than a placebo.[15]

Cayenne stimulates peripheral circulation. In Cuba, a topical tincture and cream is used to produce circulatory benefits and treat aches and pains of lumbago, arthritis and rheumatism.[16]

Cayenne is approved by the German Commission E as an external application for painful muscle spasms. Do not use it for longer than two days on the same region of tissue in order to avoid local skin inflammation.[17]

The FDA approved a cream, under the brand name Zostrix, which contains concentrated capsaicin. The company markets the cream mostly to arthritis sufferers to reduce pain, but also to reduce the pain that often lingers after an attack of shingles (a herpes-caused skin infection). A tube of Zostrix cream usually sells for about fifteen to twenty dollars. A homemade cayenne pepper cream costs pennies in comparison.[18]

CLOVE: In a study conducted in Mansoura, Egypt, patients suffering from chronic anal fissures received a preparation of clove oil 1% cream. Healing occurred in five times as many patients as in the control group. The 1% clove cream patients also experienced a greater reduction in resting anal pressure than those in the control group.[19]

A Tunisian study reported in the National Library of Medicine determined essential oil of clove extracts possessed analgesic, anti-inflammatory, antioxidant, anti-microbial, anti-fungal, anti-viral (herpes simplex –HSV and hepatitis C), anti-bacterial (including several of the multi-drug resistant Staphylococcus epidermidis) and insect repellant properties.[20]

COCOA: German scientists at the University Witten-Herdecke concluded that the long-term ingestion of cocoa with a high content of flavanols provides several markers of healthy skin. This might affect pain sensation near the skin, provide photo protection, improved blood circulation, increase skin density and hydration, and decrease skin roughness and scaling.[21]

FENNEL: The German Commission E approved fennel seeds and oil in the treatment of pain associated with: "Dyspepsia such as mild, spastic gastrointestinal afflictions, fullness, flatulence. Catarrh of the upper respiratory tract."[22]

A Kerman, Iran, study discovered that fennel extract possessed a more potent pain relief agent than mefenamic acid (such as Ponstel) in primary dysmenorrhea of high-school girls whose age averaged 13. In fact, it proved so effective that 80% of the fennel group no longer needed to rest in order to cope with aches and pains.[23] Fennel is a safe plant to use, while mefenamic acid can produce serious side effects.

GARLIC: Cubans use garlic for the treatment of inflammation, muscular pains, back pains, synovitis (inflammation of a membrane in the knee joint) and painful varicose veins.[24]

GINGER: A researcher from Durban, South Africa, supports the time-proven use of ginger by traditional African healers for its effective treatment of painful and chronic arthritic inflammatory conditions and its ability to achieve better metabolic control in patients with type-2 adult-onset diabetes.[25]

GRAINS OF PARADISE: Scientists from the University of Ibadan, Nigeria, explored this spice used in wound healing practices throughout the ages. The spice's ability to stabilize the cell membrane[26] of injured tissue sites appears to reduce the need for reconstruction and speed healing. Furthermore, scientists laud the spice's strong anti-oxidant properties, which enable the body to more effectively scavenge free radicals common in injuries.

Another study from the same Nigerian University suggests that the analgesic (pain reducing) properties of the spice are specific to sites with inflamed tissue only. They do not reduce the pain perceptions of non-inflamed tissue sites.[27]

MYRRH: German Commission E approved myrrh for the topical treatment of mucus membrane inflammation such as in sore throats.[28]

Based on traditional practice and evidence-based medicine, a researcher from Bethesda, Maryland, reported on myrrh's significant antiseptic, anesthetic, and antitumor properties most likely due to a specific alkene called furanosesquiterpene, present in essential oil of myrrh.[29]

NIGELLA: Doctors use ionizing radiation to treat many cancer patients. However, the radiation does not discriminate between cancer cells and healthy cells, resulting in massive tissue damage across the board. A study from Afyon, Turkey, using a rodent model, found that nigella sativa oil ingestion (1ml/kg body weight) and injections of glutathione might minimize the radiation damage to the healthy tissue. The study reports: "These results clearly show that NS and GSH treatment significantly antagonize the effects of radiation. Therefore, NS and GSH may be a beneficial agent in protection against ionizing radiation-related tissue injury."[30]

ROSEMARY: Cubans use an infusion of rosemary leaves to treat liver and gall bladder complaints, and to reduce painful abdominal spasms due to gas and flatulence itself.[31]

German Commission E approved for: "Internal: Dyspeptic complaints. External: Supportive therapy for rheumatic diseases, circulatory problems."

For pain due to inflammation, see also INFLAMMATORY DISEASES.
For pain due to cancer, see PAIN - (DUE TO ADVANCED CANCER).
For pain due to trauma, see INJURIES.

1 Lee WM. Acetaminophen and the U.S. *Acute Liver Failure Study Group: lowering the risks of hepatic failure.* Division of Digestive and Liver Diseases, University of Texas, Southwestern Medical Center, Dallas, 75390-9151, USA. Hepatology. 2004 Jul;40(1):6-9.

2 Green GA. *Understanding NSAIDs: from aspirin to COX-2.* Department of Family Practice, UCLA School of Medicine, Los Angeles, California, USA. Clin Cornerstone. 2001;3(5):50-60.

3 Sidney M. Wolfe, M.D., Larry D. Sasich, Pharm.D., M.P.H., Rose-Ellen Hope, R.Ph., and Public Citizen's

Health Research Group. *Worst Pills, Best Pills - A Consumer's Guide to Avoiding Drug-Induced Death or Illness.* Pocket Book, New York. 1999.

4 Moore TJ. Cohen MR, Furberg CD. *Serious Adverse Drug Events Reported to the Food and Drug Administration, 1998-2005.* Institute for Safe Medication Practices, 1800 Byberry Rd, Ste 810, Huntingdon Valley, PA 19006, USA. Arch Intern Med. 2007 Sep 10;167(16):1752-9.

5 Richard S. Weiner Ph.D., (Editor). *Pain management: a practical guide for clinicians.* American Academy of Pain Management. Chapter 31, written by Ethan B. Russo, M.D. The Role of Cannabis and Cannabinoids in Pain Management. CRC Press. Boca Raton London New York Washington, D.C.. 2002.

6 Conte A, Bettolo CM, Onesti E, Frasca V, Iacovelli E, Gilio F, Giacomelli E, Gabriele M, Aragona M, Tomassini V, Pantano P, Pozzilli C, Inghilleri M. *Cannabinoid-induced effects on the nociceptive system: A neurophysiological study in patients with secondary progressive multiple sclerosis.* Department of Neurological Sciences, University of Rome "Sapienza", Viale dell'Università 30, 00185 Rome, Italy. Eur J Pain. 2009 May;13(5):472-7.

7 Welch SP, Eads M. *Synergistic interactions of endogenous opioids and cannabinoid systems.* Department of Pharmacology and Toxicology, Box 980613, Virginia Commonwealth University, Richmond, VA 23298-0613, USA. Brain Res. 1999 Nov 27;848(1-2):183-90.

8 Sumner H. Burstein1,2 and Robert B. Zurier2. *Cannabinoids, Endocannabinoids, and Related Analogs in Inflammation.* 1Department of Biochemistry & Molecular Pharmacology, University of Massachusetts Medical School, 364 Plantation St., Worcester, Massachusetts 01605 USA. 2Department of Medicine, University of Massachusetts Medical School, 364 Plantation St., Worcester, Massachusetts 01605 USA. AAPS J. 2009 March; 11(1): 109–119.

9 Wallace M, Schulteis G, Atkinson JH, Wolfson T, Lazzaretto D, Bentley H, Gouaux B, Abramson I. *Dose-dependent effects of smoked cannabis on capsaicin-induced pain and hyperalgesia in healthy volunteers.* Department of Anesthesiology, University of California, San Diego, USA. mswallace@ucsd.edu Anesthesiology. 2007 Nov;107(5):785-96.

10 Kraft B, Frickey NA, Kaufmann RM, Reif M, Frey R, Gustorff B, Kress HG. *Lack of analgesia by oral standardized cannabis extract on acute inflammatory pain and hyperalgesia in volunteers.* Department of Anesthesiology and Intensive Care Medicine A, Medical University of Vienna, Vienna, Austria. Anesthesiology. 2008 Jul;109(1):101-10.

11 Richard S. Weiner Ph.D., (Editor). P*ain management: a practical guide for clinicians.* American Academy of Pain Management. Chapter 31, written by Ethan B. Russo, M.D. The Role of Cannabis and Cannabinoids in Pain Management. CRC Press. Boca Raton London New York Washington, D.C.. 2002.

12 Sumner H. Burstein1,2 and Robert B. Zurier2. *Cannabinoids, Endocannabinoids, and Related Analogs in Inflammation.* 1Department of Biochemistry & Molecular Pharmacology, University of Massachusetts Medical School, 364 Plantation St., Worcester, Massachusetts 01605 USA. 2Department of Medicine, University of Massachusetts Medical School, 364 Plantation St., Worcester, Massachusetts 01605 USA. AAPS J. 2009 March; 11(1): 109–119.

13 Conte A, Bettolo CM, Onesti E, Frasca V, Iacovelli E, Gilio F, Giacomelli E, Gabriele M, Aragona M, Tomassini V, Pantano P, Pozzilli C, Inghilleri M. *Cannabinoid-induced effects on the nociceptive system: A neurophysiological study in patients with secondary progressive multiple sclerosis.* Department of Neurological Sciences, University of Rome "Sapienza", Viale dell'Università 30, 00185 Rome, Italy. Eur J Pain. 2009 May;13(5):472-7.

14 Wallace M, Schulteis G, Atkinson JH, Wolfson T, Lazzaretto D, Bentley H, Gouaux B, Abramson I. *Dose-dependent effects of smoked cannabis on capsaicin-induced pain and hyperalgesia in healthy volunteers.* Department of Anesthesiology, University of California, San Diego, USA. mswallace@ucsd.edu Anesthesiology. 2007 Nov;107(5):785-96.

15 Gagnier JJ, van Tulder MW, Berman B, Bombardier C. *Herbal medicine for low back pain: a Cochrane review.* Institute of Medical Science, Faculty of Medicine, University of Toronto, Toronto, Ontario, Canada. Spine. 2007 Jan 1;32(1):82-92.

16 *Therapeutic Guide to Plant Pharmaceuticals and Honey Pharmaceuticals (Guia Terapeutica Dispensarial de Fitofarmacos y Apifarmacos* - Ministerio de Salud Publica, Ciudad de La Habana - Republica de Cuba 1992). Cuban Ministry of Public Health, Havana.

17 *Monographien der E-Kommission* (Phyto-Therapie) (380 monographs). A therapeutic guide to herbal medicine evaluating the safety and efficacy of herbs for licensed medical prescriptions in Germany. Published between 1984 and 1994 in the Bundesanzeiger (official publication by the Federal Republic of Germany). Copies of the monographs are available at the Heilpflanzen-Welt Bibliothek: http://buecher.heilpflanzen-welt.de/BGA-Commission-E-Monographs/

18 Beltran J, Ghosh AK, Basu S. *Immunotherapy of tumors with neuroimmune ligand capsaicin.* Center for Immunotherapy of Cancer and Infectious Diseases, University of Connecticut School of Medicine, 263 Farmington Avenue, Farmington, CT 06030-1601, USA. J Immunol. 2007 Mar 1;178(5):3260-4.

19 Elwakeel HA, Moneim HA, Farid M, Gohar AA. *Clove oil cream: a new effective treatment for chronic anal fissure.* Mansoura Faculty of Medicine, Surgery, Mansoura University Hospital, Mansoura, Dakahlia, Egypt. Colorectal Dis. 2007 Jul;9(6):549-52.

20 Chaieb K, Hajlaoui H, Zmantar T, Kahla-Nakbi AB, Rouabhia M, Mahdouani K, Bakhrouf A. *The chemical composition and biological activity of clove essential oil, Eugenia caryophyllata (Syzigium aromaticum L. Myrtaceae): a short review.* Laboratoire d'Analyses, Traitement et Valorisation des Polluants de l'Environnement et des Produits, Faculté de Pharmacie, rue Avicenne 5000 Monastir, Tunisie. Phytother Res. 2007 Jun;21(6):501-6.

21 Heinrich U, Neukam K, Tronnier H, Sies H, Stahl W. *Long-term ingestion of high flavanol cocoa provides photoprotection against UV-induced erythema and improves skin condition in women* .Institut für Experimentelle Dermatologie, Universität Witten-Herdecke, Germany. J Nutr. 2006 Jun;136(6):1565-9.

22 *Monographien der E-Kommission* (Phyto-Therapie) (380 monographs). A therapeutic guide to herbal medicine evaluating the safety and efficacy of herbs for licensed medical prescribing in Germany. Published between 1984 and 1994 in the Bundesanzeiger (official publication by the Federal Republic of Germany). Copies of the monographs are available at the Heilpflanzen-Welt Bibliothek: http://buecher.heilpflanzen-welt.de/BGA-Commission-E-Monographs/

23 Modaress Nejad V, Asadipour M. *Comparison of the effectiveness of fennel and mefenamic acid on pain intensity in dysmenorrhoea.* Department of Obstetrics and Gynaecology, Kerman University of Medial Sciences and Health Services, Kerman, Islamic Republic of Iran. East Mediterr Health J. 2006 May-Jul;12(3-4):423-7.

24 *Therapeutic Guide to Plant Pharmaceuticals and Honey Pharmaceuticals* (Guia Terapeutica Dispensarial de Fitofarmacos y Apifarmacos - Ministerio de Salud Publica, Ciudad de La Habana - Republica de Cuba 1992). Cuban Ministry of Public Health, Havana.

25 Ojewole JA. *Analgesic, antiinflammatory and hypoglycaemic effects of ethanol extract of Zingiber officinale (Roscoe) rhizomes (Zingiberaceae) in mice and rats.* Department of Pharmacology, Faculty of Health Sciences, University of KwaZulu-Natal, Private Bag X54001, Durban, South Africa. ojewolej@ukzn.ac.za Phytother Res. 2006 Sep;20(9):764-72.

26 Umukoro S, Ashorobi BR. *Further pharmacological studies on aqueous seed extract of Aframomum melegueta in rats.* Department of Pharmacology and Therapeutics, College of Medicine, University of Ibadan, Nigeria. J Ethnopharmacol. 2008 Feb 12;115(3):489-93.

27 Umukoro S, Ashorobi RB. *Further studies on the antinociceptive action of aqueous seed extract of Aframomum melegueta.* Department of Pharmacology and Thera peutics, University of Ibadan, Ibadan, Nigeria. umusolo@yahoo.com J Ethnopharmacol. 2007 Feb 12;109(3):501-4.

28 *Monographien der E-Kommission* (Phyto-Therapie) (380 monographs). A therapeutic guide to herbal medicine evaluating the safety and efficacy of herbs for licensed medical prescribing in Germany. Published between 1984 and 1994 in the Bundesanzeiger (official publication by the Federal Republic of Germany). Copies of the monographs are available at the Heilpflanzen-Welt Bibliothek: http://buecher.heilpflanzen-welt.de/BGA-Commission-E-Monographs/

29 Nomicos EY. *Myrrh: medical marvel or myth of the magi?* National Institute of Allergy and Infectious Diseases, National Institute of Health, Bethesda, Maryland. Holist Nurs Pract. 2007 Nov-Dec;21(6):308-23.

30 Cemek M, Enginar H, Karaca T, Unak P. *In vivo radioprotective effects of Nigella sativa L oil and reduced glutathione against irradiation-induced oxidative injury and number of peripheral blood lymphocytes in rats.* Department of Chemistry, Biochemistry Division, Faculty of Science and Arts, Afyon Kocatepe University, Afyon, Turkey. mcemek@yahoo.com Photochem Photobiol. 2006 Nov-Dec;82(6):1691-6.

31 *Therapeutic Guide to Plant Pharmaceuticals and Honey Pharmaceuticals* (Guia Terapeutica Dispensarial de Fitofarmacos y Apifarmacos - Ministerio de Salud Publica, Ciudad de La Habana - Republica de Cuba 1992). Cuban Ministry of Public Health, Havana.

Pain
Chronic Non-malignant Pains

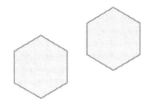

NUMBER OF STUDIES: 2

CHI VALUE: 5

Chronic non-malignant pains (CNMP's) are defined as non-cancerous pains lasting longer than three months yet significantly impairing quality of life. A study conducted in Germany surveying available data from 1995-2009 discovered that about 17% of all pain falls into this category. The most common forms of CNMP non-responsive to pharmaceutical and non-drug treatment include musculoskeletal pains of the neck, shoulder and back.[1]

CANNABIS AND CNMP

Researchers from Warsaw, Poland, conducted an animal study (2008) and discovered that cannabinoid agonists activate both endocannabinoid receptors CB1 and CB2. In addition, cannabinoids reduced sensitivity to pain in a dose dependent fashion. Furthermore, they discovered that the COX-1 inhibitors such as indomethacin (a non-steroidal anti- inflammatory drug commonly used to reduce fever, pain, stiffness) might increase these cannabinoid properties at low dosages.[2]

A human case study (2008) from Jerusalem, Israel, examined dronabinol, the synthetic version of THC, in the context of CNMP. Researchers observed: "Cannabinoids have been used for pain relief for centuries and recent studies have investigated their analgesic and anti-inflammatory mechanisms, as well as clinical efficacy, in treating chronic pain." In this study scientists wanted to examine the effects of THC on patients with CNMP unresponsive to conventional pharmacotherapy. Out of 13 participating patients, five reported an adequate response while eight patients reported an inadequate or no response to dronabinol. The authors concluded that: "...oral THC may be a valuable therapeutic option for selected patients with CNMP that are unresponsive to previous treatments, though further research is warranted to characterize those patients."[3]

STUDY SUMMARY:

Drugs	Type of Study	Published Year, Place, and Key Results	CHI
Dronabinol (synthetic isomer of THC)	Case study (13 patients)	2008 – Department of Anesthesiology, Hadassah-Hebrew University Medical Center, Jerusalem, Israel. Dronabinol is a possible therapeutic option in the treatment of chronic non-malignant pain not responsive to other analgesics.	3
CB1 and CB2 agonists	Animal study	2008 – Department of Pharmacodynamics, Medical University of Warsaw, Warsaw, Poland. May reduce pain sensitivity and may work synergistically with NSAID's.	2

Total CHI Value   5

STRAIN SPECIFIC CONSIDERATIONS

The relevant cannabinoid used in this section was dronabinol, a synthetic prescription medication, which is an isomer (same molecular formula but different structural formula) of Δ9-tetrahydrocannabinol. THC binds relatively equally with both CB1 and CB2.

Sativa and sativa dominant strains usually contain higher THC:CBD ratios.

EXPLORING MIND–BODY CONSCIOUSNESS

See PAIN IN GENERAL.

1 Wolff R, Clar C, Lerch C, Kleijnen J. *Epidemiology of chronic non-malignant pain in Germany.* Kleijnen Systematic Reviews Ltd, Unit 6, Escrick Business Park, Riccall Road, Escrick, YO196FD York, UK. Schmerz. 2011 Feb;25(1):26-44.

2 Bujalska M. *Effect of Cannabinoid Receptor Agonists on Streptozotocin-Induced Hyperalgesia in Diabetic Neuropathy.* Department of Pharmacodynamics, Medical University of Warsaw, Warsaw, Poland. mbujalska@gmail.com Pharmacology. 2008;82(3):193-200.

3 Haroutiunian S, Rosen G, Shouval R, Davidson E. *Open-label, add-on study of tetrahydrocannabinol for chronic nonmalignant pain.* Department of Anesthesiology, Hadassah-Hebrew University Medical Center, Jerusalem, Israel. J Pain Palliat Care Pharmacother. 2008;22(3):213-7.

Pain
Migraines

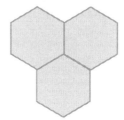

NUMBER OF STUDIES: 3

CHI VALUE: 10

Migraines are recurring headaches that range from moderate to severe. Severe migraines lasting for hours or days can be debilitating to the point where all you want to do is draw the curtains and curl up into the fetal position. One patient described it this way: "The pulse of my own heartbeat becomes a drum of pain pounding against the walls of my skull with no end in sight." The pain can induce nausea and vomiting. Other symptoms often include severe sensitivity to light and sounds.

A number of people experience sensations of paranormal flashes of light (called auras) signaling the migraine's arrival while other early indications (prodromes) might consist of a craving for chocolate, aversion to noise, sudden mood shifts to depression, anxiety or elation. Additional prodromes include sluggishness, stiff neck, gastrointestinal problems or very subjective oddities such as the sensation of a hot face yet feeling chilly or the flare-up of hemorrhoids.

Within the allopathic tradition, the cause and cure for migraines remain unknown. Physical causes considered include abnormalities in blood vessels of the scalp or brain. While scientists also hypothesize that hormonal change, stressors, weather changes[1] and food sources may play roles as triggers in migraine attacks, evidence remains inconclusive. "Menstruation had the most prominent effect, increasing the hazard of occurrence or persistence of headache and migraine by up to 96%."[2] Management of triggers through individual observations, diaries, consequent implementation of trigger avoidance, prophylaxis through supportive lifestyle choices such as nutrition and exercise has given back some sense to control in many patients.

In interview-form, doctors diagnose patients by determining the specific pain history, examining frequency of attacks, duration, specific location, presence of aura, nausea or vomiting and impact on daily routines. Treatment consists of numerous oral and injectable pharmaceuticals. Depending on some underlying physiology, sometimes blood vessel surgery provides relief. However, the overuse of pharmaceuticals (especially tricyclics and opiates) and the number of adverse effects have posed a problem in their own right.

Epidemiologically, about 75% of all adult migraine sufferers in the United States are women. Estrogen is considered as one culprit to explain the gender discrepancy.[3] Additionally, studies suggest that migraine sufferers might be at an increased risk for stroke.[4]

CANNABIS AND MIGRAINE

Ethan Russo's in-depth historical and scientific review and meta-analysis of cannabis in migraine treatment (Missoula, U.S., 2004) demonstrates the plant's effectiveness recorded throughout ancient medical literature and provides modern scientific rationale for its age-old reputation as an effective balm for headaches. Russo justifies potential use and further study of cannabinoids in the treatment of migraine based on modern biochemical discoveries that the plant constituents work through "...anti-inflammatory, serotonergic and dopaminergic mechanisms, as well as by interaction with NMDA and endogenous opioid systems."[5,6] He further suggests that certain conditions including migraines "...display common clinical, biochemical and pathophysiological patterns that suggest an underlying clinical endocannabinoid deficiency that may be suitably treated with cannabinoid medicines."[7]

In a single patient case study from New York (2006), researchers discovered that the patient's chronic frontal headaches produced by increased intracranial pressure as well as her other related symptoms of photophobia (sensitivity to light), transient blindness, enlarged blind spots, and tinnitus improved after smoking marijuana. Further experiments revealed that non-psychoactive oral dronabinol administered at 5mg twice a day relieved all of her symptoms without any reported weight gain.[8]

Researchers (1985) from Negev, Israel, obtained blood samples from patients diagnosed with migraines during an episode of migraine pain. They exposed the blood to the cannabinoids THC and CBD. Results indicated that THC, but not CBD, inhibited serotonin release from platelets (blood componant) in patients during migraine pains.[9] While the authors' discovery of THC's involvement in serotonin modulation in migraine blood plasma provided another possible clue about the exact mechanism by which cannabinoids reduce migraine pain, they acknowledged that other effects such as analgesia,[10] vasoconstriction[11] and possible migraine preventative properties[12] might all play a role.

STUDY SUMMARY:

Drugs	Type of Study	Published Year, Place, and Key Results	CHI
Cannabis and Dronabinol	One human patient	2006 – New York. Reduced all symptoms of pain, photophobia, transient blindness, enlarged blind spots, and tinnitus with both cannabis and dronabinol.	3
Cannabinoids	Meta-analysis of available studies	2004 – GW Pharmaceuticals, Missoula. Endocannabinoid deficiency may underlie migraines.	4
THC and CBD	Human patients diagnosed with migraines.	1985 – Negev, Israel. THC, but not CBD, inhibited serotonin release in patients during migraine pains.	3

Total CHI Value   10

STRAIN SPECIFIC CONSIDERATIONS

Russo's review suggests the possibility of an endocannabinoid deficiency in migraine pathology. The endogenous cannabinoid anandamide binds with both CB1 and CB2 relatively equally.

THC binds relatively equally with CB1 and CB2. Sativas and sativa dominant strains generally contain a higher THC:CBD ratio.

EXPLORING MIND–BODY CONSCIOUSNESS

The physicians Grace and Graham examined the psychosomatic underpinnings of migraines in 14 patients participating in their landmark study and wrote: "Migraine headaches occurred when an individual had been making an intense effort to carry out a definite planned program, or to achieve some definite objective. The headache occurred when the effort had ceased, no matter whether the activity had been associated with success or failure. The essential features were striving and subsequent relaxation." Typical statements were: "I had to get this done. … I had to meet the deadline. … I had a million things to do before lunch. … I was trying to get all these things accomplished."[13]

Consider the following statement from the PAMINA study: "The two days before menstruation and muscle tension in the neck, psychic tension, tiredness, noise and odors on days before headache onset increased the hazard of headache or migraine, whereas days off, a divorced marriage, relaxation after stress, and consumption of beer decreased the hazard."[14]

The significant impact of state of mind was further explored in studies, which revealed that sex and orgasmic release altered migraine pains.[15] A group of 83 women suffering from migraines participated; 28 reported no relief, 27 reported some relief; 10 noted complete relief; and 3 women reported that the pain worsened.[16] While researchers do not know the mechanism by which sex and the orgasmic experience modulates migraine pains, they speculate that it may somehow alter the genesis of migraines.

QUESTIONS

I there something or someone it hurts to think about?

AGGRAVATING FACTORS

Perception of being forced, pushed, or pressured by others or our own internal slave driver / two days before menstruation / muscle tension in the neck / psychic tension / tiredness / noise and odors on days before headache.

HEALING FACTORS

Days off / a divorced marriage / relaxation after stress / consumption of beer.

ANECDOTE

Martha was proud to be able to cram more appointments into a single day than anybody else. She worked out, took care of her family, friends and associates. Martha maintained a tight ship at her two jobs which she said she loved and still found time to take self-improvement classes. She began having debilitating migraines in her forties. Her symptoms included photophobia, phonophobia, visual hallucinations and nausea with intense vomiting that seemed to amplify her pain. Her physician tried pharmaceutical analgesia but Martha could not handle the adverse effects; it was adding to her nausea and was 'too depressing in general.' Confronted with the terrible choice of either living with her pain or the adverse effects, she went back to her doctor and asked for a cannabis prescription. Martha lowered the curtains, turned off the telephone and doorbell, and inhaled. She used an inhaler that delivered the cannabinoids without smoke, which she felt might make her cough because she dreaded the pain that would cause her. After a couple of inhalations, she noticed a pleasant relaxation and within a half an hour fell into a blissful sleep. Martha awoke from her slumber without pain. For the first time, a medicine had really worked.

1 Zebenholzer, K; Rudel, E, Frantal, S, Brannath, W, Schmidt, K, Wöber-Bingöl, C, Wöber, C (2011). *"Migraine and weather: A prospective diary-based analysis"*. Christian Wöber, Department of Neurology, Medical University of Vienna, Währinger Gürtel 18-20, 1090 Vienna, Austria. Cephalalgia March 2011 vol. 31 no. 4 391-400

2 Wöber, C; Brannath, W, Schmidt, K, Kapitan, M, Rudel, E, Wessely, P, Wöber-Bingöl, Ç (2007). *"Prospective analysis of factors related to migraine attacks: the PAMINA study"*. Christian Wöber MD, Department of Neurology, Währinger Gürtel 18-20, 1090 Vienna, Austria. Cephalalgia 27 (4): 304–314.

3 Lay CL, Broner SW (May 2009). *"Migraine in women"*. Department of Medicine, Division of Neurology, Centre For Headache, Women's College Hospital, 76 Grenville Street, Toronto, Ontario, Canada. Neurologic Clinics 27 (2): 503–11.

4 Etminan M, Takkouche B, Isorna FC, Samii A. *Risk of ischaemic stroke in people with migraine: systematic review and meta-analysis of observational studies.* Division of Epidemiology, Royal Victoria and Vancouver Hospitals, Canada. BMJ. 2005 Jan 8;330(7482):63.

5 Ethan B. Russo, M.D., *Hemp for Headache: An In-Depth Historical and Scientific Review of Cannabis in Migraine Treatment.* Russo is Clinical Child and Adult Neurologist, Clinical Assistant Professor of Medicine at the University of Washington and Adjunct Associate Professor of Pharmacy, University of Montana, 900 North Orange Street, Missoula, MT 58902. Journal of Cannabis Therapeutics, Vol. 1(2) 2001.

6 Ethan Russo. *Cannabis for migraine treatment: the once and future prescription?* An historical and scientific review. Department of Neurology, Western Montana Clinic, 515 West Front Street, Missoula, MT 58907-7609, USA. Pain 76 (1998) 3 – 8

7 Ethan B. Russo, M.D. *Clinical Endocannabinoid Deficiency (CECD): Can this Concept Explain Therapeutic Benefits of Cannabis in Migraine, Fibromyalgia, Irritable Bowel Syndrome and other Treatment-Resistant Conditions?* Senior Medical Advisor, GW Pharmaceuticals, 2235 Wylie Avenue, Missoula, MT 59802, USA. Neuroendocrinology Letters Nos.1/2, Feb-Apr Vol.25, 2004.

8 Raby WN, Modica PA, Wolintz RJ, Murtaugh K. *Dronabinol reduces signs and symptoms of idiopathic intracranial hypertension: a case report.* New York State Psychiatric Institute, Substance Abuse Division, The S.T.A.R.S. Clinic, New York, NY 10032, USA. J Ocul Pharmacol Ther. 2006 Feb;22(1):68-75.

9 Volfe Z., Dvilansky A., Nathan I. *Cannabinoids block release of serotonin from platelets induced by plasma from migraine patients.* Blood Research, Faculty of Health Sciences, Soroka Medical Center, Ben-Gurion University of the Negev, P.O. Box 151, Beer-Sheva 84101, Israel. Int J Clin Pharm. Res V (4) 243-246 (1985).

10 Kozersky S., Dewey W.L., Harris L.S. *Antipyretic analgesic and anti-inflammatory effects of delta-9-THC in the rat.* Europ. J. Pharmacol., 24, 1, 1973.

11 Adams M.D., Earnhardt J.T., Dewey W.L., Harris L.S. *Vasoconstrictor actions of delta-8 and delta-9-THC in the rat.* J. Pharmacol.l Exp. Therap., 196, 649, 1976.

12 Mikuriya T.H. *Marijuana in medicine: Past, present and future.* Calif. Med., 110, 34-40, 1969.

13 William J. Grace, M.D. and David T. Graham, M.D. *Relationship of Specific Attitudes and Emotions to Certain Bodily Diseases.* Dept. of Medicine, of the New York Hospital-Cornell Medical Center. Psychosomatic Medicine July 1, 1952 vol. 14 no. 4 243-251.

14 Wöber, C; Brannath, W, Schmidt, K, Kapitan, M, Rudel, E, Wessely, P, Wöber-Bingöl, Ç (2007). *"Prospective analysis of factors related to migraine attacks: the PAMINA study".* Christian Wöber MD, Department of Neurology, Währinger Gürtel 18-20, 1090 Vienna, Austria. Cephalalgia 27 (4): 304–314.

15 R.W. Evans,, MD, J.R. Couch MD, Ph.D. *Orgasm and Migraine.* Department of Neurology, University of Oklahoma Health Sciences Center, Oklahoma City, OK 73190-3048, USA. Headache 2001;41:512-514.

16 Couch J., Bearss C. *Relief of Migraine with Sexual Intercourse.* Headache 1990;30:302

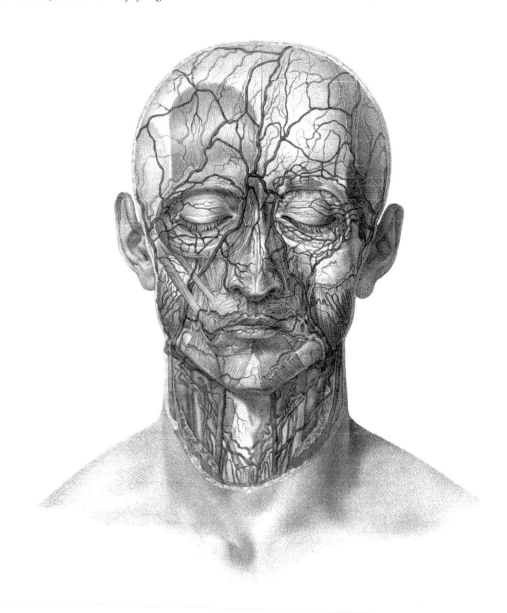

Pain
Neuropathies

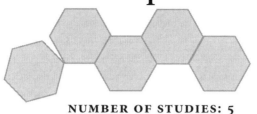

NUMBER OF STUDIES: 5

CHI VALUE: 15

Neuropathies are pains generally caused over time by nerve damage from either past traumatic events (pressure, heat, cold, chemicals, radiation) or a progression of certain diseases, toxins, pathogens, or lack of nutrients. Deformities, scar tissue, impaired tissue metabolism, impairment of nerve fiber insulation (demyelination) and inflammation all individually or together contribute to neuropathies.

Neuropathies' classifications depend on the type of nerve(s) involved. Pains from isolated nerve(s) (mononeuropathy or mononeuritis multiplex) may result from the compression of a disc in the spinal column and can produce nerve pain extending to outward lying tissue. Polyneuropathy affects larger network nerve fibers and is often seen in diabetes or amyotrophic lateral sclerosis (ALS/Lou Gehrig's disease). Autonomic neuropathies are pains involving nerves controlled by the involuntary nervous system, which can debilitate all organs, systems and functions governed by it such as the bladder, heart and blood pressure. Another type of neuropathic pain, neuritis, is an inflammation of nerve fiber(s) and is named for its underlying cause.

Symptoms correspond to the affected nerve fibers and the origin of the neuropathy. Sensory symptoms can range from mild tingling and numbness to debilitating pains shooting or burning down the path of the nerve. Motor symptoms range from mild weakness, cramps or spasms to severe tremors with loss of function. Difficulty walking, using one's of hands, and talking may be accompanied by severe pain. Impairment of autonomic functions can lead to incontinence, heart irregularities, postural hypotension or difficulty in temperature regulation.

Allopathic treatments include analgesics, antidepressants, anti-seizure drugs and synthetic cannabinoids such as nabilone. Common underlying non-traumatic causes are iotrogenic, ie., caused my allopathic treatments such as pharmaceutical drugs, surgery, chemotherapy, or radiation therapy. Other common causes include diabetes, multiple sclerosis, AIDS and shingles (herpes zoster).

With the exception of vitamin deficiency-induced neuropathies, patients typically find modern medicine's treatment of neuropathies ineffective. This often derives from the inability to cure many of the underlying illnesses. Treatment caution must also be exercised as some of the medications used can be potentially habit-forming or result in dangerous adverse effects.

CANNABIS AND NEUROPATHIES (IN GENERAL)

Th majority of randomized, placebo-controlled, crossover trial of the effects of cannabis on neuropathic pain discovered a marked therapeutic impact with few and manageable side effects. An overview of the existing studies on the subject of cannabinoids and neuropathies published between 2004-2009 mostly confirmed cannabinoids' effectiveness in relieving neuropathic pain.[1]

STUDY SUMMARY:

Drugs	Type of Study	Published Year, Place, and Key Results	CHI
Smoked Cannabis.	Human double-blinded, placebo-controlled, crossover study.	2008 – VA Northern California Health Care System, Department of Anesthesiology and Pain Medicine, University of California, Davis Medical Center, Davis, California, USA. Positive analgesic effects with peripheral neuropathic pain.[2]	5
Oral THC at an average dose of 16.6mg.	Open label prospective study on 8 patients with chronic refractory neuropathic pain.	2004 – Centre d'Evaluation et de Traitement de la Douleur, Hôpital Ambroise Paré Boulogne-Billancourt, France. No benefits observed and adverse effects noted in some patients.[3]	-5
Sativex, containing THC:CBD in an approximate 1:1 ratio, GW-2000-02, containing primarily THC and placebo delivered as oral sprays.	48 human patients with neuropathic pain. Randomized, double blind, placebo-controlled, three period crossover study.	2004 – Royal National Orthopaedic Hospital, Brockley Hill, Stanmore, Middlesex, UK. Mild reduction of neuropathic pain. Improved sleep, no major adverse effects.[4]	5
Whole-plant extracts containing CBD:THC sublingual spray 2.5-120 mg/24 hours.	A consecutive series of double-blind, randomized, placebo-controlled single-patient cross-over trials of 24 patients with MS, spinal cord injuries.	2003 – Oxford Centre for Enablement, Windmill Road, Oxford, UK. Significant pain relief.[5]	5
Synthetic cannabinoid CT-3, a potent analog of THC-11-oic acid.	21 patients with chronic neuropathic pain, a randomized, placebo-controlled, double-blind crossover trial.	2003 – Department of Anesthesiology, Pain Clinic, Hannover Medical School, Hannover, Germany. Effective in reducing chronic neuropathic pain compared with placebo. No major adverse effects observed.[6]	5

Total CHI Value 15

STRAIN SPECIFIC CONSIDERATIONS

The cannabinoids reviewed here include oromucosal spray sativex, cannabis, and THC (oral spray). Those suggesting positive results included sativex.

Sativex, a pharmaceutical plant derivative, is a cannabinoid combination containing THC and CBD in similar proportions as the strain cannabis sativa. Cannabis contains THC and CBD in different ratios depending on the strain.

Sativa or sativa dominant strains generally contain a higher THC:CBD ratio.

EXPLORING MIND–BODY CONSCIOUSNESS

Nerves communicate and connect each cell with the brain and nervous system allowing trillions of different cells to efficiently work together and in balance for the benefit of the whole being. Each cell listens and speaks. Each receives and transmits signals perceived by the seven common senses (sight, sound, touch, smell, taste, equilibrium and imagination).

The disease picture of neuropathies suggests an element of communication about one's general experience of pain. For more information, see PAIN IN GENERAL, INFLAMMATORY DISEASES OR NEUROLOGICAL DISEASES.

1 Sumner H. Burstein1,2 and Robert B. Zurier2. Cannabinoids, *Endocannabinoids, and Related Analogs in Inflammation.* 1Department of Biochemistry & Molecular Pharmacology, University of Massachusetts Medical School, 364 Plantation St., Worcester, Massachusetts 01605 USA. 2Department of Medicine, University of Massachusetts Medical School, 364 Plantation St., Worcester, Massachusetts 01605 USA. AAPS J. 2009 March; 11(1): 109–119.

2 Wilsey B, Marcotte T, Tsodikov A, Millman J, Bentley H, Gouaux B, Fishman S. *A randomized, placebo-controlled, crossover trial of cannabis cigarettes in neuropathic pain.* VA Northern California Health Care System, Department of Anesthesiology and Pain Medicine, University of California, Davis Medical Center, Davis, California, USA. blwilsey@ucdavis.edu J Pain. 2008 Jun;9(6):506-21.

3 Attal N, Brasseur L, Guirimand D, Clermond-Gnamien S, Atlami S, Bouhassira D. *Are oral cannabinoids safe and effective in refractory neuropathic pain?* INSERM E-332, Centre d'Evaluation et de Traitement de la Douleur, Hôpital Ambroise Paré, AP-HP, 92100 Boulogne-Billancourt, France. Eur J Pain. 2004 Apr;8(2):173-7.

4 Berman JS, Symonds C, Birch R. *Efficacy of two cannabis based medicinal extracts for relief of central neuropathic pain from brachial plexus avulsion: results of a randomised controlled trial.* Royal National Orthopaedic Hospital, Brockley Hill, Stanmore, Middlesex HA7 4LP, UK. Pain. 2004 Dec;112(3):299-30.

5 Wade DT, Robson P, House H, Makela P, Aram J. *A preliminary controlled study to determine whether whole-plant cannabis extracts can improve intractable neurogenic symptoms.* Oxford Centre for Enablement, Windmill Road, Oxford, UK. derick.wade@dial.pipex.com Clin Rehabil. 2003 Feb;17(1):21-9

6 Karst M, Salim K, Burstein S, Conrad I, Hoy L, Schneider U. *Analgesic effect of the synthetic cannabinoid CT-3 on chronic neuropathic pain: a randomized controlled trial.* Department of Anesthesiology, Pain Clinic, Hannover Medical School, Hannover, Germany. JAMA. 2003 Oct 1;290(13):1757-62.

Pain
Neuropathies - AIDS Related

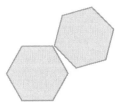

NUMBER OF STUDIES: 2

CHI VALUE   10

CANNABIS AND NEUROPATHIES (AIDS RELATED)

In 2007, researchers at San Francisco General Hospital conducted a randomized placebo-controlled human trial on cannabis and AIDS related neuropathies. Scientists discovered that HIV patients suffering from sensory neuropathies benefited equally from smoked cannabis as compared to oral pharmaceuticals used for chronic neuropathic pain. The authors concluded that: "Smoked cannabis was well tolerated and effectively relieved chronic neuropathic pain from HIV-associated sensory neuropathy."[1]

The San Francisco results were confirmed two years later by an experiment in San Diego in which researchers conducted a double blind placebo-controlled crossover trial of analgesia with smoked cannabis. Results showed a majority of enrolled HIV patients with neuropathies experienced a 30% reduction in pains when compared to the placebo.[2]

STUDY SUMMARY:

Drugs	Type of Study	Published Year, Place, and Key Results	CHI
Cannabis (smoked)	Patients with chronic neuropathic pain from HIV-associated sensory neuropathy.	2007 – Community Consortium, Positive Health Program, San Francisco General Hospital, San Francisco, California, USA. Smoked cannabis reduced daily pain by 34%.	5
Smoked Cannabis	HIV patients with neuropathies	2009 – Department of Neurosciences, University of California, San Diego, California, USA. 30% reduction in pains when compared to the placebo.	5

Total CHI Value   10

EXPLORING MIND–BODY CONSCIOUSNESS

See chapters on HIV/AIDS AND NEUROLOGICAL DISEASES IN GENERAL

1 Abrams DI, Jay CA, Shade SB, Vizoso H, Reda H, Press S, Kelly ME, Rowbotham MC, Petersen KL. *Cannabis in painful HIV-associated sensory neuropathy: a randomized placebo-controlled trial.* Community Consortium,

Positive Health Program, San Francisco General Hospital, San Francisco, CA 94110, USA. dabrams@php.ucsf.edu Neurology. 2007 Feb 13;68(7):515-21.

2 Ellis RJ, Toperoff W, Vaida F, van den Brande G, Gonzales J, Gouaux B, Bentley H, Atkinson JH. *Smoked medicinal cannabis for neuropathic pain in HIV: a randomized, crossover clinical trial.* Department of Neurosciences, University of California, San Diego, CA 92103, USA. roellis@ucsd.edu Neuropsychopharmacology. 2009 Feb; 34(3):672-80.

Pain
Pains due to Advanced Cancer

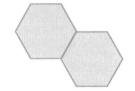

NUMBER OF STUDIES: 2

CHI VALUE: 10

CANABIS AND PAINS (DUE TO ADVANCED CANCER)

In this double blind placebo-controlled study (2010) from Shrewsbury, UK, scientists enrolled 177 patients with advanced cancers who did not fully respond to the typical opiate-based painkillers. They administered a tetrahydrocannabinol:cannabidiol extract to determine its efficacy in treating pain. The results revealed that twice as many patients taking THC:CBD experienced a reduction of more than 30% from their normal pains when compared to the placebo group. The authors noted: "This study shows that THC:CBD extract is efficacious for relief of pain in patients with advanced cancer pain not fully relieved by strong opioids."[1]

Interestingly, in a San Diego double-blind placebo-controlled crossover trial of analgesia with smoked cannabis, HIV patients with neuropathies reported similar percentage results to the Shrewsbury study.[2]

STUDY SUMMARY:

Drugs	Type of Study	Published Year, Place, and Key Results	CHI
Sativex, THC:CBD	Double blind, placebo controlled human study.	2010 – Severn Hospice, Shrewsbury, Shropshire, United Kingdom. Relief for patients not fully responding to the typical opiate based analgesics.	5
Smoked Cannabis	Double blind, placebo controlled cross-over human study.	2009 – Department of Neurosciences, University of California, San Diego. Reduction of nerve pains.	5

Total CHI Value   10

STRAIN SPECIFIC CONSIDERATIONS

The cannabinoids examined in both double blind, placebo controlled human trials included sativex and smoked cannabis. Sativex, a pharmaceutical plant derivative, is a cannabinoid combination containing THC and CBD in similar proportions as in the strain cannabis sativa. Cannabis contains cannabinoids binding with CB1 and CB2 depending on the strain.

Sativa and sativa dominant hybrids generally contain higher THC:CBD ratios.

EXPLORING MIND–BODY CONSCIOUSNESS

See relevant chapter on CANCER and PPAIN IN GENERAL.

1 Johnson JR, Burnell-Nugent M, Lossignol D, Ganae-Motan ED, Potts R, Fallon MT. *Multicenter, double-blind, randomized, placebo-controlled, parallel-group study of the efficacy, safety, and tolerability of THC:CBD extract and THC extract in patients with intractable cancer-related pain.* Severn Hospice, Shrewsbury, Shropshire, United Kingdom. J Pain Symptom Manage. 2010 Feb;39(2):167-79

2 Ellis RJ, Toperoff W, Vaida F, van den Brande G, Gonzales J, Gouaux B, Bentley H, Atkinson JH. *Smoked medicinal cannabis for neuropathic pain in HIV: a randomized, crossover clinical trial.* Department of Neurosciences, University of California, San Diego, CA 92103, USA. roellis@ucsd.edu Neuropsychopharmacology. 2009 Feb; 34(3):672-80.

Prion Diseases (Transmissible Spongiform Encephalopathies)

NUMBER OF STUDIES: 1

CHI VALUE: 3

Scientists believe prions to be infectious proteins responsible for Creutzfeldt–Jacob Disease (CJD) in humans, bovine spongiform encephalopathy (BSE or mad cow disease) in cows, and scrapie in sheep. Currently, all prion diseases are fatal. Prion diseases primarily affect the brain and the central nervous system. For clarification purposes, all types of prion diseases are also known as transmissible spongiform encephalopathies (TSEs).

The exact cause or mechanism by which patients acquire prion diseases remains the subject of ongoing debate and analysis. Some current findings focus on ingestion of prion-contaminated meat. Past feeding practices in factory farms included grinding up dead cattle and feeding the protein back to live animals, thus providing a specific route of transmission. Kuru, another prion disease similar to CJD, was found mainly among members of a cannibalistic tribe in Papua New Guinea. Kuru has been in decline since the practice of caanibalism ended.[1]

Some orthodox medical treatments have accidentally transmittted CJD: older types of growth hormones extracted from pituitary glands of cadavers, blood transfusions,[2] and certain types of surgeries (brain, eye or organ transplants). In addition, hospitals find prions extremely difficult to destroy once attached to hospital instruments and environments. Prions' resistance to normal methods of sterilization require that hospitals take extra measures to reduce the possibility of transmission.

Possibile causes of prion diseases include: hereditary genes or mutations, accumulated toxins, viral influences, fungal influences, or a combination of these factors.

It is thought that when a prion enters the organism it is able to alter the signals that produce newly formed proteins. The newly generated proteins fold into unhealthy shapes. While normally the body's own enzyme, protease, can digest old or diseased proteins, prions are resistant to the enzyme. These protease-resistant prion protein accumulations in the central nervous system claim direct responsibility for neuropathogenesis and prion infectivity.[3] Once symptoms appear, degeneration is exponential. Most patients die within a year after the onset of symptoms.

CJD symptoms are very similar to other neurodegenerative diseases such as Alzheimer's and include: confusion, forgetfulness, senility, apathy, irritability, seizures, muscle twitching, ataxia (wobbly gait) and loss of coordination. This list of common and varied indicators often leads to misdiagnoses. There is no test that can diagnose CJD. A brain biopsy can reveal the presence of the disease. However, drilling a hole into a patient's head just to confirm CJD is useless since no orthodox treatment exists.

CANNABIS AND PRIONS

Two recent factors necessitate finding a cure for the disease. First, variant forms (vCJD) have been transmitted through blood transfusions. Second, several countries have reported outbreaks of the disease due to contaminated beef consumption. Medical personnel urgently seek to determine a therapeutic agent that can slow the disease process or, preferably, effectively cure it.

Cannabinoids have known neuroprotective properties. In 2003, the US Federal Government issued a patent on a newly found property of cannabis, declaring it: "…useful in the treatment and prophylaxis of a wide variety of oxidation-associated diseases, such as ischemic, age-related, inflammatory and autoimmune diseases. The cannabinoids are found to have particular application as neuroprotectants; for example, in limiting neurological damage following ischemic insults, such as stroke and trauma, or in the treatment of neurodegenerative diseases, such as Alzheimer's disease, Parkinson's disease and HIV dementia."[4]

A 2007 experiment showed cannabidiol (CBD) not only inhibits accumulation of protease-resistant prion proteins but reducing their neurotoxic effects as well. CBD may be neuroprotective during prion infections.

To date, no studies have examined the impact of cannabinoids in humans infected with prions. However, time-proven uses of CBD rich cannabis for other neurological disorders suggest CBD may offer hope as a treatment for CJD. Cannabinoids easily cross the blood-brain barrier and can reach affected tissue with relatively few side effects. No other treatment exists and in light of the disease's dismal prognosis, any promising treatment approach warrants serious consideration.

Optimal dosage requirements and administration routes must still be determined. There are laboratory studies, however, which may prove instructive in this regard. For example, a 2007 study on mice established the neuroprotective value of CBD as follows: Mice were treated intraperitoneally three times per week for the indicated period of time, with 200 µl of 20 or 60 mg/kg CBD diluted 1:1:2 in an ethanol/cremophor/NaCl 0.9% mixture.[5]

STUDY SUMMARY:

Drugs	Type of Study	Published Year, Place, and Key Results	CHI
Injection of cannabidiol (CBD).[6]	Animal study (mice) and laboratory study	2007 – International research institutions. CBD inhibited prion accumulation. CBD inhibited the neurotoxic effects of protease-resistant prion protein. CBD may be neuroprotective during prion infection.	1+2

Total CHI Value   3

STRAIN AND FORM SPECIFIC CONSIDERATIONS

These laboratory and animal trials concluded that CBD may be the primary cannabinoid of interest in the context of prion accumulation and prion related neuroprotection. No human trials have been conducted to date.

Indicas or indica dominat hybrids tend to contain higher CBD:THC ratios when compared to sativa-based plants. Raw, fresh leaf or juice contain high concentrations of CBD in the form of CBD-acid.

EXPLORING MIND–BODY CONSCIOUSNESS

Prion diseases primarily affect the mind, the physical brain and the central nervous system. It is said there comes a time in everybody's life when the prospect of returning to the source begins to be more in the forefront of the mind. There are two ways in which most people approach the inevitable. Either they return the way of the wise wo/man or they return the way of the infant. Prion disease bares similarity to those diseases that revert people into infancy, and this may be reflective of one side of this juncture.

However, in CJD, once symptoms appear, the disease progresses more rapidly than other such diseases, like Alzheimer's, where the degeneration occur over the course of many years.

QUESTIONS

Where am I hopeless or despairing about my place in life?
Where am I helpless in my life?
Where am I refusing to let the world be as it is?
Is there a constructive way to channel my anger at life the way it is?
Why am I ready to throw in the towel?

1 Simon Mead, M.R.C.P., Jerome Whitfield, M.A., Mark Poulter, B.Sc., Paresh Shah, Ph.D., James Uphill, B.Sc., Tracy Campbell, B.Sc., Huda Al-Dujaily, B.Sc., Holger Hummerich, Ph.D., Jon Beck, B.Sc., Charles A. Mein, Ph.D., Claudio Verzilli, Ph.D., John Whittaker, Ph.D., Michael P. Alpers, F.R.S., and John Collinge, F.R.S. *A Novel Protective Prion Protein Variant that Colocalizes with Kuru Exposure.* From the Medical Research Council Prion Unit, Department of Neurodegenerative Disease, University College London Institute of Neurology (S.M., J. Whitfield, M.P., P.S., J.U., T.C., H.A.-D., H.H., J.B., M.P.A., J.C.); the Genome Centre, Barts and the London Queen Mary's School of Medicine and Dentistry, John Vane Science Centre (C.A.M.); and the Department of Epidemiology and Population Health, London School of Hygiene and Tropical Medicine (C.V., J. Whittaker) — all in London; Papua New Guinea Institute of Medical Research, Goroka, Eastern Highlands Province, Papua New Guinea (J. Whitfield, M.P.A.); and the Centre for International Health, Curtin University, Perth, WA, Australia (M.P.A.). N Engl J Med 2009; 361:2056-2065.

2 Llewelyn CA, Hewitt PE, Knight RS, Amar K, Cousens S, Mackenzie J, Will RG (2004) *Possible transmission of variant Creutzfeldt-Jakob disease by blood transfusion.* National Blood Service, Cambridge Centre, Cambridge CB2 2PT, UK. Lancet 363:417–421.

3 Sevda Dirikoc,1 Suzette A. Priola,2 Mathieu Marella,3 Nicole Zsürger,1 and Joëlle Chabry1 *Nonpsychoactive cannabidiol prevents prion accumulation and protects neurons against prion toxicity.* 1Institut de Pharmacologie Moléculaire et Cellulaire, Unité Mixte de Recherche 6097, Centre National de la Recherche Scientifique, 06560 Valbonne, France, 2Laboratory of Persistent Viral Diseases, National Institutes of Health, National Institute of Allergy and Infectious Diseases, Rocky Mountain Laboratories, Hamilton, Montana 59840, and 3Scripps Research Institute, La Jolla, California 92037. J Neurosci. 2007 Sep 5;27(36):9537-44.

4 The United States of America as represented by the Department of Health and Human Services. (Aidan J.

Hampson, Julius Axelrod and Maurizio Grimaldi) Patent No. 09/674028 filed on 02/02/2001. Patent 6630507 issued on October 7, 2003. Estimated expiration date: 2021. *Cannabinoids as antioxidants and neuroprotectants.* http://www.patentstorm.us/patents/6630507.html

5 Sevda Dirikoc,1 Suzette A. Priola,2 Mathieu Marella,3 Nicole Zsurger,1 and Joelle Chabry1. *Nonpsychoactive Cannabidiol Prevents Prion Accumulation and Protects Neurons against Prion Toxicity.* 1 Institut de Pharmacologie Moleculaire et Cellulaire, Unite Mixte de Recherche 6097, Centre National de la Recherche Scientifique, 06560 Valbonne, France, 2 Laboratory of Persistent Viral Diseases, National Institutes of Health, National Institute of Allergy and Infectious Diseases, Rocky Mountain Laboratories, Hamilton, Montana 59840, and 3Scripps Research Institute, La Jolla, California 92037. The Journal of Neuroscience, September 5, 2007 • 27(36):9537–9544

6 Mice were treated intraperitoneally three times per week for the indicated period of time with 200 μl of 20 or 60 mg/kg CBD diluted 1:1:2 in an ethanol/cremophor/NaCl 0.9% mixture. CBD was from GW Pharmaceuticals (Wiltshire, UK), dissolved at 10–2 M in ethanol, and stored at −20°C until use.

Sickle Cell Disease

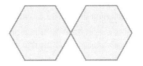

NUMBER OF STUDIES: 2

CHI VALUE: 5

Sickle Cell Disease (SCD) is a genetic illness characterized by 'flawed' red blood cells, which, instead of being round, mimic the shape of a sickle. Most likely, the body originally produced the mutation to protect itself from malaria parasites; now the disease claims responsibility for destroying one's quality of life or even shortening it. SCD is prevalent in descendents from sub-Saharan Africa and other tropical regions where malaria runs rampant. Malaria is a cyclical disease and, in that sense, SCD mirrors the cyclical nature of sickle cell crisis. Carriers of one gene of sickle cell (sickle cell trait) may enjoy some protection from the malaria parasite and avoid SCD all together. However, if both parents carry the sickle cell trait, the chances that their offspring will acquire SCD rises to one in four, and in this unlucky offspring, the disease turns chronic. The expression of the disease exists within a very wide range from relatively mild to moderate and severe. The frequency, intensity, and duration of a sickle cell crisis can also vary tremendously, but usually lasts for about five to seven days.

The disease's symptoms derive from the misshapen red blood cells' inability to carry oxygen and nutrients to the body and to the clumping of cells, which causes occlusions. Resulting symptoms include: anemia, low energy, pain, enlarged spleen, paleness of the skin, itching, infections with fever, rapid heartbeat, shortness of breath, stroke, autosplenectomy (destruction of the spleen), renal failure, and other organ damage. In addition, symptoms may progress to tissue death.

Orthodox treatments include: pain medication, anti-depressants, anti-anxiety medication, blood transfusions, surgery, other emergency care and sometimes bone marrow transplants in children. Although presently orthodox medicine provides no cure, it can diagnose the trait and, thus, give potential future parents the information they need to make informed choices.

CANNABIS AND SICKLE CELL DISEASE

A London study (2005) demonstrated that cannabis relieved pain, depression and anxiety for sickle cell patients.[1] A research team from Minnesota (2010) came to similar conclusions in the course of an animal study. They genetically altered mice to produce human sickle cell hemoglobin while creating an internal environment similar to sickle cell crisis pain. Researchers then studied the effects of morphine and cannabinoids during objectively measurable experiences of pain. Results revealed that both morphine and cannabinoids reduced sickle cell-like pain in the animals.[2] Certainly more studies could provide a better understanding as to why and how cannabinoids reduce the symptoms of SCD.

STUDY SUMMARY:

Drugs	Type of Study	Published Year, Place, and Key Results	CHI
CP 55940	Animal study (mice)	2010 – University of Minnesota. Cannabinoids reduce sickle cell like pain in mice.	2
Cannabis inhalation	Human case study	2005 – London, UK. Reduces pain, anxiety and depression associated with SCD.	3

Total CHI Value   5

STRAIN SPECIFIC CONSIDERATIONS

The drugs tested against SCD in these trials included smoked cannabis and CP 55,940. CP 55,940 is 40 times more potent than Δ9-THC and is extremely psychoactive. CP 55,940 is equally strong at CB1 and CB2 receptors.[3]

THC binds relatively equally to both CB1 and CB2. Sativas or sativa dominant strains generally contain a higher THC:CBD profile.

EXPLORING MIND–BODY CONSCIOUSNESS

Depression and anxiety among sickle cell patients is relatively common. A team of international researchers discovered that both psychological states were associated with an increased intensity and duration of pain on both crisis and non-crisis days when compared to sickle cell patients without anxiety or depression.[4]

The joy of life compares to the flow of blood coursing through the veins. Just as blood nurtures and sustains cellular life, joy feeds and sustains a healthy mind. One's capacity for joy might be destroyed by holding on to beliefs such as "You are no good; you are flawed" or, "there is something wrong with you". Sickle cells and malformed red blood cells are incapable of carrying sufficient nutrients to the body and, thus, cause much suffering.

Furthermore, constantly faced with the threat of another crisis looming somewhere in the near future, anxiety and hopelessness further impact the mental and emotional lives of patients suffering from SCD.

Blood is also related to kin (blood bonds, blood relations with family, tribe or group). SCD is physically hereditary; but since the expression of the disease varies so greatly in duration and intensity, it is likely that non-physical signals such as the impact of deep-seated shame perhaps passed down through the generations may play a role in the severity of SCD.

AGGRAVATING FACTORS

Negative affect such as anxiety and depression.

SUGGESTED BLESSING:

May you find a way to ease depression and diminish anxiety.

May they soothe your pain and aches.

May they elevate your resonance and lighten your mood.

SUGGESTED AFFIRMATION:

May the joy of life be my focus and my nourishment.

May it be a magnet for the miraculous and a lighting rod for the greatest joy of all.

Emotional release work especially related to blood relatives / changing belief(s) that produce anxiety or depression / working towards positive affect.

TAKE NOTICE

ROSEMARY • VANILLA

ROSEMARY: German Commission E approved for: "Supportive therapy circulatory problems."

VANILLA: Researchers at the Children's Hospital of Philadelphia have discovered that vanillin, a dietary compound in vanilla beans, was able to bind with sickle shaped hemoglobin in rodents and, in doing so, improved oxygen transport - a key necessity for reducing symptoms in sickle cell patients. However, since vanillin is rapidly digested before it can reach the bloodstream, scientists are working on man-made intravenous compounds based on the spice.[5]

1 Howard J, Anie KA, Holdcroft A, Korn S, Davies SC. *Cannabis use in SICKLE CELL DISEASE: a questionnaire study*. Department of Haematology, Central Middlesex Hospital, London, UK. jo.howard@nwlh.nhs.uk Br J Haematol 2005;131(1):123-8.

2 Kohli DR, Li Y, Khasabov SG, Gupta P, Kehl LJ, Ericson ME, Nguyen J, Gupta V, Hebbel RP, Simone DA, Gupta K. *Pain-related behaviors and neurochemical alterations in mice expressing sickle hemoglobin: modulation by cannabinoids*. Vascular Biology Center, Division of Hematology, Oncology & Transplantation, Department of Medicine, University of Minnesota, Minneapolis 55455, USA. Blood. 2010 Jul 22;116(3):456-65.

3 Shmist YA, Goncharov I, Eichler M, Shneyvays V, Isaac A, Vogel Z, Shainberg A. *Delta-9-tetrahydrocannabinol protects cardiac cells from hypoxia via CB2 receptor activation and nitric oxide production*. Faculty of Life Sciences, Bar-Ilan University, Ramat-Gan, Israel. Mol Cell Biochem. 2006 Feb;283(1-2):75-83.

4 James L. Levenson, MD, Donna K. McClish, PhD, Bassam A. Dahman, BS, Viktor E. Bovbjerg, PhD, MPH, Vanessa de A. Citero, MD, Lynne T. Penberthy, MD, MPH, Imoigele P. Aisiku, MD, MSCR, John D. Roberts, MD, Susan D. Roseff, MD and Wally R. Smith, MD. *Depression and Anxiety in Adults With Sickle Cell Disease: The PiSCES Project*. Department of Psychiatry, Virginia Commonwealth University, Richmond, Virginia (J.L.L., D.K.M., B.A.D., L.T.P., I.P.A., J.D.R., S.D.R., W.R.S.); Department of Psychology University of Virginia, Charlottesville, Virginia (V.E.B.); and the Department of Psychiatry Universidade Federal de Sao Paulo, Sao Paulo, Brazil (V.A.C.). Psychosomatic Medicine 70:192-196 (2008).

5 Zhang C, Li X, Lian L, Chen Q, Abdulmalik O, Vassilev V, Lai CS, Asakura T. *Anti-sickling effect of MX-1520, a prodrug of vanillin: an in vivo study using rodents*. Division of Hematology, The Children's Hospital of Philadelphia, Philadelphia, PA, USA. Br J Haematol. 2004 Jun;125(6):788-95.

Skin Diseases (in General)

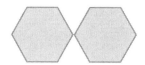 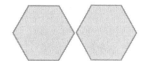

NUMBER OF STUDIES: 4

CHI VALUE: 11

Diseases affecting the skin, hair and nails are generally considered skin diseases. However, a majority of patients who seek treatment from a dermatologist also request cosmetic procedures such as hair removal, hair transplants, mole removal, wrinkle reduction or liposuction. The dermatological treatment options include the three basic tools of western medicine: pharmaceuticals, radiation (including laser, UVB) and surgeries (cryosurgery, mole removal, hair transplants).

THE ENDOCANNABINOID SYSTEM AND SKIN DISEASES

A multi-institutional study (2009) with researchers from Germany, the United States, England and Hungary identified the endocannabinoid system (ECS) in the skin as possible targeted approaches in the treatment of various skin diseases. It concluded that the main function of an endocannabinoid system (ECS) in the skin is to control and balance growth, differentiation (the process of becoming a specific skin cell), and survival of skin cells as well as to produce proper immune responses. Researchers believe that the specific manipulation of the ECS might be beneficial in a multitude of human skin diseases including acne, dermatitis, dry skin, hair loss (alopecia, effluvium), hirsutism (excessive hair growth), itching, seborrhea, skin tumors, pain and psoriasis.[1] (The following chart gives an overview of key findings).

Condition	CB1	CB2
Skin cancer	Up-regulation of both ECS receptors CB1 and CB2 produces suppression of cancer cell growth, angiogenesis and metastasis. Also induces apoptosis (cancer cell death).[2]	
Psoriasis	Up-regulation of both ECS receptors CB1 and CB2 will produce the suppression of keratinocyte proliferation and inflammation.[3]	
Hair Loss	Down-regulation of CB1 stimulates hair growth.[4]	
Hirsutism (Unwanted Hair Growth)	Up-regulation of CB1 produces the suppression of hair growth.[5]	
Seborrhea, Acne		Down-regulation of CB2 produces an inhibition of sebum/lipid production.[6]
Dry Skin		Up-regulation of CB2 increases sebum/lipid production and may remedy dry skin.[7]
Dermatitis (Eczema)	Up-regulation of both ECS CB1 and CB2 receptors produces a suppression of the immune/inflammatory process in cases of dermatitis.[8]	
Systemic Sclerosis (Scleroderma)		Up-regulation of CB2 induces a suppression of the immune/inflammatory process and fibrosis.[9]
Pain, Itching	Up-regulation of CB1 and CB2 reduces pain and itching. Also inhibits transmission of signals in the nervous system.[10]	

A therapeutic up or down regulation could be achieved by using isolated specific cannabinoids (endo- and exo-), by utilizing agonists (drugs that selectively activate CB1 or CB2 receptors) or antagonists (drugs which selectively block one or the other of these receptor types), or by using specific strains known to increase activation of these receptors.

Researchers (2007) from Debrecen, Hungary, discovered that human scalp hair follicles contain both endocannabinoid receptors and endocannabinoids, which were determined to be key players in hair growth regulation. Thus, type and dose specific cannabinoids play a significant role in regulating unwanted hair growth and unwanted hair loss.[11]

Dermatologists are aware of the very limited and often ineffective allopathic options in the treatment of chronic itching. In a case study (2006) from Münster, Germany, scientists learned that a cream containing N-palmitoyl ethanolamine, a fatty acid amide that enhances the action of anandamide, reduced the itching sensation in participating patients on an average of over 80%. The investigating neuro-dermatologists wrote: "Topical cannabinoid agonists represent a new, effective and well-tolerated therapy for refractory itching of various origins. Creams with a higher concentration may be even more effective with broader indications."[12]

A study from Miami, Florida (2002) reported on the symptoms of itching from a different origin in three patients diagnosed with pruritus due to cholestatic liver disease that failed to respond to any other form of therapy. Researchers started them on a cannabis protocol and reported that: "All patients were started on 5 mg of delta-9-THC (Marinol) at bedtime. All three patients reported a decrease in pruritus, marked improvement in sleep, and, eventually were able to return to work. Resolution of depression occurred in two of three. Side effects related to the drug included one patient experiencing a disturbance in coordination. Marinol dosage was decreased to 2.5 mg in this patient with resolution of symptoms. The duration of antipruritic effect was approximately 4-6 hrs in all three patients, suggesting the need for more frequent dosing. Delta-9-tetrahydrocannabinol may be an effective alternative in patients with intractable cholestatic pruritus."[13]

STUDY SUMMARY:

Drugs	Type of Study	Published Year, Place, and Key Results	CHI
ECS and various cannabinoids	Meta-analysis	2009 – Multi-institutional/international study. "…targeted manipulation of the ECS (…) might be beneficial in a multitude of human skin diseases."[14]	4
ECS, anandamide and THC	Laboratory	2007 – Department of Physiology, University of Debrecen, Hungary. Endocannabinoid are present in human hair follicles. CB1 agonists may reduce unwanted hair growth, while CB1 antagonists might counteract hair loss.[15]	1
An emollient cream containing N-palmitoyl ethanolamine	Human Case Study	2006 – Abteilung fur Klinische Neurodermatologie, Klinik und Poliklinik fur Hautkrankheiten, Universitatsklinikum Münster, Germany. Average of 80% reduction in itching during treatment of prurigo, lichen simplex and pruritus.[16]	3
Oral doses of Delta-9-THC 2.5mg to 5mg	Clinical Study (3 patients)	2002 – Department of Medicine, University of Miami, Florida. Decrease in itching, improvement in sleep and resolution of depression in patients with pruritus due to cholestatic liver disease.[17]	3

Total CHI Value   11

STRAIN SPECIFIC CONSIDERATIONS

See individual skin diseases.

EXPLORING MIND–BODY CONSCIOUSNESS

The skin is the largest organ of the body, sensing touch, vibration and temperature. It is semi-permeable in that it prevents fluid loss, and at the same time prevents water from washing out essential nutrients. The skin also absorbs some oxygen and small substances. Furthermore, the skin functions as a first line of defense and is in involved in temperature regulation. It is at once border, boundary and barrier determining where one begins and ends. The skin is associated with self-image, identity and individuality.

Through our skin, we present self-image, identity or individuality to the outside world. The way a person feels about their skin (blemishes) often reveals the inner image they hold of themselves. Feeling ugly, feeling hideous, embarrassed, feeling ashamed or betrayed by one's own body are common emotional themes in the self talk of patients with skin problems. Projecting these feelings onto others, thinking that everybody else feels the same way about their less than perfect skin intensifies these emotional prisons. "If I feel ugly, I look ugly." It's no surprise that acne goes hand in hand with teenagers going through a change of life, body, image and identity. Studies have confirmed that stress increases acne outbreaks.[18]

The emotional stress inflicted by a negative self image constantly reinforced by negative self-talk and internal judgments shows up in body language, facial expressions, complexion, sense of well-being and the way we carry ourselves. Stress reduces the ability of the body to heal itself[19] and worsens overall skin health in general by increasing hormone releases such as epinephrine and the steroid cortisol, which in turn over-stimulate sebaceous glands producing skin eruptions.

Tracing these feelings back to the constricting pattern that comprises a person's self image and replacing it with one that gives rise to a more positive sense of self image can yield positive results in the emotional life and may also balance hormone levels. This increases the effectiveness of whatever healing regimen is engaged.

For more Information, see individual skin diseases. If applicable see – SKIN CANCER (NON-MELANOMA) – MELANOMA (MALIGNANT SKIN CANCER) – VIRAL INFECTIONS (HERPES, KAPOSI'S SARCOMA).

TAKE NOTICE

GENERAL SKIN HEALTH: BUSH TEA • CAYENNE • CAJUPUT • COCOA • COCONUT • GARLIC • GRAINS OF PARADISE • OREGANO • ROSEMARY • TURMERIC

BUSH TEA: This South African herb has been found to contain protective abilities against skin cell mutation.[20]

CAYENNE: Scientists from the 'Big Easy' (2002), probably no strangers to wonderfully spicy foods, have determined that an isolated compound made from cayenne is effective in the laboratory against a variety of fungus, including Candida albicans.[21]

CAJUPUT: Various traditional practitioners use tee tree oil in the treatment of acne, eczema, psoriasis, dandruff, fungal infections and bacterial infections.

Scientists at the Department of Infectious, Parasitic and Immune-mediated Disease in Rome, Italy (2006) isolated a single compound found in tea tree oil believed to be the agent responsible in the destruction of candida albicans fungus (a fungus implicated in vaginal yeast infections).[22]

Another Italian study (2006) found tea tree oil effective on superficial skin infestations, which had been caused by antibacterially resistant strains of staphylococcal bacteria. Tea tree oil is thus an important addition to the limited choices available to patients afflicted with these stubborn and possibly dangerous bacteria.[23]

American doctors routinely prescribe Fluconazole, a pharmacological antifungal agent, to AIDS patients suffering from oral candida albicans (fungal infection) inflammations. However, they found it often ineffective, leaving patients with no relief. In a recent study, Detroit's Wayne State University School of Medicine (2002) scientists discovered that oral solutions of tea tree oil appeared to be effective when Fluconazole failed to work.[24]

COCOA: German scientists at the University Witten-Herdecke (2006) concluded that the long-term ingestion of cocoa with a high content of flavanols provides for several markers of healthy skin: photo protection, improved blood circulation, increased skin density and hydration, and a decrease in skin roughness and scaling.[25] Researchers from Tokyo, Japan, found that cacao bean extract, among other compounds, has protective properties against wrinkles caused by exposure to UV-light.[26]

COCONUT: "In this study from Reykjavík, Iceland researchers discovered in a laboratory experiment that medium chain fatty acids, but especially capric acid ($C_{10}H_{20}O_2$), worked effectively in killing all strains of Neisseria gonorrhea."[27]

Another laboratory study from the island determined how well medium chain fatty acids destroy or inhibit the growth of other groups of bacteria. Both lauric acid and capric acid showed strong antibacterial abilities.[28]

Again, researchers demonstrated another aspect of lauric and capric acids' broad anti-microbial properties in the laboratory; this time against a fungus associated with yeast infections.[29]

Lauric acid and capric acid were also found to effectively inactivate Chlamydia in the laboratory. This suggests that these two fatty acids found in relatively high concentrations in coconut milk and fat may play a role in the prevention of this particular bacterial infection as well.[30]

The authors of a study from Staten Island, U.S., wrote: "Lipids can inactivate enveloped viruses, bacteria, fungi, and protozoa." By adding medium chain fatty acids (MCFA) to HIV-infected blood products, the researchers learned that they could reduce the virus concentration by a very large number. Furthermore, the scientists expect that MCFA "… may potentially be used as combination spermicidal and virucidal agents."[31]

GARLIC: Allicin (allylthiosulfinate, diallyl disulfide-S-monoxide), a potent, well known and researched anti-microbial and anti-fungal is an active ingredient in garlic. A laboratory study (2007) from Ferrara, Italy, determined that concentrations of spray-dried garlic (1.5 g per 10 mL) had the strongest fungicidal reaction of those tested.[32]

GRAINS OF PARADISE: Scientists from Ibadan, Nigeria (2008) explored this spice used healing practices throughout the ages. The spice possesses the ability to stabilize the cell membrane[33] of injured tissue sites, thus reducing the need for reconstruction and speeding healing. Furthermore, scientists laud its strong anti-oxidant properties that enable the body to more effectively scavenge free radicals common in injuries.

OREGANO: Veterinarians from Bologna, Italy (2005) studied the effects of several essential oils, including oil of oregano, against candida fungal infections. They found oregano to have "maximum inhibitory activity,"[34] of which the most active phenol component (acidic chemical compound) was carvacrol.

ROSEMARY: Scientists from Harbin, China (2007) confirmed the anti-microbial activity of the essential oil of rosemary against a variety of bacterial and fungal pathogens, including those of Staphylococcus epidermidis, Escherichia coli and Candida albicans.[35]

An infusion of rosemary leaves is used in Cuba as a tonic for hair.[36]

Rosemary is approved by German Commission E for external use as a supportive therapy for circulatory problems.

TURMERIC: In a meta-study from Dallas, Texas (2007) scientists gave an overview of decades of scientific studies on turmeric. Among the long list of turmeric's potential therapeutic properties: promoter of wound-healing and psoriasis.[37]

1 Tamás Bíró,1 Balázs I. Tóth,1 György Haskó,2 Ralf Paus,3,4 and Pál Pacher5 *The endocannabinoid system of the skin in health and disease: novel perspectives and therapeutic opportunities.* 1Department of Physiology, University of Debrecen, Research Center for Molecular Medicine, Debrecen 4032, Hungary. 2University of Medicine and Dentistry, Department of Surgery, New Jersey Medical School, Newark, NJ 07103, USA.3Department of Dermatology, University Hospital Schleswig-Holstein, University of Lübeck, Lübeck 23538, Germany. 4School of Translational Medicine, University of Manchester, Manchester, M13 9PL, UK. 5Section on Oxidative Stress Tissue Injury, Laboratory of Physiological Studies, National Institutes of Health/NIAAA, Rockville, MD 20892-9413, USA. Trends Pharmacol Sci. 2009 August; 30(8): 411–420.

2 Ibid.

3 Ibid.

4 Ibid.

5 Ibid.

6 Ibid.

7 Ibid.

8 Ibid.

9 Ibid.

10 Ibid.

11 Telek A, Bíró T, Bodó E, Tóth BI, Borbíró I, Kunos G, Paus R. *Inhibition of human hair follicle growth by endo- and exo-cannabinoids.* Department of Physiology, University of Debrecen, Medical and Health Science Center, 4032 Debrecen, Hungary. FASEB J. 2007 Nov;21(13):3534-41.

12 Stander S, Reinhardt HW, Luger TA. *Topical cannabinoid agonists : An effective new possibility for treating chronic pruritus.* [Article in German]. Abteilung fur Klinische Neurodermatologie, Klinik und Poliklinik fur Hautkrankheiten, Universitatsklinikum Munster, Von-Esmarchstrasse 58, 48149 , Munster, sonja.staender@uni-muenster.de. Hautarzt. 2006 Jul 28.

13 Neff GW, O'Brien CB, Reddy KR, Bergasa NV, Regev A, Molina E, Amaro R, Rodriguez MJ, Chase V, Jeffers L, Schiff E. *Preliminary observation with dronabinol in patients with intractable pruritus secondary to cholestatic liver disease.* Department of Medicine, University of Miami, Florida, USA. Am J Gastroenterol. 2002 Aug; 97(8):2117-9.

14 Tamás Bíró,1 Balázs I. Tóth,1 György Haskó,2 Ralf Paus,3,4 and Pál Pacher5 *The endocannabinoid system of the skin in health and disease: novel perspectives and therapeutic opportunities.* 1Department of Physiology, University of Debrecen, Research Center for Molecular Medicine, Debrecen 4032, Hungary. 2University of Medicine and Dentistry, Department of Surgery, New Jersey Medical School, Newark, NJ 07103, USA.3Department of Dermatology, University Hospital Schleswig-Holstein, University of Lübeck, Lübeck 23538, Germany. 4School of Translational Medicine, University of Manchester, Manchester, M13 9PL, UK. 5Section on Oxidative Stress Tissue Injury, Laboratory of Physiological Studies, National Institutes of Health/NIAAA, Rockville, MD 20892-9413, USA. Trends Pharmacol Sci. 2009 August; 30(8): 411–420.

15 Telek A, Bíró T, Bodó E, Tóth BI, Borbíró I, Kunos G, Paus R. *Inhibition of human hair follicle growth by endo- and exo-cannabinoids.* Department of Physiology, University of Debrecen, Medical and Health Science Center, 4032 Debrecen, Hungary. FASEB J. 2007 Nov;21(13):3534-41.

16 Stander S, Reinhardt HW, Luger TA. *Topical cannabinoid agonists : An effective new possibility for treating chronic pruritus.* [Article in German]. Abteilung fur Klinische Neurodermatologie, Klinik und Poliklinik fur Hautkrankheiten, Universitatsklinikum Munster, Von-Esmarchstrasse 58, 48149 , Munster, sonja.staender@uni-muenster.de. Hautarzt. 2006 Jul 28.

17 Neff GW, O'Brien CB, Reddy KR, Bergasa NV, Regev A, Molina E, Amaro R, Rodriguez MJ, Chase V, Jeffers L, Schiff E. *Preliminary observation with dronabinol in patients with intractable pruritus secondary to cholestatic liver disease.* Department of Medicine, University of Miami, Florida, USA. Am J Gastroenterol. 2002 Aug; 97(8):2117-9.

18 Yosipovitch G, Tang M, Dawn AG, Chen M, Goh CL, Huak Y, Seng LF. *Study of psychological stress, sebum production and acne vulgaris in adolescents.* Department of Dermatology, Wake Forest University School of Medicine, Winston-Salem, North Carolina 27157, USA. gyosipov@wfubmc.edu Acta Derm Venereol. 2007;87(2):135-9.

19 Zorrilla EP, Luborsky L, McKay JR, Rosenthal R, Houldin A, Tax A, McCorkle R, Seligman DA, Schmidt K. *The relationship of depression and stressors to immunological assays: a meta-analytic review.* University of Pennsylvania, Philadelphia, Pennsylvania 19104, USA. Brain Behav Immun. 2001 Sep;15(3):199-226.

20 Marnewick J, Joubert E, Joseph S, Swanevelder S, Swart P, Gelderblom W. *Inhibition of tumour promotion in mouse skin by extracts of rooibos (Aspalathus linearis) and honeybush (Cyclopia intermedia), unique South African herbal teas.* PROMEC Unit, Medical Research Council, P.O. Box 19070, Tygerberg 7505, South Africa. Cancer Lett. 2005 Jun 28;224(2):193-202.

21 De Lucca AJ, Bland JM, Vigo CB, Cushion M, Selitrennikoff CP, Peter J, Walsh TJ. *CAY-I, a fungicidal saponin from Capsicum sp. fruit.* Southern Regional Research Center, Agricultural Research Service, US Department of Agriculture, New Orleans, LA 70124, USA. Med Mycol. 2002 Apr;40(2):131-7.

22 Mondello F, De Bernardis F, Girolamo A, Cassone A, Salvatore G. *In vivo activity of terpinen-4-ol, the main bioactive component of Melaleuca alternifolia Cheel (tea tree) oil against azole-susceptible and -resistant human pathogenic Candida species.* Department of Infectious, Parasitic and Immune-mediated Diseases, Istituto Superiore di Sanità, Viale Regina Elena 299, 00161 Rome, Italy. BMC Infect Dis. 2006 Nov 3;6:158.

23 Ferrini AM, Mannoni V, Aureli P, Salvatore G, Piccirilli E, Ceddia T, Pontieri E, Sessa R, Oliva B. *Melaleuca alternifolia essential oil possesses potent anti-staphylococcal activity extended to strains resistant to antibiotics.* Istituto Superiore di Sanita, National Centre for Food Quality, Rome, Italy. Int J Immunopathol Pharmacol. 2006 Jul-Sep;19(3):539-44.

24 Vazquez JA, Zawawi AA. *Efficacy of alcohol-based and alcohol-free melaleuca oral solution for the treatment of fluconazole-refractory oropharyngeal candidiasis in patients with AIDS.* Division of Infectious Diseases, Wayne State University School of Medicine, Detroit, Michigan, USA. HIV Clin Trials. 2002 Sep-Oct;3(5):379-85.

25 Heinrich U, Neukam K, Tronnier H, Sies H, Stahl W. *Long-term ingestion of high flavanol cocoa provides photoprotection against UV-induced erythema and improves skin condition in women.* Institut für Experimentelle Dermatologie, Universität Witten-Herdecke, Germany. J Nutr. 2006 Jun;136(6):1565-9.

26 Mitani H, Ryu A, Suzuki T, Yamashita M, Arakane K, Koide C. *Topical application of plant extracts containing xanthine derivatives can prevent UV-induced wrinkle formation in hairless mice.* Photodermatol Photoimmunol Photomed. 2007 Apr-Jun;23(2-3):86-94.

27 Bergsson G, Steingrímsson O, Thormar H. *In vitro susceptibilities of Neisseria gonorrhoeae to fatty acids and monoglycerides.* Institute of Biology, University of Iceland. gudmunb@rhi.hi.is Antimicrob Agents Chemother. 1999 Nov;43(11):2790-2.

28 Bergsson G, Arnfinnsson J, Steingrímsson O, Thormar H. *Killing of Gram-positive cocci by fatty acids and monoglycerides.* Institute of Biology, University of Iceland, Reykjavik. gudmunb@hi.is APMIS. 2001 Oct;109(10):670-8.

29 Bergsson G, Arnfinnsson J, Steingrímsson O , Thormar H. *In vitro killing of Candida albicans by fatty acids and monoglycerides.* Institute of Biology, University of Iceland, Reykjavik, Iceland. gudmunb@hi.is Antimicrob Agents Chemother. 2001 Nov; 45(11):3209-12.

30 Bergsson G, Arnfinnsson J, Karlsson SM, Steingrímsson O, Thormar H. *In vitro inactivation of Chlamydia trachomatis by fatty acids and monoglycerides.* Institute of Biology, University of Iceland, Reykjavik, Iceland. Antimicrob Agents Chemother. 1998 Sep;42(9):2290-4.

31 Isaacs CE, Kim KS, Thormar H. *Inactivation of enveloped viruses in human bodily fluids by purified lipids.* Department of Developmental Biochemistry, New York State Institute for Basic Research in Developmental Disabilities, Staten Island 10314. Ann N Y Acad Sci. 1994 Jun 6;724:457-64.

32 Tedeschi P, Maietti A, Boggian M, Vecchiati G, Brandolini V. *Fungitoxicity of lyophilized and spray-dried garlic extracts.* Department of Pharmaceutical Science, University of Ferrara, Ferrara, Italy. J Environ Sci Health B. 2007 Sep;42(7):795-9.

33 10 Umukoro S, Ashorobi BR. *Further pharmacological studies on aqueous seed extract of Aframomum melegueta in rats.* Department of Pharmacology and Therapeutics, College of Medicine, University of Ibadan, Nigeria. J Ethnopharmacol. 2008 Feb 12;115(3):489-93.

34 Tampieri MP, Galuppi R, Macchioni F, Carelle MS, Falcioni L, Cioni PL, Morelli I. *The inhibition of Candida albicans by selected essential oils and their major components.* Dipartimento di Sanità Pubblica Veterinaria e Patologia Animale, Università di Bologna, Italy. Mycopathologia. 2005 Apr;159(3):339-45.

35 Fu Y, Zu Y, Chen L, Shi X, Wang Z, Sun S, Efferth T. *Antimicrobial activity of clove and rosemary essential oils alone and in combination.* Key Laboratory of Forest Plant Ecology, Ministry of Education, Northeast Forestry University, Harbin 150040, P. R. China. Phytother Res. 2007 Jun 11.

36 *Therapeutic Guide to Plant Pharmaceuticals and Honey Pharmaceuticals (Guia Terapeutica Dispensarial de Fitofarmacos y Apifarmacos* - Ministerio de Salud Publica, Ciudad de La Habana - Republica de Cuba 1992). Cuban Ministry of Public Health, Havana.

37 Goel A, Kunnumakkara AB, Aggarwal BB. *Curcumin as "Curecumin": From kitchen to clinic.* Gastrointestinal Cancer Research Laboratory, Department of Internal Medicine, Charles A. Sammons Cancer Center and Baylor Research Institute, Baylor University Medical Center, Dallas, TX, United States. Biochem Pharmacol. 2007 Aug 19.

Skin Diseases
Acne

Acne is a common skin disease affecting both genders during puberty. An increase in androgen hormones contributes to an increase in sebaceous gland activity producing sebum (oily/waxy substance), which when not properly discharged through the pores can cause back ups, inflammation and pimples. Allopathic treatment consists of topical pharmaceuticals, pills, laser therapy, phototherapy and sometimes-localized surgical procedures. No allopathic cure for acne exists.

THE ENDOCANNABINOID SYSTEM AND ACNE

Condition	CB1	CB2
Acne		Down-regulation of CB2 will produce an inhibition of sebum/lipid production.[1]

STRAIN SPECIFIC CONSIDERATIONS

Not applicable.

EXPLORING MIND–BODY CONSCIOUSNESS

SUGGESTED BLESSING:

May you relax the stranglehold of 'feeling ugly,' for a moment so that you can fully accept yourself as a growing and maturing human being.

The results of a large human study conducted on 94 teenagers concluded that stress-related inflammation played a significant role in breakouts.[2]

Becoming a grown-up is built-in by nature. Adolescence is the process and the passage from childhood to a fully sexually capable body induced by gender specific hormonal changes. These changes force an often-dramatic change in physical image and intense internal mental and emotional landscapes, which are often difficult to embrace and own. The new and developing self-image is often disliked and rejected. For many, feeling ugly becomes a reality in the emerging pimples.

AGGRAVATING FACTORS

SUGGESTED AFFIRMATION:

I have the capacity to define and find what is unique and beautiful inside of me.

Stress.

HEALING FACTORS

Positive coping mechanisms.

1 Tamás Bíró,1 Balázs I. Tóth,1 György Haskó,2 Ralf Paus,3,4 and Pál Pacher5 *The endocannabinoid system of the skin in health and disease: novel perspectives and therapeutic opportunities.* 1Department of Physiology, University of Debrecen, Research Center for Molecular Medicine, Debrecen 4032, Hungary. 2University of Medicine and Dentistry, Department of Surgery, New Jersey Medical School, Newark, NJ 07103, USA.3Department of Dermatology, University Hospital Schleswig-Holstein, University of Lübeck, Lübeck 23538, Germany. 4School of Translational Medicine, University of Manchester, Manchester, M13 9PL, UK. 5Section on Oxidative Stress Tissue Injury, Laboratory of Physiological Studies, National Institutes of Health/NIAAA, Rockville, MD 20892-9413, USA. Trends Pharmacol Sci. 2009 August; 30(8): 411–420.

2 Gil Yosipovitch, Mark Tang, Aerlyn G. Dawn, Mark Chen, Chee Leok Goh, Yiong Huak Chan and Lim Fong Seng. Study of Psychological Stress, Sebum Production and Acne Vulgaris in Adolescents. Acta Dermato-Venereologica Vol. 87/2007 Iss. 2/March pp. 135-139.

Skin Diseases
Dermatitis (Eczema)

Dermatitis is an inflammation of the skin believed to be caused in part by coming in contact with irritants. It may also be due to underlying causes from certain diseases or allergic sensitivities. Depending on the underlying cause, western tradition uses topical and systemic pharmaceuticals such as steroids or antihistamines to reduce symptoms.

THE ENDOCANNABINOID SYSTEM AND ECZEMA

Condition	CB1 and CB2
Dermatitis (Eczema)	Up-regulation of both ECS receptors CB1 and CB2 produces a suppression of the immune/inflammatory process in cases of dermatitis.[1]

STRAIN SPECIFIC CONSIDERATIONS

THC binds with both CB1 and CB2 relatively equally. Sativas and sativa dominant strains tend to present with a higher THC:CBD ratio.

EXPLORING MIND–BODY CONSCIOUSNESS

Grace and Graham wrote: "Eczema occurred when an individual felt that he was being interfered with or prevented from doing something, and could in no way deal with the frustration. … His preoccupation was with the interference and the person or things thwarting him…" Typical statements (of 27 patients with eczema) were: "I want to make my mother understand but I can't. … I couldn't do what I wanted to but there wasn't anything I could do about it. … I was upset because it interfered with what I wanted to do. … I felt terribly frustrated." The researcher also noted themes of embarrassment and self-aggression in cases with eczema.[2]

QUESTIONS

What is the irritation that has gotten under the outer layer of your skin?
What is inflaming you?
What are you extra sensitive about?
Where are you really thin-skinned?

1 Tamás Bíró,1 Balázs I. Tóth,1 György Haskó,2 Ralf Paus,3,4 and Pál Pacher5 *The endocannabinoid system of the skin in health and disease: novel perspectives and therapeutic opportunities.* 1Department of Physiology, University of Debrecen, Research Center for Molecular Medicine, Debrecen 4032, Hungary. 2University of Medicine and Dentistry, Department of Surgery, New Jersey Medical School, Newark, NJ 07103, USA.3Department of Dermatology, University Hospital Schleswig-Holstein, University of Lübeck, Lübeck 23538, Germany. 4School of Translational Medicine, University of Manchester, Manchester, M13 9PL, UK. 5Section on Oxidative Stress Tissue Injury, Laboratory of Physiological Studies, National Institutes of Health/NIAAA, Rockville, MD 20892-9413, USA. Trends Pharmacol Sci. 2009 August; 30(8): 411–420.

2 William J. Grace, M.D. and David T. Graham, M.D. *Relationship of Specific Attitudes and Emotions to Certain Bodily Diseases.* Dept. of Medicine, of the New York Hospital-Cornell Medical Center. Psychosomatic Medicine July 1, 1952 vol. 14 no. 4 243-251.

Skin Diseases
Hair Growth – Unwanted (Hirsutism)

While male pattern hair growth in women is not an illness, it can be a great cosmetic and psychological concern. Western medicine considers an increased presence of male hormones or higher than normal levels of the hormone insulin to be causative agents. No allopathic cure is available, but suggested treatment includes pharmaceuticals and hair removal techniques.

THE ENDOCANNABINOID SYSTEM AND HIRSUTISM

Condition	CB1	CB2
Hirsutism	Up-regulation of CB1 will produce the suppression of hair growth.[1]	

STRAIN SPECIFIC CONSIDERATIONS

THC binds with both CB1 and CB2 relatively equally. Sativas and sativa dominant strains tend to present with a higher THC:CBD ratio.

EXPLORING MIND–BODY CONSCIOUSNESS

SUGGESTED BLESSING:

May you realize the power, strength and confidence of your animus (inner male energy) and let it inform your will and action in a balanced and harmonious way.

A study comparing the emotional behavior of 30 patients dealing with hirsutism with an equal number of non-hirsute women discovered that hirsute women demonstrated greater tendency to exhibit severe and sudden shifts in moods as well as display significantly more hostile and irritable emotions.[2] The appearance of male pattern hair growth in women may evokes intense emotional reactions in some while others may find that displaying a more physically male image is to their liking. Hirsutism is often discovered paired with higher than normal levels of male hormones. While some women have dealt with hirsutism since puberty (hormonal changes), many discover hairs in new places during menopause (hormonal changes). Hirsutism is primarily a cosmetic issue unless it interferes with one's body image and identity.

TAKE NOTICE

FENNEL

SUGGESTED AFFIRMATION:

I can handle what life brings my way.

I protect myself by making sure my feelings are heard and respected.

FENNEL: Fennel has been used as an estrogenic agent by traditional healers for centuries. Now scientists from Shiraz University, Iran, are looking at fennel's ability to help women who have developed hirsutism (growing hair like a male), even though they have normal menstrual cycles and normal levels of sex hormones. Researchers noted significant male type hair growth reduction when compared to the placebo. Of the two tested formulas, (1% and 2%) 2% topical fennel extract proved most effective.[3]

1 Tamás Bíró,1 Balázs I. Tóth,1 György Haskó,2 Ralf Paus,3,4 and Pál Pacher5 *The endocannabinoid system of the skin in health and disease: novel perspectives and therapeutic opportunities.* 1Department of Physiology, University of Debrecen, Research Center for Molecular Medicine, Debrecen 4032, Hungary. 2University of Medicine and Dentistry, Department of Surgery, New Jersey Medical School, Newark, NJ 07103, USA.3Department of Dermatology, University Hospital Schleswig-Holstein, University of Lübeck, Lübeck 23538, Germany. 4School of Translational Medicine, University of Manchester, Manchester, M13 9PL, UK. 5Section on Oxidative Stress Tissue Injury, Laboratory of Physiological Studies, National Institutes of Health/NIAAA, Rockville, MD 20892-9413, USA. Trends Pharmacol Sci. 2009 August; 30(8): 411–420.

2 Fava GA, Grandi S, Savron G, Bartolucci G, Santarsiero G, Trombini G, Orlandi C. *Psychosomatic assessment of hirsute women.* Department of Psychology, University of Bologna, Italy. Psychother Psychosom. 1989;51(2):96-100.

3 Javidnia K, Dastgheib L, Mohammadi Samani S, Nasiri A. *Antihirsutism activity of Fennel (fruits of Foeniculum vulgare) extract.* A double-blind placebo controlled study. Faculty of Pharmacy, Shiraz University of Medical Sciences, Shiraz, Iran. javidniak@sums.ac.ir Phytomedicine. 2003;10(6-7):455-8.

Skin Diseases
Hair Loss (Baldness)

Until relatively recently, the allopathic tradition believed that male pattern baldness occurred in 3 out of 4 cases due to a gene passed down from the maternal father. Environmental signals, in addition to genetic influences, are thought to induce hormonal changes in the remainder. The role of a male sex hormone named dihydrotestosterone (DHT), is implicated but not fully understood. No allopathic cure is available. Some pharmaceutical and surgical procedures have been used with limited success.

THE ENDOCANNABINOID SYSTEM AND BALDNESS

Condition	CB1	CB2
Hair Loss	Down-regulation of CB1 stimulates hair growth.[1]	

STRAIN SPECIFIC CONSIDERATIONS

Not applicable.

EXPLORING MIND–BODY CONSCIOUSNESS

Mythology associates hair with power, as in the biblical story of Samson and Delilah. Samson loses his supernatural strength after Delilah cuts off his hair while he sleeps. Hair is also connected to the body beautiful, virility, youthfulness, and sensuality. In the western world, 'long hair' has recently come to be associated with rebellion from 'old' and 'outdated values.' Haircuts, hair colors and styles can communicate and project a strong meaning just as hair loss due to trauma, surgery or chemotherapy may elicit intense feelings. While baldness is not a disease, it can have psychological consequences and can contribute to a negative self-image.

1 Tamás Bíró,1 Balázs I. Tóth,1 György Haskó,2 Ralf Paus,3,4 and Pál Pacher5 *The endocannabinoid system of the skin in health and disease: novel perspectives and therapeutic opportunities.* 1Department of Physiology, University of Debrecen, Research Center for Molecular Medicine, Debrecen 4032, Hungary. 2University of Medicine and Dentistry, Department of Surgery, New Jersey Medical School, Newark, NJ 07103, USA.3Department of Dermatology, University Hospital Schleswig-Holstein, University of Lübeck, Lübeck 23538, Germany. 4School of Translational Medicine, University of Manchester, Manchester, M13 9PL, UK. 5Section on Oxidative Stress Tissue Injury, Laboratory of Physiological Studies, National Institutes of Health/NIAAA, Rockville, MD 20892-9413, USA. Trends Pharmacol Sci. 2009 August; 30(8): 411–420.

Skin Diseases
Itching (Pruritis)

The itch. While physiologically similar to the experience of pain, the response to an itch is not to withdraw, but rather to scratch. Itching can be produced externally by temperature variations, slight electrical stimulation, parasites (lice, scabies) and contact with certain substances (natural or synthetic). Itching only occurs superficially on the outer layers of the skin.

Internal causes may include: psychological origins (stress, hallucinations), brain tumors, multiple sclerosis, neuropathies, diabetes, certain hereditary causes, cholestatic liver disease, skin diseases (contagious or non-contagious), nerve damage, inflammation, wound healing (skin trauma or burns), hives, allergic reactions, certain medication (pharmaceutical and holistic), fungus, parasites, eczema or hormonal changes such as occur during menopause.

Orthodox dermatologists rely on internal and topical pharmaceuticals to reduce and suppress the itch. Common anti-itch medications include antihistamines and steroids. When these do not work, the itch continues affecting quality of life and contributing to frustration, hopelessness and depression.

THE ENDOCANNABINOID SYSTEM AND ITCHING

Condition	CB1 and CB2
Pain, Itching	Up-regulation of CB1 and CB2 produces a reduction of pain and itch by suppressing pain- and itch-producing substances as well as inhibits transmission of signals in the nervous system.[1]

STRAIN SPECIFIC CONSIDERATIONS

Both indica and sativa strains contain CB1 and CB2 activating cannabinoids. Future studies may confirm positive reports of cannabis from numerous cannabis-using pruritis sufferers who prefer a topical oil of their choice infused with whole plant constituents to the use of inhaled cannabis

EXPLORING MIND–BODY CONSCIOUSNESS

Similar to the indecision underlying some neck problems, chronic complaints of itching may also represent contradicting or conflicting desires. On one end of the spectrum, the sensation of an itch or tickling is a pleasurable and even sensual experience. On the other end, itching (especially the incessant type) can make someone want to jump out of his skin. In the latter case, scratching might produce temporary relief, but as soon as one stops scratching, the itch returns with a vengeance. Furthermore, the skin can only take so much scratching before it breaks and pain replaces the sensation. In some cases, patients prefer the pain to the itch and can scratch until bloody.

"Urticaria occurred when an individual saw himself as being mistreated. This mistreatment might take the form of something said to him or something done to him. He was preoccupied entirely with what was happening to him, and was not

> **SUGGESTED BLESSING:**
>
> *May you hold and respect contradictory desires until something completely new emerges, to reolve the conflict.*

thinking of retaliation or of any solution of his problem. Typical statements were: "They did a lot of things to me and I couldn't do anything about it." "I was taking a beating." "My mother was hammering on me." "The boss cracked a whip on me." "My fiancée knocked me down and walked all over me but what could I do?"[2]

It is interesting to note that as with yawning, itching can be psychologically contagious, as evident by the observation that when one person in a group begins scratching others will soon follow their example.

QUESTIONS

Where do I see myself as mistreated or judged?
In what ways do I feel like a victim?
What am I itching to get away from?
What has gotten under my skin?
What is driving me nuts?
Do I have paradoxical (conflicting) desires?
What am I itching to change?
Where am I indecisive?
Do I want to control an irritation even if it hurts?

AGGRAVATING FACTORS

Feeling mistreated or judged / indecisiveness / feeling victimized / using pain to control an irritation.

HEALING FACTORS

Gratitude and the employment of forgiveness / making a list of priorities / sheding any victim self-image and instead developing a sense of empowerment / accepting or embracing a present irritation.

1 Tamás Bíró,1 Balázs I. Tóth,1 György Haskó,2 Ralf Paus,3,4 and Pál Pacher5 *The endocannabinoid system of the skin in health and disease: novel perspectives and therapeutic opportunities.* 1Department of Physiology, University of Debrecen, Research Center for Molecular Medicine, Debrecen 4032, Hungary. 2University of Medicine and Dentistry, Department of Surgery, New Jersey Medical School, Newark, NJ 07103, USA.3Department of Dermatology, University Hospital Schleswig-Holstein, University of Lübeck, Lübeck 23538, Germany. 4School of Translational Medicine, University of Manchester, Manchester, M13 9PL, UK. 5Section on Oxidative Stress Tissue Injury, Laboratory of Physiological Studies, National Institutes of Health/NIAAA, Rockville, MD 20892-9413, USA. Trends Pharmacol Sci. 2009 August; 30(8): 411–420.

2 William J. Grace, M.D. and David T. Graham, M.D. *Relationship of Specific Attitudes and Emotions to Certain Bodily Diseases.* Dept. of Medicine, of the New York Hospital-Cornell Medical Center. Psychosomatic Medicine July 1, 1952 vol. 14 no. 4 243-251.

Skin Diseases
Psoriasis

In the allopathic tradition, psoriasis is a chronic skin disease in which skin cells divide too rapidly, build up and cause red and white, scaly looking skin surfaces. While psoriasis can affect any area of the skin, it is often found on the elbows and knees. No allopathic cure is available. Management consists of topical medications, systemic pharmaceuticals, ultra-violet light therapy, and nutritional supplements.

THE ENDOCANNABINOID SYSTEM AND PSORIASIS

Condition	CB1 and CB2
Psoriasis	Up-regulation of both ECS receptors CB1 and CB2 produces suppression of keratinocyte proliferation and inflammation.[1]

STRAIN SPECIFIC CONSIDERATIONS

THC binds with both CB1 and CB2 relatively equally. Sativas and sativa dominant strains tend to present with a higher THC:CBD ratio.

EXPLORING MIND–BODY CONSCIOUSNESS

Constantly anticipation pain or hurt may play out on the physical stage. A cushiony build-up and thickening of the skin may occur. Areas of the body especially vulnerable are the knees and elbows, which during a fall, are used to shield more vital body parts from damage. However, by becoming more thick-skinned, the affected area also loses sensitivity and either becomes numb or itchy, painful even inflamed.

Based on the chronic expectancy of pain, shame and hurt, psoriasis patients might feel overly vulnerable. They may respond by being overly numb and aggressive in an attempt to compensate. Their projected fears may impact their dealing with others and so become self-fulfilling prophecies.

By releasing chronic anxiety with its anticipation of hurt, shame and pain and replacing underlying beliefs that constantly feed that anxiety, the patient can take responsibility for his emotional reality. He may then more easily shift from the physical arena to a mental-emotional arena, informed by a positive self-image. This shift can remove stressors and allow whatever regimen the patient chooses to be more effective in achieving a lasting cure.

TAKE NOTICE

TURMERIC

TURMERIC: In a meta-study, scientists gave an overview of decades of scientific studies on turmeric. They summarized a long list of turmeric's potential therapeutic propertie and noted is a therapeutic agent in psoriasis.[2]

SUGGESTED BLESSING:

May our flowers help you to relax and discover a healthy and balanced response to the anxieties of life.

SUGGESTED AFFIRMATION:

Anxiety is a part of life. I can learn to define and embrace anticipated feelings and emotions with confidence.

1 Tamás Bíró,1 Balázs I. Tóth,1 György Haskó,2 Ralf Paus,3,4 and Pál Pacher5 *The endocannabinoid system of the skin in health and disease: novel perspectives and therapeutic opportunities.* 1Department of Physiology, University of Debrecen, Research Center for Molecular Medicine, Debrecen 4032, Hungary. 2University of Medicine and Dentistry, Department of Surgery, New Jersey Medical School, Newark, NJ 07103, USA.3Department of Dermatology, University Hospital Schleswig-Holstein, University of Lübeck, Lübeck 23538, Germany. 4School of Translational Medicine, University of Manchester, Manchester, M13 9PL, UK. 5Section on Oxidative Stress Tissue Injury, Laboratory of Physiological Studies, National Institutes of Health/NIAAA, Rockville, MD 20892-9413, USA. Trends Pharmacol Sci. 2009 August; 30(8): 411–420.

2 Aggarwal BB, Kumar A, Bharti AC. *Anticancer potential of curcumin: preclinical and clinical studies.* Cytokine Research Section, Department of Bioimmunotherapy, University of Texas M. D. Anderson Cancer Center, 1515 Holcombe Boulevard, Box 143, Houston, TX, USA. Anticancer Research. 2003 Jan-Feb;23(1A):363-98.

Skin Diseases
Seborrhea

Seborrhea is an inflammation of the skin. It appears often in areas rich with sebaceous glands such as the face, chest, and the upper back or anywhere skin folds produce skin-to-skin contact. In the western tradition, the causes are not currently known but research has implicated stress as a possible contributing factor.[1] No allopathic cure is available. Treatment consists of using topical or systemic pharmaceuticals.

THE ENDOCANNABINOID SYSTEM AND SEBORRHEA

Condition	CB1	CB2
Seborrhea		Down-regulation of CB2 would produce an inhibition of sebum/lipid production.[2]

STRAIN SPECIFIC CONSIDERATIONS

Not applicable.

EXPLORING MIND–BODY CONSCIOUSNESS

The skin is inflamed similarly to that of dermatitis but in deeper layers. Stress is a known contributing factor in the development of seborrhea.[3]

QUESTIONS

What is the irritation that has gotten under the deeper layers of my skin?
What is deeply irritating?

1 Schwartz RA, Janusz CA, Janniger CK. *Seborrheic dermatitis: an overview.* University of Medicine and Dentistry at New Jersey-New Jersey Medical School, Newark 07103, USA. roschwar@cal.berkeley.edu Am Fam Physician. 2006 Jul 1;74(1):125-30.

2 Tamás Bíró,1 Balázs I. Tóth,1 György Haskó,2 Ralf Paus,3,4 and Pál Pacher5 *The endocannabinoid system of the skin in health and disease: novel perspectives and therapeutic opportunities.* 1Department of Physiology, University of Debrecen, Research Center for Molecular Medicine, Debrecen 4032, Hungary. 2University of Medicine and Dentistry, Department of Surgery, New Jersey Medical School, Newark, NJ 07103, USA.3Department of Dermatology, University Hospital Schleswig-Holstein, University of Lübeck, Lübeck 23538, Germany. 4School of Translational Medicine, University of Manchester, Manchester, M13 9PL, UK. 5Section on Oxidative Stress Tissue Injury, Laboratory of Physiological Studies, National Institutes of Health/NIAAA, Rockville, MD 20892-9413, USA. Trends Pharmacol Sci. 2009 August; 30(8): 411–420.

3 Schwartz RA, Janusz CA, Janniger CK. *Seborrheic dermatitis: an overview.* University of Medicine and Dentistry at New Jersey-New Jersey Medical School, Newark 07103, USA. roschwar@cal.berkeley.edu Am Fam Physician. 2006 Jul 1;74(1):125-30.

Skin Diseases
Systemic Sclerosis

Orthodox medicine remains unclear as to the causes of this skin disease. Symptoms may include tough, tight and hard skin, discolorations or tight facial tone. Possible culprits considered include irritants, microbes, or an autoimmune response where the body considers certain skin cells foreign objects and attempts to eliminate them. For many patients, no allopathic cure is available. Managing treatments include topical and systemic pharmaceuticals.

THE ENDOCANNABINOID SYSTEM AND SYSTEMIC SCLEROSIS

Condition	CB1	CB2
Systemic Sclerosis (Scleroderma)		Up-regulation of CB2 would induce a suppression of the immune/inflammatory process and fibrosis.[1]

STRAIN SPECIFIC CONSIDERATIONS

Indicas and indica dominant hybrids tend to present with a lower THC:CBD profile, thus favoring up-regulation of CB2.

EXPLORING MIND–BODY CONSCIOUSNESS

The word sclero- in sclerosis or scleroderma is derived from the Greek word for hard. Tough, thick skin and stone-faced or leathery facial expressions may reflect a belief system in which life is perceived as constantly dangerous and thus requiring a thick skin. Furthermore, emotional vulnerability displayed in facial expressions must be hidden behind a mask because it is seen as a liability rather than an asset.

1 Tamás Bíró,1 Balázs I. Tóth,1 György Haskó,2 Ralf Paus,3,4 and Pál Pacher5 *The endocannabinoid system of the skin in health and disease: novel perspectives and therapeutic opportunities.* 1Department of Physiology, University of Debrecen, Research Center for Molecular Medicine, Debrecen 4032, Hungary. 2University of Medicine and Dentistry, Department of Surgery, New Jersey Medical School, Newark, NJ 07103, USA.3Department of Dermatology, University Hospital Schleswig-Holstein, University of Lübeck, Lübeck 23538, Germany. 4School of Translational Medicine, University of Manchester, Manchester, M13 9PL, UK. 5Section on Oxidative Stress Tissue Injury, Laboratory of Physiological Studies, National Institutes of Health/NIAAA, Rockville, MD 20892-9413, USA. Trends Pharmacol Sci. 2009 August; 30(8): 411–420.

Vomiting (in General)

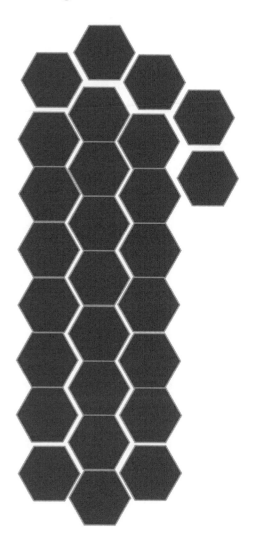

COMBINED NUMBER OF STUDIES: 27

COMBINED CHI VALUE: 111

Vomiting involves involuntary but coordinated contractions of the stomach, respiratory and esophageal muscles to forcefully eject the stomach's contents through the mouth or nose. Vomiting may occur as an autonomic response to the body's detection of poisons. Vomiting may also be induced voluntarily by stimulating the gag reflex through touch to the uvula or by taking an emetic (a substance which induces vomiting such as ipecac). Thus, vomiting can be a self-preservation mechanism; a self-induced evacuation of stomach content, or brought on by disease or injury.

For MORNING SICKNESS see OBGYN (NUMBER OF STUDIES 1, CHI VALUE 3)

Vomiting
Motion Sickness

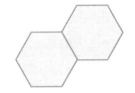

NUMBER OF STUDIES: 2

CHI VALUE: 4

Seasickness, airsickness and carsickness are associated with nausea, vomiting, dizziness and vertigo. Motion sickness occurs due to discord between the movements perceived by the eyes versus those perceived by the inner ear. If this conflict finds no resolution, nausea may progress to vomiting. An estimated 7 - 28% of travelers experience acute motion sickness.[1]

CANNABIS AND MOTION SICKNESS

While numerous studies elucidate the anti-emetic properties of cannabis, the Bradford study (2008) discovered that the cannabinoid THC prevented specific motion-induced nausea and vomiting in animals.

A multi-institutional German study (2010) on human subjects further revealed that cannabinoid-receptor (CB1) expression was significantly lower in subjects who suffered from motion sickness compared to those who felt fine indicating a relationship between reduced endocannabinoid activity and motion sickness. By extension, these discoveries represent a new possibility for treating aspects of motion sickness, mental stress, physical nausea and vomiting.

STUDY SUMMARY:

Drugs	Type of Study	Published Year, Place, and Key Results	CHI
ECS (CB1 and CB2). Anandamide	21 healthy, male volunteers	2010 – Multi-institutional German research group. CB1 expression in leucocytes 4 h after the experiment was significantly lower in volunteers with motion sickness than in participants without N&V. Anandamide levels fell in subjects who got sick but rose in subjects who felt fine.[4]	3
Cannabidiol (CBD 0.5, 1, 2, 5, 10, 20 and 40 mg/kg) Delta(9)-tetrahydro-cannabinol (THC 0.5, 3, 5 and 10 mg/kg)	Animal study (Asian house Shrew, lat. S. murinus)	2008 – The School of Pharmacy, University of Bradford, Bradford, West Yorkshire, UK. THC prevented motion induced vomiting while CBD did not.[5]	1

Total CHI Value 4

STRAIN SPECIFIC CONSIDERATIONS

The cannabinoid studies on motion sickness employed anandamide, CBD and

THC. Anandamide and THC bind with CB1 and CB2 relatively equally. CBD tends to favor CB2 expression.

Sativa and sativa dominant strains tend to contain a higher THC:CBD ratio.

EXPLORING MIND–BODY CONSCIOUSNESS

Grace and Graham wrote: "Nausea and vomiting occurred when an individual was thinking of something which he wished had never happened. He was preoccupied with the mistake he had made, rather than with what he should have done instead. Usually he felt responsible for what happened." Typical statements: "I wish it hadn't happened. … I was sorry I did it. … I wish things were the way they were before. … I made a mistake. … I shouldn't have listened to him."[2] The authors concluded that: "Vomiting is a way of undoing something which has been done. It thus corresponds with the patients' wishes to restore things to their original situation, as if nothing has ever happened."[3]

The part of the human physiology responsible for producing motion-induced nausea and vomiting is an involuntary mechanism. This particular context may be indicative of fear as a response to mismatching or opposing experiences beyond one's control.

Suddenly, the security that comes from feeling solid ground under one's feet disappears, replaced by the motion of the sea or by riding in a car down the serpentine roads of the Swiss Alps. Often the person at the helm of the sea vessel or behind the wheel of the car firmly in control of direction does not experience motion sickness to the same degree (or at all) as their passengers do.

NASA trains astronauts in parabolic flight maneuvers, in which temporary (about 30 sec.) weightlessness is achieved by flying an airplane following an elliptic flight pattern parallel to the earth. This simulation is nicknamed "the vomit comet". Roughly two-thirds of all participants experience degrees of nausea or vomiting. Researchers blame anxiety, or the anticipation of hitherto unknown sensations beyond one's control for this response.

Several factors point to the difference in participants' responses. Some found the sensation exciting while others experienced anxiety and fear. It is not unreasonable to make a connection between the blood levels of anandamide after parabolic maneuvers. In fact, levels dropped in subjects with motion sickness but rose in subjects who felt fine.[4] Those feeling fear may reject the change by ejecting the contents of their stomachs just as many warriors do before battle.

While the conscious mind sits firmly in charge of free will, this type of involuntary experience suggests a learned subconscious influence. Consider that researchers report that children born into water have an instinctive ability to swim without much effort. Bruce Lipton, Ph.D., in Developmental Cell Biology, used this example and asked: "So why do we need to teach children how to swim?" Dr. Lipton proposed that children hold a given set of negative beliefs about water due to their parents or caretakers; this in turn produces fear, trepidation and ultimately the very real inability to swim safely and easily until it is re-learned. In order to "learn" how to swim, kids must first learn to trust that they can swim with ease and without harm, but it takes time to change the mind's internal architecture.

SUGGESTED BLESSING:

May you relax and let go of fear.

May you find it as easy as 1,2,3 to let go of beliefs that produce unwarranted fear of change.

SUGGESTED AFFIRMATION:

I have complete dominion of my mind. I am the master of my belief. I can choose thoughts that make me feel safe and secure.

AGGRAVATING FACTORS

Anxiety a fearful anticipation or reaction to unfamiliar sensations beyond one's control.

HEALING FACTORS

Embracing excitement / feeding your curiosity rather than your anxiety.

TAKE NOTICE

GINGER

GINGER: Researchers from Graz, Austria, (2007) reported that while the abilities of ginger and cannabis to reduce nausea and vomiting are well established by a series of scientific studies, the focus on special receptor sites involved in nausea and vomiting remains unclear. They suggested more research.[6]

German Commission E approved ginger for the prevention of motion sickness.[7]

Researchers from Zürich, Switzerland, (1994) recruited thousands of volunteers to help determine how well seven different commonly used seasickness prophylactics worked. Researchers gathered data during whale watching tours in Norway. In the control group (who did not receiving any prophylactics), 80% showed signs of seasickness, namely nausea with vomiting and malaise. In the group receiving a prophylactic, amongst seven various agents, only about 4 – 10% of individuals experienced nausea with vomiting, and 16 – 23% experienced malaise independent of which prophylactic they took thus indicating a similar effectiveness in preventing seasickness. The agents included: ginger root, cinnarizine, cinnarizine with domperidone, cyclizine, dimenhydrinate with caffeine, meclozine with caffeine, and scopolamine, which seemed the least effective.[8]

In a double-blind placebo-controlled study from Bangkok, Thailand, (2006) ginger proved effective in preventing nausea and vomiting among patients receiving major gynecological surgery. The patients in the treatment group received two capsules of ginger taken one hour before the procedure (one capsule containing 0.5 gram of ginger powder).[9] Another study (2010) discovered that 650mg of ginger given three times daily for a total of 4 days to pregnant women experiencing morning sickness worked even better than vitamin B-6 (another natural supplement commonly used for this purpose).[10]

1 Alexander Chouker1, Ines Kaufmann1, Simone Kreth1, Daniela Hauer1, Matthias Feuerecker1, Detlef Thieme2, Michael Vogeser3, Manfred Thiel4, Gustav Schelling1. *Motion Sickness, Stress and the Endocannabinoid System*. 1 Department of Anesthesiology, Ludwig-Maximilians-University, Munich, Germany, 2 Institute of Doping Analysis and Sports Biochemistry, Dresden, Germany, 3 Department of Clinical Chemistry, Ludwig-Maximilians-University, Munich, Germany, 4 Department of Anaesthesiology and Intensive Care, Medical Faculty Mannheim, University Medical Center Mannheim, University of Heidelberg, Mannheim, Germany. PLoS ONE 5(5): e10752. doi:10.1371/journal.pone.0010752

2 William J. Grace, M.D. and David T. Graham, M.D. *Relationship of Specific Attitudes and Emotions to Certain Bodily Diseases*. Dept. of Medicine, of the New York Hospital-Cornell Medical Center. Psychosomatic Medicine

July 1, 1952 vol. 14 no. 4 243-251.

3 bid.

4 Alexander Chouker1, Ines Kaufmann1, Simone Kreth1, Daniela Hauer1, Matthias Feuerecker1, Detlef Thieme2, Michael Vogeser3, Manfred Thiel4, Gustav Schelling1. *Motion Sickness, Stress and the Endocannabinoid System.* 1 Department of Anesthesiology, Ludwig-Maximilians-University, Munich, Germany, 2 Institute of Doping Analysis and Sports Biochemistry, Dresden, Germany, 3 Department of Clinical Chemistry, Ludwig-Maximilians-University, Munich, Germany, 4 Department of Anaesthesiology and Intensive Care, Medical Faculty Mannheim, University Medical Center Mannheim, University of Heidelberg, Mannheim, Germany. PLoS ONE 5(5): e10752. doi:10.1371/journal.pone.0010752

5 Cluny NL, Naylor RJ, Whittle BA, Javid FA. *The effects of cannabidiol and tetrahydrocannabinol on motion-induced emesis in Suncus murinus.* The School of Pharmacy, University of Bradford, Bradford, West Yorkshire, UK. ncluny@ucalgary.ca Basic Clin Pharmacol Toxicol. 2008 Aug;103(2):150-6.

6 Crockett SL, Schühly W, Bauer R. *Pflanzliche antiemetika. Inhaltsstoffe, molekulare wirkmechanismen und klinische evidenz.* Bereich Pharmakognosie, Institut für Pharmazeutische Wissenschaften, Universitätsplatz 4/1, Karl-Franzens-Universität Graz, A-8010 Graz, Osterreich. Pharm Unserer Zeit. 2007;36(5):381-8.

7 *Monographien der E-Kommission* (Phyto-Therapie) (380 monographs). A therapeutic guide to herbal medicine evaluating the safety and efficacy of herbs for licensed medical prescribing in Germany. Published between 1984 and 1994 in the Bundesanzeiger (official publication by the Federal Republic of Germany). Copies of the monographs are available at the Heilpflanzen-Welt Bibliothek: http://buecher.heilpflanzen-welt.de/BGA-Commission-E-Monographs/

8 Schmid R, Schick T, Steffen R, Tschopp A, Wilk T. *Comparison of Seven Commonly Used Agents for Prophylaxis of Seasickness.* Institute of Social and Preventive Medicine of the University of Zurich, Switzerland. J Travel Med. 1994 Dec 1;1(4):203-206.

9 Nanthakomon T, Pongrojpaw D. *The efficacy of ginger in prevention of postoperative nausea and vomiting after major gynecologic surgery.* Department of Obstetrics and Gyecology, Faculty of Medicine, Thammasat University, Bangkok 12120, Thailand. J Med Assoc Thai. 2006 Oct;89 Suppl 4:S130-6.

10 Chittumma P, Kaewkiattikun K, Wiriyasiriwach B. *Comparison of the effectiveness of ginger and vitamin B6 for treatment of nausea and vomiting in early pregnancy: a randomized double-blind controlled trial.* Department of Obstetrics and Gynecology, Bangkok Metropolitan Administration Medical College and Vajira Hospital, Dusit, Bangkok, Thailand. J Med Assoc Thai. 2007 Jan;90(1):15-20.

Vomiting
Chemotherapy Induced Nausea and Vomiting (CINV)

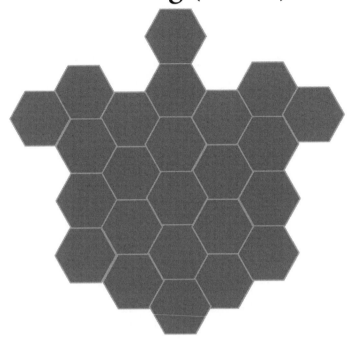

NUMBER OF STUDIES: 24

CHI VALUE: 104

Nausea and vomiting is a very common occurrence following chemotherapy, as the toxic pharmacological agents do not differentiate between cancer cells and healthy cells. Retching and vomiting occurs as a result of toxins detected by the brain. A signal travels from the vomiting center (area postrema), down cranial nerves, salivary glands, diaphragmatic and gastrointestinal muscles which initiates vomiting.

Anecdotal evidence from patients who smoked marijuana before chemotherapy and encountered significantly less nausea and vomiting as a result ultimately led to clinical trials demonstrating the therapeutic properties of cannabinoids.

The following studies are part of the foundation on which physicians, patients and advocacy groups base their recommendations that cannabinoids can greatly reduce chemotherapy induced nausea and vomiting (CINV).

CANNABIS AND CINV

THC reduces nausea and vomiting via CB1.[1] The 24 studies reviewed here examined the effectiveness of cannabinoids in the treatment of CINV. They span a period of four decades. Studies conducted in the laboratory on animal, adult and pediatric patients reached similar conclusions. Early studies focused on comparing the effectiveness of cannabinoids to the most common antiemetic pharmaceutical used at that time - prochlorperazine (generic of compazine and used as an anti-psychotic and anti-emetic). Most studies reported cannabinoids as superior.

Later studies broadened their focus and reported that cannabinoids proved more effective than other antiemetics such as metoclopramide, chlorpromazine, thiethylperazine, haloperidol, domperidone, or alizapride. Most recent studies examine the ability of cannabinoids, especially cannabidiol, to markedly reduce anticipated oxidative stress, inflammation, and cell death in the kidneys, therefore improving renal function in cancer pathologies.

CONSIDERATION:

As in most cases where cannabinoids may be helpful, research suggests that a therapeutic window exists which may depend on individual tolerance. For instance, either a very high or low dose could offer a lack of antiemetic effects or adverse-effects. To determine your optimal window, follow the advice of a licensed health care provider and your own subjective experience.

STUDY SUMMARY:

Drugs	Type of Study	Published Year, Place, and Key Results	CHI
Cannabidiol	Animal study (mice)	2009 – College of Medicine, Zhejiang University, Hangzhou, China. Cannabidiol markedly reduced the anticipated oxidative stress, inflammation, and cell death in the kidneys, and therefore improved renal function.[3]	2
Dronabinol orally starting at 2.5mg the day before chemo and on day one. From day 2 and on, 10-20 mg daily.	64 cancer patients undergoing chemotherapy	2007 – Bethesda Memorial Hospital, Comprehensive Cancer Care Center, Boynton Beach, Florida. Dronabinol proved as effective as ondansetron in reducing nausea and vomiting. Combination therapy was not more effective.[4]	3
Dronabinol and smoked cannabis	Review of selective studies	2003 – The Cleveland Clinic Taussig Cancer Center. Cannabinoids reduced chemotherapy-induced nausea and vomiting.[5]	4
Cannabinoids vs prochlorperazine, metoclopramide, chlorpromazine, thiethylperazine, haloperidol, domperidone, or alizapride	Review of selective studies	2001 – Département Anesthésiologie, Genève, Department of Anaesthetics, Churchill, Pain Management Centre Nottingham, Department of Clinical Pharmacology, Radcliffe Infirmary, Oxford. Cannabinoids were more effective antiemetics than prochlorperazine, metoclopramide, chlorpromazine, thiethylperazine, haloperidol, domperidone, or alizapride.[6]	4
THC was administered orally (18 mg in an edible oil).	Children with cancer receiving chemotherapy	1995 – Department of Pediatrics, Shaare Zedek Hospital, Jerusalem, Israel. Complete prevention of vomiting with negligible side effects.[7]	5
Oral THC (as marinol) 10 mg every 6 hr vs Prochlorperazine	67 cancer undergoing chemotherapy	1991 – Prochlorperazine better than THC, but both drugs combined were better than both alone.[8]	4
Nabilone and prochlorperazine v. metoclopramide and dexamethasone	Chemotherapy patients	1988 – Department of Medical Oncology, Royal Infirmary, Glasgow. Better control of emesis with metoclopramide. Nabilone combination better tolerated.[9]	4

Drugs	Type of Study	Published Year, Place, and Key Results	CHI
THC as oral dronabinol 15 mg/m2 (m2=per body surface area) 1 hr before chemotherapy and every 4 hr thereafter for 24 hr v. prochlorperazine	36 cancer patients undergoing chemotherapy where pharmaceutical emetics were ineffective	1988 – Division of Medical Oncology, Vincent T. Lombardi Cancer Research Center, Georgetown University, Washington, D.C. THC was able to decrease nausea and vomiting in 23 of 36 patients compared to 1 of 36 receiving prochlorperazine.[10]	4
Cannabis (inhaled)	56 cancer patients undergoing chemotherapy unresponsive to standard anti-emeticdrugs	1988 – 78% of treated patients demonstrated a positive response to marijuana.[11]	4
Nabilone and prochlorperazine	Pediatric chemotherapy patients	1987 – Hospital for Sick Children and the University of Toronto. Nabilone more effective in reducing retching and vomiting.[12]	5
Nabilone and metoclopramide	Patients undergoing radiation therapy	1987 – Department of Radiotherapy, Queen Elizabeth Hospital, Birmingham. No difference in effectiveness; more side effects noted with nabilone.[13]	0
Nabilone 1 mg every 8 hours vs IV metoclopramide (1 mg kg-1 3 hourly)	32 cancer patients undergoing chemotherapy	1986 – Oncology, Charing Cross Hospital and University College Hospital, London. No difference between nabilone and metoclopramide.[14]	5
Nabilone (oral)	18 pediatric patients	1986 – Department of Haematology, The Children's Hospital, Sheffield. Nabilone significantly reduced nausea and vomiting and two thirds of the kids expressed a preference for the drug.[15]	5
Nabilone (oral)	38 cancer patient receiving chemotherapy	1986 – Nabilone is superior to domperidone for the control of chemotherapy-induced emesis.[16]	5
Oral Nabilone 2mg X 2 daily vs prochlorperazine 15mg	24 lung cancer patients receiving chemotherapy.	1985 – Nabilone was significantly superior to prochlorperazine in the reduction of vomiting episodes.[17]	5
Nabilone v. prochlorperazine	34 patients with lung cancer	1983 – Symptom scores were significantly better for patients on nabilone for nausea, retching and vomiting.[18]	5
Oral nabilone 3 mg three times a day v. Chlorpromazine administered at a dose of 12.5 mg IM	20 patients with advanced gynecological cancer	1983 – Nabilone, when compared to chlorpromazine, did not significantly reduce vomiting, and most patients preferred nabilone.[19]	5
Synthetic cannabinoid levonantradol (0.5, 0.75 or 1mg) v. chlorpromazine (25mg)	108 cancer patients	1983 – 0.5mg levonantradol was a more effective antiemtic than 25mg chlorpromazine.[20]	5
THC v. prochlorperazine. THC was given by body surface area (BSA): BSA less than 1.4 m2 = 7.5 mg; BSA 1.4-1.8 m2 = 10- mg; and BSA greater than 1.8 m2 = 12.5 mg prochlorperazine was administered in a fixed dose of 10 mg	212 cancer patients undergoing chemotherapies	1982 – THC and prochlorperazine produced similar results but patients who felt THC in their system did better.[21]	5

Drugs	Type of Study	Published Year, Place, and Key Results	CHI
Nabilone 2mg X 2 daily vs prochlorperazine 10mg X 2 daily.	27 cancer patients undergoing chemotherapy who failed to respond to pharmacological anti-emetics	1982 – Vomiting ejections and dry retching significantly reduced by nabilone.[22]	5
Oral nabilone 2mg vs placebo.	24 cancer patients undergoing chemotherapy	1982 – "Nabilone is an effective antiemetic agent for chemotherapy-induced nausea and vomiting."[23]	5
Oral THC vs prochlorperazine vs placebo.	55 chemotherapy patients	1981 – Oral THC is far more effective than prochlorperazine and placebos.[24]	5
Nabilone vs prochlorperazine.	113 cancer chemotherapy patients	1979 – Nabilone is far more effective in reducing nausea and vomiting.[25]	5
Oral THC	20 cancer chemotherapy patients	1975 – Sidney Farber Cancer Center, Peter Bent Brigham Hospital and Harvard Medical School, Boston. "No patient vomited while experiencing a subjective "high."[26]	5

Total CHI Value   104

STRAIN SPECIFIC CONSIDERATIONS

The cannabinoids studied include nabilone (or nabilone similar drugs such as dronabinol, marinol, levonantradol) and to a lesser degree smoked cannabis, THC infused oil and lastly CBD. THC reduces nausea and vomiting via CB1.[2]

Nabilone is a synthetic cannabinoid similar to THC and binds with both CB1 and CB2 relatively equally. Smoked cannabis binds with CB1 and CB2 but at a different ratio depending on the strain. CBD has a greater affinity for CB2 expression than CB1.

Sativa and sativa dominant strains tend to have a higher THC:CBD ratios.

EXPLORING MIND–BODY CONSCIOUSNESS

The physical brain perceives a threat (a chemo-toxin) and instantly reacts to expel it. The mind's parallel might be the perception of an experience that brings great fear or even dread (such as a cancer diagnosis).

QUESTIONS

Do I express my emotions, especially those I do not like, appropriately and with intensity?
Can I release and forgive all hatred, pain, grief and disapproval that I still carry from my past?
Can I love and approve of myself, right now, just as I am?
What is the ancient hatred I still carry with me?
What is that terrible secret that eats away at the substance of my soul?
Where does my hopelessness find fertile ground?

SUGGESTED BLESSING:

May your changes strengthen your resolve to live a healthy life.

SUGGESTED AFFIRMATION:

May all poisons and all fears leave you so all that remains is forgiveness and a world in which love reigns supreme.

1 Parker LA, Rock E, Limebeer C. *Regulation of nausea and vomiting by cannabinoids*. Department of Psychology and Collaborative Neuroscience Program University of Guelph, Guelph, Ontario, Canada N1G 2W1. Br J Pharmacol. 2010 Dec 22.

2 Ibid.

3 Pan H, Mukhopadhyay P, Rajesh M, Patel V, Mukhopadhyay B, Gao B, Hasko G, Pacher P. *Cannabidiol attenuates cisplatin-induced nephrotoxicity by decreasing oxidative/nitrosative stress, inflammation and cell death*. Department of Urology, The First Affiliated Hospital, College of Medicine, Zhejiang University, Hangzhou, Zhejiang, China. J Pharmacol Exp Ther. 2009 Mar;328(3):708-14.

4 Meiri E, Jhangiani H, Vredenburgh JJ, Barbato LM, Carter FJ, Yang HM, Baranowski V. *Efficacy of dronabinol alone and in combination with ondansetron versus ondansetron alone for delayed chemotherapy-induced nausea and vomiting*. Bethesda Memorial Hospital, Comprehensive Cancer Care Center, Boynton Beach, FL 33435-7995, USA. Curr Med Res Opin 2007;23(3):533-43.

5 Walsh D, Nelson KA, Mahmoud FA. *Established and potential therapeutic applications of cannabinoids in oncology*. The Harry R Horvitz Center for Palliative Medicine, The Cleveland Clinic Taussig Cancer Center, Cleveland Clinic Foundation - M-76, Cleveland, OH 44195, USA. Support Care Cancer. 2003 Mar;11(3):137-43.

6 Martin R Tramèr, staff anaesthetist a, Dawn Carroll, senior research nurse b, Fiona A Campbell, consultant in anaesthetics and pain management c, D John M Reynolds, consultant clinical pharmacologist d, R Andrew Moore, consultant biochemist b, Henry J McQuay, professor of pain relief b. *Cannabinoids for control of chemotherapy induced nausea and vomiting: quantitative systematic review*. a Division d'Anesthésiologie, Département Anesthésiologie, Pharmacologie Clinique et Soins Intensif de Chirurgie, Hôpitaux Universitaires, CH-1211 Genève 14, Switzerland, b Pain Research, Nuffield Department of Anaesthetics, Churchill, Oxford Radcliffe Hospital, Oxford OX3 7LJ, c Pain Management Centre, Undercroft, South Block, Queen's Medical Centre, Nottingham NG7 2UH, d Department of Clinical Pharmacology, Radcliffe Infirmary, Oxford OX2 6HE. BMJ 2001;323:16-21.

7 Abrahamov A, Abrahamov A, Mechoulam R. *An efficient new cannabinoid antiemetic in pediatric oncology*. Department of Pediatrics, Shaare Zedek Hospital, Jerusalem, Israel. Life Sci. 1995;56(23-24):2097-102.

8 Lane M, Vogel CL, Ferguson J, Krasnow S, Saiers JL, Hamm J, Salva K, Wiernik PH, Holroyde CP, Hammill S, et al. Dronabinol and prochlorperazine in combination for treatment of cancer chemotherapy-induced nausea and vomiting. J Pain Symptom Manage. 1991 Aug;6(6):352-9.

9 Cunningham D, Bradley CJ, Forrest GJ, et al. A randomized trial of oral nabilone and prochlorperazine compared to intravenous metoclopramide and dexamethasone in the treatment of nausea and vomiting induced by chemotherapy regimens containing cisplatin or cisplatin analogues. Department of Medical Oncology, Royal Infirmary, Glasgow, U.K. Eur J Cancer Clin Oncol 1988;24:685–689.

10 McCabe M, Smith FP, Goldberg D, Macdonald J, Woolley PV, Warren R. Division of Medical Oncology, Vincent T. Lombardi Cancer Research Center, Georgetown University, Washington, D.C. 20007. *Efficacy of tetrahydrocannabinol in patients refractory to standard anti-emetic therapy*. Investigational New Drugs 1988;6:243-246.

11 Vinciguerra V, Moore T, Brennan E. I*nhalation marijuana as an antiemetic for cancer chemotherapy*. New York State Journal of Medicine 1988;88:525-527.

12 Chan HS, Correia JA, MacLeod SM. *Nabilone versus prochlorperazine for control of cancer chemotherapy-induced emesis in children: a double-blind, crossover trial*. From the Divisions of Hematology-Oncology and Clinical Pharmacology, Department of Pediatrics and Pharmacology, the Hospital for Sick Children and the University of Toronto, Toronto. Pediatrics 1987;79:946–52.

13 Priestman SG, Priestman TJ, Canney PA. *A double-blind randomized cross-over comparison of nabilone and metoclopramide in the control of radiation-induced nausea*. Department of Radiotherapy, Queen Elizabeth Hospital, Birmingham. Clin Radiol 1987;38:543–544.

14 Crawford SM, Buckman R. *Nabilone and metoclopramide in the treatment of nausea and vomiting due to cisplatinum: a double blind study.* Department of Medical Oncology, Charing Cross Hospital, London W6 8RF; Department of Oncology, University College Hospital, London WC1, U.K. Med Oncol Tumor Pharmacother. 1986;3(1):39-42.

15 Dalzell AM, Bartlett H, Lilleyman JS. *Nabilone: an alternative antiemetic for cancer chemotherapy.* Department of Haematology, The Children's Hospital, Sheffield. Arch Dis Child. 1986 May;61(5):502-5.

16 Pomeroy M, Fennelly JJ, Towers M. *Prospective randomized double-blind trial of nabilone versus domperidone in the treatment of cytotoxic-induced emesis.* Cancer Chemother Pharmacol 1986;17(3):285-8.

17 Niiranen A, Mattson K. *A cross-over comparison of nabilone and prochlorperazine for emesis induced by cancer chemotherapy.* American Journal of Clinical Oncology 1985 Aug;8(4):336-40

18 Ahmedzai S, Carlyle DL, Calder IT, Moran F. *Antiemeticefficacy and toxicity of nabilone, a synthetic cannabinoid, in lung cancer chemotherapy.* Br J Cancer. 1983 Nov;48(5):657-63.

19 George M, Pejovic MH, Thuaire M, Kramar A, Wolff JP. *Randomized comparative trial of a new anti-emetic: nabilone, in cancer patients treated with cisplatin.* Biomed Pharmacother. 1983;37(1):24-7.

20 Hutcheon AW, Palmer JB, Soukop M, Cunningham D, McArdle C, Welsh J, Stuart F, Sangster G, Kaye S, Charlton D, et al. *A randomised multicentre single blind comparison of a cannabinoid antiemetic(levonantradol) with chlorpromazine in patients receiving their first cytotoxic chemotherapy.* European Journal for Cancer and Clinical Oncology 1983 Aug;19(8):1087-90.

21 Ungerleider JT, Andrysiak T, Fairbanks L, Goodnight J, Sarna G, Jamison K. *Cannabis and cancer chemotherapy: a comparison of oral delta-9-THC and prochlorperazine.* Cancer 1982;50:636-645

22 Johansson R, Kilkku P, Groenroos M. *A double-blind, controlled trial of nabilone vs. prochlorperazine for refractory emesis induced by cancer chemotherapy.* Cancer Treat Rev. 1982 Dec; 9 Suppl B:25-33.

23 Jones SE, Durant JR, Greco FA, Robertone A. *A multi-institutional Phase III study of nabilone vs. placebo in chemotherapy-induced nausea and vomiting.* Cancer Treat Rev. 1982 Dec;9 Suppl B:45-8.

24 Orr LE, McKernan JF. *Antiemetic effect of delta 9-tetrahydrocannabinol in chemotherapy-associated nausea and emesis as compared to placebo and compazine.* J Clin Pharmacol 1981;21:76S–80S.

25 Herman TS, Einhorn LH, Jones SE, Nagy C, Chester AB, Dean JC, Furnas B, Williams SD, Leigh SA, Dorr RT, Moon TE. *Superiority of nabilone over prochlorperazine as an antiemetic in patients receiving cancer chemotherapy.* N Engl J Med. 1979 Jun 7;300(23):1295-7.

26 Stephen E. Sallan, M.D., Norman E. Zinberg, M.D. and Emil Frei III, M.D. *Antiemetic Effect of Delta-9-Tetrahydrocannabinol in Patients Receiving Cancer Chemotherapy.* Sidney Farber Cancer Center, Peter Bent Brigham Hospital and Harvard Medical School, Boston. N Engl J Med 1975; 293:795-797

Wound Care

Cannabis has been applied topically in the form of poultices, plasters, salves, tinctures and oils to treat of slow healing wounds and skin ulcers (as in "diabetic foot" in turn-of-the-century American medicine). Modern users have reported successful treatments of slow healing skin wounds with cannabis-infused honey and cannabis-infused oils.

CANNABIS INFUSED HONEY

Modern medicine has rediscovered honey's ancient use in the care of infected wounds.[1,2,3,4,5] Applied to slow healing skin wounds such as ulcerations, burns or infected wounds, provides numerous therapeutic benefits. Honey is antibacterial, anti-inflammatory, improves circulation, reduces swelling, stimulates formation of new capillaries and connective tissue, and reduces pain. The Cuban Ministry of Health widely recommends honey as a skin protective agent, as an anti-microbial for skin infections where it is prepared as a topical cream, as an alcohol tincture and as oral drops.[6]

While no current studies examine the combined and possibly synergistic properties of honey and cannabis in infused form, it is interesting to note that many of the therapeutic properties of honey also exist in cannabis - most notably, anti-inflammatory and pain reducing properties.

CANNABIS INFUSED HEMPSEED OIL

Oil made from hemp seed is void of any mind-altering cannabinoids and has historically been used for the treatment of dry skin, and age related skin blemishes and wounds. It is a rich and properly balanced source of omega-3 and omega-6 polyunsaturated fatty acids. Recent studies reveal that ingestion of hempseed oil positively changes fat profiles in the body and significantly reduces the symptoms of dryness, itching and inflammation in atopic dermatitis.[7]

Some patients have combined the skin healing and anti-inflammatory properties of hempseed oil by infusing the oil with cannabinoid rich cannabis to create a topical ointment. The skin is the largest organ of the body and thus provides an ideal route for the gentle delivery of biologically active substances. Many cannabis-hemp oil users report a variety of benefits, including the shrinking of moles and age spots, localized and systemic pain relief, therapeutic relaxation of tight muscles and cramps, deeper and more restful sleep, the soothing of inflammation and a subtle increase in libido, all with a gentle uplift in mood.

As with all natural biologically active substances, effects are usually optimal within a specific therapeutic window, which may vary from person to person. Taking too much may aggravate symptoms. Taking too little may have a suboptimal effect. As always, start slowly and increase application until you reach your therapeutic window.

EXPLORING MIND–BODY CONSCIOUSNESS

Few people wake up one morning and consciously choose to inflict injuries on themselves. However, within the paradigm that stipulates 'you are the generator of all of your experiences,' there are no exceptions. In cases of trauma, accidents, burns, wounds and injuries, taking a step back and looking more carefully at the complex interplay of the conscious, subconscious and unconscious often reveals free will at work.

While a person may never consciously decree "I am going to hurt myself today," they can become aware of consciously held beliefs concerning punishment. Nobody is perfect, everybody errs and makes mistakes; but with a belief in punishment, injuries will occur to meet a self-generated need. One might consider the use of guilt as motivation and its implicit demand for purification through punishment. This makes the choice for injury more clearly visible. An examination of self-hatred, inappropriately expressed anger, harbored anger, and underlying belief structures may reveal surprizing aspects of the 'why' and how of traumatic events.

TAKE NOTICE

For general immune support, see TAKE NOTICE in BACTERIAL and VIRAL INFECTIONS; for anti-inflammatory support see TAKE NOTICE in INFLAMMATORY DISEASES IN GENERAL; for pain see TAKE NOTICE in PAIN IN GENERAL; and for anti-spasmotic and neuro-protective support see NEURO-PROTECTIVE IN GENERAL.

1 Radwan S, El- Essawy A, Sarhan MM. *Experimental evidence for the occurrence in honey of specific substances active against Microorganisms.* Zentral Microbiol. 1984;139:249–255.

2 Ibrahim AS. *Antibacterial action of honey.* Bull Islam Med. 1985;1:363–365.

3 Jeddar A, Kharsany A, Ramsaroop UG, Bhamjee A, Hafejee IE, Moosa A. *The Antibacterial action of honey.* South Afri Med J. 1985;67:257–258.

4 Molan PC, Smith IM, Reid GM. *Acomparison of the antibacterial activities of some New Zealand honeys.* Journal of Agricultural Research. 1988;27:252–256.

5 Subramanyam M. T*ropical application of honey in treatment of burns.* Br J Surg. 1991;78:497–498.

6 *Therapeutic Guide to Plant Pharmaceuticals and Honey Pharmaceuticals (Guia Terapeutica Dispensarial de Fitofarmacos y Apifarmacos* - Ministerio de Salud Publica, Ciudad de La Habana - Republica de Cuba 1992). Cuban Ministry of Public Health, Havana.

7 Callaway J, Schwab U, Harvima I, Halonen P, Mykkanen O, Hyvonen P, Jarvinen T. *Efficacy of dietary hempseed oil in patients with atopic dermatitis.* J Dermatolog Treat. 2005 Apr;16(2):87-94.

Wound Care
Post-surgery Wounds

NUMBER OF STUDIES: 1

CHI VALUE: 4

Wounds caused by surgical interventions require careful attention to possible complications signaled by an increase in pain, the presence of inflammation, swelling, discharge, discoloration or heat.

CANNABIS AND POST-SURGERY WOUNDS

A Worcester, MA study (2009) casts a wide net for their meta-analysis, reviewing all cannabinoid studies "…published in the last 5 years on the activities of all classes of cannabinoids, including the endogenous cannabinoids such as anandamide, related compounds such as the elmiric acids (EMAs), and noncannabinoid components (200-250 constituents) of Cannabis that show anti-inflammatory action."[1] Results revealed that all types of cannabinoids as well as noncannabinoid parts of the plant effectively reduce pain from inflammation associated with post-surgery patients, rheumatism, rheumatoid arthritis, chronic neuropathic pain and fibromyalgia.

STUDY SUMMARY:

Drugs	Type of Study	Published Year, Place, and Key Results	CHI
All types of cannabinoids (endogeneous, plant-based and synthetic)	Meta-analysis (2004-2009)	2009 – University of Massachusetts Medical School. Cannabinoids effective in pain from post-surgery patients.	4

Total CHI Value   4

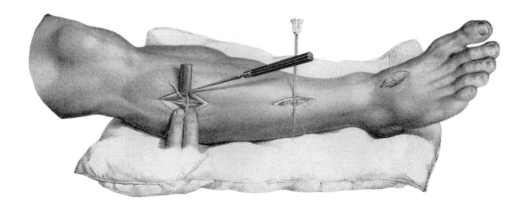

EXPLORING MIND–BODY CONSCIOUSNESS

See WOUND CARE and/or SPINALCORD INJURIES.

TAKE NOTICE

For general immune support, see TAKE NOTICE in BACTERIAL and VIRAL INFEC-TIONS; for anti-inflammatory support see TAKE NOTICE in INFLAMMATORY DISEASES IN GENERAL; for pain see TAKE NOTICE in PPAIN IN GENERAL; and for anti-spasmotic and neuro-protective support see NEURO-PROTECTIVE IN GENERAL

1 Sumner H. Burstein1,2 and Robert B. Zurier2. *Cannabinoids, Endocannabinoids, and Related Analogs in Inflammation.* 1Department of Biochemistry & Molecular Pharmacology, University of Massachusetts Medical School, 364 Plantation St., Worcester, Massachusetts 01605 USA. 2Department of Medicine, University of Massachusetts Medical School, 364 Plantation St., Worcester, Massachusetts 01605 USA. AAPS J. 2009 March; 11(1): 109–119.

Wound Care
Spinal Cord Injuries

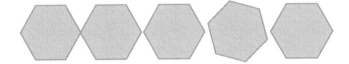

NUMBER OF STUDIES: 5

CHI VALUE: 19

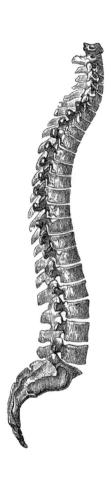

The spine is a marvel of the human body. It allows us to walk upright, bend, stretch and reach well above our heads. It is a solid load-carrying support system that is at once remarkably flexible all-the-while housing and protecting the spinal cord. Solid support is derived from vertebral bone rigidity, and flexibility is achieved by the placement of intervertebral discs (intervertebral fibrocartilage) placed between each of 26 spinal bones.[1] Furthermore, seen from the side, the spine contains four curves that further allow for support, flexion, extension and cushioning.

The brain and the spinal cord make up the central nervous system (CNS). The spinal cord is a relatively think bundle of nerves, which descends from the medulla oblongata (the lowest part of the brain) through the center of the spine. Here, spinal cord nerves junction and exit the spine between each vertebrae to ultimately connect all parts of the body in ever smaller branching nerve fibers.

An injury to the spinal column most commonly results from external trauma (car crash, gunshot, etc.), but may also result from internal trauma (stroke, aneurism) or via certain diseases (cancer). The location of damage in the spinal cord determines the degree of disability. For example, a paraplegic person is paralyzed from the waist down after sustained damage to the thoracic or lower spine. A quadriplegic person paralyzed from the neck down loses the ability to move his arms or legs after sustaining damage to the spinal cord in the neck or brain itself.

The management of spinal column injuries, where some sensation is still present, is often accompanied by chronic pain and uncontrollable muscle spasms of the back, arms and legs.

CANNABIS AND SPINAL CORD INJURIES

The time-proven anti-spasmodic properties of cannabis have been confirmed by modern science in numerous human studies (see also NEUROLOGICAL DISEASES – SPASMS). Here we look at studies specifically related to spinal cord injuries and resulting spasms. As early as 1974, VA-hospital based researchers began looking at data suggesting a practical therapeutic anti-spasmodic benefit. Later studies confirmed the efficacy of cannabinoids, especially THC. The latest of these studies (2007) from Basel, Switzerland,[2] recommends a minimum of 15-20mg daily dose to produce a therapeutic and measurable effect in reducing spinal-cord injury-related spasmodic activity.

STUDY SUMMARY:

Drugs	Type of Study	Published Year, Place, and Key Results	CHI
Oral THC average daily dose 31mg. Rectal THC average daily dose 43mg	25 patients with spinal cord injuries and regular spasms	2007 – REHAB Basel, Centre for Spinal Cord Injury and Severe Head Injury, Basel, Switzerland. THC is an effective antispasmotic. At least 15-20mg per day was needed to achieve therapeutic effect.[3]	5
Dronabinol from 2 x 5mg increased gradually to 3 x 20mg	5 patients with spinal cord injuries and regular spasms	1995 – Medical College of Georgia, Augusta, GA, USA. Reduced spasms in 2 patients.[4]	3
Placebo vs 50mg codeine p.o. (by mouth) vs 5mg THC p.o.	One single patient with spinal cord injury and subsequent pains and spasms	1990 – Psychologisches Institut für Beratung und Forschung, Zürich, Switzerland. THC produced significant reduction in spasticity.[5]	5
Inhaled cannabis	Data collected from 43 patients with spinal-cord injury and related spasms	1982 – Cannabis produced significant reduction in spinal cord injury related spasticity.[6]	3
Inhaled cannabis	10 patients with spinal cord injuries and resulting pain and spasms	1974 – Spinal Cord Injury ward of the Miami, FL V.A. Hospital. Decreased pain and spasms.[7]	3

Total CHI Value 19

STRAIN SPECIFIC CONSIDERATIONS

Clinical trials employed cannabinoids from various sources: cannabis, THC and dronabinol (synthetic THC). Scientists tested them on patients with spinal cord injuries. Cannabis binds with both CB1 and CB2. THC and dronabinol both bind with CB1 and CB2.

While both sativa and indica strains contain cannabinoids that activate CB1 and CB2, sativas or sativa heavy strains tend to produce higher THC:CBD ratios.

EXPLORING MIND–BODY CONSCIOUSNESS

The spinal cord contains neural pathways connecting a trillion cells. It is analogous to a highway for electrical signals that control the entire body. Spinal cord (SC) injuries are like a sinkhole or collapsed bridge that block traffic in both directions, isolating previously connected communities. The most common causes of SC injuries are car and motorcycle accidents followed by trauma from violence, falls and sport accidents. SC injuries usually present with some degree of paralysis, pain and/or spasms.

Paralysis patients often express an immobilizing terror or the feeling of being frozen with fear. Patients may say they are giving up external exploration of the world and focusing instead on their inner development. In that sense, SC injuries provide an opportunity to (re)-commit to a new direction. Paralysis may draw the patients attention to a prior inability to relax the affected part(s) and spur them to consider what that part represents to them. Paralyzed legs may represent issues of progress or a shift in one's priorities in life. They may also relate to steadfastness or the ability to stand up for oneself. Paralysis below the belly button involves issues of sexuality and of the release of stool and urine and so love must be raised from the genitals to the heart. Stool relates to the element of earth and discerning that which matters. Paralysis reduces vertical height by half and challenges one to ask for help and to receive help. It may require a re-assessment of the meaning of pride, humiliation, humility and self-worth.

Pain (see section on PAIN).

Spasms (in forms ranging from minor twitching to serious cramps) may be reflective of a life force trying to shake up and wake up affected body parts. It may indicate a physical manifestation of contracting and fearful thoughts or emotions and underlying beliefs.

QUESTIONS

What was the last straw that broke…?
What were the other straws that pushed me to the breaking point?
What broke my life in half?
What was the purpose of my life before?
What is the purpose of my life now?
How did I define my self-worth before?
How do I define my self-worth now?
What was I proud of before?
What am I proud of now?
Love before was…?
Love now is…?
Do I feel broken/humbled?
What is the affected body part a representation of?
What is the body function (lost) a representation of?

TAKE NOTICE

For general immune support, see TAKE NOTICE in BACTERIAL and VIRAL INFECTIONS; for anti-inflammatory support see TAKE NOTICE in INFLAMMATORY DISEASES IN GENERAL; for pain see TAKE NOTICE in PPAIN IN GENERAL; and for anti-spasmotic and neuro-protective support see NEURO-PROTECTIVE IN GENERAL.

1 There are actually 33 spinal bones. The sacral spine consists of five vertebrae fused without discs in between. The coccyx part of the spine consists of four vertebrae fused without discs in between.

2 Hagenbach U, Luz S, Ghafoor N, Berger JM, Grotenhermen F, Brenneisen R, Mader M. *The treatment of spasticity with Delta(9)-tetrahydrocannabinol in persons with spinal cord injury*. REHAB Basel, Centre for Spinal Cord Injury and Severe Head Injury, Basel, Switzerland. Spinal Cord. 2007 Aug;45(8):551-62.

3 Hagenbach U, Luz S, Ghafoor N, Berger JM, Grotenhermen F, Brenneisen R, Mader M. *The treatment of spasticity with Delta(9)-tetrahydrocannabinol in persons with spinal cord injury*. REHAB Basel, Centre for Spinal Cord Injury and Severe Head Injury, Basel, Switzerland. Spinal Cord. 2007 Aug;45(8):551-62.

4 Kogel RW, Johnson PB, Chintam R, Robinson CJ, Nemchausky BA. *Treatment of Spasticity in Spinal Cord Injury with Dronabinol, a Tetrahydrocannabinol Derivative*. Medical College of Georgia, Augusta, GA, USA. Am J Ther. 1995 Oct;2(10):799-805.

5 Maurer M, Henn V, Dittrich A, Hofmann A. *Delta-9-tetrahydrocannabinol shows antispastic and analgesic effects in a single case double-blind trial.* PSIN - Psychologisches Institut für Beratung und Forschung, Zürich, Switzerland. Eur Arch Psychiatry Clin Neurosci. 1990;240(1):1-4.

6 Malec J, Harvey RF, Cayner JJ. *Cannabis effect on spasticity in spinal cord injury.* Arch Phys Med Rehabil. 1982 Mar;63(3):116-8.

7 Dunn M, Davis R. *The perceived effects of marijuana on spinal cord injured males.* Spinal Cord Injury ward of the Miami V.A. Hospital. Paraplegia. 1974 Nov;12(3):175.

Made in the USA
San Bernardino, CA
19 April 2015